AF352193

ASTHMA

LUNG BIOLOGY IN HEALTH AND DISEASE

Executive Editor: **Claude Lenfant**

Director, National Heart, Lung, and Blood Institute
National Institutes of Health
Bethesda, Maryland

Additional Volumes in Preparation

ASTHMA
ITS PATHOLOGY AND TREATMENT

Edited by

Michael A. Kaliner
National Institute of Allergy and Infectious Disease
National Institutes of Health
Bethesda, Maryland

Peter J. Barnes
Department of Thoracic Medicine
National Heart and Lung Institute
London, England

Carl G. A. Persson
Department of Clinical Pharmacology
University of Lund Hospital
Exploratory Clinical Research
AB Draco
Lund, Sweden

MARCEL DEKKER, INC.   New York • Basel • Hong Kong

Library of Congress Cataloging-in-Publication Data

Asthma : its pathology and treatment / edited by Michael A. Kaliner,
    Peter J. Barnes, Carl G.A. Persson.
        p.   cm. — (Lung biology in health and disease ; v. 49)
    Includes bibliographical references.
    Includes indexes.
    ISBN 0-8247-8217-8 (alk. paper)
    1. Asthma—Pathophysiology. 2. Asthma—Treatment. I. Kaliner,
Michael A. II. Barnes, Peter J.,   . III. Persson, C. G. A.
IV. Series.
    [DNLM: 1. Asthma—pathology. 2. Asthma—therapy. W1 LU62 v. 49
/ WF 553 A8544]
    RC591.A8182   1991
    616.2′38—dc20
    DNLM/DLC
    for Library of Congress   90-13829
                                                                      CIP

This book is printed on acid-free paper

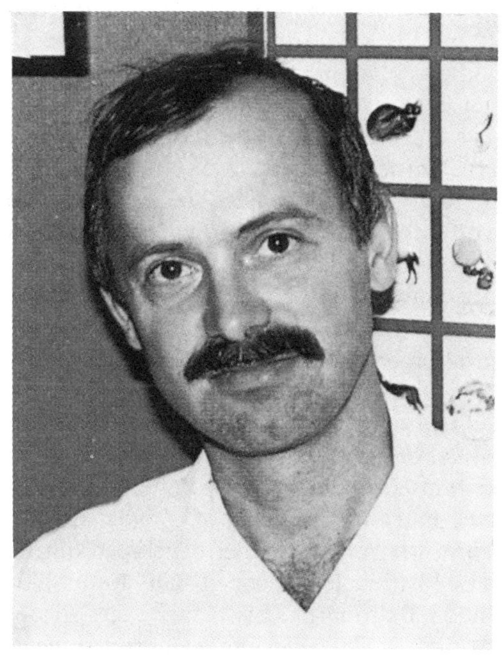

IN MEMORIAM

Ulf Pipkorn

On the morning of June 13th I had my almost daily talk with Ulf Pipkorn. It was, as always with Ulf, characterized by a free flow of thoughts and ideas where research, friends, family, colleagues, meetings, publications, everything was brought up. Discussing airway research with Ulf was a wonderful excursion into endless possibilities. Working together with Ulf was to experience a geometric progression of projects actually being realized. On this day Ulf naturally talked about the first sailing adventures experienced by his young children. He also looked forward to an imminent three weeks' travel with his family where work would "only" be a few plenary lectures at international meetings. Indeed, Ulf had just returned from a workshop on asthma and rhinitis held in Florida; a trip that, as both testified, was like a mini-honeymoon to Ulf and his wife Anne-Sofie. Ulf made good use of his new 10-year calendar and was planning to organize several meetings in the future. Next winter there was a particular priority. Ulf would have gathered colleagues and friends from both sides of the Atlantic to discuss an airway subject of great concern. This exercise was also to result in a major book, and in a few days, on June 16th Ulf was scheduled to discuss this project with Marcel Dekker's Executive Editor, Paul Dolgert, who was planning to be in Lund at that time. During our talk Ulf, not too unpleased, mentioned that he had reread his important chapter for the present book (Chapter 24). In the evening of that summer day of June 13th, Ulf Pipkorn was suddenly seized by a severe cardiac infarction and died. When we heard of this tragic event, we decided immediately to dedicate this book to Ulf.

Since 1985, Assistant Professor Ulf Pipkorn was an ENT specialist at the University Hospital of Lund, where special arrangements had been made so he could devote himself equally to research and clinical work. His 1982 thesis made a strong mark in the fields of airway diseases and actions of glucocorticoids. This interest was further developed during the years 1984-1985, when Ulf was Visiting Professor at The Johns Hopkins University School of Medicine in Baltimore. It is a fact that Ulf already was giving plenary lectures worldwide, that he had authored some 150 publications, edited a few books, and tutored several students. Ulf was an extremely creative and expeditious researcher with a richly developed global network of friends and collaborators. By any criteria, Ulf would have contributed so much more to our understanding of airway diseases and their treatment. This important field of research has now suffered a great loss. So have all those workers who knew Ulf Pipkorn and enjoyed his generosity, friendship and benefited from his enthusiasm and expertise. However, our thoughts are foremost with Ulf's young family, his three children aged from 4 to 11, and his wife, Anne-Sofie Pipkorn, who participated in so many facets of Ulf's work and was a tremendous support to him. We can meet Anne-Sofie's wish and honor Ulf by continuing, as best we can, the research that he carried out and made possible.

INTRODUCTION

> I have assigned the immediate cause of asthma to the straitness, compression, or constriction of the bronchi.

> *A Treatise of the Asthma*
> Sir John Floyer, 1698

At the time Sir John Floyer wrote his treatise, the concept of airway hyperresponsiveness did not exist, yet his words presaged today's description of the airways' reactions to endogenous and exogenous stimulation. The next historic stride toward our current understanding of asthma came in the eighteenth century when Laennec attributed asthma to a spasm of the smooth muscle fibers of the bronchi.

It is interesting that the views of Floyer met with some skepticism. M. Lieutaud, pediatrician to the Dauphin, had this to say about asthma: "It is one of these overdiagnosed diseases, and of ten so-called asthmatics only one may be real. I am not surprised that ordinary physicians be mistaken. But that Floyer, who wrote about the disease, and himself an asthmatic, could not distinguish [between real and false asthmatics] is inconceivable."

There is no longer any question that asthma is associated with airway hyperresponsiveness, but accurate diagnosis remains a significant problem. The increased prevalence of asthma reported during the past decade most assuredly suggests that there have been improvements in recognition and identification of the condition. Nevertheless, clinicians, epidemiologists, and public health officials agree that much more needs to be done, both in research and in education, to improve asthma diagnosis.

It is often said that asthma is a condition that can be treated and controlled, but not cured given our current state of knowledge. Thus, to reach that ultimate goal, we must engage actively in fundamental research to uncover basic mechanisms and therapeutic approaches that impinge upon the primary manifestation of asthma, airways hyperresponsiveness. Since Floyer's treatise, much has been written about asthma and related issues. The series of monographs Lung Biology in Health and Disease has included a number of titles that attest to the immense interest in this area of research and the productivity of the investigators involved. Two of the editors of this new volume, Drs. Michael Kaliner and Peter Barnes, previously produced a monograph on *The Airways*: *Neural Control in Health and Disease*, which is a landmark in the series. This new volume, *Asthma: Its Pathology and Treatment,* is a natural extension of the previous title and includes a new coeditor, Dr. Carl Persson of Sweden. The fact that these editors represent three countries in itself assures the participation of three schools of thought. Moreover, these editors sought and successfully obtained the contributions of researchers from many other countries. The result is an impressive list of authors who provide state-of-the-art reviews, ideas, and directions for research yet to come in the many facets of airway hyperresponsiveness. I am grateful to the editors and the contributing authors for a superb, important, and timely addition to this series of monographs.

Claude Lenfant, M.D.
Bethesda, Maryland

PREFACE

We have borrowed the title of this book, *Asthma: Its Pathology and Treatment*, from Hyde Salter's brilliant book published in 1860. It seemed appropriate to reach back for this title, as so much of what we know about asthma began with this innovative physician. Indeed, this book itself began more than 4 years ago when it became apparent that it was timely to bring together the world's best investigators to discuss asthma. We planned this book to give clinicians and scientists a series of treatises on the components of asthma, with a focus on where we are headed and what we have learned. The presentation of asthma was planned to start with the epidemiology, delve layer by layer into the airway wall, dissect each potentially important cell and its contribution to the pathophysiology, detail each of the components of the nervous system and their role in asthma, and finally look at which mediators might be contributing. The final sessions asked what lessons had been learned from our experience with pharmaceutical agents currently being used to treat asthma. Thus, asthma was divided into 24 segments, each exposing an important facet of either the underlying pathophysiology or the treatment of the disease.

The chapters are written as "state-of-the-art" reviews, but each chapter is augmented by a discussion section which is derived from an intense three-day meeting, kindly sponsored by Astra/Draco. These discussions distill the context of many heated sessions which took place after the formal presentations of these chapters. We hope that the issues raised at the meeting will make this an even more interesting book.

When we look back to Salter and his understanding of asthma, we can appreciate the state of knowledge we have today. We are blessed with immensely more information about the causes of the disease and infinitely better pharmaceutical tools to treat the disease. While there are still unanswered issues in asthma, we now have the knowledge and capacity to begin to treat asthma in a more effective manner. This book provides the basis for moving from an "era of symptomatic treatment" of asthma to an era of "specific treatment.'' In other words, the time when asthma was treated to simply reverse the airflow obstruction has passed, and the time when specific approaches to reduce the underlying disease processes is at hand.

Salter would be pleased to share his book's title with ours. His was an advanced understanding of asthma and its treatment in his day. This book is the state of our current knowledge and should be useful reading to every physician and scientist who wishes to know where we are and where we are headed in asthma research and treatment. We hope that you enjoy reading it.

Michael A. Kaliner
Peter J. Barnes
Carl G.A. Persson

CONTRIBUTORS

Jean-Claude Ameisen, M.D.   Centre D'Immunologie et de Biologie Parasitaire, Institut Pasteur, Lille, France

Claude Auriault, M.D.   Centre D'Immunologie et de Biologie Parasitaire, Institut Pasteur, Lille, France

Peter J. Barnes, M.A., D.M., F.R.C.P.   Professor and Director, Department of Thoracic Medicine, National Heart and Lung Institute, London, England

I. Berezin, M.D.   Department of Biomedical Science, McMaster University, Hamilton, Ontario, Canada

Ralph Brattsand, M.D.   Department of Pharmacology, A B Draco, Lund, Sweden

Michael F. Busk, M.D.   Department of Physiology and Biophysics, Mayo Clinic and Mayo Foundation, Rochester, Minnesota

André Capron, M.D.   Centre D'Immunologie et de Biologie Parasitaire, Institut Pasteur, Lille, France

Monique Capron, M.D.   Centre D'Immunologie et de Biologie Parasitaire, Institut Pasteur, Lille, France

Jean-Yves Cesbron, M.D.   Centre D'Immunologie et de Biologie Parasitaire, Institut Pasteur, Lille, France

Martin D. Chapman, M.D.   Department of Medicine, University of Virginia Medical Center, Charlottesville, Virginia

K.F. Chung, M.D.   Department of Thoracic Medicine, National Heart and Lung Institute, London, England

Martin K. Church, M.D.   Department of Clinical Pharmacology and Medicine I, Southampton General Hospital, Southampton, England

Donald W. Cockcroft, M.D., F.R.C.P.(C)   Division of Respiratory Medicine, University Hospital, Saskatoon, Saskatchewan, Canada

C.J. Corrigan, M.D.   Department of Allergy and Clinical Immunology, National Heart and Lung Institute, London, England

Martine Damonneville, M.D.   Institut D'Immunologie et de Biologie Parasitaire, Institut Pasteur, Lille, France

Edwin E. Daniel, Ph.D.   Department of Biomedical Science, McMaster University, Hamilton, Ontario, Canada

Jeffrey M. Drazen, M.D.   Department of Medicine, Beth Israel Hospital; Brigham & Women's Hospital; The Children's Hospital; Harvard Medical School, Boston, Massachusetts

A.J. Frew, M.D.   Department of Allergy and Clinical Immunology, National Heart & Lung Institute, London, England

Lena Håkansson   University Hospital, Uppsala, Sweden

Frederick E. Hargreave, M.D., F.R.C.P.(C)   Firestone Regional Chest and Allergy Unit, St. Joseph's Hospital, Hamilton, Ontario, Canada

James C. Hogg, M.D.   Pulmonary Research Laboratory, University of British Columbia, St. Paul's Hospital, Vancouver, British Columbia, Canada

Elliot Israel, M.D.   Department of Medicine, Beth Israel Hospital; Harvard Medical School, Boston, Massachusetts

Alan James, M.D.   Pulmonary Research Laboratory, University of British Columbia, St. Paul's Hospital, Vancouver, British Columbia, Canada

Christine R. Jenkins, M.D.   Institute of Respiratory Medicine, Royal Prince Alfred Hospital, Sydney, New South Wales, Australia

Michel Joseph, M.D.   Centre D'Immunologie et de Biologie Parasitaire, Institut Pasteur, Lille, France

Michael A. Kaliner, M.D.   National Institute of Allergy and Infectious Diseases, National Institutes of Health, Bethesda, Maryland

J-A. Karlssen   Department of Pharmacology, AB Draco, Lund, Sweden

A. Barry Kay, M.D.   Department of Allergy and Clinical Immunology, National Heart and Lung Institute, London, England

Karel F. Kerrebijn, M.D., Ph.D.   Department of Pediatric Pulmonary Medicine, Erasmus University Hospital; Department of Pediatric Pulmonary Medicine, Sophia Children's Hospital, Rotterdam, The Netherlands

Annika Laitinen, M.D.   Department of Electron Microscopy, University of Helsinki, Helsinki, Finland; Department of Medicine and Physiological Chemistry, University of Lund, Lund, Sweden

Lauri Laitinen, M.D.   Department of Lung Medicine, University of Lund; Exploratory Clinical Research, AB Draco, Lund, Sweden

Alan R. Leff, M.D.   Chief, Section of Pulmonary and Critical Care Medicine, Associate Professor, Department of Medicine, University of Chicago, Chicago, Illinois

Christina M. Luczynska, M.D.   Department of Medicine, University of Virginia Medical Center, Charlottesville, Virginia

Jan M. Lundberg, M.D.   Department of Pharmacology, Karolinska Institute, Stockholm, Sweden

William Maguire, M.D.   Department of Medicine, Beth Israel Hospital; Harvard Medical School, Boston, Massachusetts

Rodrigo Moreno, M.D.   Pulmonary Research Laboratory, University of British Columbia, St. Paul's Hospital, Vancouver, British Columbia, Canada

Paul M. O'Byrne, M.D.   Department of Medicine, McMaster University, Hamilton, Ontario, Canada

Veronique Pancré, M.D.   Centre D'Immunologie et de Biologie Parasitaire, Institut Pasteur, Lille, France

Peter Paré, M.D.   Department of Medicine, University of British Columbia, St. Paul's Hospital, Vancouver, British Columbia, Canada

Romain Pauwels, M.D.   Department of Respiratory Diseases, University Hospital, Ghent, Belgium

Carl G.A. Persson, Ph.D.   Department of Clinical Pharmacology, University Hospital of Lund; Exploratory Clinical Research, AB Draco, Lund, Sweden

Bohdan Pichurko, M.D.   Department of Medicine, Beth Israel Hospital; Harvard Medical School, Boston, Massachusetts

Ulf Pipkorn, M.D.   Department of Otolaryngology, University Hospital of Lund, Lund, Sweden

Thomas A. E. Platts-Mills, M.D. Department of Medicine, University of Virginia Medical Center, Charlottesville, Virginia

Susan M. Pollart, M.D.   Department of Medicine, University of Virginia Medical Center, Charlottesville, Virginia

Ricardo Polosa, M.D.   Department of Clinical Pharmacology and Medicine I, Southampton General Hospital, Southampton, England

S. Janet Rimmer, M.D.   Department of Clinical Pharmacology and Medicine I, Southampton General Hospital, Southampton, England

Malcolm R. Sears, M.D.   Department of Medicine, University of Otago Medical School, Dunedin, New Zealand

André-Bernard Tonnel, M.D.   Centre D'Immunologie et de Biologie Parasitaire, Institut Pasteur, Lille, France

Anne Tsicopoulos, M.D.   Centre D'Immunologie et de Biologie Parasitaire, Institut Pasteur, Lille, France

Paul M. Vanhoutte, M.D., Ph.D.   Director, Center for Experimental Therapeutics, Baylor College of Medicine, Houston, Texas

Per Venge, M.D.   Department of Clinical Chemistry, University Hospital, Uppsala, Sweden

Martha V. White, M.D.   National Institute of Allergy and Infectious Diseases, National Institutes of Health, Bethesda, Maryland

John G. Widdicombe, D.M.M.A., D.Phil., F.R.C.P.   Chairman and Head, Department of Physiology, St. George's Hospital Medical School, London, England

Barry Wiggs, M.D.   Pulmonary Research Laboratory, University of British Columbia, St. Paul's Hospital, Vancouver, British Columbia, Canada

Ann J. Woolcock, M.D.   Institute of Respiratory Medicine, Royal Prince Alfred Hospital, Sydney, New South Wales, Australia

CONTENTS

1

Epidemiological Trends in Bronchial Asthma

MALCOLM R. SEARS

University of Otago Medical School
Dunedin, New Zealand

During the last decade, a number of interrelated observations have raised interest in the epidemiology of asthma: a widespread impression that the prevalence of asthma has increased, dramatic increases in hospital admissions for asthma, an apparent increase in the severity of asthma despite improved treatments, relatively abrupt changes in the prevalence and nature of asthma in certain populations, and an increase in reported mortality from asthma in several countries. Epidemiological studies of disease prevalence, genetics, inducing and inciting factors including occupation and environment, together with trends in management and outcome, including mortality, have added considerably to our understanding of asthma. Several substantive epidemiological studies, using identical or similar methods in different countries, or in different populations within countries, have provided valuable national and international comparative data. These studies have not been without their difficulties, however, and several problems should be considered before drawing conclusions about epidemiological trends in bronchial asthma.

I. Problems in Epidemiological Measurements in Asthma

A. Definition and Recognition of Asthma

Since we cannot yet define asthma precisely in terms of its causes or pathology, its prevalence has generally been measured by reliance on recognition by the subject, physician, or epidemiologist of a characteristic pattern of symptoms as "asthma." Although Scadding (1983) defined asthma as "a disease characterized by wide variations over short periods of time in resistance to flow in intrapulmonary airways," it is the clustering of symptoms of dyspnea, chest tightness, wheeze, and cough, and their intermittent nature, which usually leads to a diagnosis of asthma.

Problems of definition and recognition of asthma are particularly apparent in children. Only one-third to one-half of children with the cluster of symptoms suggesting asthma have been diagnosed by a physician as having asthma; others are said to have bronchitis, recurrent infections, wheezy bronchitis, or simply wheezing. Legitimate confusion may arise in young children between asthmatic symptoms and those of bronchiolitis (Henderson et al., 1979), since the clinical features and subsequent cause of bronchiolitis and asthma are similar (Pullan and Hey, 1982; Carlssen et al., 1987). Some recommend that recurrent bronchiolitis be regarded as asthma (Tabachnik and Levison, 1981). Children with cystic fibrosis may develop labile airways with variable airflow rates consistent with asthma (Hordvik et al., 1985). Nocturnal or postexercise cough is a common presentation of asthma in children (Konig, 1981) but may be misdiagnosed as due to bronchitis or infection. Thus, Godfrey (1985) defined asthma in childhood using an extension of the definition of Scadding (1983) to include characteristic symptoms and response to treatment, stating that

> Asthma in childhood is a disease characterized by wide variations over short periods of time in resistance to flow in intrapulmonary airways, and manifest by recurrent attacks of cough or wheeze separated by symptom free intervals. The airflow obstruction and clinical symptoms are largely or completely reversed by treatment with bronchodilator drugs or steroids.

The identification of asthma may also be difficult in older subjects in whom symptoms of asthma may be confused with symptoms due to airflow limitation caused by smoking-related diseases. Dodge and Burrows (1980) reported marked differences in prevalence figures for "physician-diagnosed asthma" and "wheezing" in all age groups, even among young people. For example, among 20-24-year-olds in Tucson, while only 5% reported asthma, 12% had attacks of shortness of breath with wheeze, 25% had wheeze even apart from colds, and as many as 42% had experienced wheezing with colds.

Chronic bronchitis and emphysema are rare disorders in this age group; if these young wheezing subjects do not suffer from asthma, what diagnosis should they be given? In older subjects in Tucson, however, a large proportion of those with a diagnosis of asthma also carried the diagnosis of chronic bronchitis or emphysema. Differentiation between asthma and these conditions requires a carefully taken history combined with detailed investigations of pulmonary function and often a prolonged test of reversibility of airflow obstruction. Subjects who show partially reversible airflow obstruction, even when there is a history of heavy smoking and features of chronic bronchitis with dominant symptoms of recurrent cough and sputum production, may be classified by some as having asthma. The terms *asthmatic bronchitis* and *bronchial asthma*, while similar, are not synonymous, yet if used in hospital discharge documentation or death certification, both would result in the subject being coded as having "asthma."

Some investigators have chosen to record only physician-diagnosed asthma, but even this may not be valid as a guide to changing prevalences since physicians have an increasing interest in asthma, thus increasing the likelihood of significant diagnostic transfer. It is essential that what is recorded as "asthma" for epidemiological purposes is very precisely defined and reported.

B. Validity of Questionnaire Data

The American Thoracic Society (ATS) questionnaire (Ferris, 1978) and the Medical Research Council (MRC) respiratory questionnaire (1960) contain questions of relevance to the diagnosis and measurement of asthma in the population, but neither have been considered entirely satisfactory for this purpose (Samet, 1987). The MRC questionnaire asked: "Does your chest ever sound wheezy or whistling? If yes, do you get this with colds?—occasionally apart from colds?—most days or nights? Have you ever had attacks of shortness of breath with wheezing? If yes, is/was your breathing absolutely normal between attacks?" and it also asked about a past history of "bronchial asthma." The ATS questionnaire asked: "Does your chest ever sound wheezy or whistling—when you have a cold?—occasionally apart from colds—most days or nights? Have you ever had an attack of wheezing that has made you feel short of breath?" with supplementary questions relating to the onset of symptoms and their treatment. The questionnaire also asked: "Have you ever had asthma?" and if so, whether this was confirmed by a physician.

Many studies of the epidemiology of asthma have used modified MRC or ATS questionnaires, although the questions from which the most important information have been derived have been similar. The question that identified 96% of the children finally considered by the Tyneside investigators to have asthma was "Does your child have attacks of wheezing?" (Lee et al., 1983). An almost identical question was used in childhood studies in New Zealand and Australia and elsewhere, with similar results.

A new questionnaire is under development through the International Union Against Tuberculosis (IUAT), but the final form and validation studies are being awaited (Burney and Chinn, 1987).

The problem of recall bias must also be considered. Persons with minor infrequent symptoms are less likely to respond positively to symptom questionnaires than are those whose symptoms are more recent or more severe. The estimate of period prevalence (symptoms within the last month, or, more commonly, within the last 12 months) is more likely to be accurate than the estimate of cumulative prevalence, especially when the data relate to early childhood.

A further problem is the interpretation of symptoms of wheezing. Some investigators regard wheezing that occurs only in association with a "cold" as not being attributable to asthma, whereas other would argue that the apparent "cold" may in fact be asthma causing the cough and sputum production, and not an infection. In some studies, the duration of wheezing was regarded as an important arbiter of whether the symptoms are due to asthma; for example, symptoms lasting less than 1h were excluded by the Tyneside investigators (Lee et al., 1983). Since exercise-induced wheezing is generally of short duration, many subjects with only exercise-induced asthma will not be identified when such criteria are used.

Samet (1987) has recommended that questionnaires used in epidemiological studies of asthma include items relating to frequency of symptoms, exacerbating stimuli, seasonality, treatment, hospitalization, and functional limitation. Such "expanded" questionnaires have been used in studies in children in New Zealand, Australia, Canada, and the United Kingdom, and have provided useful data on both prevalence and severity of asthma. However, it is essential that the fundamental questions asked in each population be standardized and validated so that reliable comparisons between studies can be made.

C. Diagnostic Transfer in Disorders of Airflow Limitation

As interest in asthma has increased, the likelihood that an individual may recognize his or her symptoms as due to asthma, or mistakenly attribute non-asthmatic symptoms to this cause, has also increased. A trend away from the diagnosis of bronchitis and towards asthma may markedly affect the number of cases of reported asthma because, especially in older subjects, bronchitis is apparently much more prevalent than asthma. Diagnostic transfer may also have resulted from the continued development of pharmaceutical preparations for the treatment of asthma and the marketing of these products. A diagnosis of asthma may be made to justify a trial of treatment, or more probably the response to such treatment may make the diagnosis of asthma more evident. Increases due to diagnostic transfer and those due to real changes in prevalence can only be differentiated if detailed data relating to all respiratory diseases are reviewed, not just those pertaining to "asthma."

D. Classification and Coding of Asthma

The ninth revision of the World Health Organization International Classification of Diseases (World Health Organization, 1977) introduced in 1979 brought a significant alteration in the rules governing coding of conditions in which both bronchitis and asthma were said to coexist. Hospital discharge and death certificate data are coded under clearly defined rules. Under the rules governing the 8th revision of the International Classification of Diseases (ICD8), "chronic bronchitis and asthma" was coded to chronic bronchitis, whereas under ICD9 this would be coded to asthma. In addition, ICD9 introduced a new category of "airways obstruction not otherwise classified" that was not previously available for coding; this category may contain a mixture of bronchitis, emphysema, and chronic asthma. The effect of these changes in the ICD classifications has been well studied with regard to mortality (see later), but these changes in coding also affect morbidity data.

There are therefore many reasons why epidemiological measurements in asthma are subject to some uncertainty, and the reliability of recent trends in morbidity and mortality requires validation. The last decade has seen a marked increase in the use of objective measurements in epidemiological studies in an attempt to overcome some of these uncertainties.

II. Ancillary Aids in Epidemiological Measurements in Asthma

Asthma is defined as "variable airflow obstruction" or "reversible airway disease." That the symptoms of wheeze, cough, chest tightness, and dyspnea are due to asthma may be firmly established by objective documentation of variable or reversible airflow obstruction accompanying these symptoms (Venables et al., 1984). This may not be feasible in large epidemiological studies, but in smaller studies, portable peak expiratory flow rate (PEFR) meters have been used repeatedly over various periods of time. More commonly, however, objective measurements made in the quest for a more secure diagnosis of asthma have been undertaken only on a single occasion, either by administration of a bronchodilator aerosol to subjects demonstrating airflow obstruction, to document bronchodilator "reversibility," or by induction of airway narrowing by an inhaled or physical stimulus (e.g., methacholine or histamine inhalation challenge, hyperventilation with cold air, or exercise).

A. Variability in Peak Expiratory Flow Rates

An estimation of variability of airflow obstruction can be obtained using standard or portable peak expiratory flow rate meters (Hetzel and Clark, 1980). The normal (95% confidence interval) diurnal variability of PEFR in adults has been reported as 16-20%, and in children 28%, and the normal daily variability in PEFR as ±12% in adults and ±20% in children (Lebowitz, 1982; Lebowitz, personal communication). Persons with PEFR variability exceeding these limits on more than 5% of days can be regarded as having abnormal variability of PEFR, and hence, by inference, asthma.

B. Reversibility of Airflow Obstruction

In epidemiological studies, the prevalence of baseline airflow obstruction is considerably less than the prevalence of symptoms, and obstruction is therefore an insensitive tool for measuring asthma prevalence, although reversibility of airflow obstruction is highly specific. The degree of reversibility of airflow obstruction required to establish a diagnosis of asthma is usually stated to be a 20% or greater increase in airflow as measured by the forced expiratory volume exhaled in 1s (FEV_1) or in PEFR occurring either spontaneously or with treatment (Editorial, 1988). Some adult patients with chronic obstructive pulmonary disease due to smoking have objectively documented variations in airflow of this magnitude, although they do not usually achieve normal lung function. On the other hand, an asthmatic person who smokes or works in a highly polluted atmosphere may develop less reversible disease. Furthermore, some asthmatic people, even lifetime nonsmokers, develop irreversible or very poorly reversible airflow obstruction (Brown et al., 1984). Some impression of the degree of reversibility in earlier life may, however, be evident from the variability of symptoms (e.g., from severe dyspnea to total freedom from dyspnea). Measurement of current reversibility should not be confined to the response to an inhaled bronchodilator, but may need to include the response to a prolonged trial of high-dosage systemic corticosteroid therapy.

C. Detection of Airway Hyperresponsiveness

Increased responsiveness of the airways to nonallergic stimuli usually accompanies asthma symptoms (Hargreave et al., 1981) and has been used as an ancillary aid in several recent epidemiological studies. Airway hyperresponsiveness (AHR) has not, however, been demonstrated in some subjects with symptomatic evidence for asthma, and, conversely, has been identified in some children and adults without significant current or past respiratory symptoms (Lee et al. 1983; Sears et al., 1986a; Salome et al., 1987; Enarson et al., 1987). Hence the presence or absence of airway hyperresponsiveness cannot be regarded as a gold standard for the diagnosis of asthma in epidemiological measurements. In a study of Canadian children, the sensitivity of a methacholine inhalation challenge with respect to a cumulative history of respiratory symptoms consistent with asthma was 67%, and for recent symptoms 57%, while the specificity of the test was 83% (Fitzgerald et al., 1989). In adults, there was an overall agreement of 83% between a questionnaire response regarding "asthma" and AHR to histamine, and of 76% between a response regarding "wheezing" and AHR (Burney and Chinn, 1987). A questionnaire response regarding "asthma" was of lower sensitivity (50%) but greater specificity (96%) in detecting AHR than was a response regarding wheezing (sensitivity 86%, specificity 72%).

The patterns of airway responsiveness to inhalation of histamine or metacholine have been considered to be helpful in differentiating asthma from other forms of airflow obstruction. The dose-response curve to these agents does not show a plateau in the asthmatic person, whereas the patient with chronic airflow obstruction will achieve a plateau response if the dosage is increased sufficiently. The specificity of this observation has not yet been adequately assessed.

Some studies of the epidemiology of asthma have used the coexistence of symptoms consistent with asthma with a certain increase in airway responsiveness to define asthma. For instance, Woolcook et al. (1987) reported subjects as having asthma if they had airway hyperresponsiveness such that the provoking dose (PD) of histamine causing a 20% fall in FEV_1 ($PD_{20}FEV_1$) was 3.9 μmol or less, together with symptoms of wheeze, night cough, or shortness of breath at rest. However, this and other studies have shown a considerable discrepancy between "typical" symptoms of asthma and the presence of airway hyperresponsiveness. It is therefore preferable to describe these characteristics as independent variables that are closely related to each other and to the condition of "asthma" (Burney et al., 1987b).

A current difficulty in the use of measurements of airway responsiveness in making a diagnosis of asthma has been a lack of standardization of methodology. Some of the nonuniformity has related to the need to undertake the investigations in a short space of time in an epidemiological setting, while individual preferences or historical reasons have also determined the use of certain procedures. The recent trend towards standardizing methacholine and histamine inhalation tests is encouraging. When nonstandardized procedures are used, these should be validated by comparison with well-recognized and validated procedures (Sears et al., 1986a).

III. Studies of the Prevalence of Asthma

A. Prevalence of Asthma in Childhood

Despite the lack of a precise definition, the use of differing methodologies, and varying reporting of period and cumulative rates, studies of the prevalence of asthma in childhood in different countries during the last decade have produced some relatively consistent findings. Recurrent respiratory symptoms suggesting a diagnosis of asthma have been reported in 7-27% of children aged 7-10 years, with lower rates found in the United States (Weiss et al., 1980; Mak et al., 1982; Gergen et al., 1988) than in Canada (Kerigan et al., 1986; Fitzgerald et al., 1988), England (Lee et al., 1983; Anderson et al., 1983), New Zealand (Jones et al., 1987; Asher et al., 1988), or Australia (Salome et al., 1987; Hurry et al., 1988). Selected studies undertaken in the last decade are summarized in Table 1.

B. International Comparisons

Two studies have been undertaken to examine the possibility that New Zealand has a higher prevalence of childhood asthma. The studies used identical or highly comparable epidemiological methods in different countries within relatively short time intervals, although not simultaneously.

The study by Sears et al. (1986a) in 9-year-old New Zealand children was replicated in Canadian children (Fitzgerald et al., 1988). One important difference was that in New Zealand an abbreviated method for methacholine inhalation challenge was used, whereas the tidal breathing method was used in the Canadian study. However, a validation study showed close correlations between responses to both methods (Sears et al., 1986a). Of New Zealand 9-year-olds, 18.1% had 3 or more episodes of wheeze per year compared with 20.5% in Canada; the cumulative prevalence of any wheeze was 27% compared with 30%; the prevalence of diagnosed asthma was 8.6% compared with 8.9%; all differences were trivial and nonsignificant. There was, however, a greater prevalence of airway hyperresponsiveness (defined as methacholine $PC_{20}FEV_1$ less than 8 mg/ml) in Canadian children, mostly related to a greater occurrence of hyperresponsiveness in lifetime asymptomatic children.

An even closer replication of studies was undertaken by Asher et al. (1988) in New Zealand using questionnaires and methods for determining airway responsiveness identical to those used in Sydney, Australia (Britton et al., 1986). More than 1000 New Zealand children were compared with 769 children

Table 1 Selected Studies of the Prevalence of Asthma and Wheezing in Children Reported in the Last Decade

Location	Age	Prevalence	Reference
Sydney, Aust	12.6[a]	7.2% M, 4.2% F	Peat et al., 1980[a]
	8.9[a]	8.6% M, 4.4% F	
Queensland, Aust	8.1[a]	20.5% wheeze	Mitchell and Miles, 1983
	12.1[a]	18.1% wheeze	
South Australia	8	27.4% cumulative (asthma + wheeze)	Crockett et al., 1986
New Sth Wales, Aust	8-10	12.4% asthma, 24.3% wheezing	Salome et al., 1987
New Sth Wales, Aust	8-12	17.3% asthma, 26.5% wheezing	Hurry et al., 1988
Hamilton, Canada	7-10	4.4% asthma, 21.2% wheezing most days	Kerigan et al., 1986
Halton, Canada	9	20.5% wheezing (3/year or more)	Fitzgerald et al., 1989
Lower Hutt, NZ	11-13	13.5% asthma	Mitchell & Miles, 1983
Dunedin, NZ	9	18.1% wheezing (3/year or more)	Jones et al., 1987
Auckland, NZ	8-10	European 13.5%, Maori 10.8% (symptoms + AHR)	Asher et al., 1988
Oslo, Norway	7-15	1.6% current, 3.7% cumulative, 9% wheeze	Skarpaas & Gulsvik, 1985
Tyneside, UK	7	9.3% current, 11.1% cumulative	Lee et al., 1983
London, UK	9	11.1% current, 18.2% cumulative	Anderson et al., 1983
National, UK	7,11,16	Current 8.3%, 4.7%, 3.5% respectively	Anderson et al., 1987
		Cumulative 18.3%, 21.9%, 24.7%	
Boston, US	5-9	9.2% persistent wheeze	Weiss et al., 1980
Baltimore, US	Gds 1,6	7.2% current, 10.5% cumulative	Mak et al., 1982
National, US	6-11	7.6% asthma and wheeze apart from colds	Gergen et al., 1988

[a]Mean age reported rather than range.

from inland New South Wales (NSW? and 718 from coastal NSW. The prevalence of any respiratory symptom, diagnosed asthma, AHR, the concurrence of respiratory symptoms and AHR, and the severity of AHR were similar among New Zealand and inland NSW children, and only slightly higher than for coastal NSW children.

On superficial examination, the prevalence rates for childhood wheezing (15-25%) in Australia and New Zealand appear to be greater than those found in the United Kingdom, where 11.1% of 7 year old children had had symptoms suggesting asthma since starting school (Lee et al., 1983). However the criteria for including wheezing episodes were not strictly comparable, since wheeze lasting less than 1h (e.g., exercise-induced wheezing), which would have added perhaps a further 3-4% to the United Kingdom (UK) prevalence rate was excluded. Furthermore, the prevalence of asthmalike symptoms in early childhood, but not current at age 7, was known to be underestimated in the UK. Hence the corrected cumulative prevalence of wheezing symptoms in the Tyneside study would probably reach 18-20%, which is very similar to the prevalence rates determined in Australia, New Zealand, and Canada.

C. Has the Prevalence of Childhood Asthma Increased?

An uncritical review of studies of the epidemiology of childhood asthma would suggest that in some countries there has been a substantial increase in prevalence over the last 20-30 years. For instance, in New Zealand, 0.2% of children were reported to suffer from asthma as determined by school medical examinations in 1958 (Blanc, 1966), a questionnaire mailed to parents in 1961 identified 1.9% of children 5-16 years as having asthma (Blanc, 1966), and a school survey in 1968 found that 7.1% of 11-13-year-olds had required treatment for asthma (Milne, 1969). A cohort questionnaire survey in 1979 found that 7.4% of 7-year-old children were diagnosed as having asthma and another 4.8% had a history of wheezing and had atopic features strongly suggesting that the wheezing was due to asthma, giving a total cumulative prevalence of probable asthma of 12.2%. A further 22.6% were reported to have experienced wheezing but had weak or no evidence for an associated atopic disease; the diagnosis of asthma in these children was less certain (Sears et al., 1982). Although part of these upward trends with time may be real, there may also be a greater awareness and acceptance of a diagnosis of asthma. The changing epidemiological techniques, including a broadening of questions from those relating to "asthma" to those asking about "wheezing," may also account for much of the increase.

There is some evidence for the proposition that the true prevalence of childhood asthma has not changed significantly. Two studies in English general practices some 30 years ago found that 20% of children had one or more attacks of wheezing during the first decade of life (Goodall, 1958; Fry, 1961). The 1960s Melbourne study found that 19.1% of 7-year-old children had had recurrent episodes of wheezing (Williams and McNicol, 1969). The prevalence figures in most countries 20 years later do not exceed these earlier estimates. Anderson (1989) recently summarized UK studies between 1964 and 1986 reporting period prevalence of wheezing, and found no convincing evidence for an increase with time.

In most of the studies determining the prevalence of wheezing illnesses, some 60-70% of children with recurrent wheezing were not regarded by their parent as having asthma. A change in diagnostic fashion could therefore greatly alter the prevalence of reported asthma, but is unlikely to make a significant change in the prevalence of reported recurrent wheezing.

In Birmingham, the prevalence rate for "asthma" defined as recurrent wheezing was 1.8% in 1956-1957, whereas in 1968-1969, 2.3% of children were reported to have asthma and a further 3.2% had wheezing, giving a total prevalence of wheezing of 5.5% (Smith, 1961; Smith et al., 1971). In New Zealand, a repeat study in 11-13-year-old children at the same two intermediate schools a decade after the first study, using the identical questionnaire, yielded a prevalence rate for "asthma" of 13.5% compared with 7.1% (Milne, 1969; Mitchell, 1983). However in both the English and New Zealand studies, there was a significant change in the ethnic mix of the population and a change in attitude towards the diagnosis of "asthma," both of which changes may have increased the reported prevalence rate without an equal change in the true prevalence of asthma in a standardized population.

More substantive data suggesting a true increase in asthma prevalence have come from the United States, where the reported prevalence among 6-11-year-old children of ever having asthma increased significantly from 4.8% to 7.6% between the first and second National Health and Nutrition Examination Surveys (NHANES) conducted 5 years apart in the 1970s (Gergen et al., 1988). For this analysis, only physician-diagnosed asthma was included, but it seems unlikely that the 58% increase in prevalence could be due solely to a greater acceptance of the diagnostic label "asthma" for childhood wheezing. A study in England of consultations in general practice over an interval of 10 years (Fleming, 1987) suggested that between 1971 and 1981 there had been a real increase in the prevalence of asthma across all age groups; only in 5-14-year-olds could the increase in asthma be explained by a reduction in the prevalence of "acute bronchitis" by diagnostic transfer.

D. Increasing Hospital Admissions for Childhood Asthma

Hospital admissions for asthma in childhood have increased in many countries, suggesting that either the prevalence or severity of asthma has increased (Mitchell, 1985; Burr, 1987). In some regions of the United States, there has been a 300% increase in admissions due to asthma (Mullally et al., 1984), while across the whole country, the rate of hospitalization for children under 15 years with asthma increased at least 145% between 1970 and 1984 (Halfon and Newacheck, 1986). In England, hospital admissions of 5-14-year-olds increased by 167% over a period of 8 years (Anderson et al., 1980), and much larger increases have occurred in New Zealand (Jackson and Mitchell, 1983; Dawson, 1987). While some of this increase is explained by a doubling of the readmission rate (Anderson, 1978; Mullally et al., 1984; Mitchell and Cutler, 1984), suggesting an increase in the occurrence of severe episodes in the same children, the increase in first admissions is strong supportive evidence for an increase in prevalence.

Hospital admissions for asthma have increased in spite of a reduced admission rate for all respiratory admissions combined. The increase has also occurred despite the increase in the use of antiasthmatic medications (Mullally et al., 1984), which suggests either that therapy is ineffective or even compounding the problem, or that asthma has increased in severity for other reasons. In a New Zealand pediatric unit, the annual number of admissions for asthma rose dramatically over 20 years from 21 admissions of 17 patients in 1965, to 186 admissions of 122 patients in 1975, and 609 admissions of 374 patients in 1985 (Dawson, 1987). The severity of asthma on admission, judged by a retrospective scoring system based on wheezing, pulse rate, and use of accessory muscles, increased considerably between 1975 and 1985, strongly supporting the view that the increased hospitalization reflects increasing severity of asthma rather than earlier admission with the same degree of asthma.

In summary, the epidemiological evidence collected over the last decade suggest that the prevalence of childhood asthma has at least remained as high as it was 20 years ago and may have increased in some populations. In addition, there appears to have been an increase in severity of childhood asthma as judged by hospital admission data.

IV. Asthmatic Symptoms and Airway Hyper-responsiveness in Children

Children with more obvious or frequent symptoms of asthma generally show marked increases in airway responsiveness to histamine or methacholine (Hargreave et al., 1981; Lee et al., 1983; Sears et al., 1986a; Hopp et al., 1986; Salome et al., 1987), and many also show variability in airflow immediately following exercise. These children also show frequent variation in peak flow measurements and a significant diurnal variation. However, a number of studies in New Zealand (Sears et al., 1986a; Asher et al., 1988), Australia

(Salome et al., 1987), Canada (Fitzgerald et al., 1988), the United States (Weiss et al., 1984), and the United Kingdom (Lee et al., 1983) have identified a significant proportion of children who show airway hyperresponsiveness but who have no current or past symptoms suggestive of asthma. This observation was made whether the challenge test was performed using histamine, methacholine, or hyperventilation with cold air. To disturb further the relationship between symptoms and airway hyperresponsiveness, some children with a history of current symptoms strongly suggesting asthma (wheezing, coughing, and chest tightness on exercise) did not demonstrate airway hyperresponsiveness to these agents on single or repeated tests (Sears et al., 1987a). Although overall the correlation between symptoms suggesting asthma and the presence of airway hyperresponsiveness is high, the measurement has not been found to be sufficiently specific or sensitive to allow its uncritical use in epidemiological studies. Although it is useful in assessing severity and understanding the mechanisms of asthma (Hargreave et al., 1981), the false-negative and false-positive rates (if that is what they are shown to be) have reduced the usefulness of these measurements in epidemiological studies.

In the longitudinal New Zealand study of a birth cohort of 1,037 children (Sears et al., 1986a; Jones et al., 1987), there was a good correlation between chronic or frequent symptoms of wheezing requiring treatment and airway hyperresponsiveness to methacholine; 79% of such children showed a 20% fall in FEV_1 at a provoking concentration of methacholine of 8 mg/ml or less ($PC_{20}FEV_1 < 8$ mg/ml), which is usually accepted as the cut-off point between normal and increased airway responsiveness. However increased airway responsiveness was found in only 39% of those with a history of less than 12 wheezing episodes per year, even though symptoms had occurred within the last 12 months in the majority of these children. On the other hand, 32 of 480 children (6.7%) who had never had recurrent respiratory symptoms of any type showed increased airway responsiveness to methacholine.

In a larger study of school children aged 8-11 years in New South Wales (Salome et al., 1987; Peat et al., 1987a,b) airway hyperresponsiveness as defined by a 20% fall in FEV_1 at a provoking dose of histamine ($PD_{20}FEV_1$) of less than 7.8 mmol by the method of Yan et al. (1983) was found in 17.9% of the sample. However, 6.7% of the sample had hyperresponsiveness so defined without any current or past respiratory symptoms, while 5.6% had had a previous diagnosis of asthma but did not show airway hyperresponsiveness to histamine. The relationship with symptoms was most obvious in those with marked increases in airway responsiveness: all children with a $PD_{20}FEV_1 < 0.1$ mmol had wheezing symptoms and all but one had diagnosed asthma, whereas only 77% of children with a $PD_{20}FEV_1$ between 0.1 and 0.8 mmol had a history of wheeze and 64% had diagnosed asthma. In this study the total prevalence of airway hyperresponsiveness (17.9%) was higher than the prevalence of diagnosed asthma (12.8%), but less than the prevalence of wheezing (24.3%) or of any respiratory symptom (33.9%). Despite the "false negatives" and "false positives," the association between symptoms and airway hyperresponsiveness was highly significant (p < 0.001). The $PD_{20}FEV_1$ of children with diagnosed asthma and respiratory symptoms was significantly lower than that in hyperresponsive children without symptoms, or children with wheezing not diagnosed as asthma by their physician. The relationship between respiratory symptoms, diagnosed asthma, and airway responsiveness as found in this Australian study is shown in Figure 1.

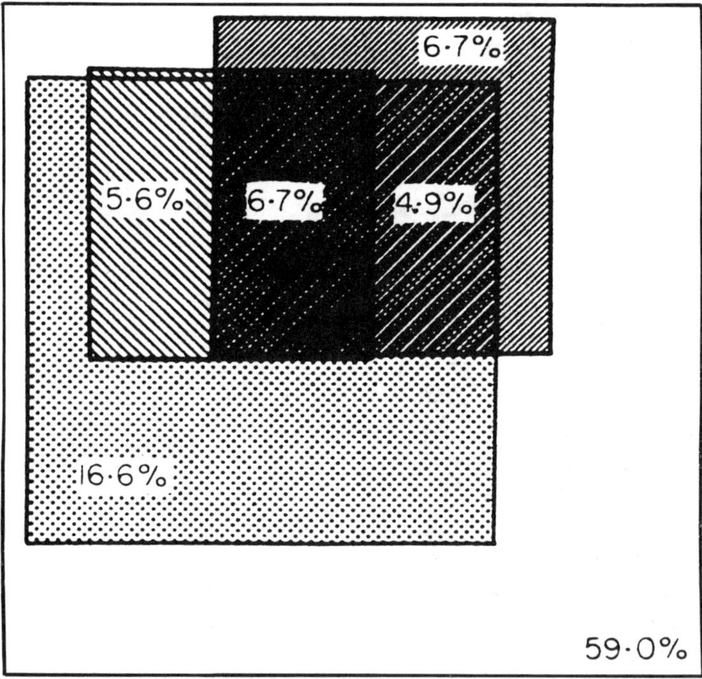

Figure 1 The degree of overlap between airway hyperresponsiveness (AHR), diagnosed asthma, and respiratory symptoms in Australian children. The outer square represents the whole sample, the lower inner square those with respiratory symptoms, the upper left square those with diagnosed asthma, and the upper right square those with AHR. The degree to which the squares overlap represents the degree to which these three factors overlap in the population (reproduced with permission from Salome et al., 1987).

In a Canadian study of 230 children, the sensitivity of a methacholine $PC_{20}FEV_1$ of 8 mg/ml or less in relation to a cumulative history of respiratory symptoms suggesting asthma was 67%, and for symptoms within the last month was 57%, while the specificity of the test was 83% (Fitzgerald et al., 1988).

V. Risk Factors for Childhood Asthma

From their analysis of data from the National Child Development Study involving a cohort of 8806 British children studied at 7, 11, and 16 years, Anderson et al. (1987) found that the subsequent onset of asthma was predicted by male sex, mother's age at birth, pneumonia, whooping cough, tonsillectomy/adenoidectomy, allergic rhinitis, eczema, and abdominal pain/vomiting attacks. Factors that were not predictive included infant feeding patterns, housing, and socioeconomic status. Maternal smoking in pregnancy increased the relative risk of asthma or wheezing in early life, but the parents' and child's smoking habits when the child was aged 16 were not related to asthma. Some of these factors have been examined in several other studies, with varying levels of agreement.

A. Male Sex

The preponderance of male children found in studies of asthma prevalence has ranged from 1.6:1 (Mak et al., 1982) to over 2:1 (Milne, 1969), with a reducing male preponderance in later childhood and early teenage years (Dawson et al., 1969). Since there is little if any difference in the distribution of atopy between male and female children, but a significant male preponderance of bronchial lability (Verity et al., 1984), the latter factor may be the more significant as a cause of childhood asthma. However the male/female (m/f) ratio reported in many studies may reflect bias if the label "asthma" is more readily applied to boys than girls. In Boston, Weiss et al. (1980) found the m/f ratio for "asthma" was 1.8:1, but for recurrent wheezing on most days or nights, whether or not labeled as asthma, the ratio was 1:1. In a New Zealand longitudinal study of children evaluated to age 15, the m/f ratio among the children with the most obvious asthma, whether or not so diagnosed by parent or doctor, was 1.5:1 (Sears et al., unpublished). Anderson et al. (1987) found male sex to be a stronger predictor of onset in later childhood or of early onset with persistence into later childhood, than of an early onset with remission.

B. Genetic Predisposition

The prevalence of asthma, hay fever, and eczema is significantly higher among relatives of patients with atopic asthma than among relatives of nonatopic asthmatics (Sibbald and Turner-Warwick, 1979). The prevalence of asthma among relatives was correlated with the prevalence of hay fever or eczema among relatives, and with the degree of atopy in the asthmatic subjects themselves. All studies suggest that the expression of asthma depends at least in part on a genetic predisposition to the condition and that the presence of atopy in genetically predisposed individuals increases the risks of developing asthma. In the New South Wales study, a history of asthma in either parent as well as the presence of atopy were key factors associated with the development of airway hyperresponsiveness in the subject (Peat et al., 1987a). Studies in twins have shown a genetic effect on serum IgE levels in adults and children (Bazaral et al., 1974); total serum IgE levels demonstrated family concordance in the Tucson population (Lebowitz, 1984).

A genetic effect on airway responsiveness was noted by Godfrey and Konig (1974) even when there was no clinical concordance for asthma. The slope of the dose-response curve to methacholine was not different between monozygotic and dizygotic twins (Zamel et al., 1984). These studies suggest that environmental factors are more important than genetic factors in determining the degree of clinical expression of airway responsiveness in any individual.

C. Ethnicity

In the United States, the prevalence of reported asthma is consistently 50% higher among black children than white children. Studies in first grade Baltimore children revealed prevalence rates in blacks of 12.0% and in whites of 7.9%, while 11.2% of black children and 8.8% of white children in sixth grade were reported to have asthma (Mak et al., 1982). The NHANES study reported the prevalence of asthma in black children as 9.4% and in white children 6.2% (Gergen et al., 1988). This persistent racial difference suggests that significant genetic and ethnic factors influence the expression of asthma, or that significant differences in lifestyle affect environmental factors despite residence in the same community. In contrast, children living within the same environment in London, England, but of different ethnic background showed very similar prevalence rates for respiratory symptoms. There were no significant differences in the proportions of children with a history of wheezing illness (15-18%), whether they were of European, African, or Indian descent, although the European children reported more whooping cough, bronchitis, and croup (Johnston et al., 1987). New Zealand studies of respiratory symptoms and airway responsiveness have shown that a similar proportion of European (13.5%) and Maori (10.8%) children have recent respiratory symptoms with concurrent airway hyperresponsiveness (Harrison et al., 1986). That environmental factors dominate over genetic and ethnic factors is strongly suggested by the increase in prevalence of atopic disease and asthma in Tokelauan Island children relocated to New Zealand, whose prevalence rates now approximate those of European New Zealand children (Waite et al., 1980).

D. Atopy

The expression of asthma in childhood is clearly related to the presence of atopy, whether documented by skin tests (Zimmerman et al., 1988) or elevated serum IgE levels (Stempel et al., 1980), although not all children with obvious and persistent asthmatic symptoms are atopic. Of children with the most obvious asthma identified in the Dunedin Multidisciplinary Study, 85% were atopic to at least one skin test allergen, and 72% to two or more allergens, whereas in the whole cohort, 45% had one or more positive skin test and 27% two or more positive tests (Sears et al., 1989). In Tucson, among children with negative skin tests, the prevalence of asthma/wheezing was 2% compared with 14% among atopic children; shortness of breath with wheezing occurred in 8.6% of skin-test-negative children compared with over 25% of atopic children (Burrows et al., 1976). The relative risk for developing asthma symptoms with concurrent airway hyperresponsiveness in the New Zealand longitudinal child development study was significantly raised in association with positive skin test responses to the house dust mite and/or cat dander (odds ratios 6.7 and 4.2 respectively), but was not significantly increased with skin test sensitivity to grass pollen (Sears et al., 1988, 1989).

The persistence of symptoms of wheezing into later childhood is strongly associated with atopy. A follow-up study of a Tasmanian birth cohort showed that the presence of atopy manifested by hay fever and eczema in 7-year-old children with wheeze was associated with a fourfold increase in risk of persistence of asthma to age 20 (Gibson et al., 1969; Giles et al., 1984). The likelihood of persistence of asthma may depend on the nature of the allergen sensitivity. In a 5 year follow-up study of 9-14-year-old Melbourne children, remission of asthma was more likely to occur in those who were sensitized to a perennial allergen to which they became hyposensitized (e.g., house dust mite), whereas sensitivity to intermittent seasonal allergen (e.g., grass pollen) was associated with more persistent clinical asthma and immunological hypersensitivity (Hill et al., 1981).

Australian children who were atopic had an increased risk of having airway hyperresponsiveness, especially those with sensitivity to more than one allergen group (Peat et al., 1987a,b). The severity of the airway hyperresponsiveness increased with the severity of atopy. Similar findings have emerged from the New Zealand longitudinal study of childhood asthma (Sears et al., unpublished). While neither study provides clear evidence for a direct causal link between atopy and airway hyperresponsiveness, there may be a common link in their development.

E. Parental Smoking

A role for passive smoking in the development of childhood asthma has been strongly suggested by several studies. Weiss et al. (1980) found that parental cigarette smoking was linearly related to the occurrence of persistent wheeze. Among a study cohort of 650 children aged 5-9 years, 9.2% had persistent wheeze; in households in which neither parent smoked, only 1.85% of children wheezed, whereas 6.85% and 11.8% of children from households in which one or both parents were smokers developed persistent wheezing. This trend was independent of a parental history of wheezing. Furthermore, there was an association between the parental smoking history and a reduction in lung function in the children of the household. Nonasthmatic children showed an association between maternal smoking and lower lung function, while there was a relationship between increased airway responsiveness and maternal smoking in subjects with asthma.

In a cohort of high-risk children born to parents of whom at least one was atopic, there was no difference in the prevalence of wheezing at age 1 year in children of parents who did or did not smoke, but by age 5 years 62% of parents who smoked had children who had experienced episodes of wheeze, compared with 37% in families among whom neither parent smoked (Cogswell et al., 1987). In another study, the prevalence of parent-reported asthma in children up to 17 years of age was increased from 5.0% to 7.7% if the mother smoked, and the prevalence of "functionally impairing asthma" was doubled from 1.1% to 2.2% (Gortmaker et al., 1982).

Charlton (1984) found a positive correlation between maternal smoking and frequent cough in nonsmoking British children aged 8-19 years; the association was more obvious in younger children, and there was no effect of socioeconomic status. The prevalence of frequent cough in sons and daughters of nonsmoking parents was 35% and 32%, respectively, compared with 42% and 40% if one parent smoked, and 48% and 52% if both parents smoked. Since childhood cough can be a manifestation of asthma and is often associated with increased airway responsiveness to nonspecific stimuli, these findings could be interpreted as indirect evidence linking parental smoking with asthma.

Martinez et al. (1988a) found an increased relative risk (4.3) for airway hyperresponsiveness in male but not female children of smoking parents; the risk was still significant after controlling for atopy and asthma. Male children of smoking parents also showed a greater reactivity to skin allergens. Lung function was lower, and airway responsiveness greater, in children of smoking mothers studied during the cold, wet months when windows were closed and children were indoors compared with the warm, dry months. In the winter, there was a dose-response relationship between the maternal cigarette consumption indoors and childhood lung function, which was not seen in the summer months (Murray and Morrison, 1988).

F. Lower Respiratory Tract Infections

Although several studies have suggested that early childhood respiratory infection predisposes to later development of asthma, it seems equally possible that children with predisposition to asthma, or with early childhood symptoms of asthma not recognized as such, are more susceptible to infections. A 7 year study of 200 children with lower respiratory tract infections in infancy showed that these children subsequently had an increased prevalence of cough, wheeze, colds going to the chest, use of medication, consultations with general practitioners, and absences from school compared with control children (Mok and Simpson, 1984a,b). There was no difference between the symptomatic children and controls with regard to atopy, but the former showed increased airway responsiveness to exercise and reduced pulmonary function. Children with bronchiolitis due to the respiratory syncytial virus (RSV) showed a greater airway lability on exercise than did control children with the same degree of atopy (Sims et al., 1978). Over half of a group of Canadian children evaluated 10 years after an admission for bronchiolitis were found to have a positive methacholine test (Gurwitz et al., 1981). In England, children with RSV bronchiolitis had a greater prevalence of wheezing, although the prevalence of recognized and treated asthma was not different from that of a control group (Pullan and Hey, 1982). The RSV bronchiolitis group also showed a greater lability to exercise and to histamine challenge, with a threefold increased prevalence of airway hyperresponsiveness but no significant difference in the prevalence of atopy. These studies do not answer the question of whether asthma was induced by bronchiolitis, or the "bronchiolitis" was an early manifestation of asthma, or the potentially asthmatic child was more susceptible to RSV infection.

Children said to have "bronchitis" before age 5 who were then subsequently found at age 11 and 14 to have symptoms consistent with asthma (Holland et al., 1978) may in fact have had asthma before age 5, with symptoms incorrectly attributed to bronchitis. This hypothesis would also fit with the data of Weiss et al. (1980), who found that children with persistent wheezing were more likely to report an early lower respiratory tract infection. The uncertainties in this area will only be resolved by rigorously controlled longitudinal studies, preferably with measurements of airway responsiveness and objective evidence of infective episodes from infancy through adulthood. Once asthma is established, viral infections are a frequent inciting factor for exacerbations (Busse, 1988), but bacterial infections are not associated. However, there is no firm evidence that viral infections induce asthma in previously normal individuals.

G. Diminished Lung Function

Martinez et al. (1988b) have recently reported a prospective study of 124 newborn infants, demonstrating a risk for wheezing illness 3.7 times higher among infants with total respiratory resistance in the lower third of values compared with infants with values in the upper two-thirds. They concluded that diminished lung function was a predisposing factor for development of a first wheezing illness in infants.

H. Socioeconomic and Psychological Factors

Some early studies suggested that asthma was more common among higher social classes (Graham et al., 1967; Peckham and Butler, 1978; Peat et al., 1980b). The United Kingdom National Cohort Study reported "asthma" to be more frequent among children whose parents did nonmanual than manual work (Peckham and Butler, 1978), but the prevalence of wheezy bronchitis showed no social class difference, suggesting that the apparently higher prevalence of asthma in upper social classes in previous studies related to a greater recognition and more accurate diagnosis of asthma rather than a true difference in prevalence rates between classes. More recently, Anderson et al. (1987) have reported a striking similarity in the prevalence of asthma in different social classes in the UK study. In Tucson, family social factors do significantly affect the presence and natural history of asthma in childhood; the incidence of new asthma was related to smaller family size, lower income, and greater residential mobility (Lebowitz et al., 1990). Andrea et al. (1988) identified a greater prevalence of symptoms suggesting bronchial hyperresponsiveness in Scandinavian children living in damp houses, especially if a parent smoked. These factors could well differ between populations, or could be overshadowed by stronger environmental factors.

No consistent psychological profile of the asthmatic child has been determined. Several studies have shown that the psychological disturbances found in asthmatic children are those found in any group of children with a chronic illness and are not specifically related to asthma.

VI. Development and Progression of Childhood Asthma

In New South Wales, the development of symptomatic airway hyperresponsiveness in 7-10-year-old children was strongly associated with a history of early respiratory illness, a history of asthma in either parent, and the presence of atopy, the latter being the most important factor (Peat et al., 1987a). If all three factors were present, the risk of a moderate or severe increase in airway hyperresponsiveness was increased sixfold, indicating that infection and/or exposure to environmental aeroallergens added additional risk over and above the inherited ability for airways to become hyperresponsive. As previously noted, the presence of atopy is a strong factor associated with the persistence of asthma into adolescence.

The frequency with which asthma progresses into adult life has been reviewed in a number of studies. Blair (1977, 1979) followed up a population of childhood asthmatics seen in a London general practice and found that 20 years later 21% of children who had had at least 3 episodes of paroxysmal dyspnoea with wheezing before age 12 had persistent asthma through into adult life, and a further 27% had recurrent asthma after a symptom-free period of 3 or more years in adolescence. The remaining 52% without persistent wheeze as adults were almost equally divided among those with occasional wheezing but no disability (24%) and those who were totally symptom free (28%). However of this latter group, one-third showed reduced pulmonary function and increased airway lability on challenge. This study suggests that the great majority of children with significant asthma before age 12 continue to show asthmatic features in adult life. Rackemann and Edwards (1952) found likewise that only 30% of 449 US children seen and treated for asthma before age 13 were symptom free and leading normal lives 20 years later (Kuzemko, 1980).

The longitudinal Melbourne study initiated by Williams and McNicol (1969) has yielded much useful information about the long-term outcome of childhood asthma and its progression into adulthood. The original investigators found no significant features that differentiated children with "bronchitis" from those with "wheezy bronchitis" or "asthma" and concluded that these conditions were all one entity, namely asthma. In following up these children, Martin et al. (1980a) reported that over one-half of the children whose childhood wheezing had been infrequent were free of wheezing in early adult life, while most of the remainder had only infrequent wheezing. However only 20% of those with frequent wheezing in childhood had undergone remission in adolescence, although half had noted a considerable improvement in symptoms by age 21. Virtually all children with persistent wheezing in childhood continue to wheeze into adult life, although many noted a significant improvement; only one-quarter were wheeze free at age 21. Those with more frequent wheezing persisting to age 21 had a higher frequency of abnormalities of pulmonary function (Martin et al., 1980b). Persistent wheeze at age 14 was highly predictive of persistence of symptoms to age 28 (Kelly et al., 1987). In addition, the condition of 44% of subjects with infrequent wheezing at 21 years had worsened by 28 years, a trend that was more evident in men than women.

Burrows et al. (1977) found that adults with chronic bronchitis or impaired airway function had a greater likelihood of a history of childhood respiratory problems, mainly "asthma-bronchitis," but because the data were retrospective and subject to preferential recall bias, the association could not be regarded as certain. In subjects aged 20-44 years, more than twice as many with a history of childhood respiratory problems reported frequent wheeze compared with those without such a history (8.6% vs. 3.8%) and there was a strikingly high prevalence of a history of any wheeze (62.9%) among those with childhood respiratory problems compared with a 33.7% prevalence rate in those without such a history.

It is tempting to hypothesize that airway hyperresponsiveness, which usually accompanies childhood asthma, may be associated with a greater tendency to airflow obstruction in adults, particularly in those who smoke, and a more rapid progression of chronic lung disease in these adults than in those without a childhood history. However, there are as yet insufficient longitudinal studies to confirm this hypothesis.

VII. Asthma in Adults

There are fewer studies of the prevalence of asthma in adults than in children, reflecting in part the difficulties in obtaining a truly random community sample of adults. A selection of adult prevalence studies undertaken in the last decade are shown in Table 2. There is some variation in age, and considerable variation in methodology, among these studies, particularly in the questions asked.

Two recent studies have suggested that asthma is underdiagnosed in adults. Of all asthmatic patients attending a hospital outpatient clinic, one-third were not diagnosed as having asthma on initial referral (Stellman et al., 1982). In a geriatric population in Wales, a 15% or greater increase in peak expiratory flow rates 5 min after inhaled salbutamol was demonstrated in over 40% of the geriatric group, but only 6% were being treated for asthma (Banerjee et al., 1987).

As in children, the possibility of an increasing prevalence of asthma has been suggested by follow-up population studies. In Busselton, Western Australia, Cullen et al. (1968), using questionnaire data only, found that 2.7% of adults suffered from asthma, whereas Woolcock et al. (1987) found that 9.1% of adults had diagnosed asthma and 6.7% were being treated for asthma. As in children, the true increase in prevalence is not possible to determine because of the effect of changes in diagnostic fashion, which may be more evident in older age groups.

Table 2 Selected Studies of the Prevalence of Asthma and Wheezing in Adults Reported in the Last Decade

Location	Age	Prevalence	Reference
Busselton, Aust	18-88	5.9% current (symptoms + AHR)	Woolcock et al., 1987
Dunedin, NZ	All	Current 4.2%, cumulative 6.2%	McQueen et al., 1979
Lebanon, US	>7	5.6% asthma, 21.3% wheeze	Schachter et al., 1984
Tucson, US	>20	3.0-7.9% asthma (age/sex related), >30% wheezing most ages	Dodge & Burrows, 1980
Po River, Italy	>20	Asthma: M 3.2% F 2.4%; shortness of breath with wheeze: M 6.4% F 3.5%	Viegi et al., 1988

On the other hand, asthma in adults may be misdiagnosed, especially in older age groups, and dyspnea and impaired lung function ascribed to bronchitis, emphysema, or cardiac failure. Attempts have been made to differentiate asthma from other forms of chronic airflow limitation by the responsiveness or otherwise of the airways to various challenge agents. In particular, the absence of a plateau in the dose-response curve to histamine or methacholine has been used to indicate the presence of an asthmatic form of airflow limitation (Woolcock et al., 1984). Although there is some evidence that this does differentiate between the two conditions, and the lesser responses to cold air, propanolol, and SO_2 in chronic nonasthmatic airflow limitation is also helpful, there is clearly overlap between these conditions. The definition of asthma therefore continues to be made somewhat arbitrarily based on the chronology of symptoms, with careful regard given to the history of smoking.

Measurements of airway responsiveness appear to be no more specific or sensitive in adults than they are in children for confirming the diagnosis of asthma. Enarson et al. (1987) found that of 1392 male workers in various industries, 38% with methacholine $PC_{20}FEV_1$ less than 8 mg/ml but greater than 2 mg/ml had no chest symptoms; 31% of workers with $PC_{20}FEV_1$ between 0.5 and .20 mg/ml had no symptoms. While workers reporting wheeze or breathlessness, and especially those with both symptoms, were more likely to show airway hyperresponsiveness, the authors concluded that identifying subjects with asthma by measurement of AHR in epidemiological surveys was not straightforward, and that priority should be given to designing and validating an asthma questionnaire. The sensitivity and specificity of the methacholine challenge test for physician-diagnosed asthma using $PC_{20}FEV_1$ < 8 mg/ml were 61% and 85%, respectively, with overall accuracy 84%; for $PC_{20}FEV_1$ < 2 mg/ml, the figures were 40%, 96%, and 95% respectively.

In an Italian study of 15-64-year-olds (Cerveri et al., 1988), there was overlap in methacholine responsiveness with those with obvious histories of asthma and those with no history, although the difference in mean airway responsiveness between the two groups was highly significant. In a study of 18-64-year-olds in England (Burney et al., 1987a), 14% of the sample had airway responsiveness to less than 8 μmol histamine; hyperresponsiveness was associated with age, smoking (the effect of which increased with age), and atopy (the effect of which decreased with age). Airway hyperresponsiveness was least obvious in midadult life (35-44 years), and increased in both older and younger subjects. Britton et al. (1988) reported associations between changes in airway responsiveness in a community population and changes in frequency of wheezing and use of asthma medications. There are consistent correlations between the presence of nonsensitizing airway hyperresponsiveness and chronic respiratory symptoms in adults (Ricjken et al., 1987; Sparrow et al., 1987) but the presence of hyperresponsiveness is not specific for asthma. Woolcock et al. (1987) found that of 916 adult subjects in Busselton, Western Australia, 83 (9.1%) had diagnosed asthma and 61 (6.7%) received asthma treatments, but fewer than two-thirds of these subjects showed airway hyperresponsiveness to histamine as determined by $PD_{20}FEV_1$ values < 3.9 μmol.

The development of true adult-onset asthma is well recognized, but the question of whether such adults have had preexisting hyperresponsive airways in childhood or early adult life cannot yet be answered. The incidence of asthma in adulthood has been studied infrequently. In the Melbourne study, 82 control children were evaluated into adulthood, 15 of whom developed asthmatic symptoms between age 14 and 21, an incidence of 2.65% per annum (Martin et al., 1980a). This is significantly higher than that found in two US studies in which the incidence rates were 0.2% and 0.25% per annum in Connecticut (Schachter et al., 1984) and Tecumseh (Broder et al., 1974), respectively. Dodge and Burrows (1980) reported an incidence of

49 new asthma cases among 3432 Tucson residents during a mean follow-up period of 3.5 years, with a peak in young children and the lowest incidence in late adolescence. Newly diagnosed asthma in persons over age 40 years occurred almost exclusively in women, suggesting that diagnostic fashion was causing men to be labeled as having chronic obstructive disease due to bronchitis or emphysema.

Among the Tucson population, Burrows et al. (1989) found that the prevalence of self-reported asthma was closely related to serum IgE levels, with no asthma being reported by subjects with IgE in the lowest portion of the age- and sex-standardized range (greater than 1.4 SD below the mean). The odds ratio for asthma increased linearly with the serum IgE level after possible confounders and the degree of skin test reactivity were controlled for. Burrows et al. concluded that asthma is almost always associated with some type of IgE-mediated reaction, even if the routine battery of skin tests give negative results. Although the association between asthma and atopy has always been regarded as much stronger in children than in adults, this study indicates that atopy may have a more important role than previously thought in adult "intrinsic" asthma, which Burrows et al. suggest is no longer appropriate.

VIII. Asthma in Migrant Populations

Interesting differences in the prevalence of asthmatic symptoms and associated atopic features have been reported in migrant children in South Africa and in the South Pacific. In South Africa, Xhosa children living in Capetown had a prevalence of exercise-induced asthma of 3.17%, compared with only 0.14% in Xhosa children remaining in rural Transkei (van Niekerk et al., 1979). Children of the Tokelauan Islands who remained in the islands had a prevalence of asthma in 11%, whereas 25% of Tokelauan children relocated to New Zealand developed asthma, a rate similar to that of normally resident New Zealand children (Waite et al., 1980). These increases in the prevalence of asthma strongly suggest that environmental factors override the genetic or ethnic factors predisposing to asthma. Whether the increase is due to exposure to different allergens, to changes in diet, air pollution, microbiological flora, or treatment of infectious diseases is as yet unknown. Studies in adults in New Guinea (Dowse et al., 1985; Turner, 1987) strongly suggest that an increased exposure to the house dust mite may be a major causative factor in increasing the prevalence of asthma (see below). The prevalences of rhinitis and eczema in the Tokelauan children living in New Zealand were 28.3% and 8.5%, respectively, compared with rates of 13.7% and 0.1% in their peers living in the islands (Waite et al., 1980), which suggests that the New Zealand environment contained more potent sensitizing allergens; this seems the most likely reason for the increased prevalence of asthma.

IX. Asthma in Developing Countries: The Role of the House Dust Mite

In contrast to the usual findings in developed countries, the prevalence of asthma in childhood in some developing countries is considerably lower than the prevalence in adults, with the usual age of onset being in adulthood rather than childhood. In an early study among the South Fore of Papua New Guinea, asthma in children was unknown, and the adult prevalence was only 0.28% (Anderson, 1974). A decade later, the prevalence in children was measured at 0.6%, but had increased markedly in adults, to 7.3% (Woolcock et al., 1983; Turner et al., 1985, 1986). The disease in adults is much more severe than elsewhere, with a 28% fatality rate in 10 years (Woolcock et al., 1988). A postulated cause for this striking increase was the exposure to house dust mite in the environment (Dowse et al., 1985), since the blanket-derived dust of the group with the greatest increase in asthma prevalence had a mite density four to five times greater than that in a similar village that had not experienced an increase in asthma prevalence (Turner, 1987; Woolcock et al, 1988; Turner et al., 1988). This adds further weight to the suggestion that the house dust mite may be one of the key factors increasing the prevalence and/or severity of asthma in western countries over the past 20 years. Other evidence relevant to this includes the studies of Platts-Mills et al. (1982), who showed that airway hyperresponsiveness was decreased on avoidance of house dust mite exposure, and the longitudinal study of New Zealand children, in which skin test sensitivity to the house dust mite was associated with a sevenfold relative risk for the development of symptoms of asthma with concurrent airway hyperresponsiveness in childhood (Sears et al., 1989).

X. Climatic Factors

Epidemics of severe asthma resulting in increased hospital admissions have been reported during or following abrupt weather changes. Outbreaks of asthma associated with thunderstorms were reported in Melbourne, Australia (Egan, 1985), and in Birmingham (Packe et al., 1983), where there was a correlation between admissions and daily spore counts measured in Derby (Brown and Jackson, 1983). The dependence of some fungi on weather for spore release (e.g., *Didymella*) gives a biological reason for the association of fungal aeroallergens with epidemics of clinical asthma, much like that seen in countries experiencing ragweed-related seasons of acute asthma (Salvaggio and Kundar, 1968). Khot et al. (1988) found no relationship between childhood asthma admissions and temperature, humidity, or wind, but there was a strong association with rainfall, low barometric pressure, and counts of basidiospores, but not with other spores or grass pollen. Correlations between asthma and weather have, however, been observed in regions where there is little air pollution or significant pollen counts, for example, in Bermuda where asthma-caused hospital attendance increased with lower relative humidity, lower ambient air temperature, and Atlantic winds from the northeast carrying no appreciable aeroallergens (Carey and Cordon, 1986). These reports suggest that there may be a more direct effect of climatic factors on the expression of asthma than simply the effect of weather changes on allergens such as fungal spores, pollens, or house dust mite. The belief, however, that chest problems including asthma are more prevalent in cold or wet climates has not yet been substantiated. Cullen (1972) compared chest disorders in children in Australasia and the United Kingdom, and found a higher prevalence of bronchitis and asthma in warmer rather than cooler regions. Children living in a temperate part of New Zealand had a similar prevalence of asthma to children in Southern Ontario, Canada, which has much greater climatic extremes (Fitzgerald et al., 1988). The prevalence of asthma in dry, desert climates is similar to that found in moist, temperature zones (Ellul-Micallef and Al-Ali, 1984; Dodge and Burrows, 1980). Some studies have reported lower prevalence rates for asthma in countries with cooler temperatures (e.g., Scandinavia; Skarpaas and Gulsvik, 1985), but the effects of methodological differences or other factors such as diet have not been excluded as resulting in these lower prevalence rates.

XI. Occupational Factors

The prevalence of occupational asthma is not clearly defined. In Japan, some 15% of adult male asthmatics have occupational-related asthma, whereas in the US, only 2% are so diagnosed (Chan-Yeung and Lam, 1986). Since affected workers often leave a given industry, the prevalence of the condition may be significantly underestimated. The prevalence of occupational asthma varies according to the nature of the inciting agent, the duration of exposure, and the atmospheric concentration. At particularly high risk for occupational asthma are animal handlers, especially in laboratory situations; workers using isocyanates; grain workers; pot-room employees in aluminum smelters; electronics industry employees exposed to colophony in solder flux; and persons handling western red cedar.

The diagnosis of occupational asthma requires a detailed occupational history, including the chronology of development of symptoms, the pattern of symptoms at work, at weekends, and on holidays, and monitoring of peak expiratory flow rates at work and away from work. Occupational asthma may frequently be manifest with late rather than early asthmatic reactions; the pattern of symptoms and peak flow rates need to be interpreted in this light. Making the diagnosis may be helped by serial measurements of airway hyperresponsiveness if responsiveness decreases with cessation of exposure. Further evidence for occupational asthma is obtained when there is a clustering of cases in the same industry, and when there is significant recovery or full remission when exposure ceases. However, in many instances, especially in the case of exposure to isocyanates and aluminum smelter fumes, remission does not occur and asthma may persist apparently indefinitely (Lozewicz et al., 1987).

XII. Has Asthma Increased in Severity?

Hospital admissions for asthma have increased significantly in most developed countries (Anderson, 1978; Anderson et al., 1980; Jackson and Mitchell, 1983, 1985; Mullally et al., 1984; Mitchell and Cutler, 1984; Halfon and Newachack, 1986), and the use of antiasthma drugs in many countries has also increased (Keating et al., 1984). Both increases are much greater than could be readily explained by any increase in the prevalence of asthma. The increase in hospital admissions could theoretically relate to earlier presentation of patients with less acute asthma; however, a retrospective study of emergency room data on the clinical status of patients attending with acute asthma over an interval of 10 years showed no difference in the degree of distress on presentation (Rea et al., 1987a).

The use of bronchodilator medications, both beta sympathomimetic and theophylline, as well as inhaled cromoglycate and inhaled corticosteroids increased in New Zealand, Australia, and the United Kingdom between 1975 and 1981; the increase was most marked in New Zealand (Keating et al., 1984). Possible reasons for the increase include an increased severity of asthma, improved treatment of asthma, or greater use of these drugs in other diseases of airflow limitation. In examining these possibilities, Sinclair et al. (1987) found that 80% of all prescriptions for salbutamol, the bronchodilator most often used in New Zealand, were for patients verified by the investigators as having asthma rather than other chronic airway diseases. Furthermore, the increase in sales of antiasthma drugs was not necessarily the result of improved treatment of asthma. Despite higher sales, inhaled corticosteroid aerosols were still underutilized; only 42% of subjects with daily symptoms of asthma received this therapy. Hence, the data lend some credence to the hypothesis that the severity of asthma may have increased.

XIII. The Natural History of Asthma

In the Tucson population, remissions of asthma were uncommon after the second decade (Bronnimann and Burrows, 1986), and especially uncommon in adults who were 30-60 years old at enrollment in the longitudinal study. Relapses of disease were common in those with a past history of asthma that had been considered quiescent on enrollment. Among 10-19-year-olds, 65% underwent remission compared with only 6% of 40-49-year-olds. Remission was more common in those with less frequent symptoms; 12% of these with wheeze on most days experienced remission compared with 35% of those with less frequent wheeze. Relapse rates increased with age to 70 years, and relapse was more likely if the subject had a history of any wheezing and of a chronic productive cough on entry to the study. Remission and relapse rates were not associated with gender, rhinitis, or serum IgE levels, but were adversely affected by smoking.

Adult asthmatics in the Busselton, Western Australia, population had a lower baseline lung function and a greater rate of decline in FEV_1 over 18 years than nonasthmatics, the mean annual loss being some 40% greater in the asthmatics (Peat et al., 1987c). The decline was variable and unrelated to age or atopic status. Airway hyperresponsiveness accounted for 9%, and airflow limitation for 10%, of the variation in the rate of decline; the relationship to treatment was not studied. Asthmatics have a much lower rate of decline in function, however, than do patients with other forms of chronic airflow limitation (Burrows et al., 1987).

XIV. Fatal Asthma

Changes in mortality rates are generally regarded as being too small to be useful in studying the epidemiology of asthma. However, on two occasions during the last three decades "epidemics" of asthma mortality have occurred and have been widely discussed and debated (Speizer et al., 1968; Gandevia, 1973; Esdaile et al., 1987; Jackson et al., 1982; Sears et al., 1985). Reported asthma mortality in young people in England and Wales, Australia, and

New Zealand increased substantially between 1964 and 1966. While many considered the increase attributable to a direct toxic effect of high-dosage sympathomimetic bronchodilator drugs (Stolley and Schinnar, 1978), others believed that the 1960s epidemic was, if related to drug therapy at all, a manifestation of delay in obtaining more effective treatment due to overreliance on partial relief of symptoms by bronchodilator therapy (Beaupré, 1987; Lanes and Walker, 1987). Other hypotheses included increased or unusual exposure to aeroallergens (Jenkins et al., 1980), or that the epidemic was in fact spurious and resulted from diagnostic transfer, especially since the availability of potent bronchodilator aerosols may have enhanced recognition of asthma (Esdaile et al., 1987). While this hypothesis could explain trends in older subjects, it seems unlikely in young people; there are relatively few causes of wheezing other than asthma in 15-34-year-olds, and the three- to fourfold increase in mortality rates in the 1960s was fairly abrupt.

Mortality rates from asthma declined in the United Kingdom and Australia in the late 1960s back to the pre-epidemic level, but in New Zealand the rate remained somewhat elevated. A second increase in asthma mortality in New Zealand commenced in young people in 1977 and resulted in mortality rates even higher than that experienced in the 1960s epidemic, exceeding 4.0:100,000 in 5-34-year-olds. A gradual increase in asthma mortality has been reported in several other countries over the last decade (Jackson et al., 1988; Buist et al., 1987), but none have experienced the same peak in mortality or the abrupt rise seen in New Zealand. Burney (1986) showed a significant increase in mortality in young people in the United Kingdom between 1974 and 1985. In Canada, mortality from asthma in 5-34-year-olds more than doubled from 0.2:100,000 in 1974 to 0.5:100,000 in 1984 (Mao et al., 1987). In the United States, reported asthma mortality rates doubled from 0.15 to 0.36:100,000 in this age group (Robin, 1988). As in New Zealand, the increase in the United States has been more obvious in nonwhites than whites and in younger rather than in older persons (Sly, 1984, 1988). Trends in national statistics for asthma mortality in young people aged 5-34-years in various countries are summarized in Table 3.

A. Could the Increase in Mortality be an Artifact?

The questions to be answered regarding trends in asthma mortality are whether they are real or an artifact, and if real, what their basis is (Sears, 1988; Buist, 1988). Reported trends are based on national asthma mortality statistics, which in turn depend on the accuracy of physician certification of the cause of death, and the extent to which false-positive and false-negative reporting of asthma mortality occurs (Sears et al., 1986c). National statistics are also influenced by changes in the rules governing the statistical coding of death certificates. The accuracy of certification of death due to asthma was studied in both major investigations into asthma mortality, in England (British Thoracic Association, 1982) and in New Zealand (Sears et al., 1985). Deaths of all 492 New Zealanders for whom the word "asthma" or a derivative was recorded in part I of the death certificate or on the coroner's report were investigated. After detailed inquiry from relatives, doctors, hospital records, and autopsy results when available, the medical reviewing panel accepted 67% of these deaths as being due to asthma (Sears et al., 1986c). There was a strong relationship between age and accuracy of certification. The reviewing panel agreed with the National Health Statistics Centre coding of asthma deaths in 100% of persons aged less than 35 years, but accuracy declined progressively with increasing age. Inaccuracies of certification did not, however, explain the New Zealand "epidemic." In adults aged 15-64 years, New Zealand statistics overestimated asthma mortality by 13%, the same extent as that determined in a similar study in England 2 years earlier (Sears et al., 1986b; British Thoracic Association Research Committee, 1984).

Inaccuracies in certification and statistical coding of apparent asthma deaths were due largely to false-positive reporting: patients said to have died from asthma had never suffered from asthma but had chronic airflow obstruction due to chronic bronchitis or emphysema, or subjects with asthma in earlier life then developed dominant smoker's bronchitis and emphysema that caused their death (Sears et al., 1986c). A third, smaller, group of subjects did have asthma, but died of other causes (e.g., myocardial ischaemia). Theirs were falsely coded as deaths from asthma because the reporting physician included "asthma" in part I of the death certificate instead of entering it more appropriately in part II as a condition suffered by the deceased but not contributing directly to death. The existence of false-negative reporting is more difficult to quantitate but was examined in England (British Thoracic Association Research Committee, 1984) and in a regional study in New Zealand (Jackson et al., 1982); false-negative reporting was found to be essentially nonexistent among death certificates for young people.

The effect of changes in the rules governing the World Health Organization International Classification of Diseases (World Health Organization, 1977) partially obscured some changes in trends in asthma mortality. Most countries introduced ICD9 in 1979, which coincided in many of those countries with a reversal of the downward trend in asthma mortality to an upward trend. The effect of the change in rules was most apparent in older subjects. Under the previous rules governing ICD 8, those deaths certified as due to asthma, but with mention of bronchitis, were coded as due to bronchitis. Under ICD 9, this linkage was broken so that these deaths were now coded as due to asthma. In older age groups, the effect of this change in linkage was to increase reported asthma mortality by 35% or more (Sly, 1984; Stewart and Nunn, 1985), but in 5-34-year-olds the effects was negligible (Jackson et al., 1988). Hence, trends in 5-34-year-olds through the last two decades can be taken at face value, but in older age groups, and in total populations, the change in rules lead to a substantial step increase in mortality in 1979. This step increase, however, cannot explain subsequent trends in mortality rates in several countries, as seen in the United States, Canada, England and Wales, and elsewhere. The continuing increase in reported mortality must be due to an increase in severity or in prevalence of asthma, a reduction in efficacy of treatment, an adverse effect of treatment, or possibly changes in diagnostic fashion particularly in relation older age groups. In young people, changes in diagnostic fashion and in accuracy of certification and coding do not appear to account for the upward trends; other reasons must be sought. In 5-34-year-old persons in the US, total deaths from all types of airflow obstruction increased as asthma deaths increased, with no reduction in deaths attributed to nonasthmatic obstructive diseases (Fig. 2). Diagnostic transfer therefore seems untenable as an explanation of the trends in younger people.

B. Factors Associated with Fatal Asthma

Most of the studies of fatal asthma have been descriptive, and although these studies yielded valuable profiles of patients who appear to be at high risk of dying of their disease, the risk associated with such factors cannot be quantitated. For this purpose, case-control studies are more helpful, although these too pose difficulties in the selection of controls adequately matching those who experience fatal attacks. Rea et al. (1986) identified several risk factors for death including a previous history of severe or life-threatening attacks, previous hospital admissions and emergency room visits, and discontinuity of physician care. An increased risk of death was not associated with the age at onset of asthma, family history of asthma, and smoking habits.

The only study of fatal asthma to include a whole population, the New Zealand National Asthma Mortality Study (Sears et al., 1985) showed a bimodal distribution of deaths by age group, with a peak in the 15-24-year-old group as well as the expected peak in later life. The younger peak was similar to the peak age of mortality in the United Kingdom, Australia, and New Zealand during the 1960s. Review of case histories in this age group suggested that an attitude of rebellion against medical and parental authority and removal of parental care were factors associated with less reliable self-care,

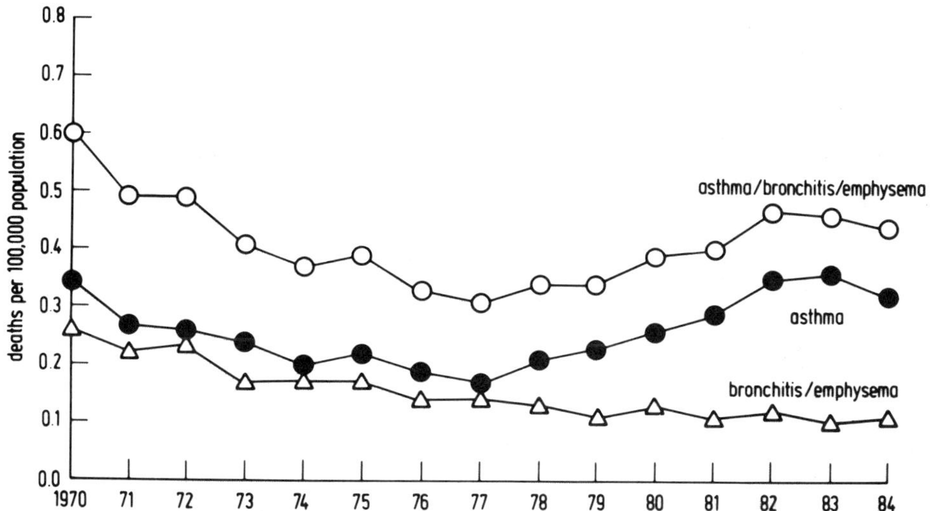

Figure 2   Mortality from asthma and chronic bronchitis/emphysema in persons aged 5-34 years in the United States, 1970-1984 (reproduced with permission from Jackson et al., *Chest*, 1988).

reduced compliance with therapy, and a fatal outcome. Similar findings were reported in a case-control study of asthma mortality on the United States (Strunk et al., 1985).

Ethnic differences in mortality have been well described. In the United States, mortality rates were significantly higher among black than white children (Sly, 1984, 1988). In New Zealand, the mortality rates for Maoris and for Pacific Island Polynesians were 5.6 and 2.8 times higher, respectively, than the rate for Europeans (Sears et al., 1985).

Although retrospective studies of fatal asthma can rarely pinpoint direct causal links between circumstances, treatments and other actions, and a fatal outcome, the major message emerging from the reviews of the circumstances of death in the English (Johnson et al., 1984), American (Barger et al., 1988), and New Zealand (Rea et al., 1987b) studies was that a fatal outcome was often associated with inadequate assessment and inappropriate treatment of severe asthma (Sears et al., 1987b; Rea et al., 1987b). A feature of this approach to asthma was overreliance on inhaled bronchodilator therapy, often to the exclusion of all other forms of therapy, and almost always insufficient use of corticosteroid therapy in the management of long-term and acute severe asthma.

Current trends in asthma mortality deserve careful attention. Studies validating the reported rates are necessary to exclude the influence of diagnostic fashion and false-negative and false-positive certification. In New Zealand, the mortality rate in young people has declined substantially since 1983, although not in an altogether smooth fashion. Provisional mortality statistics for 1987 give a mortality rate of 1.9:100,000 in 5-34-year-old persons, which is close to the pre-epidemic rate. This suggests that the intensive approach to the management of asthma advocated in New Zealand (Rea et al., 1987b; Sears, 1987b), which involves encouraging access to medical care, monitoring of lung function using portable peak flow meters, and stressing the need to use adequate corticosteroid therapy rather than relying on more bronchodilator therapy in acute attacks, is having a beneficial effect. It is particularly noteworthy that the much higher mortality rate in New Zealand Maoris has, in 1987, been reduced to approximately that of the European population. Mortality rates in young people in some other countries appear now to show a plateau after 5-7 years of gradual increase (Table 3, Fig. 3).

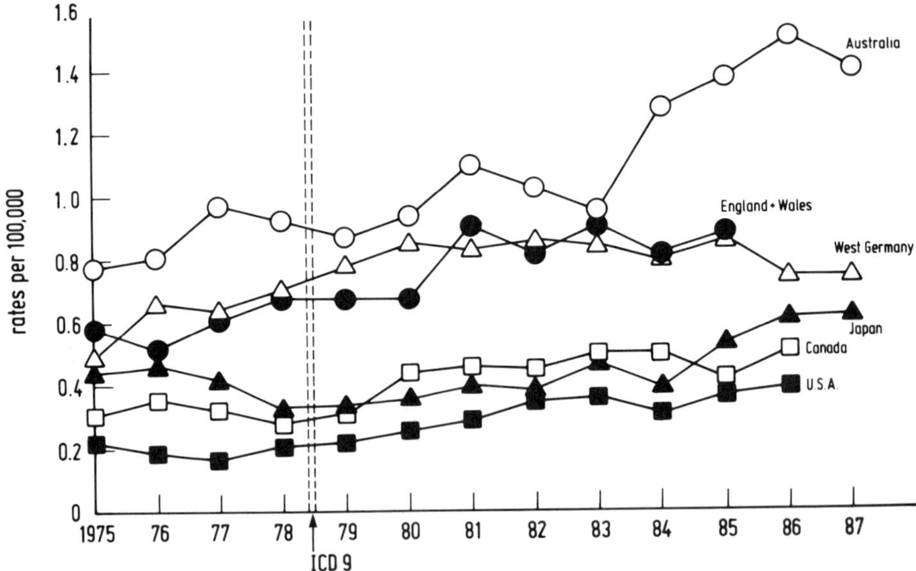

Figure 3 Trends in reported mortality from asthma in persons 5-34 years in 6 countries, 1975-1988 (per 100,000 population).

It is essential that trends in reported mortality be monitored carefully, especially in 5-34-year-olds, among whom accuracy of diagnosis of asthma is most certain, and that an open mind be maintained with regard to causes of the observed trends.

XVI. Summary

There is only weak evidence to support the view that the true prevalence of asthma has increased except in some specific populations (e.g., in developing countries and in migrants, almost certainly due to environmental influences.) It appears likely that asthma is more prevalent in Australia, New Zealand, Canada, and England than in the United States and Scandinavian countries. The sensitivity and specificity of demonstration of airway hyperresponsiveness to histamine or methacholine do not permit the use of a single measurement to define the prevalence of asthma in children or in adults. Asthma in children is associated with the male sex, atopy, family history, parental (especially maternal) smoking, and possibly respiratory illness in infancy. Persistence of asthma from childhood into adulthood is strongly associated with atopy and persistent airway hyperresponsiveness. There is fairly convincing evidence that there has been an increase in severity of asthma in many countries, possibly related to environmental factors. The upward trend in hospital admissions for asthma, and in mortality from asthma in young people, is not adequately explained by diagnostic transfer or inaccuracies in certification and coding, but appears to be real.

Discussion

Kerrebijn: There has been no rise in asthma mortality in the Netherlands over the last 20 years. This might be because of the high population density and easily available medical facilities. You mentioned three markers of asthma: symptoms, airway obstruction, and airway hyperresponsiveness (AHR). How would you define current asthma, asthma in remission, and cured asthma?

Sears: *Current* asthma is usually defined as symptoms within the last year; this is often, but not always, accompanied by AHR. *Remission* is usually clinically defined as the absence of symptoms for at least 1 year and irrespective of the degree of AHR. *Cured* asthma is not well documented but could be defined as the absence of symptoms for a prolonged period together with normal lung function and normal AHR (i.e., physiological remission).

Kay: Were the epidemiological studies standardized for point, period, or cumulative prevalence?

Sears: All such studies should define exactly the period studied and include *period prevalence* (symptoms in the last year), which is useful for comparing different age groups and populations over time. The problem of recall is far less than for *cumulative* prevalence. *Point* prevalence (abnormality or symptoms on the day of examination) is not very useful in an intermittently symptomatic condition such as asthma, and can be masked by drug therapy giving symptomatic relief.

Platts-Mills: You have made a strong case for an increase in prevalence and severity of asthma over the last 20 years. Do you think that increased treatment, or increased exposure to allergen, could account for these increases?

Sears: The *severity* of asthma may have been influenced by treatment, especially by beta-agonists, but the appropriate studies have not yet been completed. There is good evidence that house dust mite exposure is associated with increased asthma in developing countries, but many other environmental factors may be operative.

Fuller: Would not the use of objective measurements of airway function be more useful since they are not subject to diagnostic changes and perception of symptoms?

Sears: Objective measurements are helpful but have limitations. Airflow obstruction is intermittent and the use of bronchodilator responsiveness on the day of assessment will markedly underestimate the prevalence of asthma. The measurement of AHR is useful, especially if done repeatedly, but a single measurement is not sufficiently sensitive or specific to be used as the "gold standard" for diagnosing asthma.

L. Laitinen: Geographical and cultural differences in definition of asthma must be important in questionnaires.

Sears: Questionnaires must be carefully designed and then validated in different countries and different languages.

Tattersfield: It is unlikely that everyone will agree on a definition of asthma. Perhaps it would be better not to be too concerned about such a definition in epidemiological studies but to report what can be measured, for example, wheeze in the last year.

Sears: The use of the term "asthma" is increasing but it is important to include questions on wheezing in all questionnaires and not to rely solely on diagnosed asthma.

References

Anderson, H. R. (1974). The epidemiological and allergic features of asthma in the New Guinea Highlands. *Clin. Allergy* **4**:171-183.

Anderson, H. R. (1978). Increase in hospitalization for childhood asthma. *Arch. Dis. Child.* **53**:295-300.

Anderson, H. R., Bailey, P., and West, S. (1980). Trends in the hospital care of acute childhood asthma 1970-8: a regional study. *Br. Med. J.* **281**: 1191-1194.

Anderson, H. R. (1989). Is the prevalence of asthma changing? *Arch. Dis. Child.* **64**:172-175.

Anderson, H. R., Bailey, P. A., Cooper, J. S., Palmer, J. C., and West, S. (1983). Morbidity and school absence caused by asthma and wheezing illness. *Arch. Dis. Child.* **58**:777-784.

Anderson, H. R., Bland, J. M., and Peckham, C. S. (1987). Risk factors for asthma up to 16 years of age: evidence from a national cohort study. *Chest* **91**:127S-130S.

Andrea, S., Axelson, O., Bjorksten, B., Fredriksson, M., and Kjellman, N.-I. M. (1988). Symptoms of bronchial hyperreactivity and asthma in relation to environmental factors. *Arch. Dis. Child.* **63**:473-478.

Asher, M. I., Pattemore, P. K., Harrison, A. C., Mitchell, E. A., Rea, H. H., Stewart, A. W., and Woolcock, A. J. (1988). International comparison of the prevalence of asthma symptoms and bronchial hyperresponsiveness. *Am. Rev. Respir. Dis.* **138**:524-9.

Banerjee, D. K., Lee, G. S., Malik, S. K., and Daly, S. (1987). Underdiagnosis of asthma in the elderly. *Br. J. Dis. Chest* **81**:23-29.

Barger, L. W., Vollmer, W. M., Felt, R. W., and Buist, A. S. (1988). Further investigation into the recent increase in asthma death rates: a review of 41 asthma deaths in Oregon in 1982. *Ann. Allergy* **60**:31-39.

Bazaral, M., Orgel, H. A., and Hamburger, R. N. (1974). Genetics of IgE and allergy: serum IgE levels in twins. *J. Allergy Clin. Immunol.* **54**: 288-304.

Beaupre, A. (1987). Death in asthma. *Eur. J. Respir. Dis.* **70**:259-260.

Blair, H. (1977). Natural history of childhood asthma. *Arch. Dis. Child.* **52**:613-619.

Blair, H. (1979). The wheezy child. Natural hsitory of wheezing in childhood. *J. R. Soc. Med.* **72**:259-260.

Blanc, A. D. G. (1966). The prevalence of asthma. In *So You Have Asthma!* Springfield, IL, Charles C. Thomas, pp. 181-194.

British Thoracic Association. (1982). Death from asthma in two regions of England. *Br. Med. J.* **285**:1251-1255.

British Thoracic Association Research Committee. (1984). Accuracy of death certificates in bronchial asthma. *Thorax* **39**:505-509.

Britton, W. J., Woolcock, A. J., Peat, J. K., Sedgwick, C. J., Lloyd, D. M., and Leeder, S. R. (1986). Prevalence of bronchial hyperresponsiveness in children: the relationship between asthma and skin reactivity to allergens in two communities. *Int. J. Epidemiol.* **15**:202-209.

Britton, J. R., Burney, P. G. J., Chinn, S., Papacosta, A. O., and Tattersfield, A. E. (1988). The relation between change in airway reactivity and change in respiratory symptoms and medication in a community study. *Am. Rev. Respir. Dis.* **138**:530-534.

Broder, I., Higgins, M. W., Mathews, K. P., and Keller, J. B. (1974). Epidemiology of asthma and allergic rhinitis in a total community, Tecumseh, Michigan. IV. Natural history. *J. Allergy Clin. Immunol.* **54**:100-110.

Bronnimann, S., and Burrows, B. (1986). A prospective study of the natural history of asthma. Remission and relapse rates. *Chest* **90**:480-484.

Brown, H. M., and Jackson, F. (1983). Asthma and the weather. *Lancet* **2**: 630.

Brown, P. J., Greville, H. W., and Finucane, K. E. (1984). Asthma and irreversible airflow obstruction. *Thorax* **39**:131-136.

Buist, A. S. (1988). Is asthma mortality increasing? *Chest* **93**:449-450.

Buist, A. S., Sears, M. R., Reid, L. M., Boushey, H. A., Spector, S. L., and Sheffer, A. L. (1987). Asthma mortality: trends and determinants. *Am. Rev. Respir. Dis.* **136**:1037-1039.

Burney, P. G. J. (1986). Asthma mortality in England and Wales: evidence for a further increase, 1974-1984. *Lancet* **2**:323-326.

Burney, P., and Chinn, S. (1987). Developing a new questionnaire for measuring the prevalence and distribution of asthma. *Chest* **91**:Suppl. 79S-83S.

Burney, P. G. J., Britton, J. R., Chinn, S., Tattersfield, A. E., Papacosta, A. O., Kelson, M. C., Anderson, F., and Corfield, D. R. (1987a). Descriptive epidemiology of bronchial reactivity in an adult population: results from a community study. *Thorax* **38**:38-44.

Burney, P., Detels, R., Higgins, M., Peckham, C., Samet, K. M., and Tager, I. B. (1987b). Recommendations for research in the epidemiology of asthma. *Chest* **91**:Suppl 194S-195S.

Burr, M. L. (1987). Is asthma increasing? *J. Epidemiol. Commun. Health* **41**:185-189.

Burrows, B., Lebowitz, M., and Barbee, R. (1976). Respiratory disorders and allergy skin-test reactions. *Ann. Intern. Med.* **84**:134-139.

Burrows, B., Knudson, R. J., and Lebowitz, M. D. (1977). The relationship of childhood respiratory illness to adult obstructive airway disease. *Am. Rev. Respir. Dis.* **115**:751-760.

Burrows, B., Bloom, J. W., Traver, G. A., and Cline, M. G. (1987). The course and prognosis of different forms of chronic airways obstruction in a sample from the general population. *N. Engl. J. Med.* **317**:1309-1314.

Burrows, B., Martinez, F. D., Halonen, M., Barbee, R. A., and Cline, M. G. (1989). Association of asthma with serum IgE levels and skin-test reactivity to allergens. *N. Engl. J. Med.* **320**:271-277.

Busse, W. W. (1988). Respiratory infections and bronchial hyperreactivity. *J. Allergy Clin. Immunol.* **81**:770-5.

Carlsen, K. H., Larsen, S., and Orstavik, I. (1987). Acute bronchiolitis in infancy. The relationship to later recurrent obstructive airways disease. *Eur. J. Respir. Dis.* **70**:86-92.

Carey, M. J., and Cordon, I. (1986). Asthma and climatic conditons: experience from Bermuda, an isolated island community. *Br. Med. J.* **293**:843-844.

Cerveri, I., Bruschi, C., Zoia, M. C., Zanon, P., Maccarini, L., Grassi, M., and Rampulla, C. (1988). Distribution of bronchial nonspecific reactivity in the general population. *Chest* **93**:26-30.

Chan-Yeung, M., and Lam, S. (1986). Occupational asthma. *Am. Rev. Respir. Dis.* **133**:686-703.

Charlton, A. (1984). Children's coughs related to parental smoking. *Br. Med. J.* **288**:1647-1651.

Cogswell, J. J., Mitchell, E. B., and Alexander, J. (1987). Parental smoking, breast feeding, and respiratory infection in development of allergic diseases. *Arch. Dis. Child.* **62**:338-344.

Crockett, A. J., Ruffin, R. E., Schembri, D. A., and Alpers, J. H. (1986). The prevalence rate of respiratory symptoms in schoolchildren from two South Australian rural communities. *Aust. N.Z. J. Med.* **16**:653-657.

Cullen, K. J. (1972). Climate and chest disorders in schoolchildren. *Br. Med. J.* **4**:65-67.

Cullen, K. J., Stenhouse, N. S., Welbourne, T. A., McCall, M. G., and Curnow D. H. (1968). Chronic respiratory disease in a rural community. *Lancet* **2**:657-660.

Dawson, K. P. (1987). The severity of asthma in children admitted to hospital: a 20 year review. *N.Z. Med. J.* **100**:520-521.

Dawson, B., Horobin, G., Illsey, R., and Mitchell, R. (1969). A survey of childhood asthma in Aberdeen. *Lancet* **1**:827-830.

Dodge, R. R., and Burrows, B. (1980). The prevalence of asthma and asthma-like symptoms in a general population sample. *Am. Rev. Respir. Dis.* **122**:567-575.

Dowse, G. K., Turner, K. J., Stewart, G. A., Alpers, M. P., and Woolcock, A. J. (1985). The association between *Dermataphagoides* mites and the increasing prevalence of asthma in village communities within the Papua New Guinea highlands. *J. Allergy Clin. Immunol.* **75**:75-83.

Editorial. (1988). Airflow limitation—reversible or irreversible? *Lancet* **1**: 26-27.

Egan, P. (1985). Weather or not. *Med. J. Aust.* **142**:330.

Ellul-Micallef, R., and Al-Ali, S. (1984). The spectrum of bronchial asthma in Kuwait. *Clin. Allergy* **14**:509-517.

Enarson, D. A., Vedal, S., Schulzer, M., Dybuncio, A., and Chan-Yeung, M. (1987). Asthma, asthmalike symptoms, chronic bronchitis, and the degree of bronchial hyperresponsiveness in epidemiological surveys. *Am. Rev. Respir. Dis.* **136**:613-617.

Esdaile, J. M., Feinstein, A. R., and Horwitz, R. I. (1987). A reappraisal of the United Kingdom epidemic of fatal asthma. *Arch. Intern. Med.* **147**:543-549.

Ferris, B. G. (1978). Epidemiology standardization project. *Am. Rev. Respir. Dis.* **118**:(6, Part 2):1-53.

Fitzgerald, J. M., Sears, M. R., Roberts, R. S., Morris, M. M., Fester, D. A., and Hargreave, F. E. (1988). Symptoms of asthma and airway hyper-responsiveness to methacholine in a population of Canadian school-children. *Am. Rev. Respir. Dis.* **137**:285.

Fleming, D. M., and Crombie, D. L. (1987). Prevalence of asthma and hay-fever in England and Wales. *Br. Med. J.* **294**:279-283.

Fry, J. (1961). Acute wheezy chests. Clinical patterns and natural history. *Br. Med. J.* **1**:227-232.

Gandevia, B. (1973). Pressurised sympathomimetic aerosols and their lack of relationship to asthma mortality in Australia. *Med. J. Aust.* **1**:273-277.

Gergen, P. J., Mullally, D. I., and Evans, R., III. (1988). National survey of prevalence of asthma among children in the United States, 1976 to 1980. *Pediatrics* **81**:1-7.

Gibson, H. B., Silverstone, H., Gandevia, B., and Hall, G. J. L. (1969). Respiratory disorders in seven-year-old children in Tasmania. Aims, methods and administration of the survey. *Med. J. Aust.* **2**:201-205.

Giles, G. G., Gibson, H. B., Lickiss, N., and Shaw, K. (1984). Respiratory symptoms in Tasmanian adolescents: a follow up of the 1961 birth co-hort. *Aust. N.Z. Med. J.* **14**:631-637.

Godfrey, S. (1985). What is asthma? *Arch. Dis. Child.* **60**:997-1000.

Godfrey, S., and Konig, P. (1974). Exercise-induced bronchial lability in atopic children and their families. *Ann. Allergy* **33**:199-205.

Goodall, J. F. (1958). The natural history of common respiratory infection in children and some principles in its management. III. *J. R. Coll. Gen. Pract.* **1**:51-59

Gortmaker, S. L., Walker, D. K., Jacobs, F. H., and Ruch-Ross, H. (1982). Parental smoking and the risk of childhood asthma. *Am. J. Public Health* **72**:574-579.

Graham, P. J., Rutter, M. L., Yule, W., and Pless, I. B. (1967). Childhood asthma: a psychosomatic disorder? Some epidemiological considerations. *Br. J. Prev. Soc. Med.* **21**:78-85.

Gurwitz, D., Mindorff, C., and Levison, H. (1981). Increased incidence of bronchial reactivity in children with a history of bronchiolitis. *J. Pediatr.* **98**:551-555.

Halfon, N., and Newacheck, P. W. (1986). Trends in the hospitalization for acute childhood asthma, 1970-84. *Am. J. Public Health* **76**:1308-11.

Hargreave, F. E., Ryan, G., Thomson, N. C., O'Byrne, P. M., Latimer, K., Juniper, E. F., and Dolovich, J. (1981). Bronchial responsiveness to histamine or methacholine in asthma: measurement and clinical significance. *J. Allergy Clin. Immunol.* **68**:347-55.

Harrison, A. C., Asher, M. I., Pattemore, P. K., Mitchell, E. A., Rea, H. H., and Stewart, A. (1986). Do racial differences in asthma prevalence and severity account for racial differences in asthma admission and mortality rates? *Am. Rev. Respir. Dis.* **133**:A178.

Henderson, F. W., Clyde, W. A., Collier, A. M., and Denny, F. W. (1979). The etiologic and epidemiologic spectrum of bronchiolitis in pediatric practice. *J. Pediatr.* **95**:183-190.

Hetzel, M. R. and Clark, T. J. H. (1980). Comparison of normal and asthmatic circadian rhythms in peak expiratory flow rate. *Thorax* **35**:732-738.

Hill, D. J., Hosking, C. S., Shelton, M. J., and Turner, M. W. (1981). Growing out of asthma: clinical and immunological changes over 5 years. *Lancet* **2**:1359-1362.

Holland, W. W., Bailey, P., and Bland, J. M. (1978). Long-term consequences of respiratory disease in infancy. *J. Epidemiol. Commun. Health* **32**:256-259.

Hopp, R. J., Bewtra, A. K., Nair, N. M., Watt, G. D., and Townley, R. G. (1986). Methacholine inhalation challenge studies in a selected pediatric population. *Am. Rev. Respir. Dis.* **134**:994-998.

Hordvik, N. L., Konig, P., Morris, D., Kreutz, C., and Barbero, J. (1985). A longitudinal study of bronchodilator responsiveness in cystic fibrosis. *Am. Rev. Respir. Dis.* **131**:889-893.

Hurry, V. M., Peat, J. K., and Woolcock, A. J. (1988). Prevalence of respiratory symptoms, bronchial hyperresponsiveness and atopy in schoolchildren living in the Villawood area of Sydney. *Aust. N.Z. J. Med.* **18**:745-752.

Jackson, R. T., and Mitchell, E. A. (1983). Trends in hospital admission rates and drug treatment of asthma in New Zealand. *N.Z. Med. J.* **96**:727-729.

Jackson, R. T., Beaglehole, R., Rea, H. H., and Sutherland, D. C. (1982). Mortality from asthma: a new epidemic in New Zealand. *Br. Med. J.* **285**:771-774.

Jackson, R., Sears, M. R., Beaglehole, R., and Rea, H. H. (1988). International trends in asthma mortality: 1970 to 1985. *Chest* **94**:914-918.

Jenkins, P. F., Mullins, J., Davies, B. H., and Williams, D. A. (1980). The possible role of aero-allergens in the epidemic of asthma deaths. *Clin. Allergy* **11**:611-620.

Johnson, A. J., Nunn, A. J., Somner, A. R., Stableforth, D. E., and Stewart, C. J. (1984). Circumstances of death from asthma. *Br. Med. J.* **288**:1870-1872.

Johnston, I. D. A., Bland, J. M., and Anderson, H. R. (1987). Ethnic variation in respiratory morbidity and lung function in childhood. *Thorax* **42**:542-548.

Jones, D. T., Sears, M. R., Holdaway, M. D., Hewitt, C. J., Flannery, E. M., Herbison, G. P., and Silva, P. A. (1987). Childhood asthma in New Zealand. *Br. J. Dis. Chest.* **81**:332-340.

Keating, G., Mitchell, E. A., Jackson, R., Beaglehole, R., and Rea, H. (1984). Trends in sales of drugs for asthma in New Zealand, Australia and the United Kingdom, 1975-81. *Br. Med. J.* **289**:348-351.

Kelly, W. J. W., Hudson, I., Phelan, P. D., Pain, M. C. F., and Olinsky, A. (1987). Childhood asthma in adult life: a further study at 28 years of age. *Br. Med. J.* **294**:1059-1062.

Kerigan, A. T., Goldsmith, C. H., and Pengelly, L. D. (1986). A three year cohort study of the role of environmental factors in respiratory health of children in Hamilton, Ontario. *Am. Rev. Respir. Dis.* **133**:987-993.

Khot, A., Burn, R., Evans, N., Lenney, W., and Storr, J. (1988). Biometeorological triggers in childhood asthma. *Clin. Allergy* **18**:351-358.

Konig, P. (1981). Hidden asthma in childhood. *Am. J. Dis. Child.* **135**:1053-1055.

Kuzemko, J. A. (1980). Natural history of childhood asthma. *J. Pediatr.* **97**:886-892.

Lanes, S. F., and Walker, A. M. (1987). Do pressurized bronchodilator aerosols cause death among asthmatics? *Am. J. Epidemiol.* **125**:755-760.

Lebowitz, M. D., Knudson, R. J., Robertson, G., and Burrows, B. (1982). Significance of intraindividual changes in maximum expiratory flow volume and peak expiratory flow measurements. *Chest* **81**:566-570.

Lebowitz, M. D., Barbee, R., and Burrows, B. (1984). Family concordance of IgE, atopy, and disease. *J. Allergy Clin. Immunol.* **73**:259-264.

Lebowitz, M. D., Holberg, C. J., and Martinez, F. (1990). A longitudinal study of risk factors in asthma and chronic bronchitis in childhood. *Eur. J. Epidemiol.* (in press).

Lee, D. A., Winslow, N. R., Speight, A. N. P., and Hey, E. N. (1983). Prevalence and spectrum of asthma in childhood. *Br. Med. J.* **286**:1256-1258.

Lozewicz, S., Assoufi, B. K., Hawkins, R., and Newman Taylor, A. J. (1987). Outcome of asthma induced by isocyanates. *Br. J. Dis. Chest* **81**:14-22.

McQueen, F., Holdaway, M. D., and Sears, M. R. (1979). A study of asthma in a Dunedin suburban area. *N.Z. Med. J.* **89**:335-338.

Mak, H., Johnston, P., Abbey, H., and Talamo, R. C. (1982). Prevalence of asthma and health service utilization of asthmatic children in an inner city. *J. Allergy Clin. Immunol.* **70**:367-372.

Mao, Y., Semenciw, R., Morrison, H., MacWilliam, L., Davies, J., and Wigle, D. (1987). Increased rates of illness and death from asthma in Canada. *Can. Med. Assoc. J.* **137**:620-624.

Martin, A. J., McLennan, L. A., Landau, L. I., and Phelan, P. D. (1980a). The natural history of childhood asthma to adult life. *Br. Med. J.* **1**: 1397-1400.

Martin, A. J., Landau, L. I., and Phelan, P. D. (1980b). Lung function in young adults who had asthma in childhood. *Am. Rev. Respir. Dis.* **122**: 609-616.

Martinez, F. D., Antognoni, G., Macri, F., Bonci, E., Midulla, F., de Castro, G., and Ronchetti, R. (1988a). Parental smoking enhances bronchial responsiveness in nine-year-old children. *Am. Rev. Respir. Dis.* **138**: 518-523.

Martinez, F. D., Morgan, W. J., Wright, A. L., Holberg, C. J., Taussig, M. D., and the Group Health Medical Associates' Personnel (1988b). Diminished lung function as a predisposing factor for wheezing respiratory illness in infants. *N. Engl. J. Med.* **319**:1112-1117.

Medical Research Council (1960). Standardized questionaires on respiratory symptoms. *Br. Med. J.* **2**:1665.

Milne, G. A. (1969). The incidence of asthma in Lower Hutt. *N.Z. Med. J.* **70**:27-29.

Mitchell, C., and Miles, J. (1983). Lower respiratory tract symptoms in Queensland schoolchildren. The questionnaire: its reliability and validity. *Aust. N.Z. J. Med.* **13**:264-269.

Mitchell, E. A. (1983). Increasing prevalence of asthma in children. *N.Z. Med. J.* **96** 463-464.

Mitchell, E. A. (1985). International trends in hospital admissions rates for asthma. *Arch. Dis. Child.* **60**:376-378.

Mitchell, E. A., and Cutler, D. R. (1984). Paediatric admissions to Auckland Hospital for asthma from 1970-1980. *N.Z. Med. J.* **97**:67-70.

Mok, J. Y. Q., and Simpson, H. (1984a). Symptoms, atopy, and bronchial reactivity after lower respiratory infection in infancy. *Arch. Dis. Child.* **59**:299-305.

Mok, J. Y. Q., and Simpson, H. (1984b). Outcome for acute bronchitis, bronchiolitis, and pneumonia in infancy. *Arch. Dis. Child.* **59**:306-309.

Mullally, D. I., Howard, W. A., Hubbard, T. J., Grauman, J. S., and Cohen, S. G. (1984). Increased hospitalizations for asthma among children in the Washington, D. C. area during 1961-1981. *Ann. Allergy* **53**:15-19.

Murray, A. B., and Morrison, B. J. (1988). Passive smoking and the seasonal difference of severity of asthma in children. *Chest* **94**:701-708.

Packe, G. E., Archer, P. St J., and Ayres, J. G. (1983). Asthma and the weather. *Lancet* **1**:281.

Peat, J. K., Woolcock, A. J., Leeder, S. R., and Blackburn, C. R. B. (1980a). Asthma and bronchitis in Sydney schoolchildren. I. Prevalence during a six-year study. *Am. J. Epidemiol.* **111**:721-727.

Peat, J. K., Woolcock, A. J., Leeder, S. R., and Blackburn, C. R. B. (1980b). Asthma and bronchitis in Sydney schoolchildren. II. The effect of social factors and smoking on prevalence. *Am. J. Epidemiol.* **111**:728-735.

Peat, J. K., Britton, W. J., Salome, C. M., and Woolcock, A. J. (1987a). Bronchial hyperresponsiveness in two populations of Australian schoolchildren. II. Relative importance of associated factors. *Clin. Allergy* **17**:283-290.

Peat, J. K., Britton, W. J., Salome, C. M., and Woolcock, A. J. (1987b). Bronchial hyperresponsiveness in two populations of Australian schoolchildren. III. Effect of exposure to environmental allergens. *Clin. Allergy* **17**:291-300.

Peat, J. K., Woolcock, A. J., and Cullen, K. (1987c). Rate of decline of lung function in subjects with asthma. *Eur. J. Respir. Dis.* **70**:171-179.

Peckham, C., and Butler, N. (1978). A national study of asthma in childhood. *J. Epidemiol. Commun. Health* **32**:79-85.

Platts-Mills, T. A. E., Mitchell, E. B., Nock, P., Tovey, E. R., Moszoro, H., and Williams, S. R. (1982). Reduction of bronchial hyperreactivity during prolonged allergen avoidance. *Lancet* **2**:675-677.

Pullan, C. R., and Hey, E. N. (1982). Wheezing, asthma, and pulmonary dysfunction 10 years after infection with respiratory syncytial virus in infancy. *Br. Med. J.* **284**:1665-1669.

Rackemann, F. M., and Edwards, M. C. (1952). Asthma in children. A follow-up study of 688 patients after an interval of twenty years. *N. Engl. J. Med.* **246**:815-823.

Rea, H. H., Scragg, R., Jackson, R., Beaglehole, R., Fenwick, J., and Sutherland, D. C. (1986). A case-control study of deaths from asthma. *Thorax* **41**:833-839.

Rea, H., Sears, M., Mitchell, E., Garrett, J., Mulder, J., and Anderson, R. (1987a). Is asthma becoming more severe? *Thorax* **42**:736.

Rea, H. H., Sears, M. R., Beaglehole, R., Fenwick, J., Jackson, R. T., Gillies, A. J. D., O'Donnell, T. V., Holst, P. E., and Rothwell, R. P. G. (1987b). Lessons from the national asthma mortality study: circumstances surrounding death. *N.Z. Med. J.* **100**:10-13.

Rijcken, B., Schouten, J. P., Weiss, S. T., Speizer, F. E., and van der Lende, R. (1987). The relationship of nonspecific bronchial responsiveness to respiratory symptoms in a random population sample. *Am. Rev. Respir. Dis.* **136**:62-68.

Robin, E. D. (1988). Death from bronchial asthma. *Chest* **93**:614-618.

Salome, C. M., Peat, J. K., Britton, W. J., and Woolcock, A. J. (1987). Bronchial hyperresponsiveness in two populations of Australian schoolchildren. I. Relation to respiratory symptoms and diagnosed asthma. *Clin. Allergy* **17**:271-281.

Salvaggio, J. E., and Kundur, V. G. (1968). New Orleans epidemic asthma: relationship between outbreaks and influx of ragweed pollen. *J. Allergy* **41**:90.

Samet, J. M. (1987). Epidemiological approaches to the identification of asthma. *Chest* **91**(6):74S-78S.

Scadding, J. G. (1983). Definition and clinical categories of asthma. In *Asthma*. Edited by T. J. H. Clark and S. Godfrey. Chapman and Hall, London, p. 5.

Schachter, E. N., Doyle, C. A., and Beck, G. J. (1984). A prospective study of asthma in a rural community. *Chest* **85**:623-630.

Sears, M. R. (1988). Increasing asthma mortality—fact or artifact? *J. Allergy Clin. Immunol.* **82**:957-960.

Sears, M. R., Jones, D. T., Silva, P. A., Simpson, A., and Williams, S. M. (1982). Asthma in seven year old children: a report from the Dunedin Multidisciplinary Child Development Study. *N.Z. Med. J.* **95**:533-536.

Sears, M. R., Rea, H. H., Beaglehole, R., Gillies, A. J. D., Holst, P. E., O'Donnell, T. V., Rothwell, R. P. G., and Sutherland, D. C. (1985). Asthma mortality in New Zealand: a two year national study. *N.Z. Med. J.* **98**:271-275.

Sears, M. R., Jones, D. T., Holdaway, M. D., Hewitt, C. J., Flannery, E. M., Herbison, G. P., Silva, P. A. (1986a). Prevalence of bronchial reactivity to inhaled methacholine in New Zealand children. *Thorax* **41**:283-289.

Sears, M. R., Rea, H. H., Rothwell, R. P. G., O'Donnell, T. V., Holst, P. E., Gillies, A. J. D., and Beaglehole, R. (1986b). Asthma mortality: comparison between New Zealand and England. *Br. Med. J.* **293**:1342-1345.

Sears, M. R., Rea, H. H., de Boer, G., Beaglehole, R., Gillies, A. J. D., Holst, P. E., O'Donnell, T. V., and Rothwell, R. P. G. (1986c). Accuracy of certification of deaths due to asthma. A national study. *Am. J. Epidemiol.* **124**:1004-1011.

Sears, M. R., Holdaway, M. D., Hewitt, C. J., Flannery, E. M., Herbison, G. P., and Silva, P. A. (1987a). Relationships between airway hyperresponsiveness, atopy and childhood asthma: a longitudinal study. *Am. Rev. Respir. Dis.* **135**:A380.

Sears, M. R., Rea, H. H., and Beaglehole, R. (1987b). Asthma mortality: a review of recent experience in New Zealand. *J. Allergy Clin. Immunol.* **80**:319-325.

Sears, M. R., Herbison, G. P., Holdaway, M. D., Hewitt, C. J., Flannery, E. M., Silva, P. A. (1988). The relative risks of allergy to grass pollen, house dust mite and cat dander in the development of childhood asthma. *Am. Rev. Respir. Dis.* **137**:239.

Sears, M. R., Herbison, G. P., Holdaway, M. D., Hewitt, C. J., Flannery, E. M., and Silva, P. A. (1989). The relative risks of sensitivity to grass pollen, house dust mite and cat dander in the development of childhood asthma. *Clin. Exper. Allergy* **19**:419-424.

Sibbald, B., and Turner-Warwick, M. (1979). Factors influencing the prevalence of asthma among first degree relatives of extrinsic and intrinsic asthmatics. *Thorax* **43**:332-337.

Sims, D. G., Downham, M. A. P. S., Gardner, P. S., Webb, J. K. G., and Weightman, D. (1978). Study of 8-year-old children with a history of respiratory syncytial virus bronchiolitis in infancy. *Br. Med. J.* **1**:11-14.

Sinclair, B. L., Clark, D. W. J., and Sears, M. R. (1987). Use of anti-asthma drugs in New Zealand. *Thorax* **42**:670-675.

Skarpaas, I. J. K., and Gulsvik, A. (1985). Prevalence of bronchial asthma and respiratory symptoms in schoolchildren in Oslo. *Allergy* **40**:295-299.

Sly, R. M. (1984). Increases in deaths from asthma. *Ann. Allergy* **53**:20-25.

Sly, R. M. (1988). Mortality from asthma in children 1979-1984. *Ann. Allergy* **60**:433-442.

Smith, J. M. (1961). Prevalence and natural history of asthma in school children. *Br. Med. J.* **1**:711-713.

Smith, J. M., Harding, I. K., and Cumming, G. (1971). The changing prevalence of asthma in school children. *Clin. Allergy* **1**:57-61.

Sparrow, D., O'Connor, G., Colton, T., Barry, C. L., and Weiss, S. T. (1987). The relationship of nonspecific bronchial responsiveness to the occurrence of respiratory symptoms and decreased levels of pulmonary function. The normative aging study. *Am. Rev. Respir. Dis.* **135**:1255-1260.

Speizer, F. E., Doll, R., and Heaf, P. (1968). Observations on recent increase in mortality from asthma. *Br. Med. J.* **1**:335-339.

Stellman, J. L., Spicer, J. E., and Cayton, R. M. (1982). Morbidity from chronic asthma. *Thorax* **37**:218-221.

Stempel, D. A., Clyde, W. A., Henderson, F. W., and Collier, A. M. (1980). Serum IgE levels and the clinical expression of respiratory illness. *J. Pediatr.* **97**:185-190.

Stewart, C. J., and Nunn, A. J. (1985). Are asthma mortality rates changing? *Br. J. Dis. Chest* **79**:229-234.

Stolley, P. D., and Schinnar, R. (1978). Association between asthma mortality and isoproterenol aerosols: a review. *Prev. Med.* **7**:519-538.

Strunk, R. C., Mrazek, D. A., Fuhrmann, G. S. W., and LaBrecque, J. F. (1985). Physiological and psychological characteristics associated with deaths due to asthma in childhood: a case-controlled study. *J.A.M.A.* **254**:1193-1198.

Tabachnik, E., and Levison, H. (1981). Infantile bronchial asthma. *J. Allergy Clin. Immunol.* **67**:339-347.

Turner, K. J. (1987). Changing prevalence of asthma in developing countries. In *Highlights in Asthmology*. Edited by F. B. Michel, J. Bousqet, and P. Godard. Springer-Verlag, New York, pp. 37-43.

Turner, K. J., Dowse, G. K., Stewart, G. A., Alpers, M. P., and Woolcock, A. J. (1985). Prevalence of asthma in the South Fore people of the Okapa district of Papua New Guinea. Features associated with a recent dramatic increase. *Int. Arch. Allergy Appl. Immunol.* **77**:158-162.

Turner, K. J., Dowse, G. K., Stewart, G. A., and Alpers, M. P. (1986). Studies on bronchial hyperreactivity, allergic responsiveness and asthma in rural and urban children of the highlands of Papua New Guinea. *J. Allergy Clin. Immunol.* **77**:558-566.

Turner, K. J., Stewart, G. A., Woolcock, A. J., Green, W., and Alpers, M. P. (1988). Relationship between mite densities and the prevalence of asthma: comparative studies in two populations in the eastern highlands of Papua New Guinea. *Clin. Allergy* **18**:331-340.

Van Niekerk, C. H., Weinberg, E. G., Shore, S. C., de V Heese, H., and Van Schalkwyk, D. J. (1979). Prevalence of asthma: a comparative study of urban and rural Xhosa children. *Clin. Allergy* **9**:319-324.

Venables, K. M., Burge, P. S., Davison, A. G., and Newman Taylor, A. J. (1984). Peak flow rate records in surveys: reproducibility of observers' reports. *Thorax* **39**:828-832.

Verity, C. M., VanHeule, B., Carswell, F., and Hughes, A. O. (1984). Bronchial lability and skin reactivity in siblings of asthmatic children. *Arch. Dis. Child.* **59**:871-876.

Viegi, G., Paoletti, P., Prediletto, R., Carrozzi, L., Fazzi, P., Di Pede, F., Pistelli, G., Giuntini, C., and Lebowitz, M. D. (1988). Prevalence of respiratory symptoms in an unpolluted area of Northern Italy. *Eur. Respir. J.* **1**:311-318.

Waite, D. A., Eyles, E. F., Tonkin, S. L., and O'Donnell, T. V. (1980). Asthma prevalence in Tokelauan children in two environments. *Clin. Allergy* **10**:71-75.

Weiss, S. T., Tager, I. B., Speizer, F. E., and Rosner, B. (1980). Persistent wheeze. Its relation to respiratory illness, cigarette smoking, and level of pulmonary function in a population sample of children. *Am. Rev. Respir. Dis.* **122**:697-707.

Weiss, S. T., Tager, I. B., Weiss, J. W., Munoz, A., Speizer, F. E., and Ingram, R. H. (1984). Airways responsiveness in a population sample of adults and children. *Am. Rev. Respir. Dis.* **129**:898-902.

Williams, H., and McNicols, K. N. (1969). Prevalence, natural history and relationship of wheezy bronchitis and asthma in children: an epidemiological study. *Br. Med. J.* **4**:321-325.

Woolcock, A. J., Dowse, G. K., Temple, K., Stanley, H., Alpers, M. P., and Turner, K. J. (1983). The prevalence of asthma in the South Fore people of Papua New Guinea. A method for field studies of bronchial reactivity. *Eur. J. Respir. Dis.* **64**:571-581.

Woolcock, A. J., Salome, C. M., and Yan, K. (1984). The shape of the dose-response curve to histamine in asthmatic and normal subjects. *Am. Rev. Respir. Dis.* **130**:71-75.

Woolcock, A. J., Peat, J. K., Salome, C. M., Yan, K., Anderson, S. D., Schoeffel, R. E., McCowage, G., and Killalea, T. (1987). Prevalence of bronchial hyperresponsiveness and asthma in a rural adult population. *Thorax* **42**:361-368.

Woolcock, A. J., Alpers, M. P., and Hurry, V. M. (1988). An epidemic of asthma in Papua New Guinea? *Aust. N.Z. J. Med.* **18**:544.

World Health Organization. (1977). *Manual of the International Statistical Classification of Diseases, Injuries and Causes of Death: Based on the Recommendations of the Ninth Revision Conference*, 1975. Vol. 1. Geneva, World Health Organization.

Yan, K., Salome, C., and Woolcock, A. J. (1983). Rapid method for measurement of bronchial responsiveness. *Thorax* **38**:760-765.

Zamel, N., Leroux, M., and Vanderdoelen, J. L. (1984). Airway response to inhaled methacholine in healthy nonsmoking twins. *J. Appl. Physiol.* **56**:936-939.

Zimmerman, B., Feanny, S., Reisman, J., Hak, H., Rashed, N., McLaughlin, F. J., and Levison, H. (1988). Allergy in asthma. 1. The dose relationship of allergy to severity of childhood asthma. *J. Allergy Clin. Immunol.* **81**:63-70.

2

Airway Hyperresponsiveness: Definition, Measurement, and Clinical Relevance

DONALD W. COCKCROFT

University Hospital
Saskatoon, Saskatchewan, Canada

FREDERICK E. HARGREAVE

St. Joseph's Hospital
Hamilton, Ontario, Canada

Airway hyperresponsiveness has been perceived to be a usual feature of asthma (Boushey et al., 1980; Hargreave et al., 1981, 1986a; Barnes, 1987; Woolcock, 1988). It can be measured with various stimuli and by different methods with the same stimuli. Confusion and misunderstanding continue to exist regarding the measurement and significance of airway responsiveness. Interpretation of the clinical relevance of airway hyperresponsiveness is difficult because it can be measured by a number of different stimuli (the results of which do not necessarily correlate) and because the definitions of asthma and chronic bronchitis are arbitrary and not necessarily accurate in terms of diseases with different pathogeneses. Nevertheless, measurement of airway responsiveness to histamine or methacholine has improved our understanding of airway hyperresponsiveness and of asthma in a number of ways. Measurements with these and other stimuli have also highlighted issues that require further investigations.

I. Definition

A. Airway Responsiveness

Airway responsiveness is the tendency of the airways to constrict to nonsensitizing physical or chemical stimuli. Airway responsiveness probably serves a normal physiological role; two probable roles are to help match ventilation to perfusion (Crawford et al., 1987) and to help protect the pulmonary parenchyma from toxic inhaled substances.

B. Airway Hyperresponsiveness

Airway hyperresponsiveness can thus be defined as a degree of airway responsiveness greater than that observed in normal subjects. The airways are more responsive in the ease with which they constrict in response to histamine or methacholine (left shift of a dose-response curve) or in the degree to which they will constrict (elevation or disappearance of a maximal response plateau), or both (Woolcock et al., 1984; Sterk et al., 1985). To date, investigations have involved mainly the position of the curve rather than the plateau. The concept of airway hyperresponsiveness has developed from clinical and physiological observations of the disease syndrome we refer to as asthma, and antedates the wide recognition of the concept of normal airway responsiveness. Airway responsiveness to histamine appears to be distributed continuously in human subjects (Woolcock et al., 1987), probably in log normal distribution (Cockcroft et al., 1983), much as in animals (Douglas et al., 1977; Snapper et al., 1978). There is, therefore, no sharp division between normal and increased airway responsiveness. This feature has led to some confusion and emphasizes the need to measure and regulate the dosage of the stimulus to allow accurate interpretation of results.

The adjectives *nonallergic* and *nonspecific* have been used to differentiate this form of airway responsiveness from airway responses to sensitizers such as allergens and low-molecular-weight chemicals derived from occupational exposures. Since all stimuli act through specific mechanisms, the original term *nonspecific* airway responsiveness is ambiguous and should be discarded. The term *nonallergic* is also less than ideal; we therefore recommend the term *airway responsiveness to nonsensitizing stimuli* as more appropriate to describe this broad category, but ideally the stimulus should be specified (Hargreave et al., 1986b; Dolovich et al., 1986) (see below).

C. Nature of Stimuli

Airway responsiveness can be measured using many different chemical and physical stimuli (Pauwels et al., 1988). Mediators that act through the autonomic nervous system include cholinergic agonists, cholinesterase inhibitors, beta-adrenergic antagonists, and alpha-adrenergic agonists. Bronchoactive amines (histamine, seratonin), peptides (bradykinin), arachidonic acid metabolites (prostaglandin F2α, leukotrine C4, D4, E4), neuropeptides, and adenosine or adenosine monophosphate (AMP) may also be used. Exercise, cold air, hyperventilation, and combinations thereof, as well as both both hyper- and hypoosmolar stimuli are physical triggers that provoke airway constriction. Constriction is stimulated through different pathways, some of which are not completely understood. The relative sensitivity and specificity of the various stimuli, particularly with relevance to asthma, need to be better defined.

Pauwels et al. (1988) suggest that a distinction be made between "direct" stimuli, which act directly on the airway smooth muscle (e.g., methacholine and, probably, histamine), and "indirect" stimuli, which act through secondary mediator release or neural pathways, or both. Examples of stimuli that are probably indirect are exercise, cold air, hypo- or hypertonic aerosols, propranolol, neurokinin A, and AMP. Pauwels et al. (1988) predict that indirect airway hyperresponsiveness should correlate better with naturally occurring symptoms of variable airflow limitation, since natural symptoms are chiefly induced by indirect mechanisms. In view of these differences, and the possibility of different sensitivity and specificity of various stimuli relative to the presence of asthma, it is suggested that the stimulus be used to define the nature of the responsiveness under discussion (e.g., histamine airway responsiveness, exercise airway responsiveness, etc.).

II. Measurement of Airway Responsiveness

A. Choice of Stimulus

The "ideal" stimulus for measurement of airway responsiveness has not been identified. It may differ depending on the clinical or research purpose of the test.

Airway responsiveness has been measured most extensively by inhalation tests with histamine or methacholine (or occasionally other cholinergic analogues such as acetylcholine or carbachol). The use of these agents has been based partially on historical reasons, and partially on their availability. Airway responsiveness to histamine or methacholine correlates well with the presence and severity of variable airflow limitation (asthma) (Cockcroft et al., 1977a; Hargreave et al., 1981), is technically easier to measure than responses to exercise or cold air hyperventilation, is more sensitive, and tends to have better patient acceptability than either exercise or cold air hyperventilation.

B. Standardization of Inhalation Provocation Tests

Accurate and comparable measurements of airway responsiveness to histamine or methacholine depend upon well-standardized inhalation tests. The presence of a continuous distribution with a less than clearly defined "cutpoint" between normal and increased airway responsiveness emphasizes the need for proper standardization, since this is not an "all or nothing" phenomenon. The topic of standardization of airway responsiveness has been recently reviewed in depth (Hargreave and Woolcock, 1985).

The most important technical aspects that require standardization are those that will lead to a reproducible dosage of inhaled agonist. Nebulizer output and pattern of inhalation are the two important technical factors to regulate to produce a reproducible inhaled dosage; particle size within the range of 1.2-3.6 μm mass medium diameter does not appear to be an important variable (Ryan et al., 1981a).

Two acceptable types of aerosol generation and inhalation are a timed period of tidal breathing inhalation from a continuous-output jet nebulizer (Cockcroft et al., 1977a; Juniper et al., 1978), and a counted number of inspiratory capacity inhalations from an intermittent dosing device (Yan et al. 1983; Fabbri et al., 1985). For the tidal breathing technique, attention to the regulation of nebulizer output and accurate timing of the tidal breathing period lead to a reproducible dosage and uniform distribution of aerosol within the lung (Ryan et al., 1981b). For the dosing devices, similar attention must be paid to standardizing nebulizer output per puff, but in addition to the regulation of the pattern of inhalation including speed and depth of inhalation as well as breath-hold time, all of which influence deposition and retention of aerosol (Dolovich, 1985).

Aerosols of histamine or methacholine are generally administered in doubling dosages at carefully regulated intervals. The response is measured by physiological determination of airflow timed to coincide with the peak effect of the agonist, between 0.5 and 3 min for histamine or methacholine (Cartier et al., 1983). The forced expiratory volume in 1s (FEV_1) is the favored measurement for clinical purposes; despite the bronchoactive effect of the maneuver (Orehek et al., 1980), the FEV_1 appears to discriminate better between asthma and nonasthmatic conditions (Fish and Kelly, 1979; Cockcroft and Berscheid, 1983), and is an easy, reproducible, and inexpensive measurement to obtain. Other measurements may have value for research or epidemiological studies.

Depending on the dosage interval, the results are plotted on either cumulative or noncumulative log dose-response curves and are expressed as the provocation dosage or concentration that produces a given percentage reduction in the parameter measured (e.g., PD_{20} or PC_{20} in cumulative or noncumulative units) (Hargreave and Woolcock, 1985). The shape of the dose-response curve may provide an adjunct to the cutpoint. Normal subjects develop a maximal response plateau or limited airway constriction to histamine or methacholine, after which increasing dosages of agonist produce no further response (Woolcock et al., 1984; Sterk et al., 1985). This may also be seen in patients with mild asthma but not in patients with moderate or severe asthma (Woolcock et al., 1984).

Standardization principles using other inhaled agonists are essentially the same. Similar concerns underline the standardization of bronchoprovocation tests with physical stimuli such as cold air hyperventilation (Hargreave et al., 1986b), exercise (Anderson and Schoeffel, 1985a; Hargreave et al., 1986b), and the osmolar triggers (Anderson and Schoeffel, 1985b; Boulet et al., 1987).

III. Airway Hyperresponsiveness and Asthma

The use of histamine and methacholine inhalation tests have improved our understanding of asthma in a number of ways.

A. Asthma Severity

The level of airway hyperresponsiveness to histamine or methacholine correlates well with both clinical and physiological assessment of the severity of asthma or variable airflow limitation. It correlates with a score of asthma severity (Murray et al., 1981) and with the minimum medications required for control of symptoms (Cockcroft et al., 1977a; Juniper et al., 1981); these correlations, however, are far from perfect. There is also a reasonable correlation between airway responsiveness and diurnal variation in peak flow rates when asthma is controlled and stable (Ryan et al., 1982). Resting airflow limitation is usually not a feature of airway hyperresponsiveness in asthma until airway responsiveness is moderately to markedly increased (Ryan et al., 1982). The level of airway responsiveness is a determinant of airflow limitation to exercise (Anderton et al., 1979) and cold air hyperventilation (O'Byrne et al., 1982; Weiss et al., 1983; Aquilina, 1983) and the early asthmatic response to allergen (Cockcroft et al., 1979). It requires an exceptionally strong stimulus, usually to a sensitizing agent such as an allergen (Cockcroft et al., 1977b) or occupational chemical (Hargreave et al., 1984), to provoke airflow limitation in subjects with normal airway responsiveness.

B. Inducers of Airway Hyperresponsiveness and Inciters of Airway Constriction

Several agents or "inducers" may produce transient (but prolonged) heightening of airway responsiveness superimposed on a baseline either of normal or persistently increased responsiveness (Hargreave, 1986). This was first noted with inhaled allergens by Altounyan in 1964. Since then inhaled allergens have been noted to increase airway responsiveness both upon natural exposure (Altounyan, 1970; Boulet et al., 1983; Sotomayor et al., 1984; Lowhagen and Rak, 1985) and in the laboratory (Cockcroft et al., 1977b; Cartier et al., 1982). Exposure to occupational sensitizing chemicals either in the workplace (Cartier et al., 1984a,b; Hargreave et al., 1984) or in the laboratory (Lam et al., 1979; Mapp et al., 1986) likewise produces transient heightening of airway responsiveness. In the laboratory, these increases in airway responsiveness after administration of an allergen or occupational sensitizer are strongly associated with the late asthmatic response occurring between 3 and 8 h after exposure (Cockcroft et al., 1977b; Cartier et al., 1982; Mapp et al., 1986). Significant and sometimes long-lasting increases in airway responsiveness, however, do occur in the presence of clinically and measurably insignificant late responses, in the range of 5-15% FEV_1 reduction (Cockcroft et al., 1977b; Cartier et al., 1982) and occasionally can be seen in the absence of any measurable late asthmatic response after administration of either an allergen (Cockcroft et al., 1989) or an occupational sensitizer (Cartier et al., 1986; Malo et al., 1989). A late asthmatic response is seen infrequently without an increase in airway responsiveness (Malo et al., 1989). These discrepancies are in keeping with the possibility that an induced prolonged increase in airway responsiveness is a more sensitive and specific marker of the cellular phase of airway inflammation than the late asthmatic response (see below).

A transient increase in airway responsiveness is also seen in normal subjects after viral respiratory tract infections (Empey et al., 1976). The precise importance of this in naturally acquired viral infections in asthmatic persons has not yet been clearly documented.

Noxious gases such as ozone (Holtzman et al., 1979) and nitrogen dioxide (Orehek et al., 1976) also produce transient airway hyperresponsiveness in the laboratory in both normal and asthmatic subjects. The response to ozone is relatively short-lived and, unlike with allergen, tolerance develops fairly quickly (Boushey and Holtzman, 1985). The relevance of this to naturally occurring noxious agents (i.e., air pollution) has not been clearly established.

By contrast to inducers, there are a large number of clinically recognizable triggers of airway constriction. These "inciters" provoke transient short-lived airflow limitation without enhanced airway responsiveness (Dolovich and Hargreave, 1981; Cockcroft, 1987). In addition to isolated allergen-induced early asthmatic responses, they include exercise, cold air hyperventilation, most pharmacological triggers, emotions, and inhaled irritant dust, smells, and fumes including cigarette smoke (McIntyre et al., 1982).

C. Airway Hyperresponsiveness and Airway Inflammation

Increasing evidence links airway hyperresponsiveness and transient increases in airway hyperresponsiveness with airway inflammation. Asthma triggers that cause transient airway hyperresponsiveness also produce airway inflammation. This has been studied in humans using bronchoalveolar lavage (BAL) following allergen challenge (de Monchy et al., 1985; Metzger et al., 1986) and following sensitizing chemical challenge (Lam et al., 1985; Fabbri et al., 1987). Subjects with allergen-induced late asthmatic responses and, it is presumed, heightened airway responsiveness develop BAL eosinophilia (de Monchy et al., 1985; Metzger et al., 1986) whereas those with isolated early responses do not (de Monchy et al., 1985). Similar relationships exist between plicatic-acid-induced late responses and BAL eosinophils (Lam et al., 1985) and iso-cyanate-induced late responses and both BAL neutrophils and eosinophils (Fabbri et al., 1987). Allergen inhalation tests, which induce increases in airway responsiveness, are also associated with an increase in peripheral blood eosinophils, basophils, and the progenitors for these cells, whereas those that do not are not followed by increases in levels of these blood cells (Cookson et al., 1989, Gibson et al., 1989a).

These strong relationships, however, do not prove cause and effect. The inhibition of late responses and allergen-induced increases in airway responsiveness by anti-inflammatory drugs (Cockcroft and Murdock, 1987) is supportive. Animal studies have also shown strong relationships between inflammation and induced airway hyperresponsiveness after both allergen (Chung et al., 1985; Marsh et al., 1985) and ozone (Holtzman et al., 1983). Animal models have convincingly demonstrated that transient airway hyperresponsiveness requires the presence of inflammatory cells of the polymorphonuclear leukocyte series (Murphy et al., 1986; O'Byrne et al., 1984).

Recent investigations in stable asthmatic subjects with persistent airway hyperresponsiveness have also demonstrated a relationship between level of airway responsiveness and BAL recovery of both eosinophils and metachromatic (likely mast) cells (Kirby et al., 1987; Wardlaw et al., 1988), and epithelial shedding (Wardlaw et al., 1988).

It is thus a logical hypothesis that one or more types of the cellular phase of airway inflammation can cause airway hyperresponsiveness. The mechanism(s) by which the inflammatory cells are recruited into the airways, and the mechanism(s) by which these inflammatory cells induce airway hyperresponsiveness are as yet uncertain, but they may involve edematous thickening in and around the airway wall (Macklem, 1985; James et al., 1989). These are important questions with pathophysiological and therapeutic relevance.

D. Persistent Airway Hyperresponsiveness

In addition to their transient airway hyperresponsiveness, chronic asthmatics demonstrate persistent airway hyperresponsiveness that seems partially refractory to environmental control or corticosteroid treatment. The origins of this persistent airway responsiveness are not clearly understood.

Nevertheless, there is increasing evidence that exposure to those "inflammatory" asthma inducers known to produce transient heightening of airway responsiveness can lead to persistent airway responsiveness (Hargreave et al., 1986c). Data from occupational asthma provide the strongest support for this. Persistent airway hyperresponsiveness in western red cedar-induced asthma (Chan Yeung et al., 1982) and in isocyanate-induced asthma (Mapp et al., 1988) is common and appears retrospectively to be acquired as a result of the disease. The most consistent determinant appears to be the length of continued exposure after symptoms of asthma have developed (Chan Yeung et al., 1982; Mapp et al., 1988). There is anecdotal evidence that a single exposure to a toxic chemical can occasionally produce permanent airway hyperresponsiveness (Brooks et al., 1985) and similar anecdotal data surrounding single or multiple viral or *Mycoplasma* infections. Indirect evidence for the hypothesis that chronic or repeated atopic allergic airways inflammation can lead to persistent airway hyperresponsiveness comes from various population studies. In random populations, involving over 5,500 people, there is a strong correlation between the degree of atopy and the presence both of asthma and airway hyperresponsiveness (Cockcroft et al., 1984; Cookson et al., 1984; Witt et al., 1986; Peat et al., 1987; Burney et al., 1987; Cockcroft and Hargreave, 1989). These data support but do not prove that chronic/recurrent atopic airway inflammation can lead to persistent airway hyperresponsiveness.

IV. Sources of Confusion

A. Population Studies

A number of population studies of histamine airway responsiveness in unselected individuals have recently been reported (Lee et al., 1983; Cockcroft et al., 1985; Sears et al., 1986; Burney et al., 1987; Salome et al., 1987; Woolcock et al., 1987). Airway hyperresponsiveness to histamine is strongly associated with symptoms, particularly those consistent with asthma (variable wheezing). The majority of subjects with evidence from their history of current symptomatic asthma will have airway hyperresponsiveness, proving the test to be sensitive for current symptoms of asthma. This is not surprising since this is the way that cutpoints between "normal" and "increased" airway responsiveness have been arbitrarily defined from clinic populations. Nevertheless, there are a large number of individuals denying current or past symptoms of asthma or any other respiratory disease who, by arbitrary criteria, are defined as having mild airway hyperresponsiveness. In one study, the prevalence of airway hyperresponsiveness ($PC_{20} < 8$ mg/ml; Cockcroft et al., 1977a) was 4.5% in normal asymptomatic adults and 12.7% in individuals with symptoms of rhinitis but not of asthma (Cockcroft et al., 1985). Since these groups make up a large segment of the population, more than 50% of subjects with mild airway hyperresponsiveness (PC_{20} between 2 and 8 mg/ml) denied symptoms suggestive of asthma at any time. These results appear similar to those of other population studies. Woolcock et al. (1987) found that 32% of adults with airway hyperresponsiveness (histamine $PD_{20} < 3.9$ μmole; Yan et al., 1983) never had symptoms suggestive of asthma; this approached or exceeded 50% for those with mild or intermediate hyperresponsiveness (PD_{20} 3.9-7.8 μmole).

Possible explanations for the presence of mild airway hyperresponsiveness in the absence of symptoms include the following. These subjects may be those in whom the airway hyperresponsiveness is truly a "false positive." Cutpoints have been arbitrarily defined to make the test sensitive, and therefore have almost no false negatives (with regard to current asthma symptoms). As with any other biological tests, this high "sensitivity" should lead to some sacrifice in the area of "specificity" and thus be associated with at least a prevalence of false-positive tests. However, subjects with asymptomatic mild airway hyperresponsiveness do show increased diurnal variation in peak flow rates (Ramsdale et al., 1985a; Gibson et al., 1988), indicating that these subjects also have asymptomatic variable airflow limitation. These subjects with asymptomatic airway hyperresponsiveness and variable airflow limitation likely either fail to encounter stimuli strong enough to provoke symptomatic airflow limitation in their daily activities or have airflow limitation but fail to perceive it or fail to recognize it as abnormal. These same considerations are likely to be responsible for some of the overlap and variability in the correlations between asthma severity and airway hyperresponsiveness (Cockcroft et al., 1977a; Juniper et al., 1981; Murray et al., 1981).

Population studies have also identified many people who have had symptoms consistent with asthma but who have normal histamine airway responsiveness when measured. There are also a number of reasons for this discrepancy. First, most of these studies have not related the symptoms to the timing of test. Symptoms associated with airway hyperresponsiveness may have occurred in the past but may have reversed, and be absent, at the time of the test. Cockcroft et al. (1985) found that the majority of subjects with seasonal asthma (in the previous year) and past asthma (> 1 year ago) had normal histamine airway responsiveness when symptoms were absent at the time of the test. Second, it is possible to trigger airway constriction in subjects with normal histamine or methacholine airway responsiveness if the stimulus is especially strong, as can occur with a sensitizing agent. This has been demonstrated in allergen inhalation tests (Cockcroft, 1977b), and in seasonal allergic asthmatics (Boulet et al., 1983) and occupational asthmatics (Hargreave et al., 1984) before airway responsiveness has increased into the hyperresponsive range. Finally, wheezing is not specific for methacholine airway hyperresponsiveness (and, presumably, variable airflow limitation) (Adelroth et al., 1986) and should therefore not be regarded as a gold standard for asthma defined as variable airflow limitation. Furthermore, other (nonwheeze) symptoms occur in the presence of variable airflow limitation but also with other conditions.

B. Other Diseases

Airway hyperresponsiveness also occurs in other lung diseases. These include diseases in which airway limitation and inflammation may play a role, such as sarcoidosis, extrinsic allergic alveolitis, and bronchiectasis. The majority of attention in airway responsiveness in nonasthmatic lung disease, however, has been directed towards smoking-related chronic airflow limitation.

Although cigarette smoking can produce inflammation in airways in animal models (Hulburt et al., 1987), there are few data to suggest that cigarette smoking produces clinically significant airway hyperresponsiveness in adult human smokers in the absence of airflow limitation (Cockcroft, 1988). Smokers with chronic airflow limitation have airway hyperresponsiveness to both histamine and methacholine that is strongly associated with the degree of reduction in airway caliber (Ramsdale et al., 1984; Du Toit et al., 1986; Verma et al., 1988; Lim et al., 1988); this is not a feature of the airway hyperresponsiveness in asthma (Cockcroft et al., 1977a; Ramsdale et al., 1985b; Du Toit et al., 1986). There are other differences in the airway hyperresponsiveness seen in patients with asthma and chronic airflow limitation. For a given degree of resting airflow obstruction, asthmatics are much more hyperresponsive to methacholine than are subjects with chronic airflow limitation (Ramsdale et al., 1985b). A number of stimuli also appear to provoke airway constriction in patients with asthma and not in those with chronic airflow limitation. These include cold air hyperventilation (Ramsdale et al., 1984, 1985b), alpha-adrenergic agonist (Du Toit et al., 1986), and propanolol (Woolcock et al., 1986). It has also been stated (Du Toit et al., 1986) that asthmatics respond in an equimolar fashion to histamine and methacholine, whereas subjects with chronic airflow limitation are somewhat more responsive to histamine than to methacholine. The latter was not seen, however, by Bahous et al. (1984). Since the molecular weights are not that far apart, however, this difference is small and subtle and likely to be of limited clinical or diagnostic relevance. Subjects with chronic airflow limitation and airway hyperresponsiveness can have a dose-response plateau similar to normals and dissimilar to asthmatics with similar degrees of airway hyperresponsiveness (Du Toit et al., 1986).

These data suggest that the pathogenesis of histamine and methacholine airway hyperresponsiveness in patients with asthma and chronic airflow limitation is different, that certain stimuli may provoke different responses in one condition compared to another, and that some stimuli may be more specific for asthma than others. Further investigations are needed.

V. Future Directions

The preceding discussion has identified a number of areas that need more careful study. Subject characteristics need to be documented in more detail, as was recommended by the Ciba Foundation study group (Fletcher et al., 1971). The type of symptoms and their proximity to measurements of airway function need to be detailed. Measurements of airway responsiveness need to be made with indirect stimuli as well as histamine or methacholine so that their relationship to clinical characteristics can be compared. The recognition of the importance of airway inflammation in asthma indicates that the structural and functional characteristics of this need to be related to the clinical and physiological features to allow us to learn more about the nature, pathogenesis, and treatment of asthma and other airway disease. So far, only limited studies have been performed.

Airway inflammation can be studied directly by histopathological examinations of autopsy or surgical specimens or by bronchial biopsies and bronchial brushings and, providing there is no disease of the peripheral respiratory tissues, by the cytological examination of BAL, bronchial lavage, or sputum. Indirect correlates of airway inflammation include the heightening of airway responsiveness and changes in peripheral blood cells.

Studies of BAL and bronchial lavage in persons with mild stable asthma have identified small elevations of eosinophils and metachromatic cells above those seen in asymptomatic subjects with normal airway responsiveness to methacholine (Flint et al., 1985; Kirby et al., 1987; Wardlaw et al., 1988); there is also shedding of epithelial cells (Wardlaw et al., 1988). The metachromatic cells, which resemble mucosal mast cells on light microscopic examination, seemed to be an early, or the earliest, abnormality.

Gibson and co-workers (1989b) have recently examined the possibility that sputum can provide reliable information about the characteristics of the inflammatory response. A method of sample collection and handling was found to give reproducible total cell and differential cell counts not only between selected portions of the same specimen but between specimens on 2 consecutive days. This method was then used to compare the cytological appearance of one group of patients with a mild exacerbation of asthma (and no other airway disease) with another group of cigarette smokers with chronic cough and sputum (but no functional evidence of asthma). The cytological differences between the two groups were striking. The asthmatic patients had increased numbers of eosinophils and metachromatic cells, while the bronchitic patients had few or none of these cell types. No differences were observed in the other cell counts with the exception of increased numbers of macrophages in the patients with bronchitis. Treatment of the two groups with corticosteroids resulted in complete disappearance of the sputum in the asthmatic patients and return of postbronchodilator spirometry values to normal. No changes in these features were observed in the bronchitic subjects. Examination of the peripheral blood of the asthmatic subjects showed increases in levels of cells of the same lineage, specifically eosinophils, basophils, and progenitors for these cells, which fell after treatment with corticosteroids (Gibson et al., 1989c). In another study, the peripheral blood cells were studied before and 1 and 24 h after allergen inhalation (Gibson et al., 1989a). The subjects who had allergen-induced asthmatic responses with heightened methacholine airway responsiveness at 24 h, but not those who had isolated early asthmatic responses, also had increases in similar cells at 24 h. There were no changes in the other peripheral blood cell counts or in the granulocyte-macrophage progenitors. These results suggest that the airway inflammation of asthma is characterized by an increase in eosinophils and metachromatic cells and that the cytological characteristics of sputum (when there is no evidence of peripheral respiratory disease) might be used to define better airway diseases of different pathogeneses.

An example of the use of sputum cytological studies to investigate the pathogenesis of airway disease is provided by a recent study of chronic productive cough in nonsmokers (Hargreave et al., 1989). The patients had normal spirometry and methacholine airway responsiveness and so they did not have asthma as currently defined. However, their sputum, as in patients with asthma, showed increases in levels of eosinophils and metachromatic cells and was reversed by treatment with corticosteroids. Further studies to relate the histopathological appearance of airway disease and its clinical characteristics are required.

Discussion

Paré: Should we measure the maximum response as well as the sensitivity (dose causing a 20% drop in FEV_1) of subjects with inhalation challenge?

Hargreave: I agree that the measure of maximum responsiveness may provide very useful information, particularly in regards to the plateau we see in many patients with mild asthma.

Irvin: Should we be using measurements other than the FEV_1 as the reflection of airflow changes in tests of airway hyperresponsiveness?

Hargreave: If you employ a more sensitive test, such as airway conductance, you will shift the curve to the left, but the cutoff between normal and abnormal will remain relatively the same.

Platts-Mills: Have you examined nasal washings for eosinophils in patients symptomatic for asthma?

Hargreave: No.

Pipkorn: We find no relationship between nasal eosinophils and nasal hyperreactivity.

Fabbri: Have you compared cell counts in the sputum of asthmatic patients in relationship to natural exacerbations and compared the results to the cells counts reported after bronchial provocations?

Hargreave: No.

Venge: In BAL we find eosinophils to account for only 2-10% of recovered cells, yet in asthmatic sputum the eosinophils may represent 80-90% of cells. What do you think accounts for the difference?

Hargreave: We do bronchial provocation and BAL in patients with very mild asthma, while those subjects with increased symptoms and sputum eosinophilia may have much more severe degrees of asthma.

Drazen: What percentage of the cells are epithelial cells?

Hargreave: About 12%.

References

Adelroth, E., Hargreave, F. E., and Ramsdale, E. H. (1986). Do physicians need objective measurements to diagnose asthma? *Am. Rev. Respir. Dis.* **134**:704-707.

Altounyan, R. E. C. (1964). Variation of drug action on airway obstruction in man. *Thorax* **19**:406-415.

Altounyan, R. E. C. (1970). Changes in histamine and atropine responsiveness as a guide to diagnosis and evaluation of therapy in obstructive airways disease. In *Disodium Cromoglycate in Allergic Airways Disease.* Edited by J. Pepys and A. W. Franklands. London, Butterworths, pp. 47-53.

Anderson, S. D., and Schoeffel, R. E. (1985a). Standardization of exercise testing in the asthmatic patient: a challenge in itself. In *Airway Responsiveness: Measurement and Interpretation.* Edited by F. E. Hargreave and A. J. Woolcock. Mississauga, Astra Pharmaceuticals Canada Ltd., pp. 51-59.

Anderson, S. D., and Schoeffel, R. E. (1985b). The inhalation of ultrasonically nebulized aerosols as a provocation test for asthma. In *Airway Responsiveness: Measurement and Interpretation.* Edited by F. E. Hargreave and A. J. Woolcock. Mississauga, Astra Pharmaceuticals Canada Ltd., pp. 39-50.

Anderton, R. C., Cuff, M. T., Frith, P. A., Cockcroft, D. W., Morse, J. L. C., Jones, N. L., and Hargreave, F. E. (1979). Bronchial responsiveness to inhaled histamine and exercise. *J. Allergy Clin. Immunol.* **63**:315-320.

Aquilina, A. T. (1983). Comparison of airway reactivity induced by histamine, methacholine, and isocapnic hyperventilation in normal and asthmatic subjects. *Thorax* **38**:766-770.

Bahous, J., Cartier, A., Ouimet, G., Pineau, L., and Malo, J.-L. (1984). Nonallergic bronchial hyperexcitability in chronic bronchitis. *Am. Rev. Respir. Dis.* **129**:216-220.

Barnes, P. J. (1987). The changing face of asthma. *Q. J. Med.* **241**:359-365.

Boulet, L. P., Cartier, A., Thomson, N. C., Roberts, R. S., Dolovich, J., and Hargreave, F. E. (1983). Asthma and increases in nonallergic bronchial responsiveness from seasonal pollen exposure. *J. Allergy Clin. Immunol.* **71**:399-406.

Boulet, L. P., Legris, C., Thibault, L., and Turcotte, H. (1987). Comparative bronchial responses to hyperosmolar saline and methacholine in asthma. *Thorax* **42**:953-958.

Boushey, H. A., Holtzman, M. J., Sheller, J. R., and Nadel, J. A. (1980). Bronchial hyperreactivity. *Am. Rev. Respir. Dis.* **121**:389-413.

Boushey, H. A., and Holtzman, M. J. (1985). Experimental airway inflammation and hyperreactivity. *Am. Rev. Respir. Dis.* **131**:312-313.

Brooks, S. M., Weiss, M. A., and Bernstein, I. L. (1985). Reactive airways dysfunction syndrome (RADS). Persistent asthma syndrome after high level irritant exposures. *Chest* **88**:376-384.

Burney, P. F. J., Britton, J. R., Chinn, S., Tattersfield, A. E., Papacosta, A. O., Kelson, M. C., Anderson, F., and Corfield, D. R. (1987). Descriptive epidemiology of bronchial reactivity in an adult population: results from a community study. *Thorax* **42**:38-44.

Cartier, A., Thomson, N. C., Frith, P. A., Roberts, R., and Hargreave, F. E. (1982). Allergen-induced increase in bronchial responsiveness to histamine: relationship to the late asthmatic response and changes in airway caliber. *J. Allergy Clin. Immunol.* **70**:170-177.

Cartier, A., Malo, J.-L., Begin, P., Sestier, M., and Martin, R. R. (1983). Time course of bronchoconstriction induced by inhaled histamine and methacholine. *J. Appl. Physiol.* **54**:821-826.

Cartier, A., Pineau, L., and Malo, J.-L. (1984a). Monitoring of maximum expiratory peak flow rates and histamine inhalation tests in the investigation of occupational asthma. *Clin. Allergy* **14**:193-196.

Cartier, A., Malo, J.-L., Forest, F., Lafrance, M., Pineau, L., StAubin, J.-J., and Dubois, J.-Y. (1984b). Occupational asthma in snow crab-processing workers. *J. Allergy Clin. Immunol.* **74**:261-269.

Cartier, A., L'Archeveque, J., and Malo, J.-L. (1986). Exposure to sensitizing occupational agent can cause a long-lasting increase in bronchial responsiveness to histamine in the absence of significant changes in airway caliber. *J. Allergy Clin. Immunol.* **78**:1185-1189.

Chan-Yeung, M., Lam, S., and Koener, S. (1982). Clinical features and natural history of occupational asthma due to Western Red Cedar (*Thuja plicata*). *Am. J. Med.* **72**:411-415.

Chung, K. F., Becker, A. B., Lazarus, S. C., Frick, O. L., Nadel, J. A., and Gold, W. M. (1985). Antigen-induced hyperresponsiveness and pulmonary inflammation in allergic dogs. *J. Appl. Physiol.* **58**:1347-1353.

Cockcroft, D. W. (1987). Airway hyperresponsiveness: therapeutic implications. *Ann. Allergy* **59**:405-414.

Cockcroft, D. W. (1988). Cigarette smoking, airway hyperresponsiveness, and asthma. *Chest* **94**:675-676.

Cockcroft, D. W., and Berscheid, B. A. (1983). Measurement of responsiveness to inhaled histamine: comparison of FEV_1 and SGaw. *Ann. Allergy* **50**:374-377.

Cockcroft, D. W., and Hargreave, F. E. (1989). Relationship between atopy and airway responsiveness. In *Bronchitis IV.* Edited by H. J. Sluiter and R. van der Lende. Assen, The Netherlands, Van Gorcum & Co., pp. 23-32.

Cockcroft, D. W., and Murdock, K. Y. (1987). Comparative effects of inhaled salbutamol, sodium cromoglycate and beclomethasone dipropionate on allergen-induced early asthmatic response, late asthmatic responses and increased bronchial responsiveness to histamine. *J. Allergy Clin. Immunol.* **79**:734-740.

Cockcroft, D. W., Killian, D. N., Mellon, J. J. A., and Hargreave, F. E. (1977a). Bronchial reactivity to inhaled histamine: a method and clinical survey. *Clin. Allergy* **7**:235-243.

Cockcroft, D. W., Ruffin, R. E., Dolovich, J., and Hargreave, F. E. (1977b). Allergen induced increase in nonallergic bronchial reactivity. *Clin. Allergy* **7**:503-513.

Cockcroft, D. W., Ruffin, R. E., Frith, P. A., Cartier, A., Juniper, E. F., Dolovich, J., and Hargreave, F. E. (1979). Determinants of allergen-induced asthma: dose of allergen, circulating IgE antibody concentration and bronchial responsiveness to inhaled histamine. *Am. Rev. Respir. Dis.* **120**:1053-1058.

Cockcroft, D. W., Berscheid, B. A., and Murdock, K. Y. (1983). Unimodal distribution of bronchial responsiveness to inhaled histamine in a random human population. *Chest* **83**:751-754.

Cockcroft, D. W., Murdock, K. Y., and Berscheid, B. A. (1984). Relationship between atopy and bronchial responsiveness to histamine in a random population. *Ann. Allergy* **53**:26-29.

Cockcroft, D. W., Berscheid, B. A., Murdock, K. Y., and Gore, B. P. (1985). Sensitivity and specificity of histamine PC_{20} measurements in a random population. *J. Allergy Clin. Immunol.* **75**:142.

Cockcroft, D. W., Murdock, K. Y., Gore, B. P., O'Byrne, P. M., and Manning, P. (1989). Theophylline does not inhibit allergen-induced increase in airway responsiveness to methacholine. *J. Allergy Clin. Immunol.* **83**:913-920.

Cookson, W. O. C. M., Musk, A. W., and Ryan, G. (1984). Association between asthma history, atopy, and non-specific bronchial responsiveness in young adults. *Clin. Allergy* **16**:425-432.

Cookson, W. O. C. M., Craddock, C. F., Benson, M. K., and Durham, S. R. (1989). Falls in peripheral eosinophil counts parallel the late asthmatic response. *Am. Rev. Respir. Dis.* **139**:458-462.

Crawford, A. B. H., Makowska, M., and Engel, L. A. (1987). Effect of bronchomotor tone in static mechanical properties of lung and ventilation distribution. *J. Appl. Physiol.* **63**:2278-2285.

de Monchy, J. G. R., Kauffman, H. F., Venge, P., Koeter, G. H., Jansen, H. M., Sleuter, H. J., and de Vries, K. (1985). Bronchoalveolar eosinophilia during allergen-induced late asthmatic reactions. *Am. Rev. Respir. Dis.* **131**:373-376.

Dolovich, M. B. (1985). Technical factors influencing response to challenge aerosols. In *Airway Responsiveness: Measurement and Interpretation.* Edited by F. E. Hargreave and A. J. Woolcock. Mississauga, Astra Pharmaceuticals Canada Ltd., pp. 9-21.

Dolovich, J., and Hargreave, F. E. (1981). The asthma syndrome: inciters, inducers, and host characteristics. *Thorax* **36**:641-644.

Dolovich, J., Hargreave, F. E., O'Byrne, P. M., Ruhno, J., and Newhouse, M. T. (1986). Asthma terminology: troubles in wordland. *Am. Rev. Respir. Dis.* **134**:1102.

Douglas, J. S., Ridgeway, P., and Brink, C. (1977). Airway responses of the guinea pig *in vivo* and *in vitro*. *J. Pharmacol. Exp. Ther.* **202**:116-24.

Du Toit, J. I., Woolcock, A. J., Salome, C. M., Sundrum, R., and Black, J. L. (1986). Characteristics of bronchial hyperresponsiveness in smokers with chronic air-flow limitation. *Am. Rev. Respir. Dis.* **134**:498-501.

Empey, D. W., Laitinen, L. A., Jacobs, L., Gold, W. M., and Nadel, J. A. (1976). Mechanisms of bronchial hyperreactivity in normal subjects after upper respiratory tract infection. *Am. Rev. Respir. Dis.* **113**:131-139.

Fabbri, L. M., Mapp, C. E., and Hendrick, D. J. (1985). Standardization of the dosimeter method for the measurement of airway responsiveness in man. In *Airway Responsiveness: Measurement and Interpretation.* Edited by F. E. Hargreave and A. J. Woolcock. Mississauga, Astra Pharmaceuticals Canada Ltd., pp. 29-34.

Fabbri, L. M., Boschetto, P., Zocca, E., Milani, G., Pivirotto, F., Plebani, M., Burlina, A., Licata, B., and Mapp, C. E. (1987). Bronchoalveolar neutrophilia during late asthmatic reactions induced by toluene diisocyanate. *Am. Rev. Respir. Dis.* **136**:36-42.

Fish, J. E., and Kelly, J. F. (1979). Measurement of responsiveness in bronchoprovocation testing. *J. Allergy Clin. Immunol.* **64**:592-596.

Fletcher, C. M., Howell, J. B. L., Pepys, J., and Scadding, J. G. (1971). Addendum. Report of the working group on the definition of asthma. In *Identification of Asthma.* Edited by R. Porter and J. Birch. Ciba Foundation, Study Group No. 38. Edinburgh and London, Churchill Livingstone, pp. 172-174.

Flint, K. C., Leung, K. B. P., Hudspith, B. N., Brostoff, J., Pearce, F. L., and Johnson, N. M. (1985). Bronchoalveolar mast cells in extrinsic asthma: a mechanism for the initiation of antigen specific bronchoconstriction. *Br. Med. J.* **291**:923-926.

Gibson, P. G., Mattoli, S., Sears, M. R., Dolovich, J., and Hargreave, F. E. (1988). Variable airflow obstruction in asymptomatic children with methacholine airway hyperresponsiveness. *Clin. Invest. Med.* **11**:C105.

Gibson, P. G., Manning, P. J., Girgis-Gabardo, A., Hargreave, F., O'Byrne, P. M., Dolovich, J., and Denburg, J. (1989a). Progenitors during the late asthmatic response to allergen. *J. Allergy Clin. Immunol.* **83**:233.

Gibson, P. G., Girgis-Gabardo, A., Morris, M. M., Mattoli, S., Kay, J. M., Dolovich, J., Denburg, J., and Hargreave, F. E. (1989b). Cellular characteristics of sputum from patients with asthma and chronic bronchitis. *Thorax* **44**:689-768.

Gibson, P. G., Girgis-Gabardo, A., Dolovich, J., Morris, M. M., Anderson, M., and Denburg, J. (1989c). Blood eosinophils (E), basophils (B), and progenitors during asthma exacerbation and resolution (abstract). *Am. Rev. Respir. Dis.* In press.

Hargreave, F. E. (1986). Mechanisms by which environmental factors increase airway responsiveness. *Bull. Eur. Physiopathol. Respir.* **22**(Suppl 7): 209-211.

Hargreave, F. E., and Woolcock, A. J. (1985). *Airway Responsiveness: Measurement and Interpretation.* Mississauga, Astra Pharmaceuticals Canada Ltd.

Hargreave, F. E., Ryan, G., Thomson, N. C., O'Byrne, P. M., Latimer, K., Juniper, E. F., and Dolovich, J. (1981). Bronchial responsiveness to histamine or methacholine in asthma: measurement and clinical significance. *J. Allergy Clin. Immunol.* **68**:347-355.

Hargreave, F. E., Ramsdale, E. H., and Pugsby, S. O. (1984). Occupational asthma without bronchial hyperresponsiveness. *Am. Rev. Respir. Dis.* **130**:513-515.

Hargreave, F. E., Ramsdale, E. H., Kirby, J. G., and O'Byrne, P. M. (1986a). Asthma and the role of inflammation. *Eur. J. Respir. Dis.* **69**(Suppl 147):16-21.

Hargreave, F. E., Fink, J. N., Cockcroft, D. W., Fish, J. E., Holgate, S. T., Ramsdale, E. H., Roberts, R. S., Shapiro, G. G., and Sheppard, D. (1986b). Workshop 4: the role of bronchoprovocation. *J. Allergy Clin. Immunol.* **78**:517-524.

Hargreave, F. E., Dolovich, J., O'Byrne, P. M., Ramsdale, E. H., and Daniel, E. E. (1986c). The origin of airway hyperresponsiveness. *J. Allergy Clin. Immunol.* **78**:825-832.

Hargreave, F. E., Gibson, P. G., Girgis-Gabardo, A., Morris, M. M., Denburg, J., and Dolovich, J. (1989). Asthmatic airway inflammation without airway hyperresponsiveness to methacholine (abstract). *J. Allergy Clin. Immunol.* **83**:245.

Holtzman, M. J., Cunningham, J. H., Sheller, J. R., Irsigler, G. B., Nadel, J. A., and Boushey, H. A. (1979). Effect of ozone on bronchial reactivity in atopic and nonatopic subjects. *Am. Rev. Respir. Dis.* **120**:1059-1067.

Holtzman, M. J., Fabbri, L. M., O'Byrne, P. M., Gold, B. D., Aizawa, H. Walters, E. H., Alpert, S., and Nadel, J. A. (1983). Importance of airway inflammation for hyperresponsiveness induced by ozone. *Am. Rev. Respir. Dis.* **127**:686-690.

Hulburt, W. C., Walker, D. C., Jackson, A., and Hogg, J. C. (1987). Airway permeability to horseradish peroxidase in guinea pigs: the repair phase after injury by cigarette smoke. *Am. Rev. Respir. Dis.* **123**:320-326.

James, A. L., Pare, P. D., and Hogg, J. C. (1989). The mechanics of airway narrowing in asthma. *Am. Rev. Respir. Dis.* **139**:242-246.

Juniper, E. F., Frish, P. A., Dunnett, C., Cockcroft, D. W., and Hargreave, F. E. (1978). Reproducibility and comparison of responses to inhaled histamine and methacholine. *Thorax* **33**:705-710.

Juniper, E. F., Frith, P. A., and Hargreave, F. E. (1981). Airways responsiveness to histamine and methacholine: relationship to minimum treatment to control symptoms of asthma. *Thorax* **36**:575-579.

Kirby, J. C., Hargreave, F. E., Gleich, G. J., and O'Byrne, P. M. (1987). Bronchoalveolar cell profiles of asthmatic and non-asthmatic subjects. *Am. Rev. Respir. Dis.* **136**:379-383.

Lam, S., Wong, R., and Yeung, M. (1979). Nonspecific bronchial reactivity in occupational asthma. *J. Allergy Clin. Immunol.* **63**:28-34.

Lam, S., Leriche, J. C., Kijek, K., and Phillips, D. (1985). Effects of bronchial lavage volume on cellular and protein recovery. *Chest* **88**:856-859.

Lee, D. A., Winslow, N. R., Speight, A. N. P., and Hey, E. N. (1983). Prevalence and spectrum of asthma in childhood. *Br. Med. J.* **286**:1256-1258.

Lim, T. K., Taylor, R. G., Watson, A., Joyce, H., and Pride, N. B. (1988). Changes in bronchial responsiveness to inhaled histamine over four years in middle aged male smokers and ex-smokers. *Thorax* **43**:599-604.

Lowhagen, O., and Rak, S. (1985). Modification of bronchial hyperreactivity after treatment with sodium cromoglycate during pollen season. *J. Allergy Clin. Immunol.* **75**:460-467.

Macklem, P. T. (1985). Bronchial hyporesponsiveness. *Chest* **87**:158S-159S.

Malo, J.-L., L'Archeveque, J., and Cartier, A. (1989). Significant changes in nonspecific bronchial responsiveness after isolated immediate bronchospecific reactions caused by isocyanates but not after a late reaction caused by plicatic acid. *J. Allergy Clin. Immunol.* **83**:159-165.

Mapp, C. E., Di Giacomo, G. R., Omini, C., Broseghini, C., and Fabbri, L. M. (1986). Late, but not early, asthmatic reactions induced by toluenediisocyanate are associated with increased airway responsiveness to methacholine. *Eur. J. Respir. Dis.* **69**:276-284.

Mapp, C. E., Cheisara, P., de Marzo, N., and Fabbri, L. (1988). Persistent asthma due to isocyanates. *Am. Rev. Respir. Dis.* **137**:1326-1329.

Marsh, W. R., Irvin, C. G., Murphy, K. R., Behrens, B. L., and Larsen, G. L. (1985). Increases in airway reactivity to histamine and inflammatory cells in bronchoalveolar lavage after the late asthmatic response in an animal model. *Am. Rev. Respir. Dis.* **131**:875-879.

McIntyre, E. L., Ruffin, R. E., and Alpers, J. H. (1982). Lack of short-term effects of cigarette smoking on bronchial sensitivity to histamine and methacholine. *Eur. J. Respir. Dis.* **63**:535-542.

Metzger, W. J., Richerson, W. B., Worden, K., Monick, M., and Hunninghake, G. W. (1986). Bronchoalveolar lavage of allergic asthmatic patients following allergen bronchoprovocation. *Chest* **89**:477-83.

Murphy, K. R., Wilson, M. C., Irvin, C. G., Glezen, L. S., Marsh, W. R., Haslett, C., Henson, P. M., and Larsen, G. L. (1986). The requirement for polymorphonuclear leukocytes in the late asthmatic response and heightened airways reactivity in an animal model. *Am. Rev. Respir. Dis.* **134**:62-68.

Murray, A. B., Ferguson, A. C., and Morrison, B. (1981). Airway responsiveness to histamine as a test for overall severity of asthma in children. *J. Allergy Clin. Immunol.* **68**:119-124.

O'Byrne, P. M., Ryan, G., Morris, M., McCormack, D., Jones, N. L., Morse, J. L. C., and Hargreave, F. E. (1982). Asthma induced by cold air and its relation to nonspecific bronchial responsiveness to methacholine. *Am. Rev. Respir. Dis.* **125**:281-285.

O'Byrne, P. M., Walters, E. H., Gold, E. D., Aizawa, H. A., Fabbri, L. M., Alpert, S. E., Nadel, J. A., and Holtzman, M. J. (1984). Neutrophil depletion inhibits airway hyperresponsiveness induced by ozone exposure. *Am. Rev. Respir. Dis.* **130**:214-219.

Orehek, J., Massari, J. P., Gayrard, P., Grimaud, C., and Charpin, J. (1976). Effect of short-term, low-level nitrogen dioxide exposure on bronchial sensitivity of asthmatic patients. *J. Clin. Invest.* **57**:301-307.

Orehek, J., Charpin, D., Velardocchio, J. M., and Grimaud, C. (1980). Bronchomotor effect of bronchoconstriction-induced deep inspirations in asthmatics. *Am. Rev. Respir. Dis.* **121**:297-305.

Pauwels, R., Roos, G., and van der Straeten, M. (1988). Bronchial hyperresponsiveness is not bronchial hyperresponsiveness is not asthma. *Clin. Allergy* **18**:317-321.

Peat, J. K., Britton, W. J., Salome, C. M., and Woolcock, A. J. (1987). Bronchial hyperresponsiveness in two populations of Australian school children: III Effect of exposure to environmental allergens. *Clin. Allergy* **17**:291-300.

Ramsdale, E. H., Morris, M. M., Roberts, R. S., and Hargreave, F. E. (1984). Bronchial responsiveness to methacholine in chronic bronchitis: relationship to airflow obstruction and cold air responsiveness. *Thorax* **39**:912-918.

Ramsdale, E. H., Morris, M. M., Roberts, R. S., and Hargreave, F. E. (1985a). Asymptomatic bronchial hyperresponsiveness in rhinitis. *J. Allergy Clin. Immunol.* **75**:573-577.

Ramsdale, E. H., Roberts, R. S., Morris, M. M., and Hargreave, F. E. (1985b). Differences in responsiveness to hyperventilation and methacholine in asthma and chronic bronchitis. *Thorax* **40**:422-426.

Ryan, G., Dolovich, M. B., Obminski, G., Cockcroft, D. W., Juniper, E., Hargreave, F. E., and Newhouse, M. T. (1981a). Standardization of inhalation provocation tests: influence of nebulizer output, particle size and method of inhalation. *J. Allergy Clin. Immunol.* **67**:151-161.

Ryan, G., Dolovich, M. B., Roberts, R. S., Frith, P. A., Juniper, E. F., Hargreave, F. E., and Newhouse, M. T. (1981b). Standardization of inhalation provocation tests: two techniques of aerosol generation and inhalation compared. *Am. Rev. Respir. Dis.* **123**:195-199.

Ryan, G., Latimer, K. M., Dolovich, J., and Hargreave, F. E. (1982). Bronchial responsiveness to histamine: relationship to dirunal variation of peak flow rate, improvement after bronchodilator, and airway calibre. *Thorax* **37**:423-429.

Salome, C. M., Peat, J. K., Britton, W. J., and Woolcock, A. J. (1987). Bronchial hyperresponsiveness in two populations of Australian schoolchildren. I. Relation to respiratory symptoms and diagnosed asthma. *Clin. Allergy* **17**:271-281.

Sears, M. R., Jones, D. T., Holdaway, M. D., Hewitt, C. J., Flannery, E. M., Herbison, G. P., and Silva, P. A. (1986). Prevalence of bronchial reactivity to inhaled methacholine in New Zealand children. *Thorax* **41**:283-289.

Snapper, J. R., Drazen, J. M., Loring, S. H., Schneider, W., and Ingram, R. J., Jr. (1978). Distribution of pulmonary responsiveness to aerosol histamine in dogs. *J. Appl. Physiol.* **44**:738-742.

Sotomayor, H., Badier, M., Vervloet, D., and Orehek, J. (1984). Seasonal increase in carbachol airway responsiveness in patients allergic to grass pollen. *Am. Rev. Respir. Dis.* **130**:56-58.

Sterk, P. J., Daniel, E. E., Zamel, N., and Hargreave, F. E. (1985). Limited bronchoconstriction to methacholine using partial flow-volume curves in nonasthmatic subjects. *Am. Rev. Respir. Dis.* **132**:272-277.

Verma, V. K., Cockcroft, D. W., and Dosman, J. A. (1988). Airway responsiveness to inhaled histamine in chronic obstructive airways disease: chronic bronchitis vs. emphysema. *Chest* **94**:457-461.

Wardlaw, A. J., Dannette, S., Gleich, G. J., Collins, J. V., and Kay, A. B., (1988). Eosinophils and mast cells in bronchoalveolar lavage in subjects with mild asthma: relationship to bronchial hyperreactivity. *Am. Rev. Respir. Dis.* **137**:62-69.

Weiss, J. W., Rossing, T. H., McFadden, E. R., Jr., and Ingram, R. H., Jr. (1983). Relationship between bronchial responsiveness to hyperventilation with cold and methacholine in asthma. *J. Allergy Clin. Immunol.* **72**:140-144.

Witt, C., Stuckey, M. S., Woolcock, A. J., and Dawkins, R. C. (1986). Positive allergy prick skin tests associated with bronchial histamine responsiveness in an unselected population. *J. Allergy Clin. Immunol.* **77**:698-702.

Woolcock, A. J. (1988). Asthma—what are the important experiments? *Am. Rev. Respir. Dis.* **138**:730-744.

Woolcock, A. J., Salome, C. M., and Yan, K. (1984). The shape of the dose-response curve to histamine in asthmatic and normal subjects. *Am. Rev. Respir. Dis.* **130**:71-75.

Woolcock, A. J., Cheung, W., and Salome, C. (1986). Relationship between bronchial responsiveness to propranolol and histamine. *Am. Rev. Respir. Dis.* **133**:A177.

Woolcock, A. J., Peat, J. K., Salome, C. M., Yan, K., Anderson, S. D., Schoeffel, R. E., McGervage, G., and Killalea, T. (1987). Prevalence of bronchial hyperresponsiveness and asthma in a rural adult population. *Thorax* **42**:361-368.

Yan, K., Salome, C., and Woolcock, A. J. (1983). Rapid method for measurement of bronchial responsiveness. *Thorax* **38**:760-765.

3

A Model of the Mechanics of Airway Narrowing in Asthma

BARRY WIGGS, RODRIGO MORENO, ALAN JAMES,
JAMES C. HOGG, and PETER PARÉ

University of British Columbia
St. Paul's Hospital
Vancouver, British Columbia, Canada

The major abnormalities that characterize the pathophysiology of asthma are reversible airway narrowing and an excessive response to nonspecific airway challenges (Paré and Montaner, 1988). An increase in resistance means that the caliber of the airways has been reduced; this can occur in several ways: airway smooth muscle shortening; an encroachment on the lumen by an increase in the volume of tissue in the airway wall; an increase in the luminal contents produced by an inflammatory exudation or secretion; an increased surface tension at the air-liquid interface within airways; and a reduction in the external support of the airway due to changes in the structures surrounding the airways. These separate processes frequently act in combination to produce airway narrowing. In this chapter we will use a recently developed computer model of the airways to evaluate the combined effects of increased wall thickness and smooth muscle shortening. We begin by reviewing the features of normal airway smooth muscle contraction and the factors that thicken the airway wall, because our analysis suggests that these two factors acting in series can explain many of the features of asthma.

I. Airway Smooth Muscle Contraction and Shortening

Excessive airway smooth muscle contraction and shortening are often thought to be the major pathophysiological mechanisms leading to airway obstruction in asthma. The rapid changes in airway obstruction that occur in asthma and the often dramatic and rapid improvement in response to drugs that are thought to act primarily by relaxing contracted smooth muscle explain this theory. These observations have led to the widespread opinion that exaggerated airway smooth muscle shortening and increased "sensitivity" of airway smooth muscle to nonspecific pharmacological and nonpharmacological irritants are of primary importance in asthma.

Extensive in vitro studies of airway smooth muscle mechanics have been provided by Stephens and his associates (1969, 1977, 1980). They have examined the passive and active mechanical properties of airway smooth muscle from the trachea and large bronchi of the dog and have shown that canine airway smooth muscle exhibits characteristic length-tension behavior that is similar to skeletal and cardiac muscle. Although muscle form all three sites shows an optimal length at which maximal active tension can be developed, airway smooth muscle differs from skeletal and cardiac muscle in that maximal isotonic shortening from optimal length can be as much as 70%. Recent studies from our laboratory on the passive and active length-tension relationship of porcine trachealis smooth muscle have shown very similar results (Ishida et al., 1989).

These findings are summarized in Figure 1, which shows a schematic passive and active isometric length-tension relationship similar to that observed in the dog and pig. Passive tension at L max (100% optimal length) is 5% of maximal active tension, and there is a distinct length at which maximal tension can be developed. At starting lengths above and below this length, active tension decreases sharply. Isotonic shortening, indicated by the horizontal arrows (a,b,c,d), show that maximal fractional shortening occurs at L max where the muscle shortens to 30% of its starting length. As the preload on the muscle increases, the starting length increases and maximal active shortening and fractional shortening decrease. The final length-tension points of isotonic contraction lie to the right of the values generated by isometric contraction. As we shall show later, our model of the human airways suggests that 70% shortening of smooth muscle in vivo would result in occlusion of the majority of airways. Since maximal concentrations of powerful pharmacological bronchoconstricting substances do not produce airway occlusion or even major changes in airway resistance in normal subjects (Michoud et al., 1981; Guillemi et al., 1989), we must assume that 70% smooth muscle shortening does not normally occur in vivo.

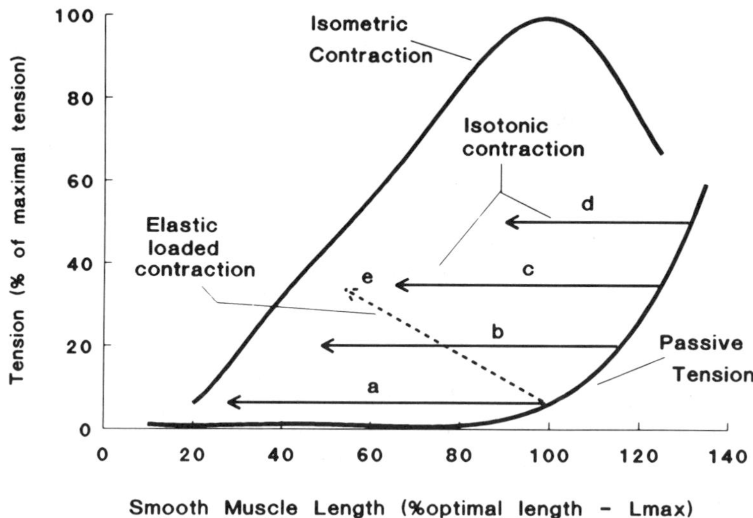

Figure 1 Schematic representation of smooth muscle length-tension relationship. The solid horizontal arrows represent isotonic contraction at varying preloads. Maximal active shortening occurs at Lmax (a) and is $\cong$ 70% in this example. In fact, smooth muscle probably contracts against elastic loads, as shown by the interrupted line (e). Less shortening and more tension will be produced by muscle contraction as the elastic load is increased.

Recent studies from our laboratory (Okazawa et al., 1988) that used sonomicrometry to measure the magnitude of shortening in the trachealis muscle of the dog in situ show that maximal activation of the smooth muscle by electrical stimulation of the vagus nerve produced variable shortening that averaged only 28.8 $\pm$ 14.2% ($\pm$ SD). This is substantially less than would be predicted if the muscle contracted isotonically from L max. In other studies performed in vitro only 30-40% maximal smooth muscle shortening occurred in porcine tracheal rings (James et al., 1987) and rabbit tracheal segments (Moreno et al., 1987) treated with supramaximal concentrations of pharmacological agonists. Similarly calculated shortening of airway smooth muscle in freshly excised human lung slices incubated with 10^{-3}m carbachol was found to range from 11 to 42% (James et al., 1988a) and the smooth muscle shortening calculated to occur in guinea pigs with a maximal increase in RL following inhalation of aerosolized agonists was approximately 40% (Hulbert et al., 1985).

The marked differences in shortening between the isolated muscle and muscle studied in situ could be explained if the airway smooth muscle contraction in vivo was not isotonic. If the only load on the muscle in vivo was the preload necessary to stretch it to optimal length, one would expect it to shorten to the same degree as it does in vitro. The fact that this does not occur suggests that airway smooth muscle in vivo must overcome loads. In the large airways the airway cartilage and other structural components in the airway wall put loads on the muscle (Moreno et al., 1986). In the more peripheral airways, the surrounding lung parenchyma provides an elastic afterload via alveolar attachments to the airway wall. In both large and small airways, an additional load may be related to the forces required to deform the submucosal and mucosal tissue. Macklem (1985) has suggested that the mode of airway smooth muscle contraction in vivo corresponds most closely to the vector e shown in Figure 1, where smooth muscle shortening is accompanied by an increase in load. The resulting shortening from any length is less than would be predicted from the maximal isotonic shortening curve because considerable additional tension must be generated to overcome the load placed on the muscle as it shortens.

Our calculations of airway smooth muscle shortening using morphometric techniques (James et al., 1988a, 1988b) assume that the smooth muscle runs circumferentially around the airways. Although the direction of the fibers in the trachea has been shown to be perpendicular to the long axis of the airway (Miller, 1913), the airway smooth muscle is known to spiral around the smaller intraparenchymal airways (Miller, 1921). If the angle of this spiral is substantial, calculations of muscle shortening based on changes in internal and external perimeters may be in error. This potential error is quantitated in Figure 2, where the internal radius of an airway expressed as a fraction of its starting radius is plotted against the angle of the spiral of the muscle around the long axis of an airway. Isopleths are shown for varying combinations of airway smooth muscle shortening (the fractional shortening of smooth muscle from starting length that occurs with a stimulus: proportion of muscle shortening, PMS) and airway wall thickness (proportion of wall [PW]: the proportion of the airway area internal to the outermost layer of smooth muscle that is occupied by airway wall: absolute airway wall area/ absolute airway wall area + luminal area). This shows that for a given wall thickness an increase in the angle of spiral will *exaggerate* the airway narrowing produced by a given amount of smooth muscle shortening, but the relationship is not significantly altered until the angle of the spiral exceeds 15 degrees. The available data suggest that the actual angle is less than this (Miller, 1921) and we have assumed that the entire effect of muscle shortening is translated into narrowing of the lumen rather than shortening of the airway length. An alternative possibility is that as a contraction shortens the muscle, there will be a change in wall thickness, airway diameter, and length

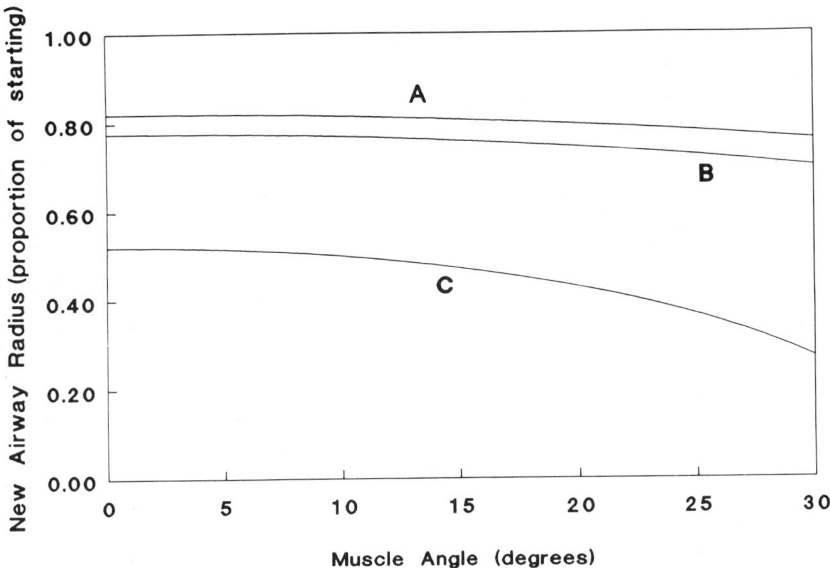

Figure 2 The effect of muscle angle on contracted radius for isopleths of PW and PMS. Curve A, PW = 0.15, PMS = 0.15. Curve B, PW = 0.30, PMS = 0.15. Curve C, PW = 0.30, PMS = 0.30.

proportional to the angle of the muscle spiral around the lumen. Unfortunately, there have been no systematic measurements made of the muscle angle of spiral and the assumptions used in our calculations are based on Miller's classic descriptive studies (Miller, 1913, 1921). These suggest that the muscle is arranged in a geodesic fashion around the lumen of the airway, allowing most of the muscle shortening to be translated into luminal narrowing rather than a reduction in airway length.

Another factor that might decrease the amount of airway smooth muscle shortening in vivo is the muscle's operating length. Maximal fractional shortening occurs at Lmax in vitro (Fig. 1), but there are few data on the operating length of airway smooth muscle in vivo. In the in vivo studies of dog trachealis muscle mentioned previously (Okazawa et al., 1988), maximal shortening occured at or near functional residual capacity (FRC). However, there was considerable variation between animals; some showed maximal active shortening at lung volumes above FRC while others showed maximal shortening at lung volumes below FRC. Shioya and associates (1987) have estimated airway smooth muscle shortening in the trachea and central bronchi, to the fifth generation, using changes in airway diameter assessed with tantalum bronchograms. The stimulus they employed was intravenous methacholine. Their data suggest that optimal shortening occurs in the trachea at FRC, but that the length of airway smooth muscle in the more peripheral bronchi is substantially below optimal length at this lung volume. Maximal airway narrowing was observed in these airways only after inflation to lung volumes above FRC (~ 18 cmH$_2$O PL in generation 5). Hahn et al. (1976) used bronchograms and electrical stimulation of the vagal nerves and calculated that the greatest narrowing occurred at FRC both in large and small airways. Since the data on resting length are inconclusive, the model to be described makes no assumptions about where airway smooth muscle is on its length-tension curve.

The degree to which airway smooth muscle contraction can narrow an airway is dependent on the geometry of that airway in relationship to the anatomical distribution and function of the airways smooth muscle. In an airway such as the trachea, where approximately 33% of airway circumference contains smooth muscle, the effect of maximal shortening is diffferent from that in a peripheral airway, where the muscle completely surrounds the airway lumen. In the trachea and major bronchi, airway smooth muscle is inserted (depending on the species) into either the inside or outside of the connective tissue surrounding the cartilaginous rings and plates. When the muscle contracts, it pulls these structures toward each other and narrows the airway lumen. Data from our laboratory (Table 1) show that the proportion of muscle in the airway circumference is approximately 33% in the trachea and mainstem bronchi, increases to 66% in lobar bronchi, and completely surrounds segmental bronchi and more distal airways. Much remains to be learned about the exact interaction between the smooth muscle and other components of the airway wall as the muscle shortens.

There is relatively little evidence that the smooth muscle of asthmatic airways behaves abnormally. In some studies the in vitro contractility of airway smooth muscle obtained from asthmatic subjects (Dahlen et al., 1983; Schellenberg and Foster, 1984; Roberts et al., 1985; Cerrina et al., 1986; Goldie et al., 1986; de Jongste et al., 1987; Whicker et al., (1988) has been examined directly. These data suggest that the "sensitivity" of asthmatic airway smooth muscle to pharmacological agonists is not different from

Table 1 Proportion of Smooth Muscle in Airway Circumference

	0	1	2	
Generation	Trachea	Main bronchi	Lobar bronchi	3 to 23
PMC	0.33	0.33	0.66	1.0

normal. This indicates that the shift of the in vivo airway dose-response curve to the left in asthmatic subjects cannot be explained by abnormal smooth muscle function. In two studies (Schellenberg and Foster, 1984; de Jongste et al., 1987) the airway smooth muscle preparations of three asthmatic patients developed two to three times the amount of tension generated by similar preparations from large groups of nonasthmatic subjects. Although these data suggest that the airway smooth muscle from asthmatics may be capable of developing more tension when stimulated maximally, the tension generated was not corrected for the cross-sectional area of smooth muscle present in these in vitro preparations. Since the amount of smooth muscle in asthmatic airways is increased, the observed increase in tension could be explained by the increased amount of smooth muscle rather than abnormal muscle function. We are not aware of a study of human asthmatic subjects' airway smooth muscle in which shortening has been measured.

In animal experiments, Antonissen et al. (1980) have shown an increase in maximal isotonic shortening in dogs sensitized and chronically exposed to ovalbumin. However, Downes et al. (1986) and Murphy et al. (1987), using a well-characterized model of airway hyperresponsiveness in the Basenji greyhound, were unable to demonstrate in vitro abnormalities of isometric or isotonic airway smooth muscle contraction. Recently Ishida et al. (1988) have demonstrated increased isotonic and isovolumetric response in tracheal segments from guinea pigs chronically exposed to an aerosol of ovalbumin.

A great many studies have shown an increased amount of airway smooth muscle in human subjects with asthma (Unger, 1945; Bullen, 1952; Houston et al., 1953; Messer et al., 1960; Dunnill, 1960; Richards and Patrick, 1965; Salvato, 1968; Dunnill et al., 1969; Takizawa and Thurlbeck, 1971; Heard and Hossain, 1971; Cudz et al., 1978). This increase in smooth muscle mass appears to be related to an increase in both number (hyperplasia) and size (hypertrophy) of the airway smooth muscle cells (Hossain, 1973). James et al. (1989) have recently examined the airway morphology in the lungs of 18 patients who died of asthma and compared this with the airway morphology in a similarly aged group of individuals who died suddenly of nonpulmonary causes. This study used the internal perimeter of airways (PI = linear distance of a line tracing the luminal border of the airway epithelium) to compare similar-sized airways in nonasthmatic and asthmatic subjects because this measure of airway size remains constant despite variable lung inflation and smooth muscle contraction (James et al., 1988a,b). James et al. (1989) found a marked increase in the thickness of the smooth muscle layer in all but the smallest airways of the asthmatic subjects but no evidence that the muscle needed to shorten excessively in order to close the airways' lumen. Although an increased quantity of smooth muscle will not necessarily increase maximal isotonic shortening, it could result in increased shortening if it were better able to overcome loads placed on the muscle to prevent excessive shortening. The other effect of increased smooth muscle thickness would be to stiffen the airway wall, but the ability of an increased mass of muscle to shorten against the additional loads produced by increased wall thickness has not been adequately investigated.

II. Airway Wall Thickening

A large number of anatomical studies of airways from asthmatic lungs show that an inflammatory process is present in the airway wall (Unger, 1945; Bullen, 1952; Houston et al., 1953; Messer et al., 1960; Dunnill, 1960; Richards and Patrick, 1965; Salvato, 1968; Dunnill et al., 1969; Takizawa and Thurlbeck, 1971; Heard and Hossain et al., 1971; Cudz et al., 1978). This process can thicken the airway wall by several mechanisms, including bronchial vascular engorgement and recruitment, exudation of fluid and cells from the vessels into the interstitial space, deposition of extracellular matrix and collagen, hypertrophy and or hyperplasia of the smooth muscle, and epithelial elements of the glands and the lining layer of the airway wall. This increased wall thickness could narrow airways simply by decreasing the cross-section of the airway lumen but, as we shall see from the results of the model, the greatest effect of the wall thickening may be to exaggerate the changes produced by smooth muscle contraction. In the studies of asthmatic airways from our laboratory in which wall thickness was quantitated and compared to the airways of control subjects with a similar PI, we calculated the proportion of the "relaxed" airway occupied by tissue (PW). As shown in Figure 3, the wall area (WA) is the tissue area between the epithelium and the outermost layer of smooth muscle. The "relaxed" airway area (AEr) is the area of a circle with a circumference equal to the relaxed external perimeter (PEr);

$$AEr = \frac{PEr^2}{4\,\pi} \tag{1}$$

James et al. (1989) found that the airway wall area of the asthmatic subjects was increased up to 2.5 times that of normal airways. They also found that this thickening consisted of an increase in the epithelial lining layer, the airway smooth muscle layer, and the submucosal tissue between the muscle and the epithelium, which included the loose connective tissue and bronchial vessels. In the model to be presented here, the effect of this increase in wall thickness on baseline airway resistance and the interaction between increased wall thickness and smooth muscle contraction will be examined.

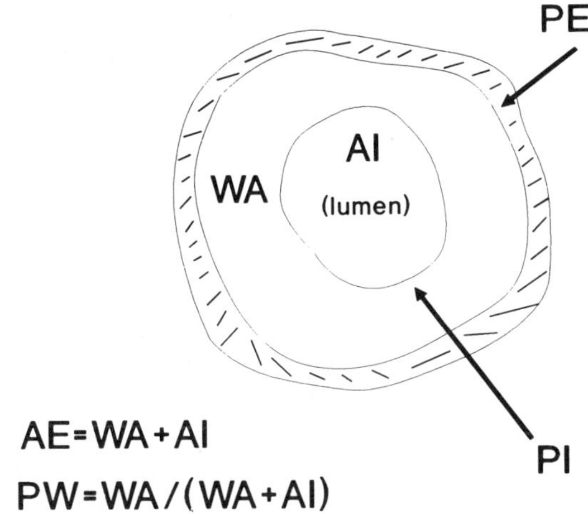

Figure 3 Cross-section of an airway. The hatched area represents the smooth muscle layer. Wall area (WA) includes the area occupied by smooth muscle, submucosa, and epithelium. External perimeter (PE) of the airway corresponds to the outermost layer of smooth muscle and internal perimeter (PI) corresponds to the luminal border of the epithelium. AI, luminal area. Experiments in animal and human lungs have shown the WA and PI remain constant at different degrees of lung inflation and after smooth muscle contraction. PW, the ratio of wall area to the sum of wall area and luminal area, varies with lung inflation and smooth muscle contraction.

The change in airway radius that occurs in a particular airway because of smooth muscle contraction is related to the magnitude of muscle shortening (PMS), where PMS = the change in length of the muscle during contraction divided by the starting muscle length; the proportion of the circumference occupied by muscle (PMC); and the airway wall thickness internal to the smooth muscle layer (PW) where PW = the airway wall area/the total wall and lumen area:

$$PW = \frac{WA}{WA + AI} \tag{2}$$

In a previous communication (Moreno et al., 1986) a simple equation for the calculation of the change in the luminal radius of an airway following smooth muscle contraction was described. If the relaxed internal radius of an airway = 1, the contracted internal radius (RIC) is:

$$RIC = \sqrt{(1\text{-}PMC \times PMS)^2 - PW} \tag{3}$$

If the resistance of the relaxed airway is 1, and we know the contracted radius and can assume the laminar flow, the airway resistance (Raw) in the contracted airway can be calculated as:

$$\text{Raw} = \left[\frac{\sqrt{(1\text{-PMC} \times \text{PMS})^2 - \text{PW})}}{\sqrt{1\text{-PW}}} \right]^{-4} \qquad (4)$$

To examine for an effect on resistance of an increase in airway wall thickness above the normal value, the abnormal value of PW (PW_A) is inserted into the numerator and the normal value (PW_N) is inserted into the denominator.

$$\text{Raw} = \left[\frac{\sqrt{(1\text{-PMC} \times \text{PMS})^2 - \text{PW}_\text{A})}}{\sqrt{1\text{-PW}_\text{N}}} \right]^{-4} \qquad (5)$$

This equation was used (James et al., 1989) to examine for the effects of alterations in PMC, PMS, and PW on the resistance in a single airway, which showed that smooth muscle contraction could couple with the increased wall thickness of asthmatic lungs to produce a very marked increase in airways resistance. We use a much more realistic airway model here to examine the influences of mechanical and geometric factors on airway resistance. This required the construction of a model based on a realistic appraisal of lung structure rather than on a single tube. To accomplish this we developed a model based on the anatomical information provided by Weibel (1963), the fluid dynamic equations described by Pedley et al. (1977), and the airway pressure-area curves of Lambert and colleagues (1982). Using a Lotus 1-2-3 spreadsheet and measurements of PMC and PW made on normal and asthmatic human airways, we have been able to examine the effects of different degrees of smooth muscle shortening on overall and regional pulmonary resistance in both normal and asthmatic lungs.

III. The Model

The data required to calculate these values for human lungs are shown in Table 2, which is an example of the Lotus spreadsheet used in the calculations. This shows the results for a single flow and the effect of a specific contraction. The model includes the effect of lung inflation obtained from Lambert's equation, but these are not shown because they would further complicate the table.

Column 1 shows airway generation number; column 2, the number of airways in that generation; column 3, the average internal diameter of airways in that generation from Weibel's data; column 4, internal perimeter of the airway; column 5, the average internal diameter of airways in that generation corrected for the appropriate transpulmonary pressure (5 cmH_2O in this example); column 6, the average length of airways in that generation; column 7, the total cross-sectional area for gas flow at that generation; column 8, the linear velocity of gas flow through that generation for a given total flow (1.25 L/s in this example); column 9, the proportion of muscle in the circumference of airways of that generation; column 10, the absolute wall area (WA = AE − internal area [AI]) for airways of that generation from our normal data (James et al., 1989); column 11, the absolute wall area for that generation from asthmatic airways (James et al., 1989); column 12, the normal wall proportion (PW_N); column 13, the abnormal wall proportion (PW_A); column 14, the dose-response curve parameter α, which determines the position of the curve relative to the y axis in that generation; column 15, the dose-response curve parameter β, which describes the slope of the dose-response curve at that generation; column 16, the maximal smooth muscle shortening achievable in that generation (PMSmax = 20% in this example); column 17, the proportion of smooth muscle shortening produced by the current dose of "agonist"; column 18, the contracted internal diameter after smooth muscle shortening; column 19, the Reynolds number for gas flow through airways of that generation; column 20, the pressure drop (cmH_2O) down that generation of airways based on an assumption of laminar flow; column 21, the factor zeta, which corrects the values of laminar flow pressure drop (column 16) for the additional pressure losses secondary to nonlaminar flow (Pedley et al., 1977); column 22, the corrected pressure drop for that generation; and column 23, the calculated resistance of all airways in parallel in that generation. Additional inputs include the total flow through the tree (A), the "dose" of agonist (B), and the density and viscosity of the gas (C). As well as the resistance at each generation, the outputs include the total resistance of the tree (D) calculated as the sum of the pressure drops divided by the total flow. The model assumes unidirectional flow on inspiration, which is adequate for modeling these pressure-flow relationships (Isabey and Chang, 1981).

To calculate the new radius of an airway following a specified muscle shortening (PMS) in an airway where the proportion of muscle in the circumference (PMC) is known, PW must be determined. It follows from Equation 2 that as the lung deflates PW will increase because luminal area decreases and WA is a constant. Figure 4 shows the linear relationship between PI and the square root of WA, which allows WA to be assigned to each generation

Table 2 Mechanics of Airway Narrowing in Asthma: A Model

Column 1	2	3	4	5	6	7	8	9
Gener	Number of Airways	Relaxed Diam cm	Inter Perim Pi cm	Volume correct Diam cm	Airway Length cm	Total XSA cm²	Linear Velocity cm/s	PMC fract
0	1	1.800	6.004	1.767	12.00	1.96	639.26	0.33
1	2	1.220	4.069	1.198	4.76	1.79	697.16	0.33
2	4	0.830	2.880	0.783	1.90	1.32	945.14	0.67
3	8	0.560	2.009	0.513	0.76	0.96	1306.74	1.00
4	16	0.450	1.291	0.403	1.27	1.15	1089.14	1.00
5	32	0.350	1.291	0.309	1.07	1.32	948.33	1.00
6	64	0.280	1.041	0.244	0.90	1.61	777.78	1.00
7	128	0.230	0.859	0.198	0.76	2.07	602.93	1.00
8	256	0.186	0.695	0.159	0.64	2.61	478.88	1.00
9	512	0.154	0.576	0.131	0.54	3.45	361.89	1.00
10	1024	0.130	0.488	0.110	0.46	4.72	264.57	1.00
11	2048	0.109	0.409	0.092	0.39	6.39	195.68	1.00
12	4096	0.095	0.357	0.080	0.33	9.38	133.27	1.00
13	8192	0.082	0.309	0.069	0.27	13.27	94.19	1.00
14	16384	0.074	0.279	0.062	0.23	20.82	60.05	1.00
15	32768	0.066	0.250	0.055	0.20	31.74	39.38	1.00
16	65536	0.060	0.226	0.050	0.17	50.73	24.64	1.00
17	131072	0.054	0.204	0.045	0.14	78.54	15.91	1.00
18	262144	0.050	0.189	0.042	0.12	129.68	9.64	1.00
19	524288	0.047	0.177	0.039	0.10	221.56	5.64	1.00
20	1048576	0.045	0.170	0.037	0.08	395.84	3.16	1.00
21	2097152	0.043	0.162	0.036	0.07	702.15	1.78	1.00
22	4194304	0.041	0.155	0.034	0.06	1235.23	1.01	1.00
23	8388608	0.041	0.155	0.034	0.05	2470.46	0.51	1.00

10	11	12	13	14	15	16	17
Normal Obs Wa mm × mm	Asthma Obs Wa mm × mm	PwN fract	PwA fract	Alpha #	Beta #	PMS max fract	PMS obs fract
24.43	57.83	0.09	0.19	−1.90	1.20	0.20	0.13
11.48	27.07	0.09	0.19	−1.90	1.20	0.20	0.13
5.91	13.98	0.11	0.22	−1.90	1.20	0.20	0.13
3.00	7.00	0.13	0.25	−1.90	1.20	0.20	0.13
2.09	4.86	0.14	0.28	−1.90	1.20	0.20	0.13
1.33	3.08	0.15	0.29	−1.90	1.20	0.20	0.13
0.91	2.08	0.16	0.31	−1.90	1.20	0.20	0.13
0.65	1.48	0.17	0.32	−1.90	1.20	0.20	0.13
0.46	1.03	0.19	0.34	−1.90	1.20	0.20	0.13
0.34	0.75	0.20	0.36	−1.90	1.20	0.20	0.13
0.26	0.57	0.21	0.38	−1.90	1.20	0.20	0.13
0.20	0.43	0.23	0.40	−1.90	1.20	0.20	0.13
0.16	0.35	0.25	0.41	−1.90	1.20	0.20	0.13
0.13	0.29	0.27	0.44	−1.90	1.20	0.20	0.13
0.12	0.25	0.28	0.45	−1.90	1.20	0.20	0.13
0.10	0.21	0.30	0.47	−1.90	1.20	0.20	0.13
0.09	0.19	0.31	0.49	−1.90	1.20	0.20	0.13
0.08	0.16	0.33	0.51	−1.90	1.20	0.20	0.13
0.07	0.15	0.35	0.52	−1.90	1.20	0.20	0.13
0.07	0.14	0.36	0.53	−1.90	1.20	0.20	0.13
0.06	0.13	0.37	0.54	−1.90	1.20	0.20	0.13
0.06	0.12	0.38	0.55	−1.90	1.20	0.20	0.13
0.06	0.12	0.39	0.56	−1.90	1.20	0.20	0.13
0.06	0.12	0.39	0.56	−1.90	1.20	0.20	0.13

Table 2 continues

Table 2 (continued)

18	19	20	21	22	23
Contracted Internal diam cm	Reynolds number #	Pressure Drop Laminar cm H_2O	Zeta #	Pressure Drop Zeta cm H_2O	Resis of gener cm H_2O/l/s
1.578	6030.681	0.01902	9.29	0.17670	1.41E-01
1.068	4453.256	0.01794	10.43	0.18719	1.50E-01
0.649	3666.439	0.02633	11.68	0.30739	2.46E-01
0.390	3048.431	0.04026	13.06	0.52557	4.20E-01
0.302	1967.925	0.09347	7.14	0.66746	5.34E-01
0.229	1298.469	0.11940	5.50	0.65688	5.26E-01
0.179	831.508	0.13512	4.24	0.57310	4.58E-01
0.144	517.672	0.13713	3.26	0.44755	3.58E-01
0.114	326.228	0.14569	2.51	0.36641	2.93E-01
0.093	200.529	0.14040	1.94	0.27182	2.17E-01
0.077	121.241	0.12785	1.48	0.18963	1.52E-01
0.063	73.729	0.11859	1.14	0.13508	1.08E-01
0.054	43.024	0.09309	1.00	0.09309	7.45E-02
0.045	25.577	0.07610	1.00	0.07610	6.09E-02
0.040	14.440	0.05270	1.00	0.05270	4.22E-02
0.035	8.269	0.03941	1.00	0.03941	3.15E-02
0.031	4.625	0.02546	1.00	0.02546	2.04E-02
0.028	2.628	0.01815	1.00	0.01815	1.45E-02
0.025	1.446	0.01105	1.00	0.01105	8.84E-03
0.023	0.782	0.00641	1.00	0.00641	5.13E-03
0.022	0.414	0.00337	1.00	0.00337	2.69E-03
0.021	0.220	0.00180	1.00	0.00180	1.44E-03
0.019	0.117	0.00098	1.00	0.00098	7.86E-04
0.019	0.059	0.00042	1.00	0.00042	3.33E-04

A....................Total flow = 1250 ml/s
B..............................Dose = 64
C.....Density of inspired gas = 0.00113 g/cm^3
     Viscosity of inspired gas = 0.00019 g/cm^2
D........Total pressure drop = 4.83 cm/H2O
     Total resistance = 3.87 cm/H2O/l/s

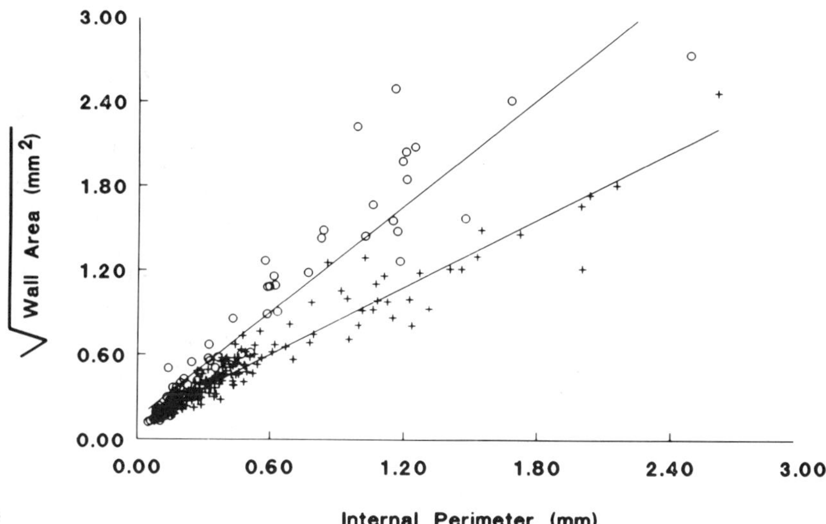

Figure 4 The relationship of airway internal perimeter and wall area. Crosses and open circles show data points for the PI and $\sqrt{(WA)}$ for individual airways from the 22 normal (*circles*) and 18 asthmatic subjects (*crosses*) studied by James et al. (1989). Plotting $\sqrt{(WA)}$ against PI produces a linear relationship.

once PI is known for both normal and asthmatic lungs. The human lung on which Weibel's measurements were made was inflated to approximately 75% of total lung capacity (TLC), which was assumed to correspond to a transpulmonary pressure of approximately 8 cmH$_2$O. Weibel gives average diameters of tracheobronchial branches that need to be corrected to TLC to ensure that the internal perimeter of the airway will be a perfect circle. This can be done using the set of equations developed by Lambert and colleagues (1982), which make it possible to calculate the relative cross-sectional area of an airway at any transpulmonary pressure, regardless of the level of inflation used for morphometric measurement. Lambert used functions of the form:

$$A = 1.0 - (1.0 - A')(1 - P/P_o)^{-N'} \tag{6}$$

where A' and N' are constants individually determined for each generation, P_o is the pressure at which morphometric measurements were recorded, and P is the pressure at which the geometry is desired. A is the correction factor by which the available data are adjusted in order to have airway measurements at the required transpulmonary pressure. The graphic solution to Lambert's equations, showing the change in airway diameter for several generations as a function of transpulmonary pressure, is shown in Figure 5.

Using Equation 6, we can then "inflate" the lung and correct the Weibel measurements obtained at 8 cmH$_2$O to 30 cmH$_2$O (TLC), where the airways were assumed to be circular in cross-section. This allows the correct PI to be assigned for each generation since it remains constant at all degrees of lung inflation (James et al., 1988b). The data in Figure 4 were than used to assign a wall area using the equation WA = $(0.121 + 0.80 \times P1)^2$ for normal and WA = $(0.147 + 1.26 \times PI)^2$ for asthmatics lungs. Then, using Lambert's equations, the appropriate lumenal area (AI) at any lung inflation can be obtained and since WA remains constant (James et al., 1988b), PW can be calculated for each generation using Equation 2.

IV. Fluid Dynamics

The pressure drop across any airway in which there is laminar flow can be calculated using the Poiseuille equation (Landau and Lifshitz, 1987).

$$P = \frac{8 * length * viscosity * flow}{\pi * radius^4}$$

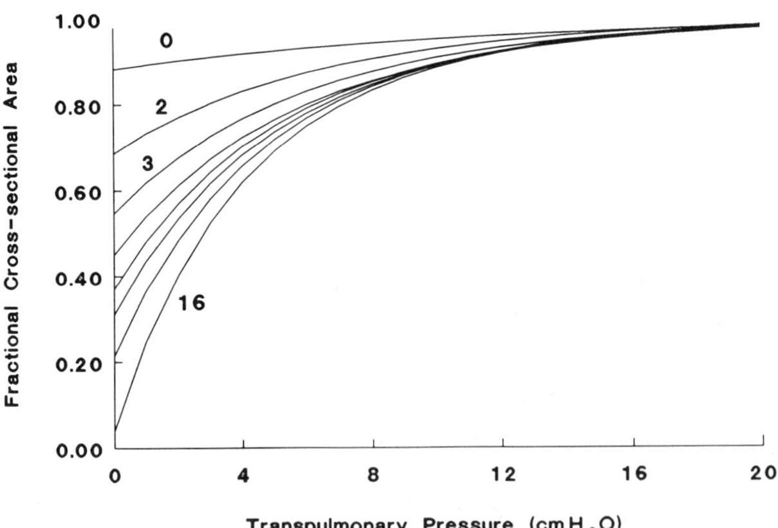

Figure 5   The effect of transpulmonary pressure on the cross-sectional area of the airways based on Equation 6 (Lambert, 1982). The lines correspond to separate generations of the tracheobronchial tree where the trachea is generation 0.

Pedley and associates (1977) derived a factor Z, which we have termed zeta, that can be used to determine the extra pressure drop related to nonlaminar flow in a bifurcating system such as the lung. Zeta is a nondimensional parameter derived empirically, which is dependent upon Reynold's number, airway length, and diameter. Column 19 (Table 2) shows the values for Reynold's number, which was calculated from the linear velocity, airway caliber, density, and viscosity of air. The values of zeta are shown in column 21. The pressure drop calculated using Poisseuille's equation is multiplied by zeta to obtain an estimate for the pressure drop in a nonlaminar bifurcating system. It can be seen (Table 2) that this correction is greatest for generations 0-10. The resistance of each generation is the corrected pressure drop divided by the flow and the total tracheobronchial resistance is obtained as the total pressure drop in the system divided by the flow.

V. Comparison of Results Obtained by the Model and Measurements Made in Human Subjects

The solid triangles in Figure 6 show the values for inspiratory pulmonary resistance for a flow of 1 L/s at different lung volumes in a 27-year-old non-smoking man seated in a volume-sensitive body plethysmograph. The solid line shows results calculated from the model at a flow of 1 L/s over the same range of transpulmonary pressures using Weibel's data for length and diameter corrected at each transpulmonary pressure using Lambert's pressure-area relationships. This shows that the data obtained from the model have the same curvilinear relationship between resistance and transpulmonary pressure as observed in this subject.

Figure 7 shows the inspiratory pressure-flow characteristics from a 64-year-old male smoker in whom flow varied between 0 and 1 L/s. The solid lines show that the results calculated from the model are close to the observed values during quiet breathing on inspiration.

Because the model uses a single geometry based on Weibel's average data, it should not be expected to fit all subjects. To date the pressure-flow characteristics from 40 normal subjects on air and helium have been examined and Figures 6 and 7 have been selected from these results because they appear to fit Weibel's geometry very well. By altering values for airway geometry in the model, it should be possible to obtain an extremely good fit for every subject.

VI. Calculation of the Dose-Response Characteristics of the Airway

The model also allows the calculation of a dose-response to a progressively increasing concentration of a bronchoconstricting agent. This was done using a function of the form:

$$\frac{10^{\alpha + \beta * \log\ \mathrm{dose}}}{1 + 10^{\alpha + \beta * \log\ \mathrm{dose}}} \tag{7}$$

which was described by Woolcock and associates (1984) and which we chose because it rises from 0 to a maximum of 1 following the S shape of a dose-response curve. The difficulty with Equation 7 is that a true zero response occurs at the log of 0, which is negative infinity, and makes the equation awkward to use. By modifying equation 7 to the form shown in Equation 8, this problem is avoided:

$$\frac{\dfrac{10^{\alpha + \beta * \log\ \mathrm{dose}}}{1 + 10^{\alpha + \beta * \log\ \mathrm{dose}}} - \dfrac{10^{\alpha}}{1 + 10^{\alpha}}}{1 - \dfrac{10^{\alpha}}{1 + 10^{\alpha}}} \tag{8}$$

Although Equation 8 appears more complicated than Equation 7, it has the same S shape between 0 and 1 and has the advantage that the response is zero at a log dose 0 rather than negative infinity.

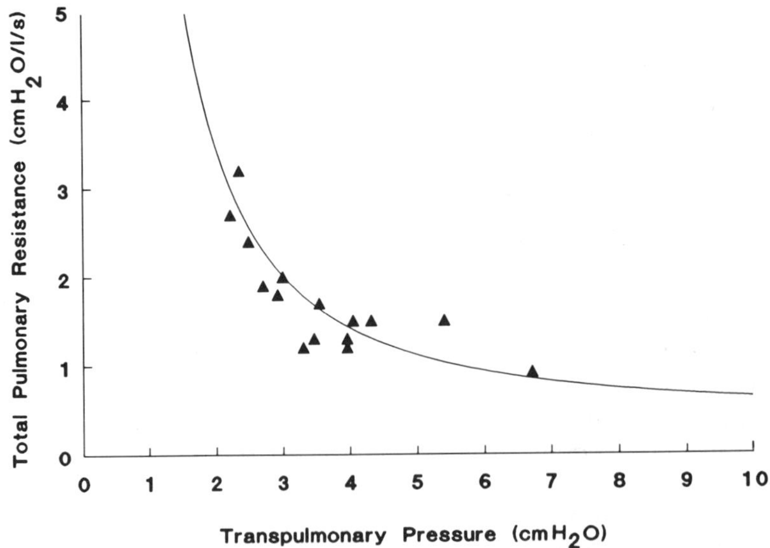

Figure 6 Pulmonary resistance versus transpulmonary pressure. The solid triangles represent individual measurements of resistance obtained at a variety of lung volumes from a 27-year-old nonsmoking man. The line is the predicted relationship from the model.

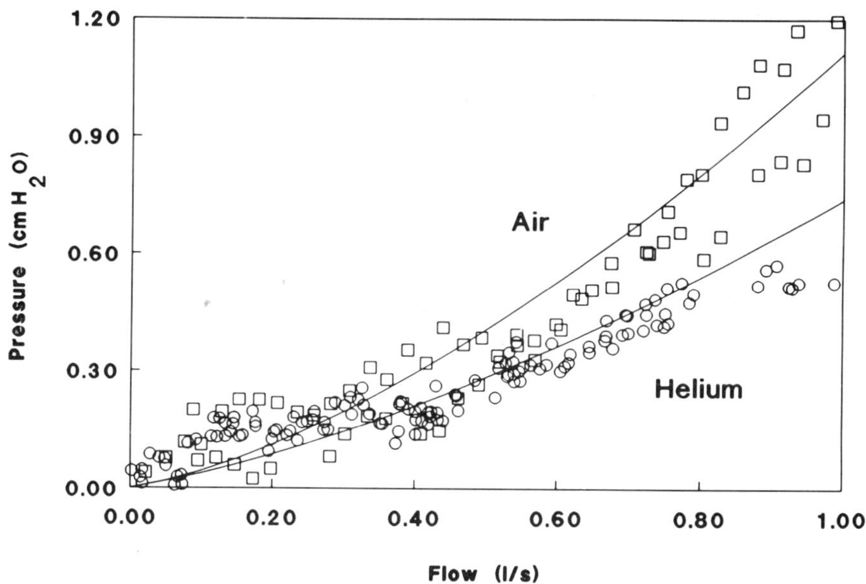

Figure 7 Actual and calculated pressure-flow curves. The open squares (air) and circles (helium-oxygen) represent averaged inspiratory pressure flow data in a 64-year-old male smoker. The lines represent pressure-flow relationships generated using the model. The fact that the model accurately predicts the curvilinearity and density dependence of actual pressure flow curves suggests that the fluid dynamic assumptions are reasonable.

Figures 8a and b show the effect of the parameters α and β on the shape of the dose response generated by Equation 8. In Figure 8a the value of β is held constant at 1.2 while α is varied from -3.0 to -1.9 to -1.0, which result in parallel shifts in the dose-response curve, with more negative values shifting the curve to the right. Figure 8b has α constant at -1.9 and β is given the values 2.0, 1.2, and 0.6. This shows that β alters the rate of response where smaller values produce a slower rise in the dose-response. The values of $\alpha = 1.9$ and B $= 1.2$ give a 50% response when the dosage has been increased by 1.5 log or 30 times.

In the example shown in Table 2, the maximal amount of smooth muscle shortening (PMSmax) allowed was set at 20% (column 16). The observed PMS (PMSobs, column 17) was obtained by multiplying PMSmax by the result of Equation 8 and is constant in Table 2 because these results are from a single dose where α, β, and PMSmax have been set the same for all generations. Equation 3 was used to calculate the contracted internal diameter (column 18, Table 2), which depends on the amount of smooth muscle shortening

Wiggs et al.

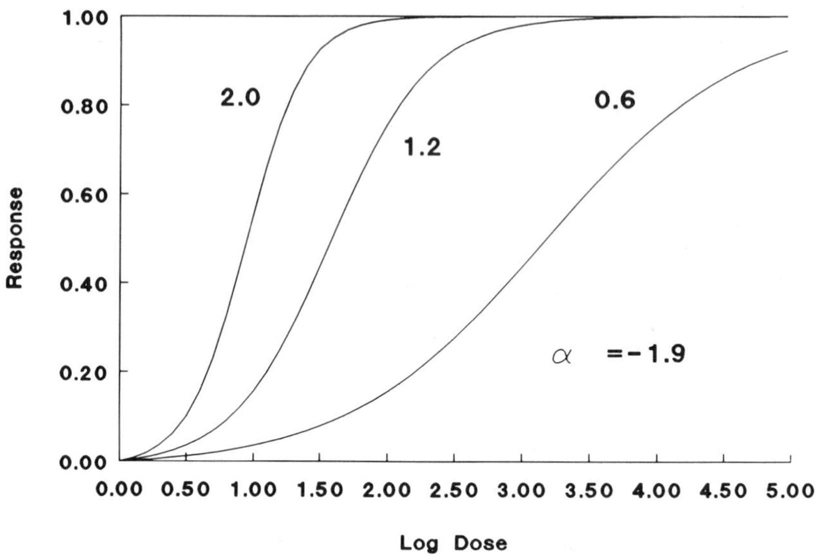

(a)

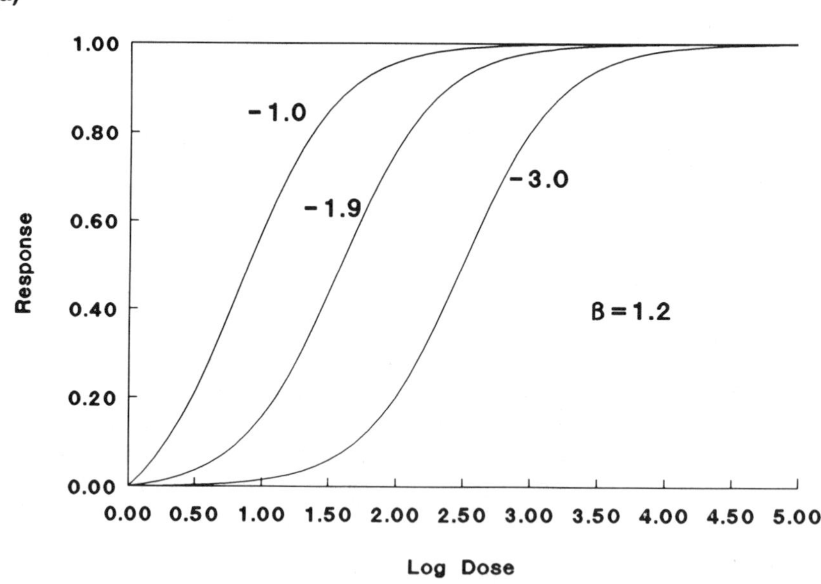

(b)

Figure 8 (a) Effect of parameter α in dose-response Equation 8. The parameter β is set to 1.2 for each curve and α is given the indicated values. More negative values of α shift the curves to the right. (b) Effect of parameter β in dose-response Equation 8. The parameter α is set to -1.9 for each curve and β is given the indicated values. Larger values of β give a faster response.

(PMS), the amount of muscle in the circumference (PMC), and PW. PW was obtained using Equation 2, after the wall area and lumen area were calculated for each generation.

Since we have assumed a constant flow and know that the cross-sectional area decreases as the muscle shortens, the pressure drop associated with laminar flow will increase. The linear velocity of the gas will also increase as cross-sectional area decreases and this will increase Reynold's number and therefore the zeta-corrected pressure drop. The combined effect of all of these factors provides the overall increase in airways resistance that can be easily tracked using the Lotus 1-2-3 program.

Figure 9 shows the measured response of total pulmonary resistance for two subjects during a methacholine challenge in which sequential doubling dosages from 0.032 to 256 mg/ml were administered to the airways as an aerosol. The solid circles are the measured values obtained from a 31-year-old nonsmoking male and line B shows the computer-predicted values obtained from the model by iteratively fitting the parameters α, β, and PMS max at an inspiratory flow of 1 L/s until a good visual fit was obtained. The final values obtained for equation 8 were $\alpha = -1$, $\beta = 2.0$, and PMSmax = 0.2. The solid squares are the measured response obtained from a 24-year-old ex-

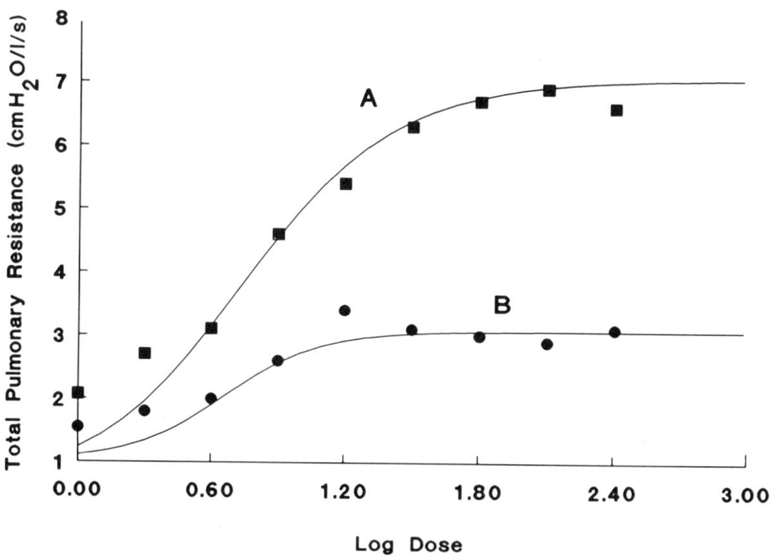

Figure 9 Methacholine dose-response curves are shown for two subjects: a 31-year-old nonsmoking man (solid circles) and a 24-year-old exsmoking woman (squares). Curves A and B are the model results after the dose-response parameters α, β, and PMSmax are iteratively fitted to produce the best visual fit to the data.

smoking woman, which are compared to the computer-derived values in line A obtained with Equation 8 using $\alpha = 0.2$, $\beta = 1.2$, and PMSmax $= 0.3$. The fitted curves correspond to the measured values extremely well, except for slightly underestimating the intial resistance. This underestimation is a function of the geometry and could be corrected by altering the diameters and lengths of the airways in the model.

Dose-response curves were generated for normal and asthmatic airways using the morphometric data for airway dimensions from James et al. (1989). Figure 10 shows the dose-response curve obtained using the normal values for wall area showing the effect of increasing the maximal smooth muscle shortening from 20% in A to 25% in B and 35% in C. Figure 11 shows the results obtained by the same procedure when the values for wall area of asthmatic lungs were used. The dose-response for the normal lung with 20% maximal muscle shortening is included for reference (curve A). Curve B shows the effect of 20% shortening in the asthmatic lung and C the effect of marginally increase muscle shortening to 25%. These curves are similar to the dose-response curves for normal subjects and subjects with (mild and moderate) asthma (Michoud et al., 1981; Woolcock et al., 1984; Guillemi et al., 1989).

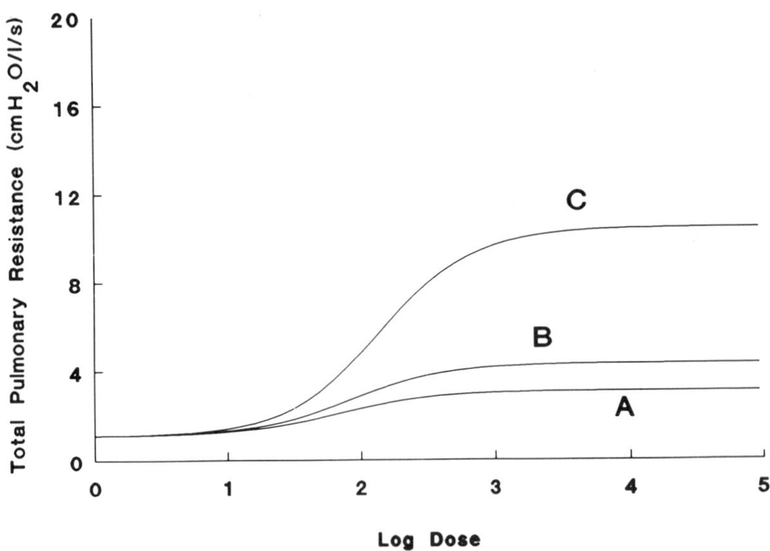

Figure 10   Effect of graded values of PMSmax on the dose-response curve in normal lungs. Each curve uses WA values measured from nonasthmatic lungs (James et al., 1989) for all generations. The three curves, A, B, and C correspond to 20%, 25%, and 35% maximal smooth muscle shortening, respectively.

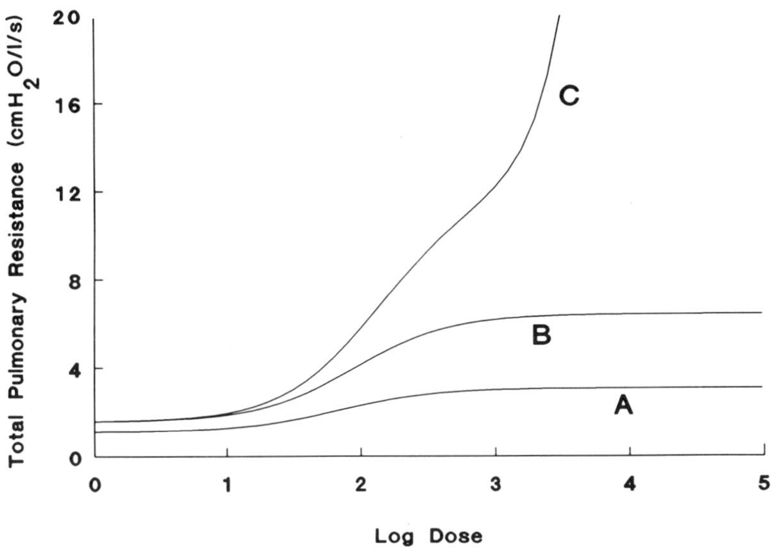

Figure 11   Effect of graded values PMSmax on the dose-response curve in lungs with thickened walls. The curves B and C use WA values obtained from asthmatic lungs (James et al., 1989) for all generations. PMSmax is 20% for curve B and 25% for curve C. For reference, curve A from Figure 10 is also shown.

These data suggest that in the presence of thickened airway walls a conversion from mild to severe airway "hyperresponsiveness" can occur with modest increases in muscle shortening that are well within the "normal" range.

The model also makes it possible to examine the effect of restricting the asthmatic changes in the airway wall to certain regions of the tracheobronchial tree. When the data for increased wall thickness from the asthmatic airways are used for only the central airways (generation 0-15) and normal values for wall thickness are entered for the peripheral airways, the results are as shown in Figure 12: 20% and 25% muscle shortening resulted in a dose-response curve with a moderate increase in resistance and a definite plateau. However, when the data from asthmatic subjects are applied only in the peripheral airways (generations 16-23), a very different response is obtained (Fig. 13). When maximal muscle shortening is 20%, there is only a small increase in total resistance beyond normal data. However, 25% muscle shortening results in a rapid increase in resistance that does not show a plateau and R_L increases well beyond the physiological range.

These calculations suggest that the increase in airways responsiveness of mild asthma could be produced by changes in the central airways, where

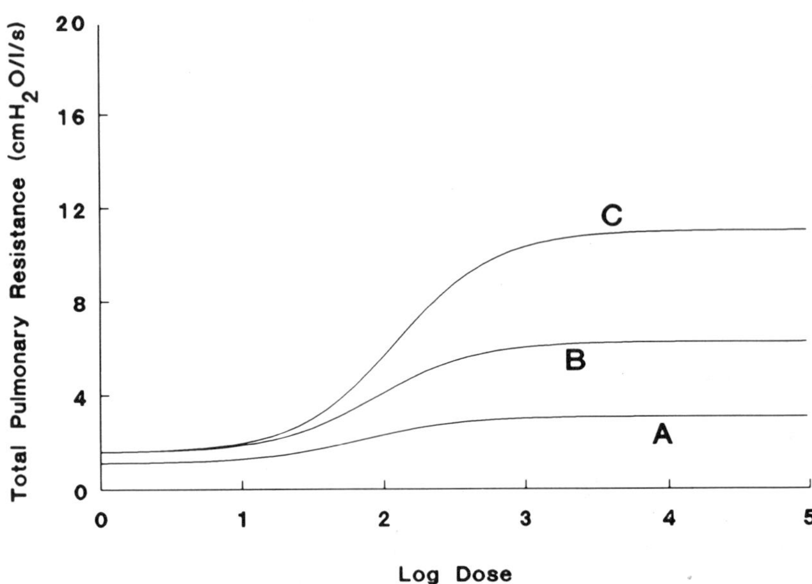

Figure 12 Effect of increased central airway wall area. Curves B and C have normal WA values for generations 16-23 and asthmatic values for generations 0-15. PMSmax is 20% in curve B and 25% in curve C. Curve A from Figure 10 is shown for reference.

smooth muscle shortening combined with thickened airway walls produces moderate increases in R_L. However, in patients with moderate or severe asthma, the wall thickening might extend to the peripheral airways, which can produce much more marked increases in airways responsiveness with only moderate increases in smooth muscle shortening. These data suggest that although the reversal of muscle shortening is important for the immediate relief of airway obstruction, long-term therapy should be designed to reduce the wall thickness produced by the chronic inflammatory response.

Discussion

Kaliner: What accounts for the cell wall thickness in asthmatic airways?

Paré: In our studies, the increased airway wall thickness was due to proportionate increases in smooth muscle area, submucosal area, and airway epithelial area.

Sybrecht: What are the effects of variations in lung volume, laminar flow, and collateral ventilation?

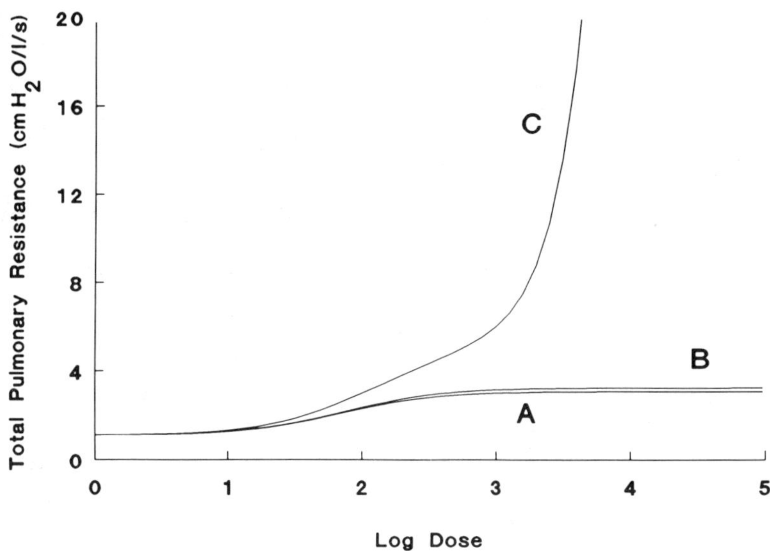

Figure 13 Effect of increased peripheral airway wall area. Curves B and C have asthmatic WA values for generations 16-23 and normal values for generations 0-15. PMSmax is 20% in curve B and 25% for curve C. Curve A from Figure 10 is shown for reference.

Paré: The calculations all employed a simulated transpulmonary pressure of 5 cmH$_2$O. Airway narrowing would surely lead to hyperinflation and the resultant increase in lung volume would attenuate the effects of smooth muscle shortening. We can examine these effects on the calculations, but have not done so as yet. We did not assume laminar flow, but have instead employed the zeta factor described by Pedley to account for nonlaminar flow. Collateral resistance probably plays a minor role in total pulmonary resistance in asthma.

Leff: My concern about the model is that it only allows you to examine one variable at a time, while asthma involves dynamic changes involving many features.

Drazen: Your model shows that increasing wall thickness will not shift the dose-response curve to the left but will increase the plateau value reached.

Paré: You are correct. We think that an increase in the maximum airway narrowing may be a more important feature of airway hyperresponsiveness than an increase in "sensitivity."

Persson: Your model must underestimate if it cannot account for hyperemia or the presence of sticky secretions.

Paré: Yes, I agree. Secretions would have the same effect as airway wall thickness in exaggerating the actions of airway muscle contraction.

Kerribijn: What are the effects of elastic forces?

Paré: Less elastic recoil would increase the actions of muscle contraction and there is evidence of reduced elastic recoil in asthma.

References

Antonissen, L. A., Mitchell, R. W., Kroeger, E. A., Kepron, W., Stephens, N. L., and Bergen, J. (1980). Histamine pharmacology in airway smooth muscle from a canine model of asthma. *J. Pharmacol. Exp. Ther.* **213**: 150-155.

Bullen, S. S. (1952). Correlation of clinical and autopsy findings in 176 cases of asthma. *J. Allergy* **23**:193-203.

Cerrina, J., Le Roy, Ladurie, M., Labat, C., Raffestin, B., Bayol, A., and Brink, C. (1986). Comparison of human bronchial muscle responses to histamine *in vivo* with histamine and isoproterenol agonists in vitro. *Am. Rev. Respir. Dis.* **134**:57-61.

Cudz, E., Levison, H., and Cooper, D. M. (1978). Ultrastructure of airways in children with asthma. *Histopathology* **2**:407-421.

Dahlen, S.-E., Hansson, G., Hedqvist, P., Bjorck, T., Granstrom, E., and Dahlen, B. (1983). Allergen challenge of lung tissue from asthmatics elicits bronchial contraction that correlates with the release of leukotrienes C4, D4, and E4. *Proc. Natl. Acad. Sci.* **80**:1712-1716.

de Jongste, J. C., Mons, H., Bonta, I. L., and Kerrebijn, K. F. (1987). Human asthmatic airway responses *in vitro*—a case report. *Eur. J. Respir. Dis.* **70**:23-29.

Downes, H., Austin, D. R., Parks, C. M., and Hirshman, C. A. (1986). Comparison of drug responses *in vivo* and *in vitro* in airways of dogs with and without airway hyperresponsiveness. *J. Pharmacol. Exp. Ther.* **237**: 214-219.

Dunnill, M. S. (1960). The pathology of asthma with special reference to changes in the bronchial mucosa. *J. Clin. Pathol.* **13**:27-33.

Dunnill, M. S., Massarella, G. R., and Anderson, J. A. (1969). A comparison of the quantitative anatomy of the bronchi in normal subjects, in status asthmaticus, in chronic bronchitis and in emphysema. *Thorax* **24**:176-179.

Goldie, R. G., Spina, S., Henry, P. J., Lulich, K. M., and Paterson, J. W. (1986). *In vitro* responsiveness of human asthmatic bronchus to carbachol, histamine, β-adrenoceptor agonists and theophylline. *Br. J. Clin. Pharmacol.* **22**:669-676.

Guillemi, S., James, A. L., and Paré, P. D. (1989). Effect of breathing pattern during inhalation challenge on the shape and position of the dose-response curve. *Lung* **167**:95-106.

Hahn, N. L., Graf, P. D., and Nadel, J. A. (1976). Effect of vagal tone on airway diameters and lung volume in anesthetized dogs. *J. Appl. Physiol.* **41**:581-589.

Heard, B. E., and Hossain, S. (1971). Hyperplasia of bronchial muscle in asthma. *J. Pathol.* **110**:319-31.

Hossain, S. (1973). Quantitative measurement of bronchial muscle in men with asthma. *Am. Rev. Respir. Dis.* **107**:99-109.

Houston, J. C., De Navasquez, S., and Trounce, J. R. (1953). A clinical and pathological study of fatal cases of status asthmaticus. *Thorax* **8**:207-213.

Hulbert, B., McLean, T., Wiggs, B., Paré, P., and Hogg, J. (1985). Histamine dose response curve in guinea pigs. *J. Appl. Physiol.* **58**:625-634.

Isabey, D., and Chang, H. K. (1981). Steady and unsteady pressure-flow relationships in central airways. *J. Appl. Physiol.* **51**:1338-1348.

Ishida, K., Paré, P. D., and Schellenberg, R. R. (1988). Hyperresponsiveness of isolated trachea from guinea pigs with airway hyperresponsiveness *in vivo. FASEB* **2**:A1697.

Ishida, K., Schellenberg, R. R., Blogg, T., and Paré, P. D. Effects of elastic loading upon porcine trachealis muscle mechanics. *J. Appl. Physiol.* (Accepted, 1990).

James, A., Paré, P. D., Moreno, R. H., and Hogg, J. C. (1987). Quantitative measurements of smooth muscle shortening in isolated pig trachea. *J. Appl. Physiol.* **63**:1360-1365.

James, A. L., Hogg, J. C., Dunn, L. A., and Paré, P. D. (1988a). The use of the internal perimeter to compare airway size and to calculate smooth muscle shortening. *Am. Rev. Respir. Dis.* **138**:136-139.

James, A. L., Paré, P. D., and Hogg, J. C. (1988b). Effects of lung volume, bronchoconstriction, and cigarette smoking on morphometric airway dimensions. *J. Appl. Physiol.* **64**:913-919.

James, A. L., Paré, P. D., and Hogg, J. C. (1989). Mechanisms of airway narrowing in asthma. *Amer. Rev. Respir. Dis.* **139**:242-246.

Lambert, R. K., Wilson, T. A., Hyatt, R. E., and Rodarte, J. R. (1982). A computational model for expiratory flow. *J. Appl. Physiol.* **52**:44-56.

Landau, L. D., and Lifshitz, E. M. (1987). Viscoud fluids. In *Fluid Mechanics,* 2nd. ed. New York, Pergamon Press, pp. 44-94.

Macklem, P. T. (1985). Bronchial hyperresponsiveness. *Chest* **87**:158S-159S.

Messer, J., Peters, G. A., and Bennet, W. A. (1960). Cause of death and pathological findings in 304 cases of bronchial asthma. *Dis. Chest* **38**:616-624.

Michoud, M. C., Lelorien, J., and Amyot, R. (1981). Factors modulating the interindividual variability of airway responsiveness to histamine. The influence of H1 and H2 receptors. *Bull. Eur. Physiopathol. Respir.* **17**:807-821.

Miller, W. S. (1913). The trachealis muscle. Its arrangement at the carina tracheae and its probable influence on the lodgement of foreign bodies in the right bronchus and lung. *Anat. Rec.* **7**:375-385.

Miller, W. S. (1921). The musculature of the finer divisions of the bronchial tree and its relation to certain pathological conditions. *Am. Rev. Tuberc.* **V**:689-704.

Moreno, R. H., Hogg, J. C., and Paré, P. D. (1986). Mechanics of airway narrowing. *Am. Rev. Respir. Dis.* **133**:1171-1180.

Moreno, R. D., McLean, T., Hogg, J. C., and Pare, P. D. (1987). Isovolume and isobaric rabbit tracheal contraction *in vitro. J. Appl. Physiol.* **62**: 82-90.

Murphy, T. M., Munoz, N. M., Hirshman, C. A., Blake, J. S., and Leff, A. R. (1987). Mechanisms of airway hypercontractility in Basenji-greyhound dogs. *J. Appl. Physiol.* **63**:2008-2014.

Okazawa, M., Paré, P. D., and Road, J. (1988). Tracheal smooth muscle mechanics—*in vivo. FASEB* **2**:A1700.

Pare, P. D., and Montaner, J. S. G. (1988). Asthma. In *Textbood of Internal Medicine*. Edited by W. N. Kelly. Philadelphia, J. B. Lippincott, pp. 1873-1881.

Pedley, T. J., Schroter, R. C., and Sudlow, M. F. (1977). Gas flow and mixing in the airways. In *Bioengineering Aspects of the Lung*. Edited by J. B. West. New York, Marcel Dekker, pp. 163-266.

Richards, W., and Patrick, J. R. (1965). Death from asthma in children. *Am. J. Dis. Child* **110**:4-21.

Roberts, J. A., Rodger, I. W., and Thomson, N. C. (1985). Airway responsiveness to histamine in man: effect of atropine on *in vivo* and *in vitro* comparison. *Thorax* **40**:261-267.

Salvato, G. (1968). Some histological changes in chronic bronchitis and asthma. *Thorax* **23**:168-172.

Schellenberg, R. R., and Foster, A. (1984). In vitro responses of human asthmatic airway and pulmonary vascular smooth muscle. *Int. Arch. Allergy Appl. Immunol.* **75**:237-241.

Shioya, T., Munoz, N. M., and Leff, A. R. (1987). Effect of resting smooth muscle length on contractile response in resistance airways. *J. Appl. Physiol.* **62**:711-717.

Stephens, N. L., Kroeger, E., and Metha, J. A. (1969). Force-velocity characteristics of respiratory airway smooth muscle. *J. Appl. Physiol.* **26**: 685-92.

Stephens, N. L., and Van Niekerk, W. (1977). Isometric and isotonic contractions in airway smooth muscle. *Can. J. Physiol. Pharmacol.* **55**: 833-838.

Stephens, N. L., and Kroeger, E. A. (1980). Ultrastructure, biophysics, and biochemistry of airway smooth muscle. In *Physiology and Pharmacology of the airways.* Edited by J. A. Nadel. New York, Marcel Dekker, pp. 31-121.

Takizawa, T., and Thurlbeck, W. M. (1971). Muscle and mucous gland size in the major bronchi of patients with chronic bronchitis, asthma, and asthmatic bronchitis. *Am. Rev. Respir. Dis.* **104**:331-336.

Unger, L. (1945). Pathology of bronchial asthma. *South Med. J.* **38**:513-522.

Weibel, E. R. (1963). *Morphometry of the Human Lung.* New York, Academic Press, p. 139.

Whicker, S. D., Armour, C. L., and Black, J. L. (1988). Responsiveness of bronchial smooth muscle from asthmatic patients to relaxant and contractile agonists. *Pulmon. Pharmacol.* **1**:25-31.

Woolcock, A. J., Salome, C. M., and Yan, K. (1984). The shape of the dose-response curve to histamine in asthmatic and normal subjects. *Am. Rev. Respir. Dis.* **130**:71-75.

4

Pathology of Human Asthma

LAURI A. LAITINEN

University of Lund and AB Draco
Lund, Sweden

ANNIKA LAITINEN

University of Helsinki
Helsinki, Finland
and University of Lund
Lund, Sweden

I. Introduction: Studying the Pathology of Human Asthma

The hallmark of asthma is the functional change associated with airways obstruction. At least in the early stages, the bronchial obstruction is a function of smooth muscle tone, and it has been suggested that there even may not be early morphological changes. There have been many indirect approaches to the examination of airway structure, especially its connections with airway inflammation and airway hyperresponsiveness (Lee et al., 1977; Hinson et al., 1984; Hulbert et al., 1985) but few studies have been conducted in living patients. One difficulty lies in obtaining representative specimens of the human airways. There have been some attempts to overcome this problem.

Several investigators (Cohen and Prentice, 1959; Naylor, 1962; Sanerkin and Evans, 1965; Frigas et al., 1981) have been studying the sputum of asthmatic patients. The presence of respiratory epithelial cells in sputum was one of the first pathological abnormalities noticed in asthma and was described by Curschmann in 1885. Naylor (1962) paid attention to the tendency of the bronchial epithelium to exfoliate during acute asthmatic attacks by studying the sputum of asthmatics. He introduced the term "Creola body" to describe large sheets of exfoliated epithelium that condense to form spherical or elongated masses in the overlying mucous layer. Sputum from asthmatic patients frequently contains eosinophils and occasional Charcot-Leyden crystals derived from eosinophils (Dor et al., 1984), but they are not specific for asthma and may also be seen in patients with allergic bronchopulmonary aspergillosis, chronic eosinophilic pneumonia, some drug reactions and parasitic infestations (Schatz et al., 1981). Recent studies have been concentrated on measuring levels of immunoglobulins (Turnbull et al., 1978) and eosinophil-derived proteins (Dor et al., 1984) in the sputum.

The histological structure of the bronchial mucosa has been studied in patients dying in an asthmatic attack or from other natural or violent causes (Huber and Koessler, 1922; Dunnill, 1975; Cutz et al., 1978; Sobonya, 1984). Classic dogma equates asthma with mucous pluggings, bronchial smooth muscle hyperplasia, eosinophilia, and thickening of the epithelial basement membrane. However, these characteristics are those seen at autopsy of lungs obtained from asthmatic persons dying from status asthmaticus and they neither reflect the changes in early disease nor relate to disease severity (Dunnill et al., 1969; Thurlbeck et al., 1970). So far the fatal cases have contributed most to our understanding of the pathological changes in asthma.

Because asthmatic patients seldom undergo lung surgery, fresh specimens can most often be obtained with bronchoscopy. However, until recent years it has been uncommon to see biopsy material from asthmatic persons (Glynn and Michaels, 1960; Cutz et al., 1978; Laitinen et al., 1985c; Lundgren et al., 1988; Beasley et al., 1989). Developments in bronchoscopic and electron microscopic techniques have been essential for the current increase in knowledge of airway morphology in living asthmatic subjects. Additional information on the bronchial airways is gained by bronchoalveolar lavage (BAL) (Wardlaw et al., 1988).

To make quantitative studies, the bronchial biopsy specimens should be taken and processed using a standardized method (Laitinen et al., 1985c). Along with introduction of new techniques, special attention has to be paid to careful patient characterization in future research. An electron microscopic method has been developed to study greater areas of airway mucosa, using slot grids without bars and making photomontages of the adjacent electron micrographs (Fig. 1). This method allows a whole thin section measuring 1 mm $\times$ 1 mm to be examined and depicted photographically. By improving this method, the number of mast cells, neutrophils, and eosinophils in the airway mucosa, with ultrastructural recognition of the cells even under different stages of degranulation, can be quantitated per mm^2 (Laitinen, 1989).

Bronchial biopsy findings, especially in the airway epithelium, are reviewed here first in relation to the present knowledge in airway structure.

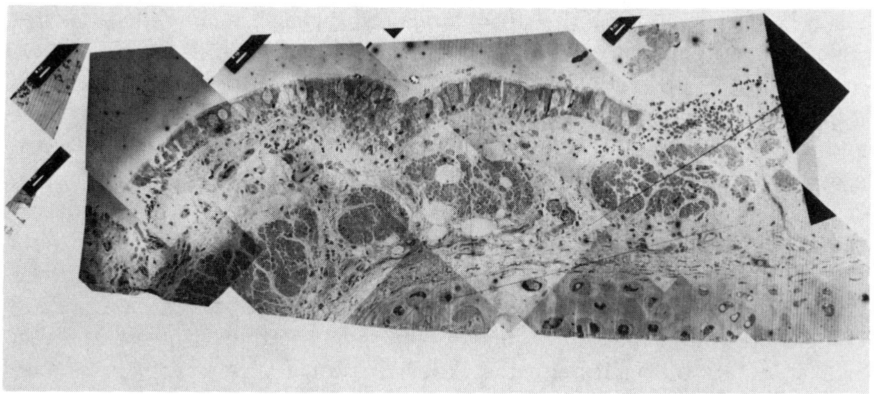

Figure 1 Photomontage combining adjacent low-power transmission electron micrographs covering the whole ultrathin section. The airway specimen seen in the picture is approximately 1 mm long in reality. The airway structures are clearly visualized: the epithelium on the top, the cartilage near the base of the montage. In between is seen the lamina propria with blood vessels and transversely cut smooth muscle bundles (original magnification, 2000).

Other airway structures in the subepithelial tissue (i.e., smooth muscle, nerves, and bronchial circulation) are also described.

II. Bronchial Mucosal Inflammation in Asthmatic Patients Between Attacks

The increase in the number of inflammatory cells, the edema formation, and the cell destruction found in the bronchial mucosa of asthma patients are only a part of the whole inflammatory process (Laitinen et al., 1985c; Beasley et al., 1989). Inflammation also includes increase in the bronchial blood flow and extravasation. In experimental animal studies it has been shown that inflammatory cell mediators, histamine, methacholine, bradykinin, prostaglandin (D_2, E_1, $F_2\alpha$), platelet-activating factor, and some neuropeptides such as substance P, vasoactive intestinal peptide, neurokinin A, calcitonin gene-related peptide, peptide histidine isoleucine, and tyrosine can cause dosage-related decreases in the airway vascular resistance, referring to the increase in the blood flow (Laitinen et al., 1987a,b). After inflammatory mediators were injected into the airway vascular bed in the dog, the histologic appearance of the extravascular mucosal space is similar to the airway changes in some asthmatic patients, showing extravasation of erythrocytes and neutrophils (Laitinen et al., 1986, 1987b).

It has been proposed that from airway epithelial damage follows neurogenic inflammation, which, due to antidromic nerve stimulation, causes smooth muscle contraction, leakage of airway blood vessels, and stimulation of bronchial glands (Barnes, 1986). The pathways of the axon reflexes have not been established histologically. The mediator for axon reflexes is suggested to be substance P (Jansco et al., 1967; Lundberg et al., 1979; Lundberg and Saria, 1983), and these reflexes have been shown to cause contraction of airway smooth muscle. There is only one study showing the presence of axon reflex in airways (Kröll et al., 1989). McDonald (1987, 1988) has studied the effects of respiratory tract infection on neurogenic inflammation in rat trachea. He found that respiratory infections of certain viruses and direct vagal stimulation, to a lesser extent, caused leakage of postcapillary venules and increased leucocyte adherence in the vessel wall. The airway epithelium showed changes such as increase in the epithelial height, widening of intercellular spaces, and increase in the number of goblet cells. No counts of inflammatory cells in the airway epithelium were made. The increase in the epithelial height and widening of intercellular spaces have also been found in asthmatic subjects (Laitinen et al., 1985c, 1988). These findings may result from increased exudation (Persson 1986, 1988). The endothelium of the bronchial vessels may have wide gaps in asthmatic subjects (Figure 2) (Laitinen and Laitinen, 1988).

A. Pathological Changes in Epithelial Structure

The epithelium of the mammalian tracheobronchial tree is of the ciliated pseudostratified columnar type in the larger airways (trachea and proximal bronchi) and turns into a simple cuboidal type inside the lung (distal bronchi and bronchioli). The cell types forming the bronchial epithelium differ somewhat in different species. In the normal human bronchial epithelium, four main cell types, which all rest on a basement membrane, are most often seen (Rhodin, 1974; Heino, 1987): ciliated cells, basal cells, secretory (mucous or goblet) cells, and Kulchitsky (neuroendocrine, amine-containing, APUD, or K) cells. The ciliated, secretory, and some of the K cells reach the lumen. There are three to five ciliated cells for every mucous cell. The epithelium also contains a few lymphocytes and nerve profiles near the lumen and basement membrane (Heino et al., 1982; Laitinen, 1985). The so-called intermediate cell type referred to in the literature is actually either a preciliated or presecretory cell according to ultrastructural criteria, although an indeterminant cell type may exist.

Examination of airway epithelial structure is especially important since this area serves as a primary target organ for exogenous irritants such as allergens. Its structural changes, such as shedding, may also greatly modify the passage of the irritants to deeper mucosa.

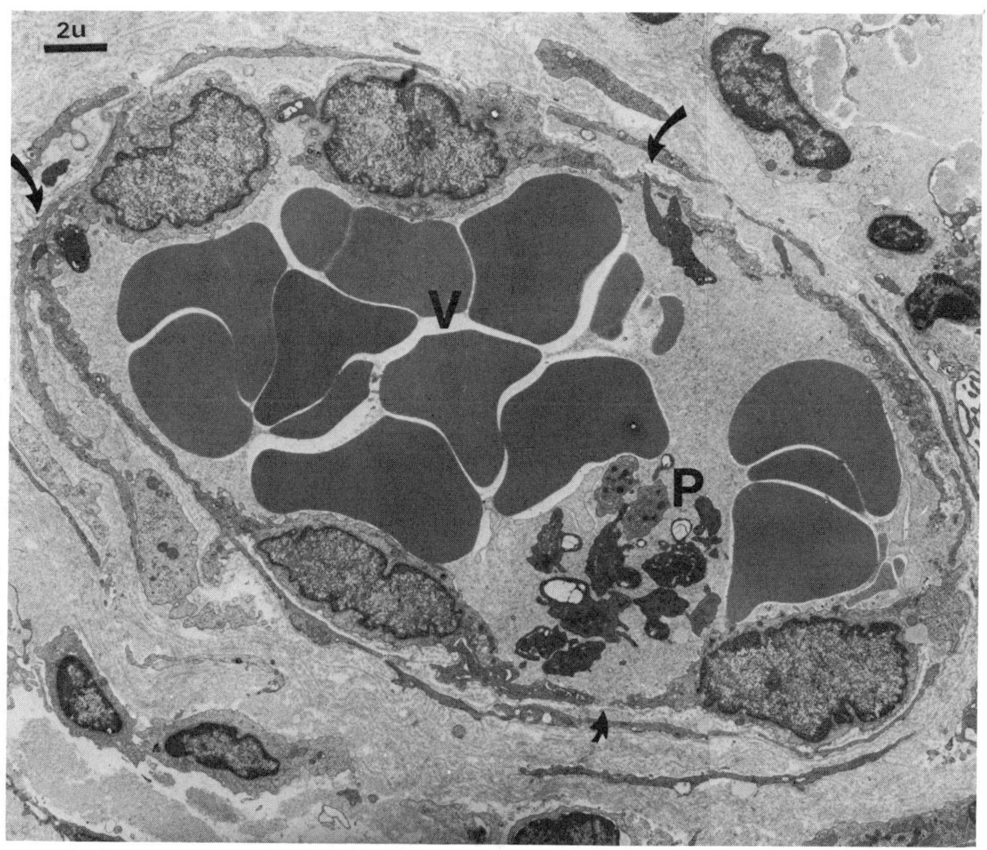

Figure 2 Specimen from the upper lobe bronchus of a patient with newly detected asthma. The electron micrograph shows a postcapillary venule (v) in the lamina propria under the epithelium and basement membrane. In addition to erythrocytes, several platelets are seen in the vascular lumen. Two platelets are penetrating the vascular endothelium (curved arrows). A cluster of platelets (p) is seen close to an endothelial disruption, gap formation (arrow head) (original magnification, 6500; bar = 2 µm).

According to the literature, at the end stage of asthma in specimens from patients dying in status asthmaticus, it is extremely difficult to find normal areas of bronchial mucosa (Dunnill, 1982). A prominent feature described is a marked airway edema with separation of the epithelial cells, leaving behind in many areas only a layer of basal or reserve cells (Dunnill, 1960). More recently, similar changes have been described in bronchial biopsies from living stable asthmatic patients examined with light and electron microscopy (Laitinen et al., 1985c; Lundgren et al., 1988).

The airway epithelium in asthmatic patients can show a clearly fragile appearance, caused either by shedding of the columnar epithelial cells or by intracellular signs of destruction, including vacuolization of the endoplasmic reticulum. In areas of shedding, there is accumulation of homogenous mass, probably edema fluid, in the widened intercellular spaces at the base of the epithelium (Fig. 3). The homogenous mass pushing the uppermost columnar cells away can often be seen close to areas of extensive epithelial destruction, for example, in areas where only the basal cells were present or where the basement membrane is totally denuded. Despite this structurally destructive separation process, the columnar epithelial cells could have quite a normal appearance, still being attached to each other at the luminal side by the tight junctions (Laitinen et al., 1985c). Epithelial shedding seems to be a commonly described feature in asthma. It is also one of the first features described in airway pathological changes of asthma (Naylor, 1962). Other not so specific changes in asthmatic airway epithelium are goblet cell hyperplasia and epithelial cell metaplasia. Hyperplasia and metaplasia may be related to airway epithelial degeneration and regeneration processes.

B. Nerves, Neuroepithelial Bodies, and Neuroendocrinelike Cells in the Epithelium

Nerves are usually seen in the epithelium near the basal lamina (Reid, 1974). Only a few reports are available on the superficial location of nerves (Das et al., 1978; Fillenz and Woods, 1970; Reid, 1974; Richardson, 1979; Heino et al., 1982; Laitinen, 1985; Laitinen et al., 1985c). The possible functional role of nerves cannot be judged based on the morphological data only. On the basis of suggested ultrastructural criteria, nerve profiles containing many mitochondria resemble nerve endings classically considered to be afferent (King et al., 1974). The exposure of superficially located nerves by sloughing of epithelial cells in asthma is possible. At places where the bronchial epithelium is missing because of shedding of the airway epithelium, a direct passage exists between the lumen and the subepithelial tissue; the latter also harbors nerves. Consequently, the exposure of mucosal afferent nerves to nonspecific stimuli or released mediators could partly explain bronchial hyperresponsiveness in patients with asthma.

The airway epithelium contains both individual granule-containing cells and also groups of cells defined as neuroepithelial bodies (NEB) (Lauweryns and Peuskens, 1972). Various names have been given to these cells based on morphological and cytochemical characteristics. The single cells have been referred to as Feyrter cells; Kulchitsky cells; argyrophil, fluorescent, and granulated (AFG) cells; neuroendocrine-like cells; and APUD cells (diAugustine and Sonstegard, 1984). Both solitary cells and neuroepithelial bodies

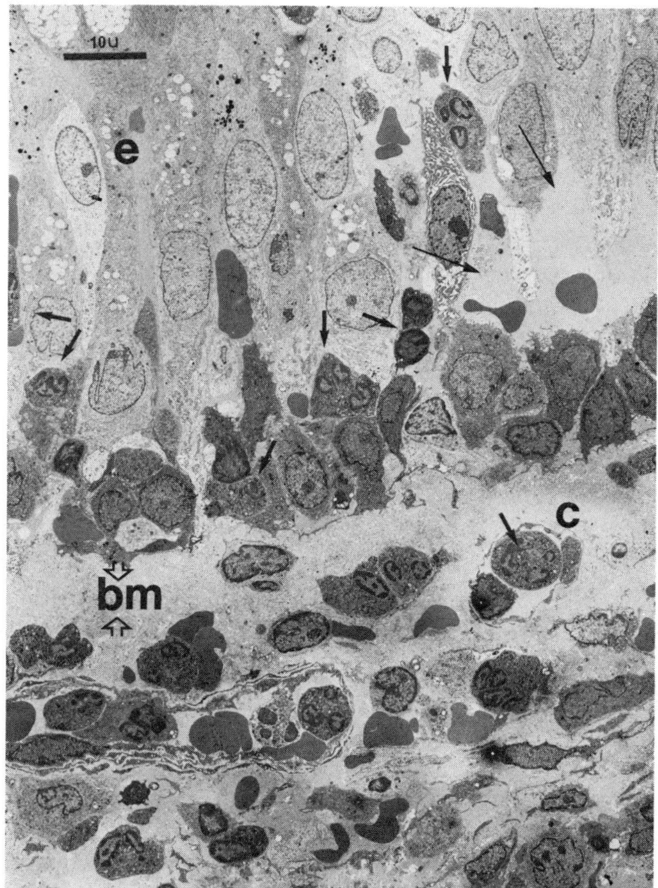

Figure 3 Electron micrograph shows airway epithelium in a patient with intrinsic-type asthma who had had clinically severe asthma for 12 years. The airway epithelium showed destructive changes: widening of intercellular spaces and shedding of the epithelium focally. The ciliated and goblet cells were separated from the base by homogeneously staining material (long thin arrows). The epithelium was highly infiltrated, especially by neutrophils (short thick arrows). The neutrophils can be seen throughout the epithelium, penetrating the basement membrane as well as close to the luminal border. e, epithelium; bm, basement membrane; c, capillary (original magnification, 2000; bar = 10 μm).

have been identified in many species, including humans (Lauweryns and Peuskens, 1972; DiAugustine and Sonstegard, 1984; Laitinen, 1988). The cells usually have a triangular shape that rests on the basement membrane. The larger basal part of the cells contains many dense-cored vesicles. Often a fenestrated capillary in the lamina propria opposes the basement membrane at the point where the granule-containing cells is located (Laitinen, 1988).

Nerve profiles have been observed close to single granule-containing cells (Laitinen, 1988) and NEBs (Lauweryns et al., 1985). The function of these nerves has not been established physiologically but experimental degeneration studies show that the majority of them are afferent (Lauweryns et al., 1985), and the most detailed investigations indicate that the NEBs may be stimulated to release their mediators under the influence of hypoxia (Lauweryns et al., 1983).

The apical pole of the cells could contact the airway lumen (Laitinen, 1988). The granule-containing cells, by releasing their dense core vesicles, may produce their effects via either the nervous system or the blood circulation. Thus, either a neural stimulation or a stimulus from the airway lumen to the amine-containing cells may release amines and possibly also neuropeptides into the local bloodstream to be carried into the deeper mucosa and smooth muscle. Both intraepithelial nerves and neuroendocrine cells are described in asthmatic airways (Laitinen et al., 1985c), but no quantitative studies of their number exist.

C. Inflammatory Cells in the Epithelium

Asthmatic patients show great individual variability in the number of mast cells, eosinophils, and neutrophils in their mucosa.

The regular occurrence of mast cells in the airway epithelium, even in patients with mild asthma and a short duration of the disease, supports the idea that these cells may be important in the initial stage of the disease (Salvato, 1968; Laitinen and Laitinen, 1988). The degranulation of the mast cells and the destruction of the surrounding tissue in the bronchial epithelium of asthmatic patients point to the active status of the cells (Fig. 4). The special cytoplasmic granules of the mast cell are associated with initiating inflammatory responses to specific stimuli. The ability of the activated mast cell to cause allergic inflammation has been studied extensively in the skin (Solley et al., 1976; Tannenbaum et al., 1980; Oertel and Kaliner, 1981). In the nasal mucosa, mast cells are related to allergic but not to infectious inflammation (Melen and Pipkorn, 1985). Several mediators in the granules have been shown experimentally to generate chemotactic factors and to call up other inflammatory cells. Mast-cell mediators with chemotactic activity for neutrophils have been described (Phillips et al., 1982; Goetzl et al., 1983). Following mast-cell degranulation, chemotactic factors, such as eosinophil chemotactic factors of anaphylaxis (Goetzl and Austen, 1975) and intermediate molecular-weight eosinophil chemotactic factors (Boswell et al., 1978), are released.

The findings in bronchoalveolar lavage (BAL) studies are in agreement with the biopsy-based observations. Significant increases in the percentage of mast cells have been found in asthmatic patients compared with healthy controls (Wardlaw et al., 1988), but the counts were no more different than those previously reported in patients with sarcoidosis or fibrosing alveolitis. Wardlaw et al. (1988) suggested that the mast cells found in asthmatics' airways are activated, releasing more mediators. This has also been shown in atopic nonasthmatic subjects (Wenzel et al., 1988).

For more than 80 years it has been known that bronchial asthma is sometimes associated with *eosinophilia* of the blood and lung (Ellis, 1908). Later it was reported that peripheral blood eosinophilia was inversely correlated with the severity of asthma, as measured by FEV_1 (Horn et al., 1975). These associations may have stimulated studies of a toxic protein released from the eosinophil granule, the major basic protein (MBP), by the respiratory epithelial damage (Gleich et al., 1975; Frigas et al., 1981; Venge et al., 1987). There are three other principle basic proteins in the eosinophil granule: eosinophil-derived neurotoxin (Durack et al., 1981) eosinophil cationic protein (Venge et al., 1980; Gleich and Adolphson, 1986), and eosinophil peroxidase (Carlson et al., 1985). In addition, eosinophils release a variety of mediators, including leukotriene C4 (Weller et al., 1983) and platelet-activating factor (Lee et al., 1984). The epithelial damage and desquamation caused by MBP are similar to the pathological changes in asthma (Dunnill, 1960; Laitinen et al., 1985c). Immunofluorescent staining of specimens from patients dying from asthma have shown MBP deposited at sites of damage to bronchial epithelium, in mucus plugs, and in amorphous deposits beneath the epithelium (Filley et al., 1982).

Even though eosinophil infiltration is a characteristic feature of asthmatic airways in necropsy specimens (Flint et al., 1985), eosinophils occurred in the airway epithelium of only a few of the patients with stable asthma taking various medications (Laitinen, 1989). The influx of eosinophils into the airway mucosa (Fig. 5) beneath the epithelium may be a characteristic feature of asthma (Glynn and Michaels, 1960; Salvato, 1968; Cutz et al., 1978; Laitinen and Laitinen, 1988; Beasley et al., 1989). Allergen inhalation results in a marked increase in eosinophils in BAL fluids obtained at the time of the late reaction (Frigas and Gleich, 1986). An increased number of eosinophils was found only in the asthmatic subjects with evidence of disease activity (Wardlaw et al., 1988). Increase in the number of eosinophils has been shown to correlate with the severity of the change in lung function (Frigas et al., 1981). This is in agreement with the finding that the increase in the number of eosinophils in the bronchial mucosa was related to the deterioration of the asthma symptoms (Laitinen et al., 1990). Eosinophils may thus contribute

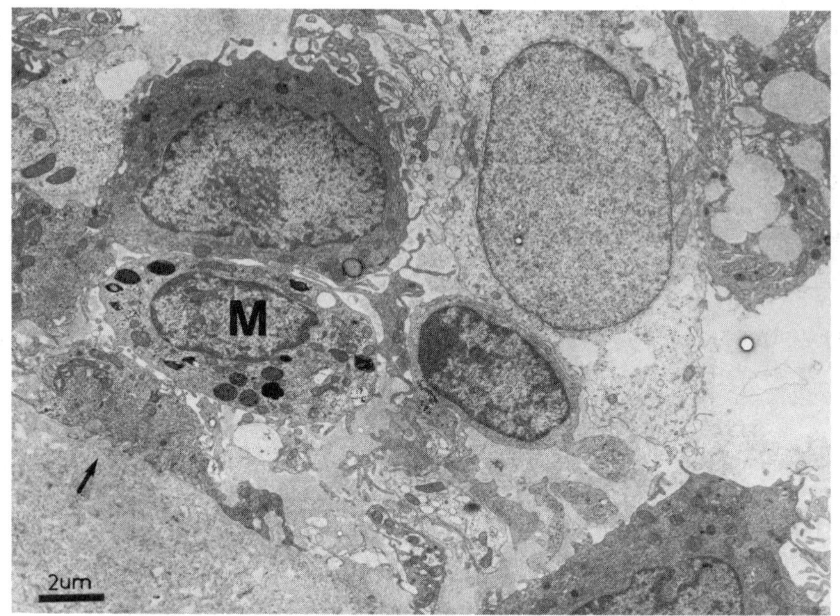

(A)

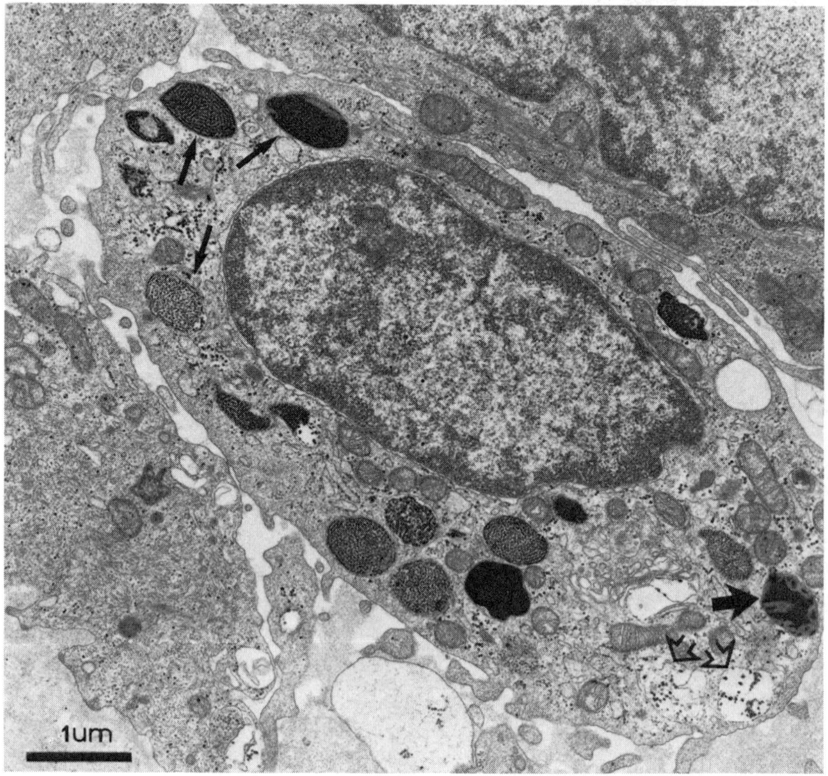

(B)

to the pathophysiological process responsible for the change of stable asthma into an asthma attack. However, several lavage studies have shown that eosinophils are also present in BAL of patients with day-to-day asthma (Godard et al., 1982; Tomioka et al., 1984; Flint et al., 1985). Wardlaw et al. (1988) also measured the amount of the eosinophilic major basic protein and suggested that it is a more specific indicator of the increased eosinophil activity than is the eosinophil count.

Neutrophils have been associated with acute (transient) bronchial hyperresponsiveness in many studies (Nadel, 1984; Boushey and Holtzmann, 1985). According to Holtzmann et al. (1983), neutrophils are active participants in epithelial damage. However, other findings do not agree. Murlas and Roum (1985a) described tracheal epithelial changes in guinea pigs that developed hyperreactive airways 2 h after ozone exposure. In a further study (Murlas and Roum, 1985b), they showed that the pathogenesis of ozone-induced bronchial hyperreactivity in guinea pigs is not dependent on inflammatory cell infiltration of the airway mucosa, which is in agreement with finding by Hulbert et al. (1985), who showed bronchial hyperreactivity but no neutrophilic infiltration in guinea pigs 30 min after exposure to cigarette smoke..

The presence of a few neutrophils in the epithelium is probably a normal phenomenon; neutrophils may even be found in the lavage fluid of normal subjects (Crystal et al., 1986). Neutrophils were even more numerous in the control specimens in a recent biopsy study in patients with mild asthma (Beasley et al., 1989). Increased numbers of both neutrophils and eosinophils have been associated with late asthmatic response in allergen challenge tests (De Moncy et al., 1985; Fabbri et al., 1987). The late response has been thought to mimic day-to-day asthma with symptoms.

In the bronchial specimens from some mild and moderate asthmatic patients, no neutrophils were found in the epithelium (Laitinen, 1989). However, in patients with severe asthma of long duration, the neutrophil counts were very high. Thus, it seems that chronic asthma of long duration and lung function impairment are associated with epithelial and mucosal neutrophil influx, probably reflecting a far advanced, severe stage of the inflammatory process or even infection in the airways.

Figure 4 Electron micrographs from the upper lobe bronchus of a patient with mild asthma. A partly degranulated mast cell is seen near the basement membrane (arrow) in damaged airway epithelium. Figure 4B shows with greater magnification the typical granules with scroll-type substructures (thick arrow) in the mast cells. Some of the granules in the mast cell are empty (open arrows). Most of the granules contain electron dense digitated material (thin arrows), probably representing an intermediate form during the degranulation. M, mast cell (original magnification, 7800 in A, 19,500 in B).

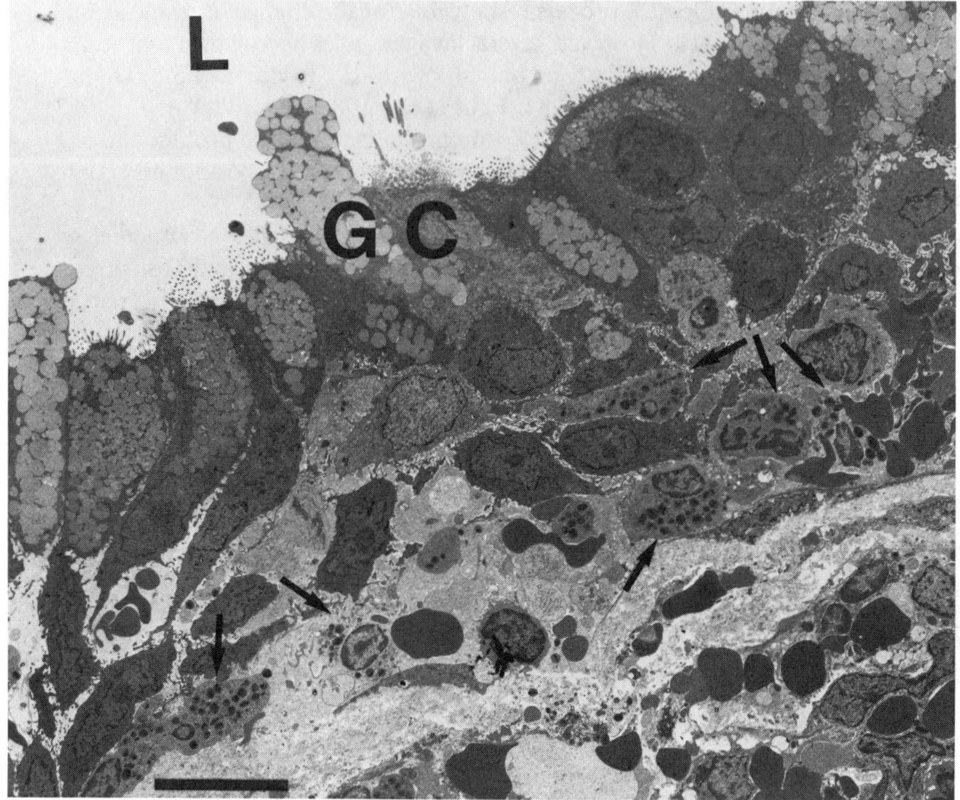

Figure 5   Electron micrograph from the upper lobe bronchus of an asthmatic patient. The epithelium shows goblet cell hyperplasia. Only few ciliated cells could be detected between the goblet cells. Many eosinophils can be seen both in the epithelium and lamina propria. Arrow, eosinophils; L, airway lumen; G, goblet cell; C, ciliated cell (original magnification, 2000; bar = 10 μm).

D. Basement Membrane

The basement membrane has usually (Fig. 6), but not always been described as thickened in patients with asthma (Dunnill, 1960; Glynn and Michaels, 1960; Cutz et al., 1978; Laitinen and Laitinen, 1988; Beasley et al., 1989).

The fibronectin location in the mucosa of nonsmoking asthmatic patients and controls has been studied using immunofluorescence techniques (Laitinen et al., 1989a). Fibronectin (FN) refers to a group of structurally and immunologically related high-molecular-weight glycoproteins present in plasma and

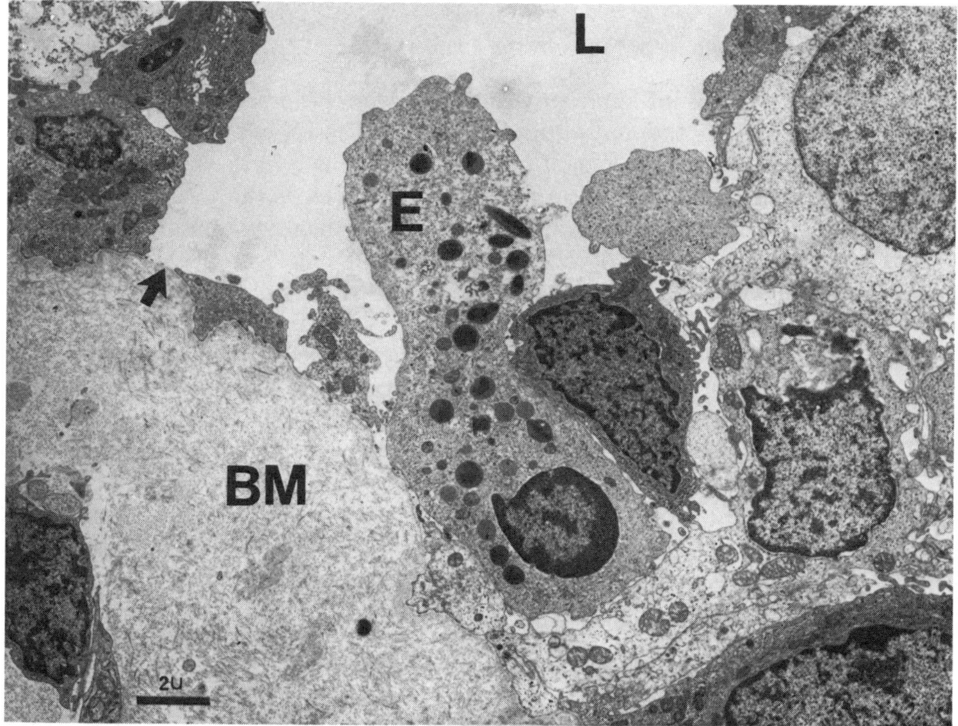

Figure 6 Specimen from a patient with mild extrinsic type asthma for 3 months. An eosinophil (E) is seen in the epithelium close to epithelial cell destruction, where the cells are apart from each other and the basal lamina is seen denuded (arrow). The basement membrane (BM) is thickened to several micrometers. L, airway lumen; BM, basement membrance (original magnification, 7800; bar = 2 μm).

extracellular matrix. It is important in cell-to-cell and cell-to-matrix interactions (Yamada and Olden, 1978; Hynes and Yamada, 1982; Vaheri et al., 1985). Cellular secretion of fibronectin mediates adhesion of cultured cells to nonbiological materials (Yamada and Olden, 1978). After tissue injury, FN appears at the site of injury (Clark et al., 1981; Grinnel et al., 1981; Saksela et al., 1981; Vaheri et al., 1983). Fibrin and FN are temporary components of the extracellular matrix in the basement membrane during healing of the epithelial wound in vivo. In specimens from asthmatic subjects, the basement membrane had a thickened structure. Fibronectin showed a bright reaction in the basement membrane at the bottom of an ulcer in the epithelium or adjacent to the edge of ulcerated epithelium. In control subjects, the fibronectin reaction was negative (Laitinen et al., 1989a).

E. Pathological Changes in the Lamina Propria

Varying degrees of inflammatory cell infiltration have been observed in the lamina propria in patients with mild asthma (Beasley et al., 1989). In that study the active recruitment of inflammatory cells into the bronchial wall was reflected in the finding of numerous leukocytes in the vascular lumina and adherent to the vessel walls of the bronchial microvasculature. In addition to eosinophils, neutrophils, monocytes, and platelet aggregates were all found adherent to the vascular endothelium. The presence of eosinophils in the lamina propria was exclusive to patients with asthma. The mast cells in the bronchial lamina propria exhibited various stages of degranulation in asthmatic but not control subjects. Beasley et al.'s (1989) finding in patients with mild asthma supports the suggestion that mast cell degranulation and mediator release occur continuously within the bronchial lamina propria of atopic persons with asthma. Mast cells obtained at BAL from such subjects exhibit increased spontaneous release of histamine (Flint et al., 1985).

III. Bronchial Mucosal Inflammation During an Asthma Attack

Data on bronchial mucosal changes during an asthma attack are extremely limited. It is known that allergen inhalation results in a marked increase in eosinophils in BAL fluids obtained at the time of late reaction and that a close relationship exists between peripheral eosinophils (Wardlaw et al., 1988) and bronchial hyperresponsiveness (Frigas and Gleich, 1986).

Bronchial biopsy specimens from one asthmatic patient during both a stable phase and an asthma attack have been taken and analyzed. During a spontaneous asthma attack, there was a 100-fold increase in the number of eosinophils in the bronchial mucosa (Laitinen et al., 1990).

IV. Repair of Inflammatory Changes in the Bronchial Mucosa

The mechanisms behind the turnover and repair of the airway epithelium are not well known. After epithelial cell detachment, the basal or reverse cells left on the basement membrane may serve as a source for regeneration of bronchial mucosa. Much of the metaplastic epithelium noticed in asthmatic patients has been of the simple, stratified, nonciliated variety exhibiting mitoses (Dunnill, 1982). This change has commonly been seen in patients dying of an asthmatic attack. However, the appearance is very similar to epithelia found in experimental animals during the wound healing process after experimentally induced trauma (Wilhelm, 1953; Fujikawa et al., 1981).

Nonciliated stratified epithelium has also been described both under light and electron microscopy in living asthmatic subjects' bronchial biopsies (Glynn and Michaels, 1960; Laitinen et al., 1985c; Lundgren et al., 1988). There is no direct evidence in asthmatic subjects that this kind of epithelial change represents regeneration or damage.

When the tracheobronchial epithelium is damaged, mucous cells and basal cells proliferate in response to the injury. It is widely assumed that basal cells are responsible for regeneration of the tracheobronchial epithelium following injury. However, according to the recent literature (see McDowell and Beals, 1987) mucous cells may play the dominant proliferative role. Resulting from a marked increase in the mitotic rate, pathological lesions including "goblet" cell hyperplasia, stratification, and noncornifying and cornifying epidermoid (squamous) metaplasias may be produced (Fig. 7). Although morphologically dissimilar, these lesions are brought about by the wide and varied spectrum of the phenotypic expression of mucous cells. Depending on the nature and extent of the injury, one or more of these lesions may be present simultaneously in the same specimen, and one lesion may change into another (Fig. 8). Mitotic activity is very low in undisturbed tracheobronchial epithelium. Both basal cells and mucous cells synthesize DNA and undergo mitosis. It is not yet resolved in humans or animals to which extent each cell type normally participates to replace damaged cells, thereby maintaining the mucociliary state (see McDowell and Beals, 1987).

Ciliated cells are easily damaged. When an epithelial injury persists or is severe, ciliated cells are lost from the epithelium. Ciliated cells are end-stage cells: they neither synthesize DNA nor divide. They are not replaced in the regenerative process until before the adverse situation is terminated. Loss of ciliated cells is an early response to many forms of injury (McDowell et al., 1979; Keenan et al., 1982a,b). Stimulated ciliogenesis may be one step in the regeneration of the epithelium. The number of cells with fibrogranular areas, which are precursors in the cilia formation, has been noted as increased in asthmatic subjects treated with oral prednisolone (Heino et al., 1988).

It has been suggested that fibronectin may play an important role in the healing process of some epithelial ulcers. The detection of fibronectin in asthmatic subjects at the site of the possible zone for bronchial epithelial regeneration, which is identical to the fibronectin location in other ulcerated human epithelia, gives evidence of a wound-healing process in the airways (Laitinen et al., 1989a).

V. Airway Smooth Muscle

Some investigators have reported airway smooth muscle hypertrophy and/or hyperplasia in asthmatic subjects (Dunnill et al., 1969; Heard and Hassain,

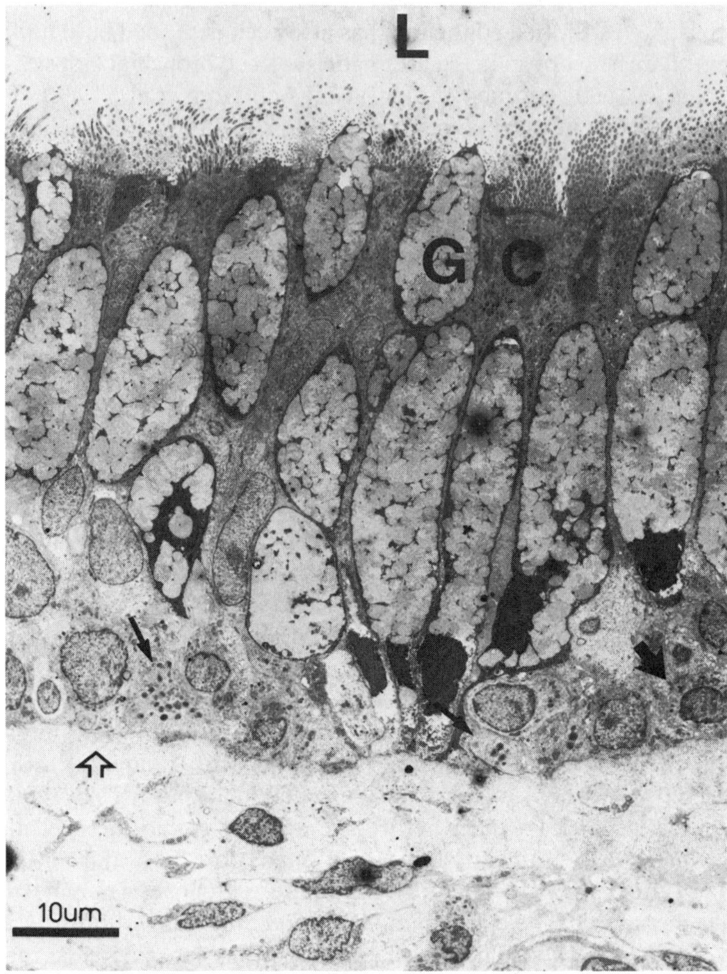

Figure 7 Low-power transmission electron microscopic image from a patient with asthma for less than 1 year. Ciliated pseudostratified epithelium shows an increased number of goblet cells; every second cell is a goblet cell. Some inflammatory cells, such as eosinophils (thin arrow) and lymphocytes, were observed in the airway epithelium as well as highly degranulated mast cells (short thick arrow). The basement membrane (open arrow) beneath the epithelium is thickened. L, lumen; C, ciliated cell; G, goblet cell (original magnification, 2000; bar = 10 μm).

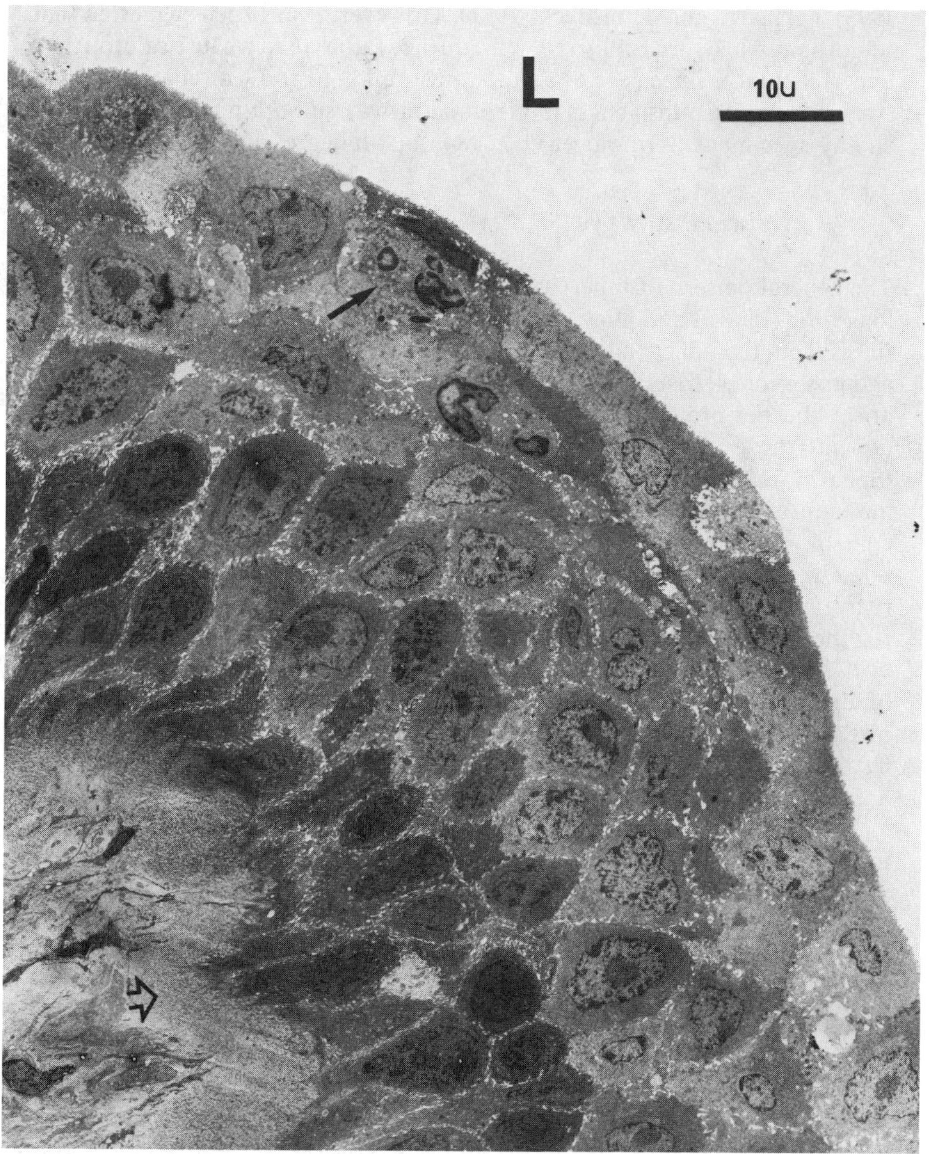

Figure 8 Specimen from a segmental bronchus of a patient with newly detected asthma. The electron micrograph shows airway metaplasia with total loss of ciliated cells. The epithelium is multilayered with polygonal cells. A neutrophil (arrow) is seen close to the flattened surface cells. L, lumen; open arrow, basement membrane (original magnification, 2000; bar = 10 μm).

1973; Takizawa and Thurlbeck, 1971). However, it has been suggested that smooth muscle hypertrophy is a consequence rather than a cause of bronchial hyperreactivity, since several studies have failed to show a relationship between airway responsiveness in vivo and airway smooth muscle quantity in airway specimens (Armour et al., 1984a,b; Mullen et al., 1986).

VI. Neural Pathways

The general pattern of innervation of human airways has been known for a long time (Larsell and Dow, 1933; Richardson, 1979). The vagus nerves and fibres from the upper four to five thoracic sympathetic ganglia form anterior and posterior plexuses at the hilum, from which the two main nerve networks arise: the peribronchial and periarterial plexuses. Nerves supply airways down to the level of respiratory bronchioles and also supply bronchial vessels (Spencer and Leof, 1964). In addition to classic cholinergic and adrenergic mechanisms (Laitinen et al., 1985a), there exists a third component of neural control, which is neither adrenergic nor cholinergic and is thus called the nonadrenergic noncholinergic nervous system (NANC) (Barnes, 1984). Current evidence has implicated neuropeptides as possible neurotransmitters for the NANC system in airways (Barnes, 1984; Laitinen et al., 1985b).

The autonomic nervous system may influence, in addition to regulation of airway smooth muscle tone, secretion from submucosal glands, transport of fluid across airway epithelium, permeability and blood flow in the bronchial circulation, and release of mediators from inflammatory cells (Nadel and Barnes, 1984).

The neural control of the human airways is complex. Because changes in the bronchomotor tone in asthma are rapid, it has been proposed that neurally mediated mechanisms are involved in the pathogenesis of asthma.

The precise relationship among neural pathological changes, bronchial hyperresponsiveness, and clinical symptoms of asthma is not known. Many chapters of this book cover innervation in detail, and therefore it is not further discussed here.

VII. Nerves and Other Airway Structures

Eosinophils and mast cells can be seen under the electron microscope in the smooth muscle layer between the cells. These cells are also seen close to nerve fibers in the mucosa (Laitinen and Laitinen, 1987), both in normal tissue and in diseases such as bronchial asthma.

Control of the airway smooth muscle and glands may depend on diverse interactions of sensory stimuli from afferent nerve receptors, by mediators released from the neuroendocrine cells, or mediators released from nonfixed cells such as leukocytes and mast cells. These mechanisms may be disturbed in disease states such as asthma.

VIII. Bronchial Circulation

In humans and several other species, such as the dog, the bronchial arteries arise from multiple sites (Suslov, 1895; Daly and Hebb, 1966; McLaughlin, 1983). They have been described as originating from the aorta, intercostal arteries, and internal mammary or pericardial arteries (Cudkovicz and Armstrong, 1951; Florange, 1960). The bronchial arteries supply not only the walls of the bronchi but also the adventitia or large pulmonary vessels, the nerves, and some of the pleura (Daly and Hebb, 1966; Cudkowicz, 1979). The arteries in the peribronchial connective tissue give rise to smaller branches that reach the submucosa and form venous plexuses there (Pietra et al., 1971).

Venous return from the larger bronchi is via bronchial veins to the azygos and hemiazygos veins. From more peripheral airways, bronchial blood is drained by tributaries of the pulmonary veins (Miller, 1947; Liebow, 1960; Pietra and Magno, 1978; Charan et al., 1984; Deffebach et al., 1987). The structure of the bronchial circulation in humans (Fig. 9) is similar to that of the dog. A rich network of capillaries runs close to the epithelium at all levels of the lower airways. The capillaries converge to form venules extending to a deeper plexus of larger venules and arterioles. The networks are continuous around and along the airways. Capillovenular structures are most frequent at the luminal edge of the mucosa, with only a few arterioles in the mucosa. Transmission electron microscopy shows capillaries very close to the epithelial basement membrane, but not in the epithelium itself (Laitinen et al., 1989a; Laitinen and Laitinen, 1990).

The function of the airway vascular bed is not limited to providing nutrition to the structures it invests (Daly and Hebb, 1966). The bronchial circulation may play a significant role in controlling the clearance of chemical mediators from the airways, regulating the interstitial fluid volume of the airway wall, and participating in airway heat exchange (Baier et al., 1985), which has been proposed to be important in exercise-induced asthma. The role of extravasation of bronchial circulation is further discussed in chapters on that subject in this book.

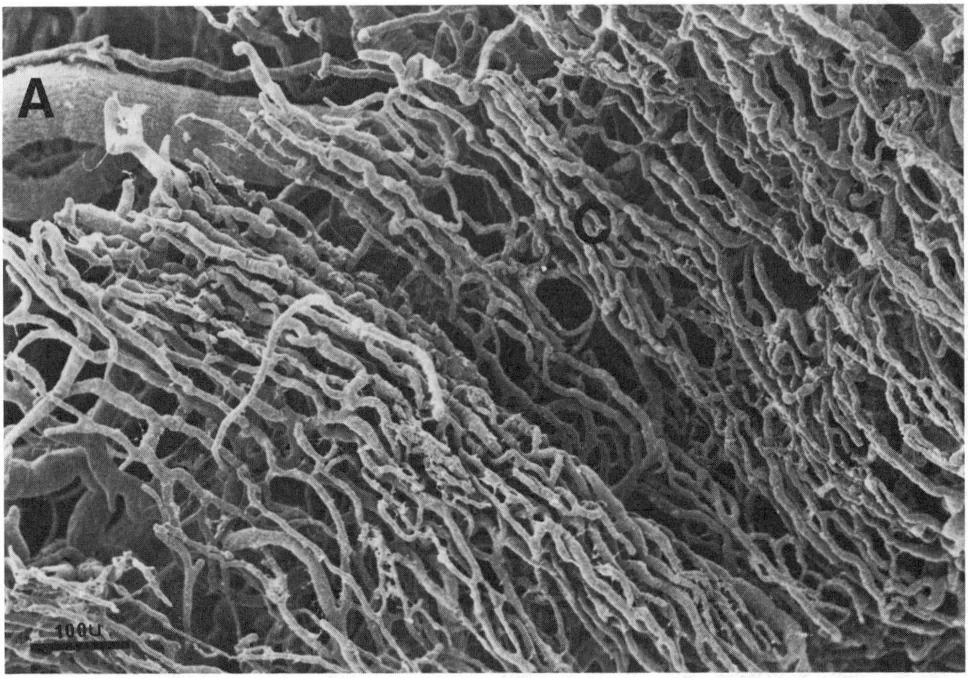

A
C
100u
(A)

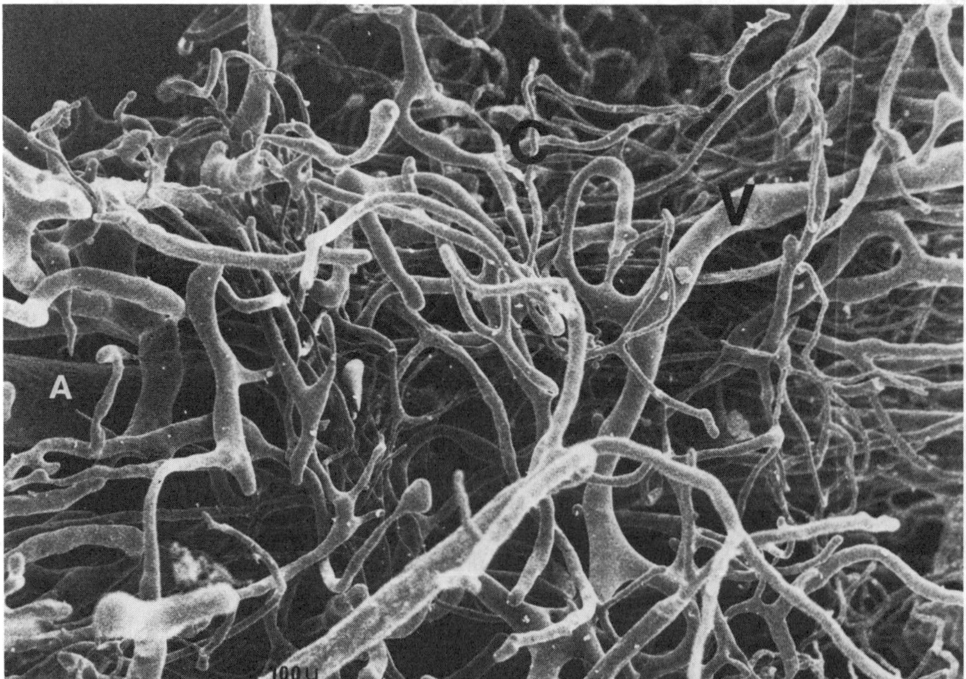

C
V
A
100u
(B)

IX. Summary

In experimental animal studies, direct injection of the tracheobronchial arteries with inflammatory mediators, neuronal stimulation, and viral respiratory tract infections results in histological features resembling recent pathological findings in human asthma. The experimental models may help us to understand the mechanisms and the sequence of events in the development and progress of asthma disease. Viral upper respiratory tract infection causes profound epithelial destructive changes in humans (Hers, 1966). Otherwise healthy humans can develop transient bronchial hyperresponsiveness during upper viral respiratory tract infection (Laitinen, 1974; Empey et al., 1976). Asthmatic patients in whom bronchial hyperresponsiveness is a more or less constant feature can show profound bronchial epithelial changes (Laitinen et al., 1985c). Asthmatic subjects with severe symptoms in particular can show features of the classic inflammatory reaction in the airways: destruction of the tissue, vascular permeability changes with edema formation, and inflammatory cell influx.

Airway epithelial damage may be the initial or the end stage to cause increased bronchial responsiveness. When, why, and how the disease in the airways does proceed to fully developed irreversible inflammatory reaction described at the beginning of our chapter (e.g., with eosinophilia, mucous plugging, and edema in the autopsy specimen is not known. Could the process be interrupted with treatment? So far, the disease has mainly been monitored with clinical observations and respiratory function tests. With recent bronchoscopic studies in living asthmatic subjects, we have evidence that there are already morphological changes at a clinically early stage of the disease. Morphological studies will give important information on functional abnormalities in asthmatic subjects' airways and of the progress of the changes leading to the fully developed inflammatory process in the airways. Knowing

---

Figure 9A Microvascular network in the mucosa of a 3 mm diameter bronchus in the dog. The cast was prepared by injecting the bronchial artery with polymerizing compound and subsequently digesting away other structures with potassium hydroxide. The capillaries run longitudinally along the course of the bronchus. A, arteriole; C, capillaries (bar = 100 μm; from Laitinen et al., 1989a).

Figure 9B Scanning electron micrograph of a cast of human airway microcirculation prepared as in A. The bronchial artery was catheterized and injected after lobectomy in a patient with lung cancer. The network of capillaries (c) runs closest to the airway surface and drains to venules (v) deeper in the mucosa. Many capillaries end as cul-de sacs indicative of unfilled vessels. The difference between the dog and human cast was caused by the delay in injecting the bronchial artery in the human patient because of the operation, the dog was heparinized to prevent blood clots in the vessels. A, arteriole (bar = 100 μm).

the sequence of these events will lead to greater progress in the treatment of patients with asthma.

Acknowledgment

The authors thank Mr. Simo Lehtinen, M.Sc. and Mrs. Mervi Lindman, Department of Electron Microscopy, University of Helsinki for their technical assistance in electron microscopy and Mrs. Eva Engberg for her excellent secretarial assistance in the preparation of the manuscript.

Discussion

Irvine: Do you see a similar decrease in granules in the other granular inflammatory cells, in particular the neutrophil and eosinophil?

A. Laitinen: Yes. Specimens from patients with exacerbation of symptoms contain high numbers of eosinophils, and these eosinophils are often degranulated (they have lost their crystalloid granules).

Sertl: Did you see glandular hyperplasia after β-agonist treatment?

Persson: The dosages at which β-agonists cause increases in goblet cells are too large to be of likely relevance to the treatment of asthmatic subjects with these drugs.

Hargreave: The cellular characteristics of the inflammation in asthma need to be compared in bronchial biopsies, bronchial brush biopsies, BAL, and sputum. However, the features in your biopsies are similar to those found in other examinations of BAL and of sputum.

Laitinen: I agree with Professor Hargreave. That kind of comparative studies should be done.

Widdicombe: Did you see the four patterns of epithelial structure in the same patient? Could you correlate the epithelial pathological changes with underlying patterns (e.g., cell infiltrations)?

Laitinen: We have not seen any correlation between the type of epithelial changes and the type or the number of inflammatory cell, but our method has limitations.

Schleimer: Among the inflammatory cells have you observed any basophils in your studies?

Laitinen: We did not see basophils.

Capron: There have been recent reports pointing to platelet accumulation both in human biopsies and in experimental models after antigen challenge. Did you observe such an accumulation?

Laitinen: Platelets are mainly seen inside the vessels and even coming out of the vessels. However, in the tissue the platelets are morphologically difficult to identify.

Fish: We have heard descriptions of edematous airways in autopsy specimens from patients dying with asthma. In your population of patients with stable asthma, was mucosa edema a prominent feature?

Laitinen: Bronchial mucosa edema is typical of asthma. However, it is difficult to quantify.

Chung: Are there any differences in pathological findings at different levels of the airway within the same asthmatic patient?

Laitinen: We have analyzed only the specimens taken from the central airways. We have some transbronchial specimens from the peripheral airways in asthmatic subjects. It will be interesting to get more information from all levels of the airways.

Paré: In your morphometric studies, have you measured an increase in the number or size of the bronchial microvessels in the lamina propria of the airway?

Laitinen: Regarding the number and size of bronchial vessels, we have data in the computer; thus, we can answer this point in the near future.

Church: Studies by Drs. Beasley, Holgate, and Locke in Southamptom have suggested that the "basement membrane thickening" is the deposition of types 3 and 5 collagen below the basement membrane, probably occurring as a result of fibroblast activation. The rigidity that this would impose on an airway would make it more amenable to the influence of edema but less to smooth muscle contraction. Does this, therefore, occur in all generations of airways?

Laitinen: We have not done measurements of the different collagen types. Basement membrane may have some other interesting functions in addition to its supportive role. It may, for instance, take part in the regeneration of the epithelium.

References

Armour, C. L., Black, J. L., Berend, N., and Woolcock, A. J. (1984a). The relationship between bronchial hyperresponsiveness to methacholine and airway smooth muscle structure and reactivity. *Respir. Physiol.* **58**: 223-233.

Armour, C. L., Lazar, N. M., Schellenberg, R. R., Taylor, S. M., Chan, N., Hogg, J. C., and Pare, P. D. (1984b). Comparison of in vivo and in vitro human airway reactivity to histamine. *Am. Rev. Respir. Dis.* **129**:907-910.

Baier, H., Long, W. M., and Wanner, A. (1985). Bronchial circulation in asthma. *Respiration* **48**:199-205.

Barnes, P. J. (1984). The third nervous system in the lung: physiology and clinical perspectives. *Thorax* **39**:561-567.

Barnes, P. J. (1986). Airway inflammation and autonomic control. *Eur. J. Respir. Dis.* **69** suppl. **147**:80-87.

Beasley, R., Roche, W. R., Roberts, J. A., and Holgate, S. T. (1989). Cellular events in the bronchi in mild asthma and after bronchial provocation. *Am. Rev. Respir. Dis.* **139**:806-817.

Boswell, R. N., Austen, K. F., and Goetzel, E. J. (1978). Intermediate molecular weight eosinophil factor in rat peritoneal mast cells; immunologic release, granule association, and demonstration of structural heterogeneity. *J. Immunol.* **120**:15-20.

Boushey, H. A., and Holtzmann, M. J. (1985). Experimental airway inflammation and hyperreactivity. *Am. Rev. Respir. Dis.* **13**:312-313.

Carlson, M. G. C., Peterson, C. G. B., and Venge, P. (1985). Human eosinophil peroxidase: purification and characterization. *J. Immunol.* **134**:1875-1879.

Charan, N. B., Turk, G., and Dhand, R. (1984). Gross and subgross Anatomy of bronchial circulation in sheep. *J. Appl. Physiol.* **57**:658-664.

Clark, R. A. F., Dvorak, H. F., and Colvin, R. B. (1981). Fibronectin in delayed-type hypersensitivity skin reactions. *J. Immunol.* **262**:497-500.

Cohen, R. C., and Prentice, A. I. D. (1959). Metaplastic cells in sputum of patients with pulmonary eosinophilia. *Tubercle* **40**:44-46.

Crystal, R. G., Reynolds, H. Y., and Kalica, A. R. (1986). Bronchoalveolar lavage. The report of an international congress. *Chest* **90**:122-128.

Cudkowicz, L. (1979). Bronchial arterial circulation in man: normal anatomy and response to disease. In *Lung Biology in Health and Disease*, Vol. 14: *Pulmonary Vascular Diseases*. Edited by K. M. Moser, New York, Marcel Dekker, pp. 111-232.

Cudkowicz, L., and Armstrong, J. B. (1951). Observations on the normal anatomy of the bronchial arteries. *Thorax* **6**:343-358.

Curschmann, H. (1885). Einege Bemerkungen über die im Bronchialsecret vorkommenden Spiralen. *Dtsch. Arch. Klin. Med.* **36**:578-585.

Cutz, E., Levison, H., and Cooper, D. M. (1978). Ultrastructure of airways in children with asthma. *Histopathology* **2**:407-421.

Daly, M. de B., and Hebb, C. (1966). *Pulmonary and Bronchial Vascular Systems*. London, Edward Arnold Ltd.

Das, R. m., Jefferey, P. K., and Widdicombe, J. G. (1978). The epithelial innervation of the lower respiratory tract of the cat. *J. Anat.* **126**:123-31.

De Moncy, J. G. R., Kauffman, H. F., Venge, P., et al. (1985). Bronchoalveolar eosinophilia during allergen-induced late asthmatic reactions. *Am. Respir. Dis.* **131**:373-377.

Deffebach, M. E., Charan, N., Lakshminarayan, F., and Butler, J. (1987). The bronchial circulation; small, but a vital attribute of the lung. *Am. Rev. Respir. Dis.* **135**:463-481.

DiAugustine, R. P., and Sonstegard, K. S. (1984). Neuroendocrine-like (small granule) epithelial cells of the lung. *Environ Health Perspect.* **55**:271-295.

Dor, P. J., Ackerman, S. J., and Gleich, G. J. (1984). Charcot-Leyden crystal protein and eosinophil granule major basic protein in sputum of patients with respiratory diseases. *Am. Rev. Respir. Dis.* **130**:1072-1077.

Dunnill, M. S. (1960). The pathology of asthma with special reference to changes in the bronchial mucosa. *J. Clin. Pathol.* **13**:27-33.

Dunnill, M. A. (1975). *The Morphology of the Airways in Bronchial Asthma.* Park Ridge Ill: American College of Chest Physicians.

Dunnill, M. S. (1982). *Pulmonary Pathology.* Edinburgh/London/Melbourne/New York, Churchill Livingstone.

Dunnill, M. S., Massarella, G. R., and Anderson, J. A. (1969). A comparison of the quantitative anatomy of the bronchi in normal subjects, in status asthmaticus, in chronic bronchitis, and in emphysema. *Thorax* **24**:176-179.

Durack, D. T., Ackerman, S. J., Loegering, D. A., and Gleich, G. J. (1981). Purification of human eosinophil-derived neurotoxin. *Proc. Natl. Acad. Sci. USA* **78**:5165-5169.

Ellis, A. G. (1908). The pathological anatomy of bronchial asthma. *Am. J. Med. Sci.* **136**:407.

Empey, D. W., Laitinen, L. A., Jacobs, L., Gold, W. M., and Nadel, J. A. (1976). Mechanism of bronchial hyperreactivity in normal subjects after upper respiratory tract infections. *Am. Rev. Respir. Dis.* **113**:131-139.

Fabbri, L. M., Boschetto, P., and Zocca, E. (1987). Bronchoalveolar neutrophilia during late asthmatic reactions induced by toluene di-isocyanate. *Am. Rev. Respir. Dis.* **136**:36-42.

Fillenz, M., and Woods, R. I. (1970). Sensory innervation of the airways. In *CIBA Foundation Symposium: Breathing.* Hering-Breuer Centenary Symposium. Edited by E. Porter. London, Churchill Livingstone, pp. 101-107.

Filley, W. C., Holley, K. E., Kephart, G. M., and Gleich, G. J. (1982). Identification by immunofluorescence of eosinophil granule major basic protein in lung tissues of patients with bronchial asthma. *Lancet* **2**:11-15.

Flint, K. C., Leung, K. B. P., Hudspith, B. N., et al. (1985). Bronchoalveolar mast cells in extrinsic asthma: a mechanism for the initiation of antigen specific bronchoconstriction. *Br. Med. J.* **291**:923.

Florange, W. (1960). Anatomie und Pathologie der Arteria bronchialis. *Ergeb. Pathol. Anat.* **39**:152-213.

Frigas, E., and Gleich, G. J. (1986). The eosinophil and the pathology of asthma. *J. Allergy. Clin. Immunol.* **77**:527-537.

Frigas, E., Loegering, D. A., Solley, G. O., Farrow, G. M., and Gleich, G. J. (1981). Elevated levels of eosinophil granule major basic protein in the sputum of patients with bronchial asthma. *Proc. Mayo Clin.* **56**: 345-353.

Fujikawa, L. S., Foster, C. S., Harrist, T. J., Lanigan, J. M., and Colvin, R. B. (1981). Fibronectin in healing rabbit corneal wounds. *Lab. Invest.* Vol. 45, No. 2:120-129.

Gleich, G. J., and Adolphson, C. R. (1986). The eosinophilic leukocyte: structure and function. *Adv. Immunol.* **39**:177.

Gleich, G. J., Frigas, E., Loegering, D. A., Wassom, D. L., and Steinmuller, D. (1975). Cytotoxic properties of eosinophil major basic protein. *J. Immunol.* **123**:2925.

Glynn, A. A., and Michaels, L. (1960). Bronchial biopsy in chronic bronchitis and asthma. *Thorax* **15**:142-153.

Godard, P., Chaintreuil, J., Damon, M., et al. (1982). Functional asessment of alveolar macrophages: comparison of cells from asthmatics and normal subject. *J. Allergy Clin. Immunol.* **70**:88-94.

Goetzl, E. J., and Austen, K. F.)1975). Purification and synthesis of eosinophilotactic tetrapeptides of human lung tissue: identification as eosinophil chemotactic factor of anaphylaxis. *Proc. Natl. Acad. Sci. USA* **72**: 4123-4127.

Goetzl, E. J., Phillips, M. J., and Gold, W. M. (1983). Stimulus specificity of the generation of leukotrienes by dog mastocytoma cells. *J. Exp. Med.* **158**:731-737.

Grinnel F., Billingham, R. E., and Burgess, L. (1981). Distribution of fibronectin during wound healing in vivo. *J. Invest. Dermatol.* **76**:181-189.

Heard, B. E., and Hassain, S. (1973). Hyperplasia of bronchial muscle in asthma. *J. Pathol.* **110**:319-331.

Heino, M. (1987). Morphological changes related to ciliogenesis in the bronchial epithelium in experimental conditions and clinical course of disease. *Eur. J. Respir. Dis.* **151**(suppl):1-39.

Heino, M., Mönkäre, S., Haahtela, T., and Laitinen, L. A. (1982). An electronmicroscopic study of the airways in patients with farmer's lung. *Eur. J. Respir. Dis.* **36**:52-61.

Heino, M., Karjalainen, J., Ylikoski, J., et al. (1988). Bronchial ciliogenesis and oral steroid treatment in patients with asthma. *Br. J. Dis. Chest* **82**: 175-178.

Hers, J. F. P. H. (1966). Disturbances of the ciliated epithelium due to influenza virus. *Am. Rev. Respir. Dis.* **93**:162-171.

Hinson, J. M., Hutchinson, A. A., Brigham, K. L., Meyrick, B. O., and Snapper, J. R. (1984). Effects of granulocyte depletion on pulmonary responsiveness to aerosol histamine. *J. Appl. Physiol.* **56**:411-417.

Holtzmann, M. J., Fabbri, L. M., and O'Byrne, P. M. (1983). Importance of airway inflammation for hyperresponsiveness induced by ozone. *Am. Rev. Respir. Dis.* **127**:686-690.

Horn, B. R., Robin, E. D., Theodore, J. A., and Van Kessel, A. (1975). Total eosinophil counts in the management of bronchial asthma. *N. Engl. J. Med.* **292**:1152.

Huber, H. L., and Koessler, K. K. (1922). The pathology of bronchial asthma. *Arch. Intern. Med.* **30**:687-760.

Hulbert, V. M., McLean, T., and Hogg, J. C. (1985). The effect of acute airway inflammation on bronchial reactivity in guinea-pigs. *Am. Rev. Respir. Dis.* **132**:7-11.

Hynes, R. O., and Yamada, K. M. (1982). Fibronectins: multifunctional modular glycoproteins. *J. Cell Biol.* **95**:369-377.

Jancso, N., Jancso-Gabor, A., and Szolcsanyi, J. (1967). Direct evidence for neurogenic inflammation and its prevention by denervation and by pretreatment with capsaicin. *Br. J. Pharmacol.* **31**:131-151.

Keenan, K. P., Combs, J. W., and McDowell, E. M. (1982a). Regeneration of hamster tracheal epithelium after mechanical injury. I. Focal lesions: quantitative morphologic study of cell proliferation. *Virchows Arch. B. (Cell Pathol.)* **41**:193-214.

Keenan, K. P., Combs, J. W., and McDowell, E. M. (1982b). Regeneration of hamster tracheal epithelium after mechanical injury. II. Multifocal lesions: stathmokinetic and autoradiographic studies of cell proliferation. *Virchows Arch. B. (Cell Pathol.)* **41**:215-229.

King, A. S., McLelland, J., Cook, R. D., King, D. Z., and Walsh, C. (1974). The ultrastructure of afferent nerve endings in the avian lung. *Respir. Physiol.* **22**:21-40.

Kröll, F., Karlsson, J.-A., Lundberg, J. M., and Persson, C. G. A. (1989). Capsaicin-induced bronchoconstriction and neuropeptide release in a perfused guinea-pig bronchopulmonary in vitro preparation. *J. Appl. Physiol.* (submitted).

Laitinen, A. (1985). Ultrastructural organization of intraepithelial nerves in the human airway tract. *Thorax* **40**:488-492.

Laitinen, A., Partanen, M., Hervonen, A., and Laitinen, L. A. (1985a). Electron microscopic study of the innervation of the human lower respiratory tract. Evidence of adrenergic nerves. *Eur. J. Respir. Dis.* **67**:209-215.

Laitinen, A., Partanen, M., Hervonen, A., Pelto-Huikko, M., and Laitinen, L. A. (1985b). VIP-like immunoreactive nerves in human respiratory tract. *Histochemistry* **82**:313-319.

Laitinen, A., Laitinen, L. A., Moss, R., and Widdicombe, J. G. (1989a). Organization and structure of the tracheal and bronchial blood vessels in the dog. *J. Anat.* **165**133-140.

Laitinen, A., Tervo, K., Haahtela, T., Tervo, T., and Laitinen, L. A. (1989b). Fibronectin may take part in healing of bronchial epithelial damage in asthmatic patients. *Eur. Respir.*

Laitinen, L. A. (1974). Histamine and methacholine challenge in the testing of bronchial reactivity. *Scand. J. Respir. Dis.* **86**(Suppl:1-48).

Laitinen, L. A. (1988). Detailed analysis of neural elements in human airways. In *Neural Regulation of the Airways in Health and Disease*. Edited by M. Kaliner and P. Barnes. New York, Marcel Dekker, pp. 35-56.

Laitinen, L. A. (1989). Epithelial damage. In *Glucocorticoids and Mechanisms of Asthma*. Edited by F. E. Hargreave, J. C. Hogg, J. L. Malo, J. H. Toogood. Amsterdam, Excerpta Medica, pp. 215-229.

Laitinen, L. A., Heino, M., Laitinen, A., Kava, T., and Haahtela, T. (1985c). Damage of the airway epithelium and bronchial reactivity in patients with asthma. *Am. Rev. Respir. Dis.* **131**:599-606.

Laitinen, L. A., and Laitinen, A. (1987). Innervation of airway smooth muscle. *Am. Rev. Respir. Dis.* **136**:S38-57.

Laitinen, L. A., and Laitinen, A. (1990). Histology and Electronmicroscopy. In *The Bronchial Circulation in Health and Disease*. Edited by J. Butler, New York, Marcel Dekker.

Laitinen, L. A., Robinson, N. P., Laitinen, A., Widdicombe, J. G. (1986). Relationship between mucosal thickness and vascular resistance in dogs. *J. Appl. Physiol.* **61**(6):2186-2193.

Laitinen, L. A., Laitinen, A., Salonen, R. O., and Widdicombe, J. G. (1987a). Vascular actions of airway neuropeptides. *Am. Rev. Respir. Dis.* **136**: S59-64.

Laitinen, L. A., Laitinen, A., and Widdicombe, J. G. (1987b). Efffects of inflammatory and other mediators on airway vascular beds. *Am. Rev. Respir. Dis.* **135**(6):S67-70.

Laitinen, L. A., Laitinen, A., Heino, M., and Haahtela, T. (1990). The effect of inhaled corticosteroid on airway inflammation in an asthmatic patient. *Am. Rev. Respir. Dis.* (submitted).

Larsell, G., and Dow, L. S. (1933). The innervation of the human lung. *Am. J. Anat.* **52**:125-146.

Lauweryns, J. M., and Peuskens, J. C. (1972). Neuro-epithelial bodies (neuro-receptor or secretory organs?) in human infant bronchial and bronchiolar epithelium. *Anat. Rec.* **172**:471-482.

Lauweryns, J. M., De Boc, V., Guelinckx, P., and Decramer, M. (1983). Effects of unilateral hypoxia on neuroepithelial bodies in rabbit lungs. *J. Appl. Physiol.* **55**:1665-1668.

Lauweryns, J. M., Van Lommer, A. T., and Dom, R. J. (1985). Innervation of rabbit intrapulmonary neuroepithelial bodies. Quantitative and qualitative ultrastructural study after vagotomy. *J. Neurol. Sci.* **67**:81-92.

Lee, L.-Y., Bleecker, E. R., and Nadel, J. A. (1977). Effect of ozone on bronchometer response to inhaled histamine aerosol in dog. *J. Appl. Physiol.* **43**:626-631.

Lee, T-C., Lenihan, D. J., Malone, B., Roddy, L. L., Wasserman, S. I. (1984). Increased biosynthesis of platelet-activating factor in activated human eosinophils. *J. Biol. Chem.* **259**:5526-5530.

Liebow, A. A. (1960). The bronchopulmonary venous collateral circulation with special reference to emphysema. *Am. J. Pathol.* **37**:361-380.

Lundberg, J. M., and Saria, A. (1983). Capsaicin-induced desensitization of airway mucosa to cigarette smoke, mechanical and chemical irritants. *Nature* **302**:251-253.

Lundberg, J. M., Hökfelt, T., Kewenter, J., Pettersson, G., Ahlman, H., Edin, R., Dahlström, A., Nilsson, G., Terenius, L., Uvnäs-Wallenstein, K., and Said, S. (1979). Substance P-, VIP- and enkephalin-like immunoreactivity in the human vagus nerve. *Gastroenterology* **77**:469-471.

Lundgren, R., Söderberg, M., Hörstedt, and Stenling, R. (1988). Morphological studies of bronchi mucosal biopsies from asthmatics before and after ten years of treatment with inhaled steroids. *Eur. Respir. J.* **1**:883-889.

McDonald, D. M. (1987). Neurogenic inflammation in the respiratory tract: actions of sensory nerve mediators on blood vessels and epithelium of the airway mucosa. *Am. Rev. Respir. Dis.* **136**:65-72.

McDonald, D. M. (1988). Respiratory tract infections increase susceptibility to neurogenic inflammation in the rat trachea. *Am. Rev. Respir. Dis.* **137**:1432-1440.

McDowell, E. M., and Beals, T. F. (1987). *Biopsy Pathology of the Bronchi.* Philadelphia, W. B. Saunders.

McDowell, E. M., Becci, P. J., Schürch, W., and Trump, F. F. (1979). The respiratory epithelium. VII. Epidermoid metaplasia of hamster tracheal epithelium during regeneration following mechanical injury. *J. Natl. Cancer Inst.* **62**:995-1008.

McLaughlin, R. F., Jr. (1983). Bronchial artery distribution in various mammals and humans. *Am. Rev. Respir. Dis.* **128**:S57-58.

Melen, J., and Pipkorn, U. (1985). Mast cells on the surface of the mucous membrane—a general features in inflammatory reactions in the nose? *Rhinology* **23**:187.

Miller, S. W. (1947). *The Lung,* 2nd ed. Springfield Il, Charles C. Thomas.

Mullen, J. B. M., Wiggs, B. R., Wright, J. L., Hogg, J. C., and Pare, P. D. (1986). Nonspecific airway reactivity in cigarette smokers. *Am. Rev. Respir. Dis.* **133**:120-125.

Murlas, C., and Roum, J. H. (1985a). Bronchial hyperreactivity occurs in steoidtreated guinea-pigs depleted of leukocytes by cyclophosphamide. *J. Appl. Physiol.* **58**:1630-1637.

Murlas, C., and Roum, J. H. (1985b). Sequence of pathological change in the airway mucosa of guinea-pigs during ozone induced bronchial hyperreactivity. *Am. Rev. Respir. Dis.* **131**:314-320.

Nadel, J. (1984). Inflammation and asthma. *J. Allergy. Clin. Immunol.* **73**: 651-653.

Nadel, J. A., and Barnes, P. J. (1984). Autonomic regulation of the airways. *Annu. Rev. Med.* **35**:451-467.

Naylor, B. (1962). The shedding of the mucosa of the bronchial tree in asthma. *Thorax* **17**:69-72.

Oertel, H. L., and Kaliner, M. A. (1981). The biological activity of mast cell granules. III. Purification of inflammatory factors of anaphylaxis (IF-A) responsible for causing late-phase reactions. *J. Immunol.* **112**: 1398-1402.

Persson, C. G. A. (1986). Role of plasma exudation in asthmatic airways. *Lancet* **2**:1126-1128.

Persson, C. G. A. (1988). Plasma exudation and asthma. *Lung* **166**:1-23.

Phillips, M. J., Calonico, L., and Gold, W. M. (1982). Morphological and pharmacological characterization of dog mastocytoma cells. *Am. Rev. Respir. Dis.* **125**:63A.

Pietra, G. G., and Magno, M. (1978). Pharmacologic factors influencing permeability of the bronchial microcirculation. *Fed. Proc.* **37**:2466-2470.

Pietra, G. G., Szidon, J. P., Leventhal, M. M., and Fisherman, A. P. (1971). Histamine and interstitial pulmonary edema in the dog. *Circ. Res.* **29**: 323-337.

Reid, L. (1974). Histological aspects of bronchial secretion. *Scand. J. Respir. Dis.* **90**Suppl:9-15.

Rhodin, J. A. G. (1974). Respiratory system. In *Histology*. New York/London/Toronto, Oxford University Press, pp. 607-645.

Richardson, J. B. (1979). Nerve supply to the lungs. *Am. Rev. Respir. Dis.* **119**:785-802.

Saksela, O., Alitalo, K., Kiistala, U., and Vaheri, A. (1981). Basal lamina components in experimentally induced skin blisters. *J. Invest. Dermatol.* **77**:283-286.

Salvato, G. (1968). Asthma and mast cells of bronchial connective tissue. *Experientia* **18**:330-331.

Sanerkin, N. G., and Evans, D. M. D. (1965). The sputum in bronchial asthma: pathognomic patterns. *J. Pathol.* **89**:535-541.

Schatz, M., Wasserman, S., and Patterson, R. (1981). Eosinophils and immunologic lung disease. *Med. Clin. North Am.* **65**:1055-1071.

Sobonoya, R. E. (1984). Concise clinical study: quantitative structural alterations in long standing allergic asthma. *Am. Rev. Respir. Dis.* **130**:289.

Solley, G. O., Gleich, G. J., and Jordan Scroeter, A. L. (1976). Late phase of the immediate sheal and flare skin reaction: its dependence on IgE antibodies. *J. Clin. Invest.* **58**:408-420.

Spencer, H., and Leof, D. (1964). The innervation of the human lung. *J. Anat.* **98**:599-609.

Suslov, K. I. (1895). Some investigators on the anatomy of the bronchial arteries in man. Thesis, St Petersburgh, USSR. (translated from Russian).

Takizawa, T., and Thurlbeck, W. M. (1971). Muscle and mucous gland size in the major bronchi of patients with chronic bronchitis, asthma and asthmatic bronchitis. *Am. Rev. Respir. Dis.* **104**:331-336.

Tannenbaum, S., Oertel, H., Henderson, W. R., and Kaliner, M. (1980). The biologic activity of mast cell granules. I. Elicitation of inflammatory responses in rat skin. *J. Immunol.* **125**:325-335.

Thurlbeck, W. M., Henderson, J. A., Fraser, R. G., and Bates, D. V. (1970). Chronic obstructive lung disease. A comparison between clinical, roentgenologic functional and morphologic criteria in chronic bronchitis, emphysema, asthma and bronchiectasis. *Med.* **49**:81-147.

Tomioka, M., Ida, S., Shondoh, Y., et al. (1984). Mast cells in bronchoalveolar lumen of patients with bronchial asthma. *Am. Rev. Respir. Dis.* **129**:1000-1005.

Turnbull, L. S., Turnbull, L. W., Crofton, L. W., and Kay, A. B. (1978). Immunoglobulins, complement and arylsulphatase in sputum from chronic bronchitis and other pulmonary diseases. *Clin. Exp. Immunol.* **32**:226-232.

Vaheri, A., Salonen, E.-M., Vartio, T., Hedman, K., and Stenman, S. (1983). Fibronectin and tissue injury. In *Biology and Pathology of the Vessel Wall.* Edited by N. Woolf. Eastbourne, Praeger, p. 161.

Vaheri, A., Salonen, E.-M., and Vartio, T. (1985). Fibronectin in formation and degradation of the pericellular matrix. In *Fibrosis, Ciba Foundation Symposium.* Edited by D. Evered and J. Whelan. London, Pitman, p. 111.

Venge, P., Dahl, R., Hällgren, R., and Olsson, I. (1980). Cationic proteins of human eosinophils and their role in the inflammatory reaction. In *The Eosinophil in Health and Disease.* Edited by A. A. F. Mahmoud and K. F. Austen. New York, Grune & Stratton, pp. 131-144.

Venge, P., Hakansson, L., and Peterson, C. G. B. (1987). Eosinophil activation in allergic disease. *Int. Arch. Allergy Appl. Immunol.* **82**:333-337.

Wardlaw, A. J., Dunnette, S., Gleich, G. J., Collins, J. V., and Kay, A. B. (1988). Eosinophils and mast cells in bronchoalveolar lavage in subjects with mild asthma. *Am. Rev. Respir. Dis.* **137**:62-69.

Weller, P. F., Lee, C. W., Foster, D. W., Corey, E. J., Austen, K. F., and Lewis, R. A. (1983). Generation and metabolism of 5-lipoxygenase pathway leukotrienes by human eosinophils: predominant production of leukotriene C_4. *Proc. Natl. Acad. Sci. USA* **80**:7626-7630.

Wenzel, S. E., Fowler, A. A., and Schwartz, L. B. (1988). Activation of pulmonary mast cells by bronchoalveolar allergen challenge. *Am. Rev. Respir. Dis.* **137**:1002-1008.

Wilhelm, D. L. (1953). Regeneration of tracheal epithelium. *J. Pathol. Bacteriol.* **65**:543-550.

Yamada, K. M., and Olden, K. (1978). Fibronectin-adhesive glycoproteins of cell surface and blood. *Nature* **275**:179-184.

5

Epithelium-Dependent Responses in Airways

MICHAEL F. BUSK

Mayo Clinic and Mayo Foundation
Rochester, Minnesota

PAUL M. VANHOUTTE

Baylor College of Medicine
Houston, Texas

I. Introduction

The respiratory epithelium may play an important role in regulating airway reactivity and damage to it could contribute to the abnormal responses characteristic of asthma. Indeed, there is in vitro evidence that removal of the epithelium increases the sensitivity of the smooth muscle to various stimuli and that this effect is not due to the simple loss of a protective barrier but may involve the release of epithelium-derived bronchoactive factor(s) (Cuss and Barnes, 1987; Farmer, 1987; Vanhoutte, 1987a, 1988b; Fedan et al., 1988; Goldie et al., 1988; Stuart-Smith and Vanhoutte, 1989). An analogous situation exists in the vascular system, where endothelial cells release relaxing and contracting factors that modulate the tone of the underlying smooth muscle (e.g., Furchgott, 1984; Rubanyi and Vanhoutte, 1985; Vanhoutte et al., 1986; Vanhoutte, 1987b,c; Furchgott and Vanhoutte, 1989). This chapter will summarize the data accumulated since the first observations that demonstrated the influence of the epithelium on the responsiveness of bronchial smooth muscle, and discuss the concept that epithelial cells release relaxing and contracting factor(s) that contribute to the regulatory functions of the respiratory tract in health and disease.

II. Initial Method of Investigation of the Phenomenon

The initial experiments were designed to determine whether the emerging principle of the modulation of vascular tone by endothelium-derived factors also applied to another tubular structure, the bronchus, and the cells lining its lumen, the epithelium (Aarhus et al., 1984; Flavahan and Vanhoutte, 1984; Flavahan et al., 1985). The first step was to see if it was possible to remove only the epithelial cell layer without disturbing the underlying structures. This procedure was accomplished by gentle rubbing of the luminal surface of an isolated canine bronchus with stainless steel forceps. The epithelial cells were removed without obvious morphological distortion of the underlying layers, in particular the smooth muscle, at the light microscopic level (Fig. 1; Flavahan et al., 1985). Furthermore, removal of the epithelium did not alter the length-tension characteristics of the bronchial rings, suggesting that the integrity of the bronchial smooth muscle was not affected.

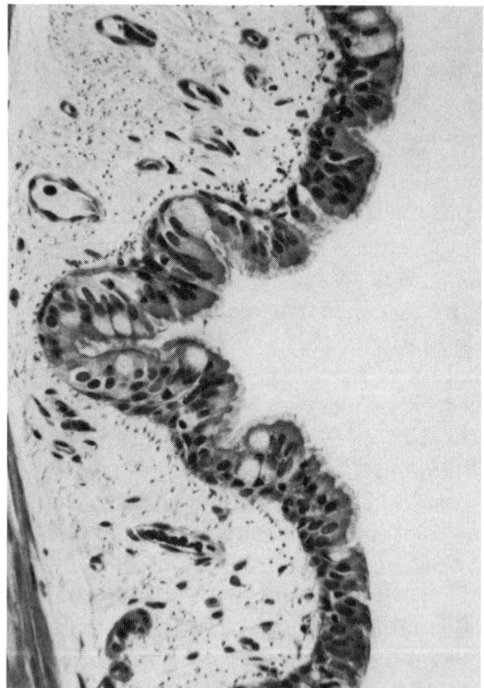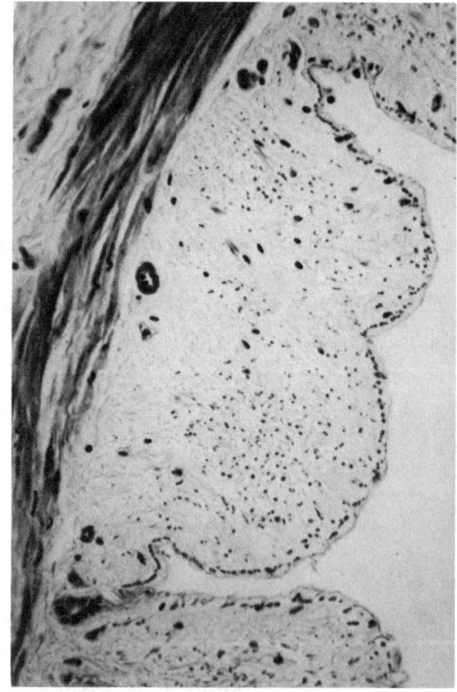

Figure 1   Histological section demonstrates that gentle rubbing of the luminal surface of canine bronchi removes epithelial cells (right) (reprinted from Gao and Vanhoutte, 1988, by permission).

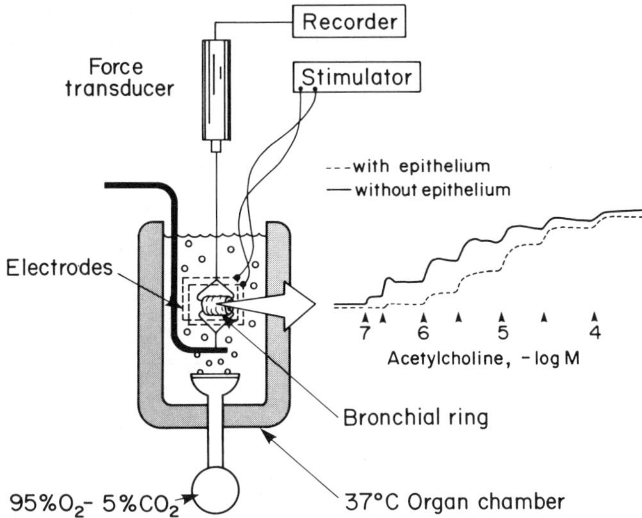

Figure 2 Organ chamber for the study of isolated airways. Arrow points to isometric tension recordings in a ring with epithelium (lower) and a ring without epithelium (upper) of the trachea of the same dog. The preparations were contracted with increasing concentrations of acetylcholine. Note that the ring with epithelium contracts to a lesser degree than the ring without epithelium (reprinted from Stuart-Smith and Vanhoutte, 1989, by permission).

Thus, the responsiveness of isolated bronchi (or tracheas) with or without epithelium to various pharmacological agents could be investigated in vitro (Fig. 2).

In the canine bronchus, removal of the epithelium shifted the concentration-response curves to acetylcholine (Fig. 3), histamine (Fig. 4), and 5-hydroxytryptamine (Fig. 4) to the left, without affecting the maximal response to the agonists (Flavahan et al., 1985). These observations suggest that the loss of the epithelial cell layer in the canine bronchus potentiates the reactivity of the underlying smooth muscle to various bronchoconstrictors. Variations of this experimental method with similar observations have been extended to other species, including isolated airways from cattle, cats, guinea pigs, pigs, rabbits, rats and humans (see Tables 1-3).

Table 1 Epithelium Removal and Response of Airway Smooth Muscle to Contractile Agents in Vitro

Reference	Species	Tissue	Contractile Agent	Sensitivity (ED_{50})	Maximal Response
Aarhus et al., 1984	Dog	Bronchus (3° & 4°)	Acetylcholine	↑	—
			Histamine	—	—
			5-hydroxytryptamine	↑	—
			Potassium chloride	—	—
Flavahan et al., 1985	Dog	Bronchus (3° & 4°)	Acetylcholine	↑	—
			Histamine[a]	↑	—
			5-hydroxytryptamine	↑	—
Hay et al., 1987c	Dog	Bronchus (2°)	Methacholine	↑	—
			Histamine	↑	↑
			Potassium chloride	—	—
		Bronchus (3°)	Methacholine	—	—
			Histamine	—	—
			Potassium chloride	—	—
Stuart-Smith and Vanhoutte, 1987	Dog	Bronchus (2°)	Acetylcholine	↑	—
			Histamine[a]	↑	—
			5-hydroxytryptamine	↑	—
			Potassium chloride	—	—
		Bronchus (3°)	Acetylcholine	↑	—
			Histamine[a]	↑	—
			5-hydroxytryptamine	↑	—
			Potassium chloride	—	—
		Bronchus (4°)	Acetylcholine	—	—
			Histamine[a]	—	—

Reference	Species	Tissue	Agonist		
			5-hydroxytryptamine	—	—
			Potassium chloride	—	—
Barnes et al., 1985	Bovine	Trachea	Acetylcholine	↑	↑
			Histamine	↑	↑
			5-hydroxytryptamine	↑	↑
			Potassium chloride	—	—
Thompson et al., 1988	Cat	Trachea	Acetylcholine	—	—
			5-hydroxytryptamine	—	—
		Bronchus	Acetylcholine	—	—
			5-hydroxytryptamine	↑	—
Thompson et al., 1985	Guinea Pig	Trachea	Acetylcholine	↑	—
			Histamine	↑	—
Finnen et al., 1986	Guinea Pig	Trachea	Acetylcholine	↑	↑
			5-hydroxytryptamine	↑	NR
	Ovalbumin-sensitized guinea pig	Trachea	Acetylcholine	—	NR
Goldie et al., 1986	Guinea Pig	Trachea	Acetylcholine	—	—
			Carbachol	—	—
			Histamine	↑	—
			Potassium chloride	—	—
Hay et al., 1986a	Guinea Pig	Trachea	Methacholine	↑	—
			Histamine	↑	↑
			Potassium chloride	—[b]	—[b]

Table 1 Continued Epithelium Removal and Response of Airway Smooth Muscle to Contractile Agents in Vitro

Reference	Species	Tissue	Contractile Agent	Sensitivity (ED$_{50}$)	Maximal Response
Hay et al., 1986b	Guinea Pig	Trachea	Methacholine	↑	—
			Histamine	↑	↑
			Potassium chloride	—[b]	—[b]
	Ovalbumin-sensitized guinea pig	Trachea	Ovalbumin	↑	—
			Methacholine	↑	—
			Histamine	↑	—
			Potassium chloride	↑	—
Holroyde, 1986	Guinea Pig	Trachea	Acetylcholine	↑	—
			Histamine	↑	—
			5-hydroxytryptamine	↑	—
			Potassium chloride	↑	—
Murlas, 1986	Guinea Pig	Trachea	Acetylcholine	↑	—
			Histamine	↑	—
			K$^+$	—	—
Tschirhart and Landry, 1986	Guinea Pig	Trachea	Substance P	↑	NR
Hay et al., 1987a	Guinea Pig	Trachea	Leukotriene C$_4$	↑	—
			Leukotriene D$_4$	↑	—
			Leukotriene E$_4$	—	—
			5-hydroxytryptamine	—	—
			U-44069[c]	—	—
	Ovalbumin-sensitized guinea pig	Trachea	Leukotriene C$_4$	↑	—
			Leukotriene D$_4$	↑	—

Table 1 continues

Reference	Species	Tissue	Agonist		
			Leukotriene E$_4$	—	—
			5-hydroxytryptamine	—	—
			U-44069[c]	—	—
Tschirhart et al., 1987	Guinea pig	Trachea	Histamine	↑	—
			Carbachol	—	—
Undem et al., 1987	Ovalbumin-sensitized guinea pig	Trachea	Ovalbumin	↑	—
			Histamine	↑	—
Braunstein et al., 1988	Guinea pig	Trachea	Histamine	↑	↑
Devillier et al., 1988	Guinea pig	Trachea	Substance P	↑	—
			Neurokinin A	↑	—
			Neurokinin B	↑	—
Frossard et al., 1988	Guinea pig	Trachea	Substance P	↑	↑
			Neurokinin A	↑	↑
			Neurokinin B	NR	↑
Grandordy et al., 1988	Guinea pig	Trachea	Substance P	↑	NR
			Neurokinin A	↑	NR
			Neurokinin B	↑	NR
			L 363851[d]	—	NR
Lundblad and Persson, 1988	Guinea pig	Trachea	Carbachol	—	↓
			Substance P	—	—
			Capsaicin	—	—
Stuart-Smith and Vanhoutte, 1988b	Pig	Bronchus (3°)	Acetylcholine	↑	—
			Histamine	↑	—
			Potassium chloride	—	↓
		Bronchus (4°)	Acetylcholine	↑	—
			Histamine	—[e]	—
			Potassium chloride	—	↓

Reference	Species	Tissue	Agonist		
		Bronchus (5°)	Acetylcholine	—[e]	↓
			Histamine	↑	—
			Potassium chloride	—	—
Raeburn et al., 1986a	Rabbit	Trachea	Methacholine	—	—
			Potassium chloride	—	—
		Bronchus (1°)	Methacholine	↑	—
			Potassium chloride	—	↓
		Bronchus (2°)	Methacholine	↑	—
			Histamine	—[e]	—
Butler et al., 1987	Rabbit	Bronchi	Bethanechol	↑	NR
Frossard and Muller, 1986	Ovalbumin-sensitized rat	Trachea	5-hydroxytryptamine	↑	NR
			Carbachol	—	—
Raeburn et al., 1986b	Human	Trachea	Methacholine	↑	—
Aizawa et al., 1988	Human	Bronchi	Acetylcholine	↑	—
			Histamine	↑	—
			Prostaglandin $F_{2\alpha}$	↑	—

— = No effect.
↑ = Increased sensitivity or maximal response after epithelium removal.
↓ = Decreased sensitivity or maximal response after epithelium removal.
NR = Not reported.
ED_{50} = Concentration producing 50% of the maximal response.
1° = Primary bronchus (rabbit)
2° = Secondary bronchus (rabbit).

2° = Lobar bronchus (dog).
3° = Segmental bronchus (dog, pig).
4° = Subsegmental bronchus (dog, pig).
5° = Subsegmental bronchus (pig).
[a]In presence of atropine (10^{-8} M).
[b]Increased sensitivity at low concentration and decreased maximal response in five of eight preparations.
[c]Thromboxane mimetic.
[d]A selective NK_2-receptor agonist.
[e]Increased sensitivity at low concentrations.

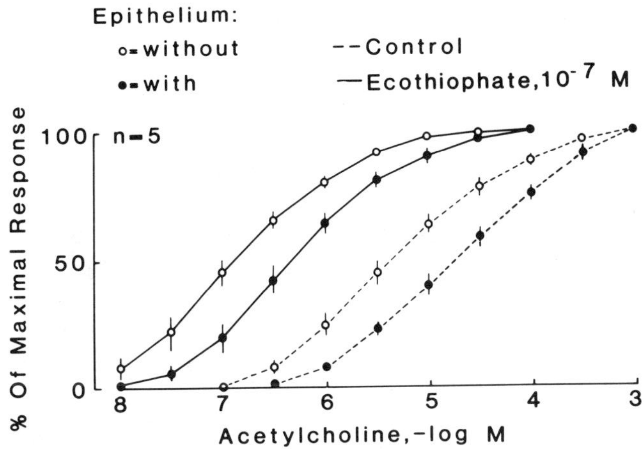

Figure 3 Effect of removal of the epithelium on concentration-response curves to acetylcholine in canine bronchi. Closed circles, rings with epithelium; open circles, rings without endothelium; dashed lines, responses under control conditions; solid lines, responses after inhibition of acetylcholinesterase (the major enzyme responsible for the breakdown of the cholinergic transmitter). Note in both cases a marked shift to the left of the concentration-response curve after removal of the epithelium (reprinted from Flavahan et al., 1985, by permission).

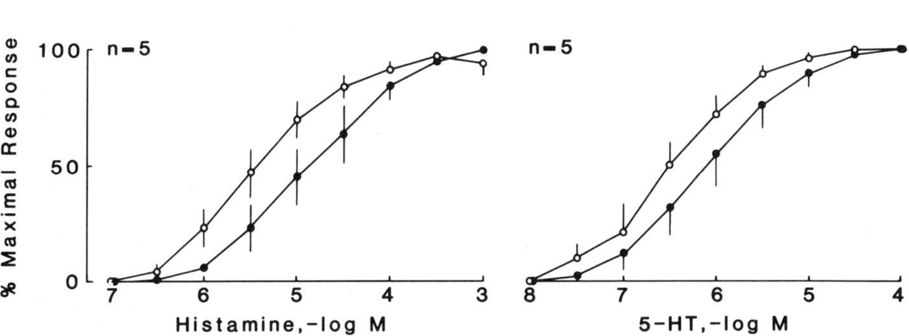

Figure 4 Effects of removal of the epithelium on concentration-response curves to histamine and 5-hydroxytryptamine (5-HT) in canine bronchi. Closed circles, bronchial rings with epithelium; open circles, rings without epithelium (reprinted from Flavahan et al., 1985, by permission).

III. Mechanisms for the Hyperresponsiveness Evoked by Epithelium Removal

The phenomenon of potentiation of bronchoconstriction by removal of the epithelium has been well established and the action of epithelium-derived relaxing factor(s) has been proposed as the mechanism. However, there are other possible explanations for the phenomenon.

A nonspecific change in the sensitivity of the airway smooth muscle could be one explanation for the hyperresponsiveness evoked by removal of the epithelium. However, this mechanism seems unlikely because contractions evoked by increasing concentrations of potassium ions are not affected by removal of the epithelium (Fig. 5, top; Aarhus et al., 1984; Barnes et al.,

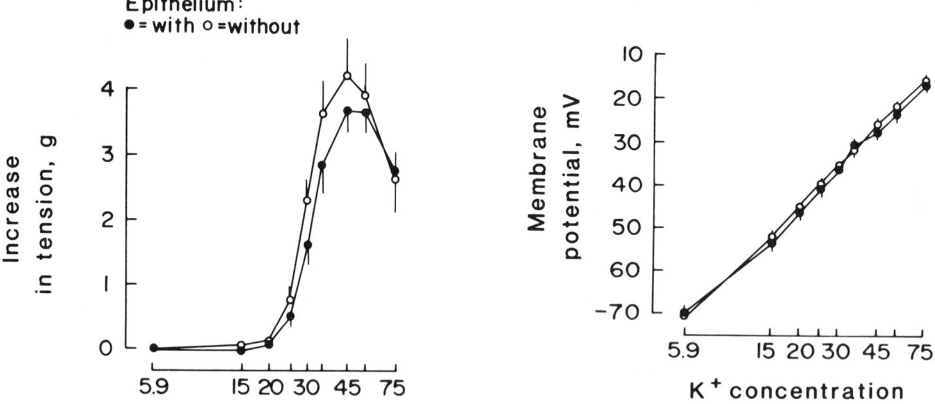

Figure 5 Responsiveness of canine bronchial strips to increasing concentrations of potassium chloride (K^+) in rings with (closed circles) and without (open circles) epithelium. Top: tension; each group contains seven preparations from different animals. Bottom: membrane potential; each group contains 8-14 successful impalements of cells from the same 7 preparations. The data are shown as means ± SEM. No significant differences were noted between the two groups, which implies that the procedure to remove the epithelium has not altered the ability of the bronchial smooth muscle to be activated directly (reprinted from Gao and Vanhoutte, 1988, by permission).

1985; Goldie et al., 1986; Murlas, 1986; Hay et al., 1987c; Stuart-Smith and Vanhoutte, 1987; Gao and Vanhoutte, 1988). Furthermore, removal of the epithelium does not affect the resting membrane potential in canine bronchial smooth muscle and does not affect the concentration-depolarization curve to potassium ions (Fig. 5, bottom; Gao and Vanhoutte, 1988). This implies that the procedure to remove the epithelium does not alter the ability of the bronchial smooth muscle to be activated directly.

Another possible explanation is a reduced enzymatic breakdown of the bronchoconstrictor agonists. This is certainly not the case for acetylcholine and 5-hydroxytryptamine, because after incubation with inhibitors of acetyl-cholinesterase and monoamine oxidase, respectively, the removal of the epithelium still augments the response to these agonists (Fig. 3; Aarhus et al., 1984; Flavahan et al., 1985). However, the epithelium of the guinea pig may play a role in the inactivation of adenosine (Advenier et al., 1988) and the tachykinins (Frossard et al., 1988; Devillier et al., 1988), and in the ex-traneuronal uptake of isoproterenol (Farmer et al., 1986).

The disappearance of a diffusion barrier has also been suggested as an explanation for the potentiation induced by the removal of the epithelium, mainly because of the negative results of superfusion-cascade bioassay ex-periments (Holroyde, 1986; Undem et al., 1988). Theoretically, this is a very logical explanation since the epithelium serves as a protective barrier (Gao and Vanhoutte, 1989a). This mechanism may possibly contribute to the aug-mentation of antigen-induced contractions by removal of the epithelium (Undem et al., 1988). However, several reasons argue against this being the sole and primary mechanism underlying the phenomenon. First, in canine bronchi, the inhibitory effect of the epithelium is present not only during contractions of the bronchial smooth muscle with exogenous acetylcholine but also during electrical stimulation of the cholinergic nerve endings, a situation in which the cholinergic transmitter is released in the immediate vicinity of the bronchial smooth muscle and thus epithelial diffusion bar-riers do not exist (Fig. 6; Flavahan et al., 1985; Vanhoutte and Flavahan, 1987). Furthermore, the depolarization of the cell membrane of bronchial smooth muscle exposed to exogenous acetylcholine is greater in preparations without epithelium; when the same degree of contraction is compared, the extent of the depolarization in the absence of epithelium is still greater than that observed in bronchi with epithelium (Figs. 7, 8; Gao and Vanhoutte, 1988). Moreover, the role of the epithelium as a diffusion barrier appears unlikely in view of the fact that the hyperresponsiveness on removal of the epithelium has been demonstrated in rings of airways where the broncho-constrictors reach the bronchial smooth muscle from the outside rather than the luminal surface (Fig. 2; Flavahan et al., 1985). A further argument against

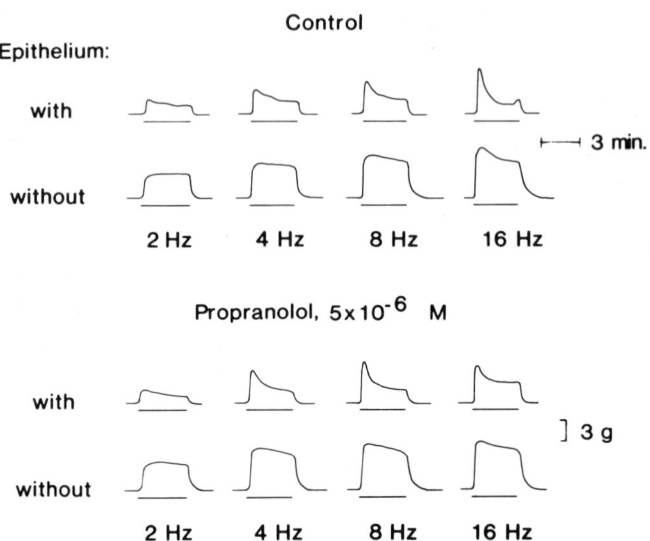

Figure 6 Comparison of the response to electrical activation of the cholinergic nerve endings of two rings, with (upper) and without (lower) epithelium, of the same canine bronchus, (top) under control conditions and (bottom) following propranolol (5 × 10^{-6} M). Note that, particularly at higher frequencies, the initial response of the ring with epithelium is followed by a secondary decrease (fade) in tension during sustained stimulation. In the ring without epithelium, the initial peak response is large and the delay of the response on sustained stimulation (fade) is less pronounced (reprinted from Flavahan et al., 1985, by permission).

the hypothesis that the epithelium acts only as a passive diffusion barrier to bronchoconstrictor agonists is provided by the observations that the hyperresponsiveness associated with epithelium removal is agonist-selective; the reactivity is either affected or unaffected by epithelium removal depending on the substance used to contract or relax the airways (Goldie et al., 1986; Farmer et al., 1986; Hay et al., 1987a; Thompson et al., 1988). Finally, the observations that removal of the epithelium attenuates the relaxation of airways induced by beta-adrenergic agonists (Flavahan and Vanhoutte, 1984; Barnes et al., 1985; Flavahan et al., 1985; Goldie et al., 1986; Ruff et al., 1987; Stuart-Smith and Vanhoutte, 1987, 1988b), arachidonic acid (Flavahan et al., 1986; Nijkamp and Folkerts, 1987; Butler et al., 1987; Farmer et al., 1987; Tschirhart et al., 1987; Braunstein et al., 1988; Stuart-Smith and Vanhoutte, 1988a), the calcium ionophore A 23187 (Flavahan et al., 1986); the calcium antagonist verapamil (Raeburn et al., 1986a,b), the methylxanthines (Busk and Vanhoutte, 1988, 1989), or changes in osmolarity (Munakata et

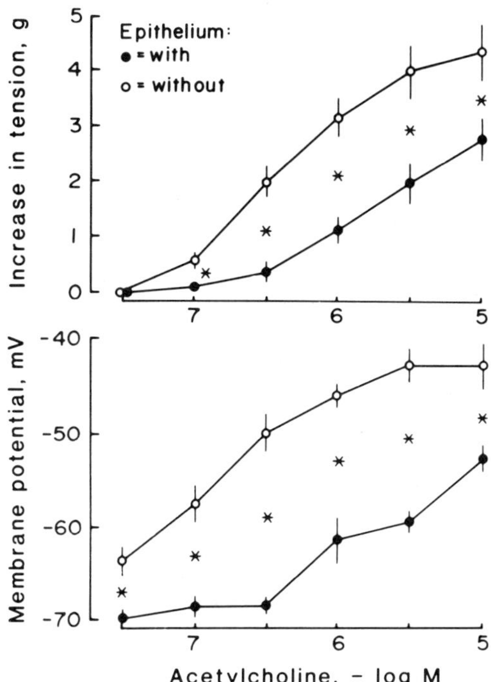

Figure 7 Responses of canine bronchial strips to increasing concentrations of acetylcholine. Closed circles, bronchial strips with epithelium; open circles, bronchial strips without epithelium. Top: changes in tensions; each group contains seven preparations from different animals. Bottom: changes in membrane potential; each group contains 7-14 successful impalements of cells from the same 7 preparations. The asterisk denotes a statistically significant difference between the two groups (reprinted from Gao and Vanhouette, 1988, by permission).

al., 1988a) argue strongly against the removal of either a metabolic sink or a diffusion barrier.

Thus, the most logical explanation for the differences in reactivity between airways with and without epithelium is that the epithelial cells release an inhibitory factor(s) (epithelium-derived relaxing factor[s]) that modulates the tone of the underlying smooth muscle. This conclusion is consistent with results of several bioassay experiments that suggest that the epithelium does indeed secrete a diffusible factor(s) that relaxes bronchial or vascular smooth muscle (Flavahan and Vanhoutte, 1985; Ilhan and Sahin, 1987; Tschirhart and Landry, 1986; Hay et al., 1987b; Aizawa et al., 1988; Guc et al., 1988; Manning et al., 1988; Busk et al., 1989; Fernandes et al., 1989). The ability

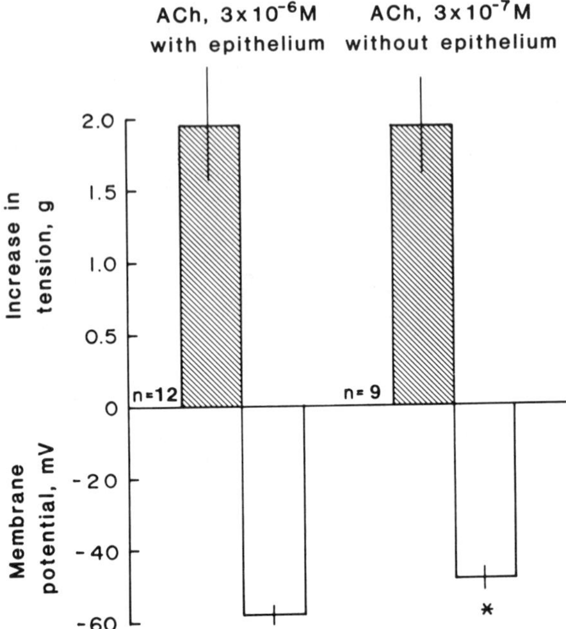

Figure 8 Canine bronchial strips with and without epithelium contracted to the same degree by exposure to 3×10^{-6} and 3×10^{-7} M acetylcholine, respectively. The asterisk denotes a statistically significant difference between the two groups (reprinted from Gao and Vanhoutte, 1988, by permission).

to bioassay an inhibitory factor(s) and the agonist-selectivity of the potentiation upon removal of the epithelium also argue against the possibility that the hyperresponsiveness is part of an inflammatory response triggered by mechanical rubbing of the mucosa.

IV. Epithelium Removal and Response of Isolated Airways in Organ Chamber Studies

This section reviews the effects of epithelium removal on the responses to different stimuli (both contracting and relaxing) in various species and isolated airways. It will illustrate that, in general, the epithelium-dependent inhibition of smooth muscle is explained best by the release of a common relaxing factor(s), with few species-dependent variations, although a heterogeneity in the response exists in airways of different diameters. In addition, data will be discussed that suggest the existence of epithelium-derived contracting (excitatory) factor(s). In order to analyze the reported data, the sensitivity or potency expressed as the concentration of the agonist producing 50% of the maximal response (ED_{50}) and the maximal response to the contractile stimulus will be compared in airways with and without epithelium.

A. Contractile Agents

Removal of the epithelium increases the sensitivity to muscarinic agonists (acetylcholine, methacholine, or bethanechol), histamine, and 5-hydroxytryptamine without an alteration in the maximal response to these agents in the canine bronchus (Aarhus et al., 1984; Flavahan et al., 1985; Hay et al., 1987c; Stuart-Smith and Vanhoutte, 1987), the cat bronchus (Thompson et al., 1988), the guinea pig trachea (Thompson et al., 1985; Finnen et al., 1986; Goldie et al., 1986; Hay et al., 1986a,b; Holroyde, 1986; Murlas, 1986; Tschirhart et al., 1987), the ovalbumin-sensitized guinea pig trachea (Hay et al., 1986b; Undem et al., 1988), the ovalalbumin-sensitized rat trachea (Frossard and Muller, 1986), the porcine bronchus (Stuart-Smith and Vanhoutte, 1988b), the rabbit bronchus (Raeburn et al., 1986a; Butler et al., 1987), and the human bronchus (Raeburn et al., 1986b; Aizawa et al., 1988). Removing the epithelium also enhances the sensitivity and increases the maximal response to acetylcholine, histamine, and 5-hydroxytryptamine in the bovine trachea (Barnes et al., 1985), to histamine in the canine bronchus (Hay et al., 1987c), and to acetylcholine (Finnen et al., 1986) and histamine (Hay et al., 1986a,b; Braunstein et al., 1988) in the guinea pig trachea. These observations suggest that the epithelium from different species may release an inhibitory factor(s) (epithelium-derived relaxing factor[s]) that partially counteracts the activation of the airway smooth muscle by contractile agents. However, an opposite effect occurs in the small-diameter bronchi of the pig. In this species, removal of the epithelium results in a reduction in the maximal response to high concentrations of acetylcholine; thus, this implies the release of a contracting factor(s) from the epithelium that potentiates the maximal response to the contractile agonist and attenuates any effect of epithelium-derived relaxing factor(s) (Stuart-Smith and Vanhoutte, 1988b).

In general, contractions evoked by increasing concentrations of potassium ions in various species and types of airways are not affected by removal of the epithelium (Aarhus et al., 1984; Barnes et al., 1985; Goldie et al., 1986; Murlas, 1986; Hay et al., 1987c; Stuart-Smith and Vanhoutte, 1987). The effect of epithelium removal on potassium-induced contractions in the guinea pig also results in an increased sensitivity at low concentrations only (Hay et al., 1986a, 1986b) and a small potentiation of the response at the ED_{50} (Hay et al., 1986b; Holroyde, 1986). In contrast, removal of the epithelium reduces the maximal response to potassium ions in the airways of the guinea pig (Hay et al., 1986a,b), pig (Stuart-Smith and Vanhoutte, 1988b), and rabbit (Raeburn et al., 1986a), which suggests an excitatory or a contracting influence by the epithelium in these species.

The epithelium of the guinea pig may affect the contractile response of the smooth muscle to antigens and the tachykinins not only by the release of epithelium-derived factor(s). In the antigen-sensitized guinea pig, the sensitivity to ovalbumin in the epithelium-denuded trachea is increased without a difference in the maximal response when compared with intact preparations (Hay et al., 1986b; Undem et al., 1988). This effect has been attributed in part, to the role of the epithelium as a diffusion barrier that can limit the rate of influx of antigen molecules and thereby influence the activation of mast cell in the tissue (Undem et al., 1988). Removal of the epithelium from the guinea pig trachea significantly enhances the sensitivity without affecting the maximal response to the tachykinins and related peptides (Tschirhart and Landry, 1986; Frossard et al., 1988; Grandordy et al., 1988; Devillier et al., 1988), although in one study the response to substance P was not altered (Lundblad and Persson, 1988). The potentiation may involve, in part, the absence of enzymatic degradation of the tachykinins by the epithelium (Frossard et al., 1988; Devillier et al., 1988).

B. Electrical Field Stimulation

Because the neurotransmitter is released in the immediate vicinity of the smooth muscle, electrical field stimulation of airway preparations provides direct evidence that the epithelium modulates the responsiveness of the underlying smooth muscle (Flavahan et al., 1985; Vanhoutte and Flavahan, 1987) (Table 2). Transmural nerve stimulation in the airways causes activation of cholinergic (leading to contraction), adrenergic (leading to relaxation), and nonadrenergic noncholinergic (leading to relaxation) nerve fibers (Altiere et al., 1984; Coburn and Tomita, 1973; Russell, 1978, 1980; Vermeire and Vanhoutte, 1979). In the canine bronchus, the effect of nonadrenergic noncholinergic stimulation leading to relaxation is minor (Russell, 1980). Following beta-adrenoreceptor blockade, removal of the epithelium from the canine bronchus augments the initial contractile response evoked by low-frequency stimulation of the cholinergic nerve endings and reduces the fade of the contractile response during continuous, sustained stimulation (Fig. 6; Flavahan et al., 1985). Removing the epithelium increases the sensitivity of the initial response to electrical field stimulation also in the guinea pig trachea (Murlas, 1986), although not all studies in the guinea pig agree (Holroyde, 1986; Thompson et al., 1988). The initial response to electrical stimulation was not affected by epithelium removal either in the cat airway (Thompson et al., 1988) or the bovine trachea (Barnes et al., 1985), in the presence and

Table 2 Epithelium Removal and Response of Airway Smooth Muscle to Electrical Field Stimulation

Reference	Species	Tissue	Stimulation	Sensitivity	Maximal Response
Flavahan et al., 1985	Dog	Bronchus (3° & 4°)	Initial response[a] (18 s)	—[b]	—
			Sustained response[a] (3 min)	↑	↑
Barnes et al., 1985	Bovine	Trachea	Initial response (20 s)	—	—
Thompson et al., 1988	Cat	Trachea	Initial response[a] (5 s)	—	—
		Trachea	Initial response[c] (5 s)	—	—
		Bronchus	Initial response[a] (5 s)	—	—
		Bronchus	Initial response[c] (5 s)	—	—
	Guinea pig	Trachea	Initial response[a,d] (5 s)	—	—
		Trachea	Initial response[c,d] (5 s)	—	—
Holroyde, 1986	Guinea pig	Trachea	Initial response (10 s)	—	—
Murlas, 1986	Guinea pig	Trachea	Initial response (20 s)	↑	—
		Trachea[b]	Initial response[d] (20 s)	↑	↑

Table 2 Continued

Reference	Species	Tissue	Stimulation	Sensitivity	Maximal Response
Stuart-Smith and Vanhoutte, 1988b	Pig	Bronchus (3°)	Initial response (30 s)	↓	—
			Sustained response[e] (3 min)	—	—
		Bronchus (4°)	Initial response (30 s)	↓	—
			Sustained response[e] (3 min)	—	—
		Bronchus (5°)	Initial response (30 s)	—[b]	—
			Sustained response[e] (3 min)	NR	↑f

— = No effect.

↑ = Increased sensitivity or maximal response after epithelium removal.

↓ = Decreased sensitivity or maximal response after epithelium removal.

NR = Not reported.

3° = Segmental bronchus (dog, pig).

4° = Subsegmental bronchus (dog, pig).

5° = Subsegmental bronchus (pig).

[a]In presence of adrenergic blockade.

[b]Significant only at low frequency.

[c]In presence of adrenergic and muscarinic cholinoceptor blockade.

[d]In presence of indomethacin.

[e]Not affected by β-adrenergic antagonist.

[f]Increase at two highest frequencies.

absence of beta-adrenoreceptor antagonists, respectively. Removing the epithelium also has no significant effect on nonadrenergic noncholinergic relaxations in isolated airways of the cat and guinea pig (Thompson et al., 1988). Removing the epithelium from the porcine bronchus decreases the sensitivity of the initial response; however, in the smaller bronchi without epithelium of that species, the fade of the contractile response is reduced during sustained stimulation (Stuart-Smith and Vanhoutte, 1988b). These data suggest that the effect of the epithelium on neuronal responses may be dependent on the duration of the electrical stimulus applied and may involve both inhibitory and excitatory components.

C. Relaxing Agents

The effect of the epithelium has been determined on the response to various relaxing agents (Table 3). A consideration of importance is the degree of activation of the smooth muscle prior to the addition of the relaxing agent, since the potency and even the direction (contraction or relaxation) of the effect of mediators may depend on the tone present when the effect of a mediator is evaluated (Persson and Karlsson, 1987). Another complicating factor is that in preparations such as the guinea pig trachea, spontaneous tone develops that is not altered by epithelium removal (Lundblad and Persson, 1988) but is inhibited by indomethacin (Orehek et al., 1975; Brink et al., 1981; Hay et al., 1986a; Braunstein et al., 1988).

In canine bronchi, the relaxation induced by the beta-adrenergic agonist, isoproterenol, is enhanced by the presence of the epithelium (Flavahan and Vanhoutte, 1984; Flavahan et al., 1985; Stuart-Smith and Vanhoutte, 1987). A reduction of the relaxation in response to isoproterenol upon removal of the epithelium has also been observed in the bovine trachea (Barnes et al., 1985), the guinea pig trachea (Goldie et al., 1986), and the porcine bronchus (Stuart-Smith and Vanhoutte, 1988b), and it may be present in the human bronchus (Aizawa et al., 1988). These results imply that either an epithelium-derived relaxing factor(s) is released by the beta-adrenergic agonist or that the presence of a background secretion of the factor(s) facilitates the action of the bronchodilator.

The influence of the epithelium on the relaxations induced by beta-adrenergic agonists in the canine bronchus depends on the contractile agent used to induce active force and the degree of contraction achieved. For example, during contraction to low concentrations of acetylcholine (less than the ED_{40} for the contractile agonist), relaxations induced by the beta-adrenergic agonist, isoproterenol, are not different between canine bronchi with and without epithelium (Flavahan and Vanhoutte, 1984; Stuart-Smith and Vanhoutte, unpublished observations, 1988). At a higher degree of cholinergic tone (ED_{50} or

Table 3 Epithelium Removal and Relaxations of Airway Smooth Muscle in Vitro

Reference	Species	Tissue	Degree of Tone			Sensitivity (IC$_{50}$)	Maximal Response
			Contractile Agent	ED$_X$	Relaxant		
Flavahan and Vanhoutte, 1984	Dog	Bronchus (3° & 4°)	Acetylcholine	ED$_{30}$	Isoproterenol[a]	NR	—
			Acetylcholine	ED$_{70}$	Isoproterenol[a]	NR	↓
Flavahan et al., 1985	Dog	Bronchus (3° & 4°)	Acetylcholine	ED$_{50}$	Isoproterenol[a]	NR	↓
Flavahan et al., 1985	Dog	Bronchus (3° & 4°)	5-hydroxytryptamine	ED$_{30}$	A 23187[b]	NR	↓
			5-hydroxytryptamine	ED$_{30}$	Arachidonic Acid	NR	↓
Ruff et al., 1987	Dog	Bronchus (3°)	Acetylcholine	ED$_{50}$	Tulobuterol	NR	↓
Stuart-Smith and Van-houtte, 1987	Dog	Bronchus (2°)	Acetylcholine	ED$_{50}$	Isoproterenol[a]	NR	↓
		Bronchus (3°)	Acetylcholine	ED$_{50}$	Isoproterenol[a]	NR	↓
		Bronchus (4°)	Acetylcholine	ED$_{50}$	Isoproterenol[a]	NR	↓↓
Busk et al., 1988,	Dog	Bronchus (2°)	Acetylcholine	ED$_{50}$	S 9795[c]	NR	↓
		Bronchus (4°)	Acetylcholine	ED$_{50}$	S 9795[c]	NR	↓
Stuart-Smith and Van-houtte, 1988a	Dog	Bronchus (2°)	5-hydroxytryptamine	ED30	Arachidonic Acid	NR	↓
			5-hydroxytryptamine	ED30	Prostaglandin E$_2$[d]	—	—
			5-hydroxytryptamine	ED30	Prostaglandin I$_2$[d]	—	—
		Bronchus (3°)	5-hydroxytryptamine	ED30	Arachidonic Acid	NR	↓
			5-hydroxytryptamine	ED30	Prostaglandin E$_2$[d]	—	—
			5-hydroxytryptamine	ED30	Prostaglandin I$_2$[d]	—	—

Reference	Species	Tissue	Agonist	Dose	Relaxant		
		Bronchus (4°)	5-hydroxytryptamine	ED30	Arachidonic Acid	NR	↓
			5-hydroxytryptamine	ED30	Prostaglandin E$_2$[d]	—	—
			5-hydroxytryptamine	ED30	Prostaglandin I$_2$[d]	—	—
Busk and Vanhoutte, 1989	Dog	Bronchus (2°)	Acetylcholine	ED$_{50}$	Theophylline	NR	↓
		Bronchus (4°)	Acetylcholine	ED$_{50}$	Theophylline	NR	↓
Barnes et al., 1985	Cow	Trachea	Acetylcholine	ED$_{80}$	Isoproterenol	—	NR
			Histamine	ED$_{80}$	Isoproterenol	—	NR
			5-hydroxytryptamine	ED$_{80}$	Isoproterenol	↓	NR
Farmer et al., 1986	Guinea pig	Trachea	Spontaneous tone		Isoproterenol	↑	—
			Methacholine	ED$_{60}$	Isoproterenol	↑	—
			Methacholine	ED$_{60}$	Salbutamol	—	—
			Spontaneous tone		Sodium nitroprusside	—	—
			Methacholine	ED$_{60}$	Sodium nitroprusside	↑	—
			Spontaneous tone		Papaverine	—	—
			Methacholine	ED$_{60}$	Papaverine	—	—
			Spontaneous tone		Adenosine	—	↑
Goldie et al., 1986	Guinea pig	Trachea	Carbachol	ED$_{50}$	Isoproterenol	—	—
			Carbachol	$4 \times$ED$_{90}$	Isoproterenol	—	↓
			Carbachol	ED$_{50}$	Forskolin	—	—
			Carbachol	$4 \times$ED$_{90}$	Forskolin	—	↓
			Carbachol	ED$_{50}$	Theophylline	—	—
			Carbachol	$4 \times$ED$_{90}$	Theophylline	—	↓
			Carbachol	ED$_{50}$	Nitroglycerin	—	—
			Carbachol	$4 \times$ED$_{90}$	Nitroglycerin	—	—

Table 3 continues

Table 3 (Continued) Epithelium Removal and Relaxations of Airway Smooth Muscle in Vitro

Reference	Species	Tissue	Degree of Tone		Relaxant	Sensitivity (IC_{50})	Maximal Response
			Contractile Agent	ED_X			
Hay et al., 1986b	Guinea pig	Trachea	Methacholine	ED_{30}	Isoproterenol	↑	—
			Methacholine	ED_{70}	Isoproterenol	↑	—
	Ovalbumin-sensitized guinea pig	Trachea	Methacholine	ED_{30}	Isoproterenol	↑	—
			Methacholine	ED_{70}	Isoproterenol	↑	
Holroyde, 1986	Guinea pig	Trachea	1 g tension		Isoproterenol	↑	—
			1 g tension		Lanthanum chloride	—	—
			1 g tension		Adenosine[e]	↑	
Nijkamp and Folkerts, 1986	Guinea pig	Trachea	Spontaneous tone		Arachidonic Acid	NR	↓[f]
			Potassium chloride	20mM	Arachidonic Acid	NR	↓[f]
Butler et al., 1987	Guinea pig	Trachea	Bethanechol	ED_{75}	Arachidonic Acid	NR	↓
			Bethanechol	ED_{75}	Prostaglandin E_2	—	—
Farmer et al., 1987	Guinea pig	Trachea	Spontaneous tone		Arachidonic Acid	NR	↓[f]
Tschirhart et al., 1987	Guinea pig	Trachea	2 g tension		Arachidonic Acid	NR	↓[f]
			Histamine	ED_{50}	Arachidonic Acid	NR	↓
			Histamine	ED_{70}	Arachidonic Acid	NR	↓
			Carbachol	ED_{50}	Arachidonic Acid	NR	↓
Advenier et al., 1988	Guinea pig	Trachea	Histamine	10^{-5}M	Adenosine	↑	NR
			Spontaneous tone		Adenosine	↑	NR
Braunstein et al., 1983	Guinea pig	Trachea	Spontaneous tone		Arachidonic Acid	NR	↓[f]
			Histamine	50uM	Arachidonic Acid	NR	↓
			Spontaneous tone		Prostaglandin E_2	NR	↓[f]
			Histamine	50uM	Prostaglandin E_2	—	—

Reference	Species	Tissue	Contractile stimulus	Concentration	Relaxant		
Lundblad and Persson, 1988	Guinea pig	Trachea	Spontaneous tone		Adenosine[g]	NR	↑
			Spontaneous tone		Arachidonic acid	NR	—
			Potassium chloride	20mM	Arachidonic acid	NR	—
			Spontaneous tone		Theophylline	—	↓
			Spontaneous tone		Enprofylline	—	—
			Spontaneous tone		Tulobuterol	↓	—
			Spontaneous tone		Isoproterenol	↑	—
Stuart-Smith and Vanhoutte, 1988b	Pig	Bronchus (3°)	Acetylcholine	Ed_{50}	Isoproterenol[a]	NR	↓
		Bronchus (4°)	Acetylcholine	ED_{50}	Isoproterenol[a]	NR	↓
		Bronchus (5°)	Acetylcholine	ED_{50}	Isoproterenol[a]	NR	↓
Frossard and Muller, 1986	Ovalbumin-sensitized rat	Trachea	5-hydroxytryptamine	NR	Substance P	NR	↓
Aizawa et al., 1988	Human	Bronchi	Acetylcholine	10^{-3}M	Isoproterenol	—	—
			Histamine	10^{-3}M	Isoproterenol	—	—

— = No effect.
↑ = Increased sensitivity or maximal response after epithelium removal.
↓ = Decreased sensitivity or maximal response after epithelium removal.
NR = Not reported.
ED_x = Concentration producing x% of the maximal response.

2° = Lobar bronchus (dog).
3° = Segmental bronchus (dog, pig).
4° = Subsegmental bronchus (dog, pig).
5° = Subsegmental bronchus (pig).

[a]In presence of cocaine (5×10^{-6}M), hydrocortisone (3×10^{-5}M), and phentolamine (10^{-6}M).
[b]Calcium ionophore.
[c]Methyl xanthine derivative.
[d]In presence of indomethacin (10^{-5}M) and atropine (10^{-6}M).
[e]At low concentrations, adenosine contracted tissue without epithelium only. At higher concentrations, it relaxed the tissue.
[f]Arachidonic acid produced contractions in tissue without epithelium.
[g]Low concentrations of adenosine produced slight contractions in trachea with and without epithelium.

greater), the relaxations in response to isoproterenol in canine bronchi without epithelium are reduced (Torphy et al., 1983, 1985; Flavahan and Vanhoutte, 1987; Flavahan et al., 1985; Stuart-Smith and Vanhoutte, 1987; Stuart-Smith and Vanhoutte, 1990b). In contrast, the responses of the bronchi with epithelium to isoproterenol are not attenuated by the increased tone of the smooth muscle; as a consequence, the relaxations are more pronounced than those of the denuded bronchi (Flavahan and Vanhoutte, 1984; Flavahan et al., 1985; Stuart-Smith and Vanhoutte, 1987; Stuart-Smith and Vanhoutte, 1990b). However, during contractions evoked by 5-hydroxytryptamine at either the ED_{40} or the ED_{80} level, the relaxations induced by isoproterenol are not different between canine bronchi with and without epithelium (Stuart-Smith and Vanhoutte, 1990b). Thus, in the canine bronchus, the action of epithelium-derived relaxing factor(s) in facilitating the relaxations to isoproterenol is apparent only with high degrees of cholinergic activation of the smooth muscle. An opposite effect has been observed in the guinea pig trachea, where the removal of the epithelium enhances relaxations to isoproterenol (Holroyde, 1986; Farmer et al., 1986; Hay et al., 1986b; Lundblad and Persson, 1988); this was attributed to extraneuronal uptake of isoproterenol by the epithelium, because corticosterone (a blocker of the extraneuronal uptake of catecholamines) abolished the effect of epithelium removal on the sensitivity to the beta-adrenergic agonist (Farmer et al., 1986). With another beta-adrenergic agonist, salbutamol (which is not a substrate for extraneuronal uptake, the relaxations in the guinea pig trachea were not affected by the presence of the epithelium or corticosterone (Farmer et al., 1986). However, this explanation is not plausible in canine and porcine bronchus because the experiments performed with these tissues were done in the presence of inhibitors of both neuronal and extraneuronal uptake of catecholamines (Flavahan and Vanhoutte, 1984; Flavahan et al., 1985; Stuart-Smith and Vanhoutte, 1987, 1988b). Likewise, the sensitivity to or the maximal relaxation induced by tulobuterol is enhanced in airways with an intact epithelium from both the dog and the guinea pig (Ruff et al., 1987; Lundblad and Persson, 1988).

The maximal response to other relaxing stimuli (theophylline, S 9795, a xanthine derivative; forskolin; and A23187, a calcium ionophore) is also enhanced in airways with an intact epithelium when the tone of the smooth muscle is increased first with contractile agents (Flavahan et al., 1986; Goldie et al., 1986; Busk and Vanhoutte, 1988, 1989, 1990b). In addition, when assessed against the spontaneous tone of the guinea pig trachea, the maximal response to theophylline is more pronounced in the trachea with an intact epithelium (Lundblad and Persson, 1988). In contrast to its effect in other species, substance P causes relaxations in the trachea of the ovalbumin-sensitized rats and the effect is greater when the epithelium is present (Frossard and Muller, 1986). These data suggest the involvement of an epithelium-derived relaxing factor(s) facilitating the relaxation of the airways. On the other hand, the relaxations in response to nitroglycerin, lanthanum chloride, papaverine, enprofylline (a xanthine derivative), and prostaglandin E_2 and I_2 are not affected by the presence of the epithelium in isolated airways of various species (Goldie et al., 1986; Holroyde, 1986; Farmer et al., 1986; Butler et al., 1987; Lundblad and Persson, 1988; Stuart-Smith and Vanhoutte, 1988a).

In the guinea pig trachea, at low concentrations of adenosine, three different actions have been observed: contractions only in the absence of epithelium (Holroyde, 1986), equal contractions in trachea with and without epithelium (Lundblad and Persson, 1988), and relaxations in both types of preparations (Farmer et al., 1986; Advenier et al., 1988). Higher concentrations of adenosine consistently cause relaxations; however, the effect of epithelium removal is to increase the sensitivity without a difference in the maximal response (Holroyde, 1986; Advenier et al., 1988), to enhance the relaxations at the highest concentrations tested (Lundblad and Persson, 1988), or not to affect the sensitivity of the tissues but to increase the maximal response (Farmer et al., 1986). In the latter study, with the addition of dipyridamole and erythro-9-2 hydroxy-3-nonyl adenine (EHNA; blockers of adenosine uptake and deamination, respectively), epithelium removal increased the sensitivity to adenosine without affecting the maximal response, suggesting an excitatory effect related to presence of the epithelium (Farmer et al., 1986). However, another study reports that the increased sensitivity of the epithelium-denuded tissue is abolished by the presence of dipyridamole; thus, the airway epithelium may be involved instead in the uptake and metabolism of adenosine (Advenier et al., 1988).

Variable results have also been observed with sodium nitroprusside. In the guinea pig trachea, removal of the epithelium increases the sensitivity of the smooth muscle to sodium nitroprusside in tissue contracted with the ED_{50} of methacholine but not when tested against the basal tone (Farmer et al., 1986). These observations with sodium nitroprusside prompted the suggestion that it may release an excitatory factor(s) from the epithelium (Farmer et al., 1986). This may be the case in the guinea pig, but there is no difference in the relaxations to sodium nitroprusside between canine bronchi with and without epithelium during contractions to either the ED_{40} of acetylcholine or ED_{40} and ED_{80} of 5-hydroxytryptamine; although at the ED_{80} level of acetylcholine, bronchi with epithelium showed a significantly greater relaxation to sodium nitroprusside than bronchi without epithelium (Stuart-Smith and Vanhoutte, 1990b).

Several studies in different species have demonstrated that arachidonic acid causes epithelium-dependent relaxations (Flavahan et al., 1986; Nijkamp and Folkerts, 1986; Butler et al., 1987; Farmer et al., 1987; Tschirhart et al., 1987; Braunstein et al., 1988; Stuart-Smith and Vanhoutte, 1988a). In canine airways, during contractions evoked by 5-hydroxytryptamine, exogenous arachidonic acid causes relaxations that depend on the presence of the epithelium (Flavahan et al., 1986; Stuart-Smith and Vanhoutte, 1988a). Epithelium-dependent relaxations in response to the fatty acid are observed during contractions evoked by potassium chloride, carbachol, bethanechol, or histamine, as well as on a background of basal tone in the guinea pig trachea (Nijkamp and Folkerts, 1986; Farmer et al., 1987; Tschirhart et al., 1987; Braunstein et al., 1988) and in the bronchi of the rabbit (Butler et al., 1987). In contrast, when the epithelium of the guinea pig trachea is removed, the smooth muscle contracts in response to arachidonic acid. (Nijkamp and Folkerts, 1986; Farmer et al., 1987; Tschirhart et al., 1987; Braunstein et al., 1988). One study failed to observe, however, a difference in the response to arachidonic acid between the two preparations of guinea pig trachea with and without epithelium (Lundblad and Persson, 1988).

D. Heterogeneity in Epithelium-Dependent Responses

In the canine bronchial tree, as the diameter decreases the potentiating effect of epithelium removal on the reponse to bronchoconstrictor agonists is reduced (Fig. 9; Hay et al., 1987c; Stuart-Smith and Vanhoutte, 1987). In contrast, with decreasing diameter, the influence of the epithelium on beta-adrenergically mediated relaxations becomes more prominent (Fig. 10; Stuart-Smith and Vanhoutte, 1987). With relaxations to arachidonic acid, an opposite relationship exists (Stuart-Smith and Vanhoutte, 1988a). Epithelium dependent responses contingent on the generation of the airway also exist in the cat (Thompson et al., 1988), pig (Stuart-Smith and Vanhoutte, 1988b), and rabbit (Raeburn et al., 1986a). Thus, if airway epithelium releases a factor (or factors) that promotes relaxation of airway smooth muscle, there is considerable heterogeneity in the release or the effect of the factor(s) along the bronchial tree. This heterogeneity may reflect the variation in the epithelial cell type and secretory properties within airways of different size and function (Weibel, 1985).

E. Agonist Selectivity of the Epithelium to Contractile and Relaxing Agents

An agonist selectivity in the modulatory influence of the epithelium on the reactivity of the smooth muscle to contractile agents may also exist (Goldie et al., 1986; Hay et al., 1987a; Thompson et al., 1988). This agonist selectivity is evident in both ovalbumin-sensitized and nonsensitized guinea pigs, where the sensitivity of the denuded trachea to leukotriene C_4 and leukotriene D_4 is increased without alteration in the maximal response, but the responses to leukotriene E_4, the thromboxane mimetic, U-44069, and 5-hydroxytryptamine

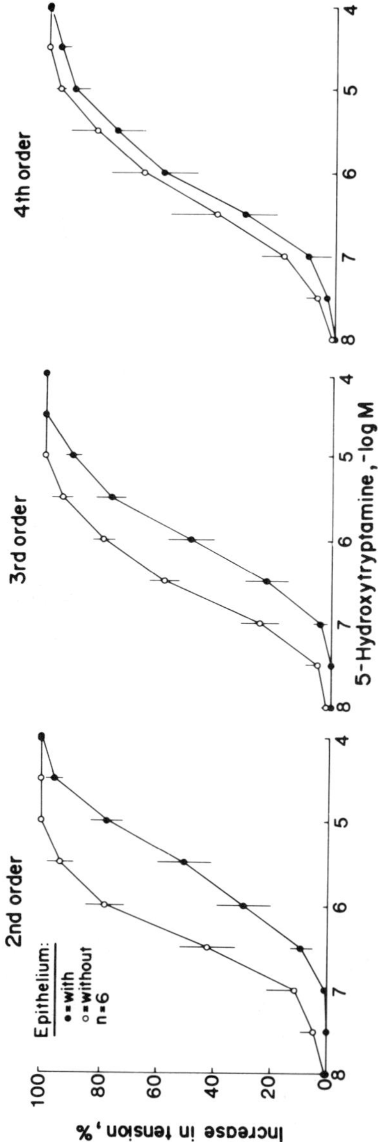

Figure 9 Comparison in lobar (second order), segmental (third order), and subsegmental (fourth order) bronchi of the same dogs of the effect of epithelium removal on the contractions evoked by increasing concentrations of 5-hydroxytryptamine. Note that with decreasing diameter of the bronchus, the potentiating effect of the removal is progressively reduced. These studies support the hypothesis that the basal release of epithelium-derived relaxing factor(s) is greater in larger than in smaller airways (reprinted from Stuart-Smith and Vanhoutte, 1987, by permission).

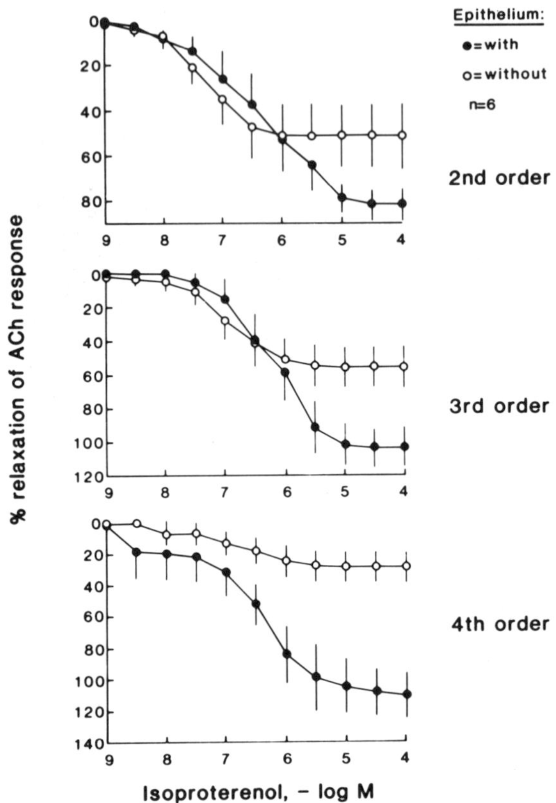

Figure 10 Comparison in lobar (second order), segmental (third order), and subsegmental (fourth order) bronchi of the same dogs of the effect of epithelium removal on the relaxations evoked by increasing concentrations of isoproterenol. Note that with decreasing diameter of the bronchus the potentiating effect of the removal is progressively augmented. These studies support the hypothesis that the triggered release of epithelium-derived relaxing factor(s) is less in larger than in smaller airways (reprinted from Stuart-Smith and Vanhoutte, 1987, by permission).

are unaffected (Hay et al., 1987a). Likewise, an agonist selectivity in the modulatory influence of the epithelium to bronchodilators has been observed in the trachea of guinea pig (Goldie et al., 1986; Farmer et al., 1986). Agonist selectivity may also explain why epithelium removal does not affect the response to certain agents in various species, such as acetylcholine in the guinea pig trachea (Goldie et al., 1986) and feline airway (Thompson et al., 1988), and carbachol in the guinea pig trachea (Goldie et al., 1986; Tschirhart et al., 1987) or the ovalbumin-sensitized rat trachea (Frossard and Muller, 1986).

Because of the agonist selectivity in epithelium-dependent responses and the heterogeneity in response along the bronchial tree, an absence of potentiation of the bronchoconstrictor effects with removal of the epithelium or of bronchodilator effects in the presence of the epithelium in a given airway preparation cannot be used to argue against the hypothesis that the epithelium controls the underlying bronchial smooth muscle.

V. Other Methods to Investigate the Phenomenon

A. Electrophysiological Studies

In electrophysiological studies, simultaneous recordings of mechanical and electrical activity were made in paired circumferential strips (with and without epithelium) from the canine bronchus (Gao and Vanhoutte, 1988). In the presence of antagonists of muscarinic and adrenergic receptors, the resting tension and membrane potential, and the levels of contraction and depolarization of the smooth muscle in response to potassium ions, are unaltered by the removal of the epithelium (Fig. 5; Gao and Vanhoutte, 1988). In contrast, echothiopate, an inhibitor of cholinesterase, does not alter the resting membrane potential of the intact tissues, but causes depolarization in bronchi without epithelium. Furthermore, in the presence of echothiophate, removal of the epithelium not only augments the contraction but also significantly increases the degree of depolarization of the cell membrane induced by acetylcholine, even when matched contractions are compared (Figs. 7, 8; Gao and Vanhoutte, 1988). These results imply that the canine respiratory epithelium generates an inhibitory factor(s) that reduces the depolarization and the contraction of bronchial smooth muscle caused by acetylcholine (Gao and Vanhoutte, 1988). The mechanism for such an effect is not known. The epithelial factor(s) may influence the sodium/potassium pump in the smooth muscle (Lamport and Fedan, 1988). Therefore, it could be postulated that the epithelium produces its inhibitory effect on the membrane potential through this mechanism. In addition, acetylcholine itself might stimulate release of the epithelium-derived relaxing factor(s), since atropine causes a depolarization in bronchi with epithelium, but has no effect in tissues without epithelium (Gao and Vanhoutte, 1988). This suggests that a tonic release of the cholinergic agonist stimulates or enhances the release of the relaxing factor(s), but the site of origin for acetylcholine (i.e., smooth muscle, nerve, or epithelium) is unknown.

B. Independent Stimulation of the Inner Epithelial Surface and the Outer Serosal Surface

Isolated airways can be cannulated and perfused at constant flow with a solution that is in direct contact with the inner epithelial-lined surface, while the outer serosal surface of the trachea is immersed within the same solution; responses are assessed by measuring the change in pressure between the tracheal inlet and outlet (Munakata et al., 1988a). This method allows stimulation of the inner (epithelial) and the outer (serosal) surfaces of the airway independently. In the guinea pig trachea contracted with carbachol or potassium chloride, the addition of hyperosmolar stimuli (potassium chloride, mannitol, urea, or sodium chloride) to the inner epithelial surface produces a concentration-dependent relaxation; removal of the epithelium reduces or abolishes the relaxation (Munakata et al., 1988a). In addition, a relaxation is not produced when isotonic potassium chloride is applied to the inner surface and a contraction is evoked when the hyperosmolar stimuli are applied to the serosal surface (Munakata et al., 1988a). With use of a similar method with the canine bronchus, epithelium-dependent relaxations to hypotonic solutions are also obtained (Gao and Vanhoutte, 1989b). Thus, the airways respond with epithelium-dependent relaxations to both hyperosmotic and hypotonic stimuli through the possible release of the epithelium-derived relaxing factor(s) (Munakata et al., 1988a; Gao and Vanhoutte, 1989b).

By using the same method in the guinea pig trachea, the sensitivity of the contractile response to both acetylcholine and histamine is decreased when the agonists are applied on the inner epithelial surface compared with application to the serosa; removal of the epithelium abolishes the difference between the inner and outer surfaces (Munakata et al., 1988b). Likewise in another study, the contractions in response to methacholine, histamine, and the relaxation in response to isoproterenol are decreased when the agonist is given on the epithelial surface (Fedan and Frazer, 1988). In perfused canine bronchi, the epithelium substantially limits the access of intraluminally administered bronchoactive agents to the airway smooth muscle (Gao and Vanhoutte, 1989a). Thus, these studies imply that the epithelium has a protective role against bronchoconstrictors present in the lumen that may involve one or a combination of the following functions: the continuous release of epithelium-derived relaxing factor(s), the activated release of relaxing factor(s) by the bronchoconstrictor agents that act on the basolateral surface of the epithelial cell, or the function as a passive and/or metabolic barrier to the actions of these agonists (Fedan and Frazer, 1988; Munakata et al., 1988b; Gao and Vanhoutte, 1989a).

C. Bioassay of Epithelium-Derived Relaxing or Inhibitory Factor(s)

Superfusion-Cascade System

Superfusion-cascade bioassay studies in canine bronchi demonstrate that epithelial cells release a factor(s) that relaxes airway smooth muscle (Fig. 11;

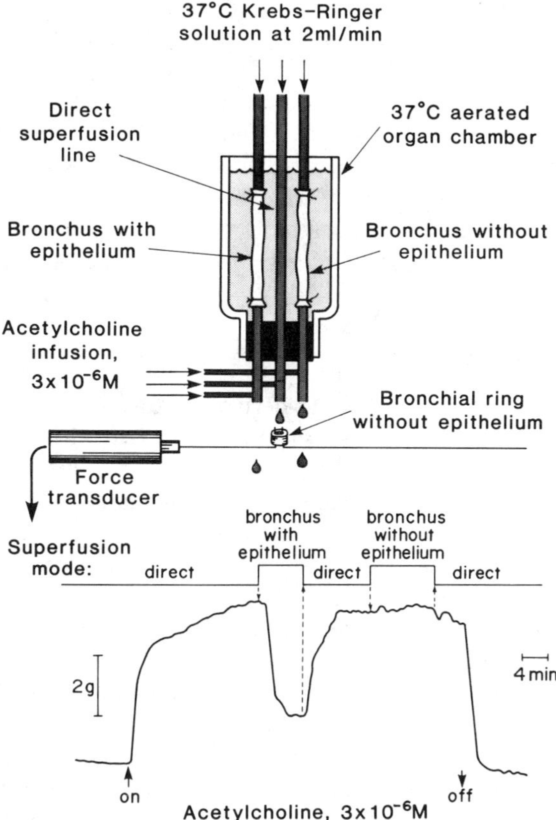

Figure 11   Bioassay experiment in which a ring of canine bronchus without epithelium (contracted with acetylcholine) is superfused with Krebs-Ringer bicarbonate solution flowing either through a bronchus with epithelium (first arrow: note the marked relaxation), a stainless steel tube (second arrow: note the reversal of the relaxation), or a bronchus without epithelium (third arrow: note the absence of relaxation). This demonstrates that the bronchial epithelium can release a potent inhibitory factor(s) (reprinted from Vanhoutte, 1987a, by permission).

Flavahan and Vanhoutte, 1985; Vanhoutte, 1987a; Vanhoutte and Flavahan, 1987). There is additional evidence using this system that an epithelium-derived factor(s) inhibits vascular smooth muscle (Vanhoutte, 1988a). However, this type of bioassay with airway smooth muscle from intact bronchi or tracheas yields variable results. Furthermore, superfusion-cascade studies with the guinea pig trachea do not provide evidence for the existence of an inhibitory factor released from the epithelium (Holroyde, 1986; Undem et al.,

1987). This could be explained if the epithelial cells, which are highly polarized, release the factor(s) preferentially toward the underlying smooth muscle rather than into the airway lumen. The factor(s) may also be catalyzed rapidly. In addition, mucus may be a major source of inactivation, which could explain why relaxing activity cannot be bioassayed in perfusate from infected airways (Vanhoutte, 1987a). The superfusion-cascade system also has several design problems, including a relatively long transit time between the two preparations, fluctuations in the temperature, and dilution of the perfusate. If epithelium-derived relaxing factor(s) is labile and has a very short half-life, this may explain the technical difficulty in bioassaying it.

Direct Transfer of an Epithelium-Derived Factor(s)

The direct transfer of an epithelium-derived factor(s) has been obtained using "sandwich" preparations, similar to that described with the vascular endothelium (Furchgott and Zawadzky, 1980). With this method, two tracheal pieces, one intact (donor) and one without epithelium (recipient), are mounted in one organ bath with the two luminal surfaces facing. By using this method, the hyperresponsiveness to substance P observed in denuded trachea of the guinea pig is reduced by applying the luminal surface of an intact airway to that of the denuded tissue (Tschirhart and Landry, 1986). The hyperresponsiveness to acetylcholine and histamine of the canine trachea without epithelium is reduced when a strip of canine mucosa is placed close, but not in contact with the smooth muscle (Manning et al., 1988). The sensitivity to the contractile effect of acetylcholine in the canine trachea without epithelium is decreased when chopped epithelium is added to the organ bath (Aizawa et al., 1988). These different studies all suggest the existence of a relaxing factor(s), generated by the epithelial cell layer and capable of diffusing to the airway smooth muscle (Tschirhart and Landry, 1986; Aizawa et al., 1988; Manning et al., 1988).

Coaxial Bioassay

In the coaxial bioassay studies, a tubular airway structure either with or without epithelium (the donor tissue) surrounds the bioassay tissue, and both are contained in the same closed system. Using this type of bioassay eliminates many of the design problems associated with the superfusion-cascade bioassay. In the first such study, the bioassay tissue, a strip of rabbit aorta without endothelium, was passed through a tubular segment of guinea pig trachea either with or without epithelium, the donor tissue (Ilhan and Sahin, 1986). In the presence of a trachea with epithelium, the aorta relaxed in a concentration-dependent manner to acetylcholine; however, when the epithelium was absent, the blood vessel did not relax in response to the cholinergic agonist (Ilhan and Sahin, 1986). Similar results have been obtained using donor airway and deendothelialized bioassay arteries from other species. For example, the denuded rat aorta relaxes to histamine and methacholine in the presence of either a guinea pig tracheal or human bronchial tube with epithelium; removal of the intact airway tube or of the epithelium from the airway abolishes the relaxation (Fernandes et al., 1989). Likewise, the potency and efficacy of the left circumflex artery of the dog to the beta-adrenergic agonist, isoproterenol, are increased when the surrounding canine brachial segment has an intact epithelium (Busk et al., 1989). Thus, the coaxial system demonstrates that the airway may release a diffusible factor(s) that influences the responses of vascular smooth muscle (Ilhan and Sahin, 1986; Fernandes et al., 1989; Busk et al., 1989). The same conclusion has been reached using the rat anococcygeus muscle as the bioassay preparation (Guc et al., 1988). In another coaxial system, a strip of guinea pig trachea without epithelium is placed inside a tube of tracheal tissue either with or without epithelium (Hay et al., 1987b). In this study, the sensitivity and maximal response of the denuded tracheal strip to ovalbumin are decreased when it is placed inside a tracheal tube with epithelium, compared with results obtained in the presence of an deepithelialized tube (Hay et al., 1987b). These results further strengthen the interpretation that an inhibitory substance(s) released from the epithelium is able to diffuse to and modulate airway smooth muscle lying in close proximity (Hay et al., 1987b). However, when bioassay tissues other than airway smooth muscle are used, it is uncertain whether the relaxing activity measured truly reflects the release of epithelium-derived relaxing factor(s).

VI. Eosinophils and Epithelium-Dependent Responses

The eosinophil, through its complement of toxic granule proteins, can cause damage to and desquamation of bronchial epithelial cells. (Gleich and Loegering, 1984; Gleich et al., 1985; Gleich, 1990). The damage to the epithelial cell may in turn contribute to the bronchial hyperreactivity associated with asthma by interfering with the action of epithelium-derived factor(s) (see Gleich et al., 1988; Gleich, 1990). Using this hypothesis, studies were done to investigate the effect on the epithelium by the toxic cationic eosinophil granule protein, the major basic protein (MBP). In one such study, the sensitivity to histamine and acetylcholine of rings of guinea pig trachea, some with and some without epithelium, was determined under control conditions and after incubation with MBP (100 mg/ml), which is a similar concentration to that found in the sputum of asthmatics (Flavahan et al., 1988). MBP did not affect the contractile activity to acetylcholine in rings of guinea pig trachea that had previously been denuded of the epithelium (Fig. 12, bottom). Thus, at this concentration, the protein is not cytotoxic to smooth muscle cells. However, when MBP was incubated with tracheal rings with an intact epithelium, MBP caused augmentation of the contractile responses to acetylcholine (Fig. 12, top). Similar results were observed with histamine. Although these functional studies suggest that MBP interferes with the function of the epithelial cells, light microscopic analysis revealed that MBP (100 μg/ml) did not cause epithelial desquamation. Therefore, the results suggest that MBP, in concentrations that do not cause epithelial denudation, may cause

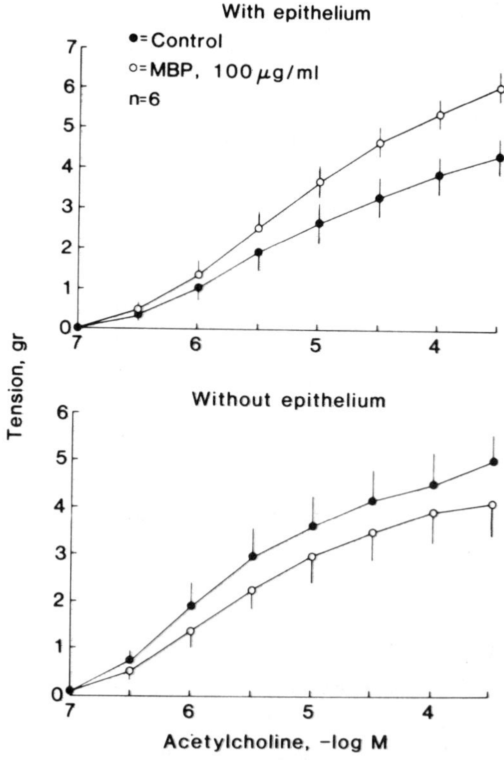

Figure 12 Effect of human MBP (100 μg/ml) on the concentration-effect curve to acetylcholine in rings of guinea pig trachea with (upper panel) and without epithelium (lower panel). Data are presented as means ± SEM for the number of observations shown. Asterisk indicates the effect of MBP is statistically significant. In rings of trachea with epithelium, the effect of human MBP is consistent with an upward shift in the concentration-effect curve, increasing the maximal response evoked by acetylcholine but not significantly affecting the ED_{50} value. In denuded rings, MBP was without effect and no change was observed in the maximal response or in the ED_{50} values (reprinted from Flavahan et al., 1988, by permission).

interruption of the release of epithelium-derived relaxing factor(s), interfere with the diffusion and/or action of the factor(s), or alter the metabolism of the epithelial cells from the production of relaxing factor(s) to the generation of contracting factor(s) (Flavahan et al., 1988).

Support for the release of contracting factor(s) comes from observations on the effect of epithelial cell removal and intraepithelial MBP injection on the contractility of underlying canine tracheal smooth muscel in vivo, utilizing a dual in situ tracheal preparation (Brofman et al., 1989). The results demonstrate that the response to intraarterial administration of acetylcholine was augmented in dogs receiving 200 μg of MBP by intraepithelial instillation; a similar augmentation was not observed in homologous tracheal segments in the same animal receiving vehicle only. In contrast, instillation of MBP directly into the subepithelial tracheal smooth muscle had no effect on its responsiveness. To assess whether MBP interfered with epithelium-derived relaxing factor(s), the epithelium was excised from one of the two tracheal segments. Removing the epithelium had no effect on the contractile response to acetylcholine or on the relaxation in response to isoproterenol. These results suggest that MBP causes the epithelium to release a substance that augments the responsiveness of airway smooth muscle (Brofman et al., 1989). Taken in conjunction, these two studies imply that the eosinophils, by releasing MBP, can alter the contractility of respiratory smooth muscle in virtue of its effects on epithelial cells.

VII. Nature of Epithelium-Derived Factor(s)

In the preceding sections, evidence has been presented to support the existence of epithelium-derived relaxing factor)s). Its identity remains unknown and may well differ between species and type of smooth muscle affected. In the vascular system, nitric oxide has been identified as one of the endothelium-derived relaxing factors (Palmer et al., 1987). This substance is released from endothelial cells and initiates relaxation via the accumulation of cyclic guanosine 3', 5'-monophosphate (GMP) (Ignarro et al., 1988). Epithelium-derived relaxing factor(s) is not likely to be identical to endothelium-derived relaxing factor or nitric oxide, since inhibitors of these substances do not affect the shift of the concentration-response curve to acetylcholine in the canine bronchus and since nitric oxide is an extremely poor relaxant of airway smooth muscle (Lorenz et al., 1989; Stuart-Smith and Vanhoutte, 1990b). Furthermore, although the relaxation to sodium nitroprusside is greater in fourth order bronchi with epithelium during contrations to the ED_{80} of acetylcholine, this effect does not appear mediated via cyclic GMP (Stuart-Smith and Vanhoutte, 1990b). Likewise, the effect of the inhibitory substance(s) released from the epithelium of the guinea pig trachea that modulates vascular smooth muscle and the anococcygeus muscle is not blocked by inhibitors of cyclic GMP or endothelium-derived relaxing factor (Ilhan and Sahin, 1986; Guc et al., 1988; Fernandes et al., 1989). As mentioned already, as long the chemical nature of the factor(s) is not known, caution should be exerted when assuming that the factor(s) derived from the epithelium that can be bioassayed with isolated blood vessels is the same as that producing relaxation of airway smooth muscle. Furthermore, in the preparations that permit independent stimulation from either the epithelial or serosal surfaces, the release of the epithelium-derived relaxing factor(s) induced by hypotonic stimulation is not inhibited by gossypol (a known inhibitor of the endothelium-derived relaxing factor with the additional properties of being a lipoxygenase and cyclooxygenase inhibitor and a scavenger of oxygen-derived free radicals) (Gao and Vanhoutte, 1989b). By contrast, gossypol attenuates the release of the epithelium-derived relaxing factor(s) in the guinea pig trachea induced by hyperosmolar stimuli (Teeter et al., 1988).

The relationship between the epithelial cell and epithelium-dependent responses of the underlying smooth muscle with products of both the cyclooxygenase and lipoxygenase is complex and the results obtained with inhibitors of these pathways differ according to the species studied. The metabolites of arachidonic acid influence the responsiveness of airway smooth muscle (Bakhle and Ferreira, 1985; Morris, 1985). Prostaglandins E_1, E_2, and I_2 (prostacyclin) induce relaxation (Shore et al., 1985; Gardiner, 1986; Stuart-Smith and Vanhoutte, 1988a); leukotrienes C_4 and D_4 (bioactive components of slow-reacting substance of anaphylaxis; Lewis et al., 1980; Murphy et al., 1979) evoke constriction of the airways (Drazen et al., 1980; Burka and Saad, 1984; Samhorn and Piper, 1986). Arachidonic acid is metabolized by isolated and cultured epithelial cells of the trachea from rats, rabbits (Xu et al., 1986), dogs (Eling et al., 1986; Holtzman et al., 1983a; Barnett et al., 1988), and humans (Leikauf et al., 1985; Hunter et al., 1985). In addition, cyclooxygenase has been localized in the epithelial cells of intact airways in the rabbit (Butler et al., 1987). Thus, epithelium may play an important role in the generation of eicosanoids that modulate the reactivity of the underlying airway smooth muscle.

A possible mechanism for the modulation of the responsiveness of the airways to arachidonic acid may involve the release of an inhibitory prostanoid by the epithelial cell. In the presence of indomethacin, the epithelium-dependent relaxations in response to arachidonic acid in intact airways are either reversed to a contraction (Farmer et al., 1987b; Nijkamp and Folkerts, 1987) or abolished (Flavahan et al., 1986; Butler et al., 1987; Tschirhart et al., 1987; Smith and Vanhoutte, 1988a). Thus, a product of cyclooxygenase, in particular prostaglandin E_2, could be the epithelial factor released in response to arachidonic acid (Bulter et al., 1987; Braunstein et al., 1988). Prostaglandin E_2 is produced in the epithelial cell of several species: dog (Smith et al.,

1982; Leikauf et al., 1986; Welsh, 1987), cow (Leikauf et al., 1988), rabbit (Butler et al., 1987). In the dog, addition of arachidonic acid stimulates the release of prostaglandin E_2 from second (lobar) and fourth order (subsegmental) bronchi with epithelium; bronchi without epithelium do not release this prostanoid when stimulated (Fig. 13; Stuart-Smith and Vanhoutte, 1988a). This suggests that prostaglandin E_2 maybe the mediator of the epithelium-dependent relaxation to arachidonic acid in canine airways. However, there is a difference in the response to fatty acid depending on the location and diameter of the bronchus studied. Thus, second and third (segmental) order bronchi with epithelium show a marked relaxation to the substance, whereas the response is smaller in fourth-order tissues (Fig. 14; Stuart-Smith and Vanhoutte, 1988a). This heterogeneity in response is not because of a reduced sensitivity in the smaller airways to prostaglandin E_2, since the relaxation induced by exogenous prostaglandin E_2 is similar in the three orders of dog bronchi (Stuart-Smith and Vanhoutte, 1988a). Fourth-order bronchi with

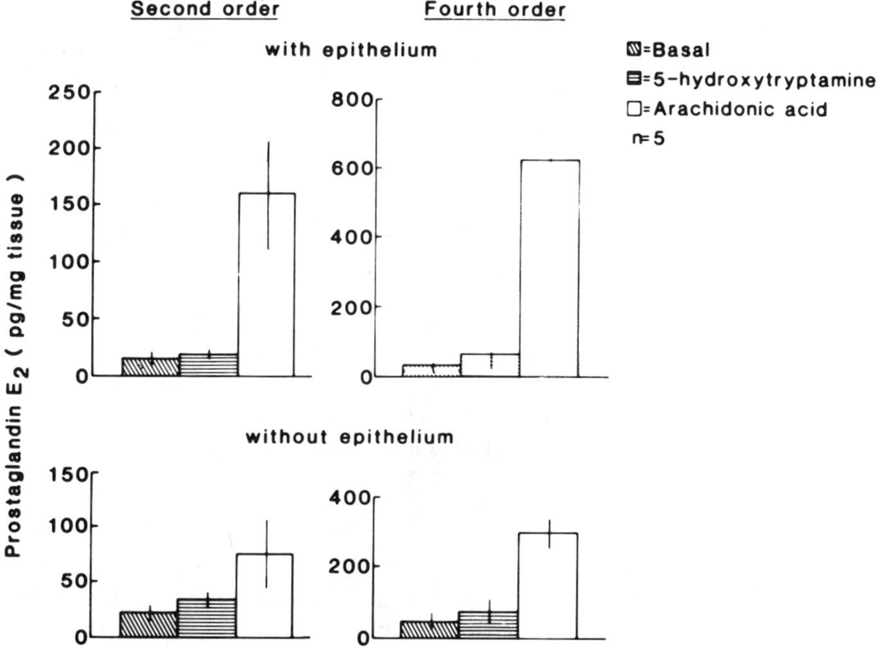

Figure 13   Release of prostaglandin E_2 under basal conditions and when evoked by 5-hydroxytryptamine and arachidonic acid in perfused second and fourth order canine bronchi (adapted from Stuart-Smith and Vanhoutte, 1988a, by permission).

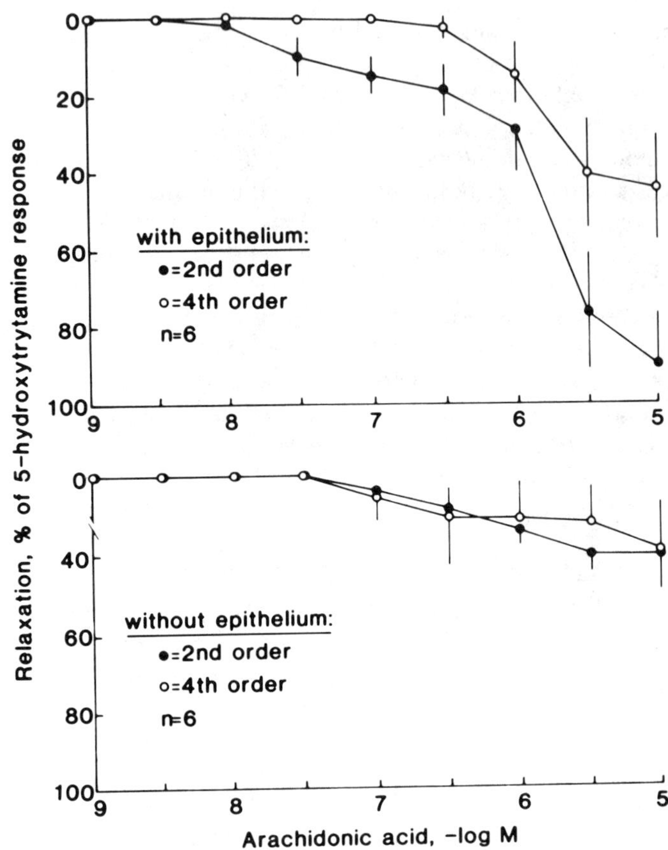

Figure 14   Effect of epithelium removal on concentration-effect curve to arachidonic acid in second order and fourth order canine bronchi. Rings were contracted using 30% effective dose for 5-hydroxytryptamine. Values (means ± SEM) are expressed as percent of response to 5-hydroxytryptamine. Upper panel: rings with epithelium; lower panel: rings without epithelium (reprinted from Stuart-Smith and Vanhoutte, 1988a, by permission).

epithelium release significantly more prostaglandin E_2 in response to arachidonic acid than do second-order tissues (Fig. 13; Stuart-Smith and Vanhoutte, 1988a). The heterogeneity in response to arachidonic acid cannot therefore be explained entirely by the differences in the release of, and sensitivity to, prostaglandin E_2.

Airway epithelial cells also release metabolites of arachidonic acid other than prostaglandin E_2 (Holtzman et al., 1983a; Eling et al., 1986; Leikauf et al., 1988). These metabolites, both of the cyclooxygenase and lipoxygenase pathways, could play a part in modulating the response of airway smooth muscle. Specifically, leukotrienes, either generated by the epithelium or non-epithelial structures in response to exogenous arachidonic acid, evoke contractions, which are greater in smaller airways (Bakhle and Ferreira, 1985). Therefore, a possible explanation for the reduced relaxation to arachidonic acid in the smaller bronchi of the dog could be the opposing effect of leukotrienes on the relaxations induced by prostaglandin E_2 (Stuart-Smith and Vanhoutte, 1988a). A similar phenomenon may exist in the trachea of the guinea pig (Nijkamp and Folkerts, 1986; Farmer et al., 1987b; Tschirhart et al., 1987). In the presence of indomethacin, the guinea pig trachea with epithelium contracts in response to arachidonic acid; this contraction is inhibited by noredihydroguaiarectic acid (NDGA; a 5-lipoxygenase antagonist), suggesting the involvement of products of lipoxygenase, most likely leukotrienes (Farmer et al., 1987b). In addition, the arachidonate-induced contractions of the trachea without epithelium are probably mediated by products of lipoxygenase, implicating leukotrienes formed outside of the epithelium in the response (Nijkamp and Folkerts, 1986; Farmer et al., 1987b). Furthermore, in the presence of only NDGA, arachidonic acid caused contractions that depended on the presence of the epithelium; this suggests another possible role for the products of lipoxygenase, namely to antagonize the action or formation of epithelium-derived contracting prostanoid (Farmer et al., 1987b). However, this effect of NDGA was not observed in another study (Tschirhart et al., 1987). Thus, the epithelium-dependent relaxations in response to arachidonic acid probably are mediated by prostaglandin E_2, but also involve complex interactions of other prostanoids and leukotrienes released by the epithelium and nonepithelial structures.

The possible relationship of eicosanoids with the increased sensitivity and/or the maximal response of the smooth muscle to contractile stimuli in airways without epithelium has also been investigated. Studies done in the guinea pig trachea conclude that to some degree indomethacin mimics the effects of epithelium removal on the responses to methacholine and leukotriene C_4, which may be due to the release of an epithelium-derived product of cyclooxygenase that could either cause relaxation directly or regulate the synthesis and release of another relaxing factor (Hay et al., 1986a, 1987a). In particular, the epithelial release of prostaglandin E_2 has been linked to epithelial regulation of the response to bethanechol in the intrapulmonary bronchi of the rabbit (Butler et al., 1987) and to that of basal tone and the response to histamine in the guinea pig trachea (Braunstein et al., 1988). In addition, cultured epithelial cells from the dog trachea when stimulated by bradykinin release a cyclooxygenase-dependent factor, probably prostaglandin E_2, that inhibits contractions of smooth muscle induced by electrical stimulation (Barnett et al., 1988). It has also been suggested that the hyper-reactivity of the airways induced by endotoxin may be caused by a disturbed ability of epithelial cells to synthesize prostaglandin E_2 (Folkerts et al., 1989). Furthermore, part of the epithelium-dependent response to tachykinins in the guinea pig can be attributed to the release of relaxing prostanoids (Frossard et al., 1989).

However, the epithelial release of relaxing prostanoids does not occur in every situation. For example, indomethacin does not affect the augmented response of epithelium removal to acetylcholine in the bronchi of the dog (Lorenz et al., 1988), to histamine in the trachea of the guinea pig (Hay et al., 1986a; Holroyde, 1986) or to acetylcholine in the trachea of the cow (Barnes et al., 1985). In similar fashion, the influence of the epithelium on the responses to isoproterenol in canine airways is not prevented by indomethacin (Stuart-Smith and Vanhoutte, 1990b). The epithelium-derived factor(s) released by hyperosmotic and hypotonic stimuli (Munakata et al., 1988a; Gao and Vanhoutte, 1989) and that relaxes vascular smooth muscle and the anococcygeus muscle is not a product of cyclooxygenase (Ilhan and Sahin, 1986; Guc et al., 1988; Fernandes et al., 1989). Other metabolites of arachidonic acid, specifically the leukotrienes, are not involved in the epithelium-dependent response to acetylcholine in the bronchi of the dog (Lorenz et al., 1988) and in the trachea of the cow (Barnes et al., 1985). Moreover, leukotrienes, which contribute to the relaxations and contractions evoked by histamine and carbachol in the guinea pig trachea, act independently of the presence of the epithelium (Tschirhart et al., 1987).

The evidence discussed in the preceding sections also supports the existence of epithelium-derived contracting (excitatory) factor(s), but the nature of it is also unknown (Frossard and Muller, 1986; Hay et al., 1986a; Raeburn et al., 1986; Farmer et al., 1987b; Flavahan et al., 1988; Stuart-Smith and Vanhoutte, 1988b; Brofman et al., 1989).

VIII. Physiological Role

Two major possibilities exist regarding the potential physiological role of the epithelium-derived factor(s). First, the similar parallel shift to the left of the concentration-response curves to acetylcholine, histamine, and 5-hydroxytryptamine (Figs 9, 15) evoked by the removal of the epithelium implies that the release of the relaxing factor(s) is continuous (basal release), rather than due to activation of specific epithelial receptors. The second possibility is the occurrence of the evoked (triggered) release of the epithelium-derived factor(s). Thus, the increased responsiveness to beta-adrenergic agonists in intact compared with epithelium-denuded bronchi (Flavahan and Vanhoutte,

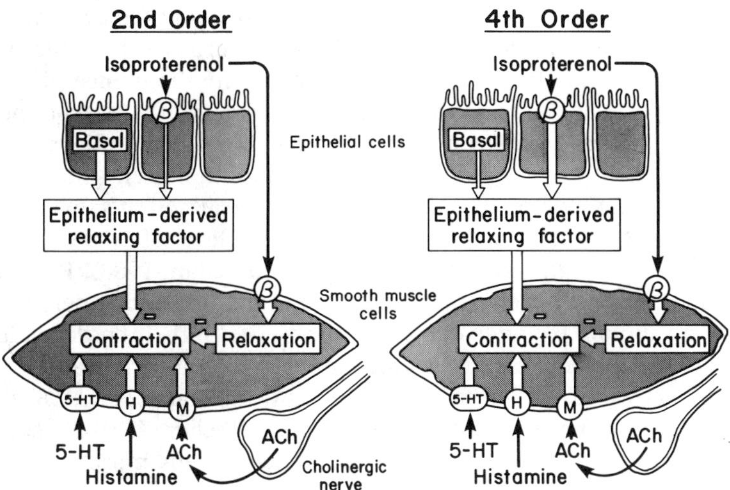

Figure 15 Diagrammatic representation of the potential physiological role of the respiratory epithelium in modulating the responsiveness of the underlying smooth muscle in large (left) and small (right) bronchi. ACh, acetylcholine; b, beta-adrenoceptor; H, histamine receptor; 5-HT, 5-hydroxytryptamine, serotonergic receptor; M, muscarinic receptor (reprinted from Vanhoutte, 1988b, by permission).

1984; Flavahan et al., 1985; Barnes et al., 1985; Goldie et al., 1986; Ruff et al., 1988; Stuart-Smith and Vanhoutte, 1988) suggests that activation of beta-adrenoceptors on the epithelial cells (which have a high density of beta-adrenoceptors compared to airway smooth muscle; Xue et al., 1983; Carstairs et al., 1984, 1985; Goldie et al., 1986; Argarawal et al., 1987) triggers the active release of epithelium-derived relaxing factor(s) (Figs. 10, 15). A similar conclusion can be reached for arachidonic acid (Flavahan et al., 1986; Nijkamp and Folkerts, 1986; Butler et al., 1987; Farmer et al., 1987; Tschirhart et al., 1987; Braunstein et al., 1988; Stuart-Smith and Vanhoutte, 1988a), platelet-activating factor (Brunelleschi et al., 1987), and methylxanthines (Goldie et al., 1986; Busk and Vanhoutte, 1988, 1989). Another important trigger for the release could be changes in osmolarity (Munakata et al., 1988a; Gao and Vanhoutte, 1989b).

A few studies have examined the mechanism by which the epithelium-derived relaxing factor(s) modulates the reactivity of the smooth muscle. It seems to be temperature sensitive and to require extracellular calcium (Lev et al., 1988), although the increase in responsiveness of airway smooth muscle observed with epithelium removal is not the result of a facilitation of the calcium entry into the muscle cells (Raeburn et al., 1987). Another possible mechanism of action of the epithelium-derived relaxing factor(s) may be to affect the agonist-induced phosphatidylinositol turnover by inhibiting the pathway (Hay et al., 1988). The factor(s) affecting the guinea pig trachea may act, in part, by reducing the endogenous release of acetylcholine from intramural cholinergic nerve terminals (Murlas, 1986). Part of its action may be to inhibit the depolarization of bronchial smooth muscle (Gao and Vanhoutte, 1988). The sodium/potassium pump has been implicated in epithelium-dependent phenomena, but whether this is at the level of epithelium or the smooth muscle remains uncertain (Lamport and Fedan, 1988). Propranolol (a beta-adrenergic blocker) and tetrodotoxin (an inhibitor of nerve activity by blocking sodium channels) failed to inhibit the epithelium-dependent relaxation to hyperosmolar stimuli which implies that these relaxations do not depend on activation of the adrenergic nerves (Munakata et al., 1988a). Propranolol also does not inhibit the effect of the epithelium-derived factor that relaxes vascular smooth muscle and the anococcygeus muscle (Ilhan and Sahin, 1986; Guc et al., 1988).

IX. Clinical Implications

In patients with asthma, prominent epithelial destruction has been observed at all levels of the respiratory tract (Laitinen et al., 1985). Furthermore, the hyperresponsiveness found in vivo in asthmatic patients cannot be explained entirely in terms of sensitivity of the smooth muscle (Armour et al., 1984). In animals and humans, exposure to stimuli such as ozone, toluene diisocyanate, plicatic acid, abietic acid, allergen, or respiratory virus can induce hyperresponsiveness of the airways and also cause acute inflammation of the epithelium (Empey et al., 1976; Cockcroft et al., 1977; Laitinen et al., 1976; Holtzman et al., 1983b; Murlas and Roum, 1985; Fabbri et al., 1987; Lam et al., 1987; Ayars et al., 1989). The eosinophils, as part of the response to inflammation, can degranulate, liberating a toxic cationic granule protein, the major basic protein, that causes desquamation and damage to ciliated epithelial cells (Gleich et al., 1979; Frigas and Gleich, 1986). Thus, damage to or malfunction of respiratory epithelial cells could explain in part the bronchial hyperreactivity observed in asthma and airway infections (Nadel, 1983; Hogg and Eggleston, 1984). This statement is supported strongly by the findings discussed in this chapter. Indeed, the absence or the dysfunction of the epithelial cell obtained by mechanical rubbing or exposure to the major basic protein augments the responsiveness of isolated airways. This augmentation can be explained by the decreased generation of epithelium-derived relaxing factor(s) or the abnormal production of epithelium-derived contracting factor(s). The loss or dysfunction of the epithelium could also lead to the abnormal metabolism of arachidonic acid, which may additionally contribute to the hyperresponsiveness of the airways in asthma. Furthermore, the epithelium-mediated partial inhibition of contraction to bronchoconstrictors and enhancement of relaxation to the bronchodilators, although relatively small in vitro, may be magnified in vivo because resistance to airflow increases in proportion to the fourth power of the radius of the airway.

The asthmatic state may represent an abnormal response to osmotic stimuli, such as dry air or hyperventilation, that tend to disrupt the epithelial cell (Hogg and Eggleston, 1984). In the normal individual, epithelial cells, in response to osmotic stimuli, might generate an epithelium-derived relaxing factor that would protect the airway. On the other hand, the epithelium of an asthmatic individual might be altered, such that no relaxing factor(s) is present and an asthmatic attack follows the exposure to the osmotic stimulus. In a complex system of tubes like the bronchial tree with its many branches, changes in caliber, and irregular wall surfaces, sheer stress could also constitute an important natural stimulus. In larger airways, the diameter may be a function of flow through them. Since the epithelial cells release a substance(s) that also affects vascular smooth muscle, the factor(s) may work by acting on other subepithelial structures (for example, sensory nerves, blood vessels), in turn, indirectly modulating the responsiveness of the airway smooth muscle. In this way, the plasma exudate of the airway may be an important source of epithelium-derived factor(s) and a medium for its transfer and metabolism (Persson, 1986). In addition to the direct effect on the bronchial smooth muscle, a facilitatory role of the epithelial cells on the response to beta-adrenergic agonists (Flavahan and Vanhoutte, 1984; Barnes et al., 1985; Flavahan et al., 1985; Goldie et al., 1986; Ruff et al., 1987; Stuart-Smith and Vanhoutte, 1987; Stuart-Smith and Vanhoutte, 1988b) and methylxanthines (Busk and Vanhoutte, 1988, 1989, 1990) could be of particular importance when these therapeutic agents are administered by aerosol.

The airway epithelium functions as a protective barrier to the subepithelial structures, but possibly is as important in controlling the tone of the underlying smooth muscle through the release of epithelium-derived factor(s). An inappropriate balance in the release and action of the epithelium-derived factor(s) may be one part of the mechanism underlying the bronchospasm of asthma.

Acknowledgment

This work was supported in part by NIH grant HL 39423.

Discussion

Barnes: Is it possible that epithelium-derived relaxing factor could be acting indirectly on smooth muscle, for example by affecting the vasculature, which might release factors influencing the smooth muscle?

Busk: It is a possibility that epithelium-derived relaxing factor works indirectly.

Widdicombe: Is it possible that the superficial vasculature could take up epithelial derived factors and transport them deeper into the tissues, for example, to muscles?

Leff: Is it possible that the phenomenon is an artifact of tissue preparation?

Busk: No. This area is addressed in detail in my chapter, and all the evidence indicates that this is not an artifact.

Dahl: Could the reasons that inhaled theophylline are ineffective bronchodilators and inhaled beta agonists effective be due to the capacity of beta agonists to generate epithelium-derived relaxing factor?

Persson: Inhaled theophylline is cleared rapidly from the lungs while beta agonists bind to receptors and stay in the airways for some time. Thus, the lack of effectiveness of inhaled theophylline is more likely due to its short residence time.

O'Byrne: What is the effect of epithelial removal on K+ actions?

Busk: Epithelial removal has little effect on the actions of K+.

Karlsson: What are the effects of partial removal of the epithelium?

Busk: We have not studied this.

Woolcock: Is the dog an adequate model of human asthma?

Busk: Several experiments utilizing human tissues demonstrate that this phenomena occurs in humans as well.

Widdicombe: Does field stimulation act through the release of neuropeptides?

Busk: Removal of the epithelium does enhance neuropeptide actions, but this is thought to be due to the removal of neuropeptide-degrading enzymes.

References

Aarhus, L. L., Rimele, T. J., and Vanhoutte, P. M. (1984). Removal of the epithelium causes bronchial supersensitivity to acetylcholine and 5-hydroxytryptamine. *Fed. Proc.* **43**:955.

Advenier, C., Devillier, P., Matran, R., and Naline, E. (1988). Influence of epithelium on the responsiveness of guinea-pig isolated trachea to adenosine. *Br. J. Pharmacol.* **93**:295-302.

Aizawa, H., Miyazaki, N., Shigematsu, N., and Tomooka, M. (1988). A possible role of airway epithelium in modulating hyperresponsiveness. *Br. J. Pharmacol.* **93**:139-145.

Altiere, R. J., Szarek, J. L., and Diamond, L. (1984). Neural control of relaxation in cat airways smooth muscle. *J. Appl. Physiol.* **57**:1536-1544.

Argarwal, D. K., Schugel, J. W., and Townley, R. G. (1987). Comparison of beta adrenoceptors in bovine airway epithelium and smooth muscle cells. *Biochem. Biophys. Res. Commun.* **148**:178-183.

Armour, C. L., Black, J. L., Berend, N., Woolcock, A. J. (1984). The relationship between bronchial hyperresponsiveness to methacholine and airway smooth muscle structure and reactivity. *Respir. Physiol.* **58**:223-233.

Ayars, G. H., Altman, L. C., Frazier, C. E., and Chi, E. Y. (1989). The toxicity of constituents of cedar and pine woods to pulmonary epithelium. *J. Allergy Clin. Immunol.* **83**:610-618.

Bakhle, Y. S., and Ferreira, S. H. (1985). Lung metabolism of eicosanoids, prostaglandins, prostacyclin, thromboxane and leukotrienes. In *Handbook of Physiology*, Section 3: The Respiratory System. Vol. I, Circulatory and Non-respiratory Functions. Edited by A. P. Fishman and A. B. Fisher. Bethesda, MD, American Physiological Society, p. 365.

Barnes, P. J., Cuss, F. M., and Palmer, J. B. (1985). The effect of airway epithelium on smooth muscle contractility in bovine trachea. *Br. J. Pharmacol.* **86**:684-691.

Barnett, K., Jacoby, D. B., Nadel, J. A., and Lazarus, S. C. (1988). The effects of epithelial cell supernatant on contractions of isolated canine tracheal smooth muscle. *Am. Rev. Respir. Dis.* **138**:780-783.

Boushey, H. A., Holtzman, M. J., Sheller, J. R., and Nadel, J. A. (1980). Bronchial hyperreactivity. *Am. Rev. Respir. Dis.* **121**:389-413.

Braunstein, G., Labat, C., Brunelleschi, S., Benveniste, J., Marsac, J., Brink, C. (1988). Evidence that the histamine sensitivity and responsiveness of guinea pig isolated trachea are modulated by epithelial prostaglandin E_2 production. *Br. J. Pharmacol.* **95**:300-308.

Brink, C., Duncan, P. G., and Douglas, J. S. (1981). The response and sensitivity to histamine of respiratory tissues from normal and ovalbumin-sensitized guinea-pigs: effects of cyclooxygenase and lipoxygenase inhibition. *J. Pharmacol. Exp. Ther.* **217**:592-601.

Brofman, J. D., White, S. R., Blake, J. S., Munoz, N. M., Gleich, G. J., and Leff, A. R. (1989). Epithelial augmentation of trachealis contraction caused by major basic protein of eosinophils. *J. Appl. Physiol.* **66**:1867-1873.

Brunelleschi, S., Haye-Legrand, I., Lebat, C., Norel, X., Benveniste, J., and Brink, C. (1987). Platelet-activating factor-acether-induced relaxation of guinea pig airway muscle: role of prostaglandin E_2 and the epithelium. *J. Pharmacol. Exp. Ther.* **243**:356-363.

Burka, J. F., and Saad, M. H. (1984). Mediators of arachidonic acid-induced contractions of indomethacin-treated guinea pig airways: leukotrienes C_4 and D_4. *Br. J. Pharmacol.* **81**:465-473.

Busk, M., and Vanhoutte, P. M. (1988). The methylxanthine, S 9795, causes the release of an epithelium-derived relaxing factor. *Clin. Res.* **36**:590A.

Busk, M. F., and Vanhoutte, P. M. (1989). Theophylline causes the release of an epithelium-derived relaxing factor. *FASEB J.* **3**:A274.

Busk, M. F., Flavahan, N. A., and Vanhoutte, P. M. (1989). Bioassay of epithelium-derived relaxing factor(s). *Am. Rev. Respir. Dis.* **139**:A354.

Busk, M. F., and Vanhoutte, P. M. (1990). Effects of the methyl xanthine, S 9795, on isolated bronchi of the dog. *J. Pharmacol. Exper. Ther.* (in press).

Butler, G. B., Adler, K. B., Evans, J. N., Morgan, D. W., and Szarek, J. L. (1987). Modulation of rabbit airway smooth muscle responsiveness by respiratory epithelium. *Am. Rev. Respir. Dis.* **135**:1099-1104.

Carstairs, J. R., Nimmon, A. J., and Barnes, P. J. (1984). Autoradiographic localization of β-adrenoceptors in human lung. *Eur. J. Pharmacol.* **103**:189-190.

Carstairs, J. R., Nimmon, A. J., and Barnes, P. J. (1985). Autoradiographic visualization of β-adrenoceptor subtypes in human lung. *Am. Rev. Respir. Dis.* **132**:541-547.

Coburn, R. F., and Tomita, T. (1973). Evidence for nonadrenergic inhibitory nerves in guinea pig trachealis muscle. *Am. J. Physiol.* **224**:1072.

Cockcroft, D. W., Ruffin, R. E., and Hargreave, R. E. (1977). Allergin-induced increase in non-allergic bronchial reactivity. *Clin. Allergy* **7**:503-513.

Cuss, F. M., and Barnes, P. J. (1987). Epithelial mediators. *Am. Rev. Respir. Dis.* **136**:S32-S35.

Devillier, P., Advenier, C., Drapeau, G., Marsal, J., and Regoli, D. (1988). Comparison of the effects of epithelium removal and of an enkephalinase inhibitor on the neurokinin-induced contractions of guinea-pig isolated trachea. *Br. J. Pharmacol.* **94**:675-684.

Drazen, J. M., Austen, K. F., Lewis, R. A., Clark, D. A., Goto, G., Marfat, A., and Corey, E. J. (1980). Comparative airway and vascular activities of leukotrienes C-1 and D in vivo and in vitro. *Proc. Natl. Acad. Sci. USA* **77**:4354-4358.

Eling, T. E., Danilowicz, R. M., Henke, D. C., Sivarajah, K., Yankaskas,

J. R., and Boucher, R. C. (1986). Arachidonic acid metabolism by canine treacheal epithelial cells. *J. Biol. Chem.* **261**:12841-12849.

Empey, D. W., Laitinen, L. A., Jacobs, L., Gold, W. M., and Nadel, J. A. (1976). Mechanisms of bronchial hyperreactivity in normal subjects after upper respiratory tract infection. *Am. Rev. Respir. Dis.* **113**:131-139.

Fabbri, L. M., Boschetto, P., Zocca, E., Milani, G., Pivirotto, F., Plebani, M., Burlina, A., Licata, B., and Mapp, C. E. (1987). Bronchoalveolar neutrophilia during late asthmatic reactions induced by toluene diisocyanate. *Am. Rev. Respir. Dis.* **136**:36-42.

Farmer, S. G. (1987). Airway smooth muscle responsiveness: modulation by the epithelium. *Trends in Pharmacol. Sci.* **8**:8-10.

Farmer, S. G., Fedan, J. S., Hay, D. W. P., and Raeburn, D. (1986). The effects of epithelium removal on the sensitivity of guinea-pig isolated trachealis to bronchodilator drugs. *Br. J. Pharmacol.* **89**:407-417.

Farmer, S. G., Hay, D. W. P., Raeburn, D., and Fedan, J. S. (1987). Relaxation of guinea-pig tracheal smooth muscle to arachidonate is converted to contraction following epithelium removal. *Br. J. Pharmacol.* **92**:231-236.

Fedan, J. S., and Frazer, D. G. (1988). Comparison of reactivity of intact guinea pig trachea (GPT) in vitro to intraluminal vs. extraluminal bronchoactive agents. *Physiologist* A97.

Fedan, J. S., Hay, D. W., Farmer, S. G., and Raeburn, D. (1988). Epithelial cells: modulation of airway smooth muscle reactivity. In *Asthma: Basic Mechanisms and Clinical Management.* Edited by P. J. Barnes, I. W. Rodger, and N. C. Thomson. London, Academic Press, pp. 143-159.

Fernandes, L. B., Paterson, J. W., and Goldie, R. G. (1989). Co-axial bioassay of a smooth muscle relaxant factor released from guinea pig tracheal epithelium. *Br. J. Pharmacol.* **96**:117-124.

Finnen, M. J., Flowers, R. J., Lashenko, A., and Williams, K. I. (1986). Airway epithelium influences responsiveness of guinea-pig tracheal strips. *Br. J. Pharmacol.* **88**:407.

Flavahan, N. A., and Vanhoutte, P. M. (1984). Epithelial-dependent attenuation of bronchial smooth muscle tone. *Fed. Proc.* **43**:429.

Flavahan, N. A., and Vanhoutte, P. M. (1985). The respiratory epithelium releases a smooth muscle relaxing factor. *Chest* **87**(suppl.):189S-190S.

Flavahan, N. A., Aarhus, L. L., Rimele, T. J., and Vanhoutte, P. M. (1985). The respiratory epithelium inhibits bronchial smooth muscle tone. *J. Appl. Physiol.* **58**:834-838.

Flavahan, N. A., Danser, A. J., and Vanhoutte, P. M. (1986). Arachidonic acid and calcium ionophore cause epithelium-dependent relaxation of canine bronchial smooth muscle. *Proceedings, International Union of Physiological Sciences.* Vancouver, B. C., Canada, July 13-18, p. 148.

Flavahan, N. A., Slifman, N. R., Gleich, G. J., and Vanhoutte, P. M. (1988). Human eosinophil major basic causes hyperreactivity of respiratory smooth muscle. *Am. Rev. Respir. Dis.* **138**:685-688.

Folkerts, G., Engels, F., and Nijkamp, F. P. (1989). Endotoxin-induced hyperreactivity of the guinea pig isolated trachea coincides with decreased prostaglandin E_2 production by the epithelial layer. *Br. J. Pharmacol.* **96**:388-394.

Frigas, E., and Gleich, G. J. (1986). The eosinophil and pathophysiology of asthma. *J. Allergy Clin. Immunol.* **77**:527-537.

Frossard, N., and Muller, F. (1986). Epithelial modulation of tracheal smooth muscle responses to antigenic stimulation. *J. Appl. Physiol.* **61**:1449-1456.

Frossard, N., Rhoden, K. J., and Barnes, P. J. (1988). Influence of epithelium on guinea pig airway response to tachykinins: role of endopeptidase and cyclooxygenase. *J. Pharmacol. Exp. Ther.* **248**:292-298.

Furchgott, R. F. (1984). The role of endothelium in responses of vascular smooth muscle to drugs. *Annu. Rev. Pharmacol. Toxic.* **24**:175-197.

Furchgott, R. F. and Vanhoutte, P. M. (1989). Endothelium-derived relaxing and contracting factors. *FASEB J.* **3**:2007-2018.

Furchgott, R. F., and Zawadzki, J. V. (1980). The obligatory role of endothelial cells in the relaxation of arterial smooth muscle by acetylcholine. *Nature* **288**:373-376.

Gao, Y., and Vanhoutte, P. M. (1988). Removal of the epithelium causes depolarization of canine bronchial smooth muscle. *J. Appl. Physiol.* **65**:2400-2405.

Gao, Y., and Vanhoutte, P. M. (1989a). Influence of the epithelium on the accessibility of intraluminal bronchoactive agents to canine airway smooth muscle. *FASEB J.* **3**:A972.

Gao, Y., and Vanhoutte, P. M. (1989b). Hypotonic solutions induced epithelium-dependent relaxation of canine bronchi. *Am. Rev. Respir. Dis.* **139**:A354.

Gardiner, P. J. (1986). Characterization of prostanoid relaxant/inhibitory receptors (4) using a highly selective agonist, TR4979. *Br. J. Pharmacol.* **87**:45-56.

Gleich, G. J. (1990). The eosinophil and bronchial asthma: current understanding. *J. Allergy Clin. Immunol.* **85**:422-436.

Gleich, G. J., and Loegering, D. A. (1984). Immunobiology of eosinophils. *Annu. Rev. Immunol.* **2**:429-459.

Gleich, G. J., Frigas, E., Loegering, D. A., Wassom, D. L., and Steinmuller, D. (1979). Cytotoxic properties of eosinophil major basic protein. *J. Immunol.* **123**:2925-2927.

Gleich, G. J., Loegering, D. A., and Adolphson, C. R. (1985). Eosinophils and bronchial inflammation. *Chest* **87**(Suppl. 1):10s-13s.

Gleich, G. J., Flavahan, N. A., Fujisawa, T., and Vanhoutte, P. M. (1988). The eosinophil as a mediator of damage to respiratory epithelium: a model for bronchial hyperreactivity. *J. Allergy Clin. Immunol.* **81**:776-781.

Goldie, R. G., Papadimitriou, J. M., Paterson, W. J., Rigby, P. J., Self, H. M., and Spina, D. (1986). Influence of the epithelium on responsiveness of guinea-pig isolated trachea to contractile and relaxant agonists. *Br. J. Pharmacol.* **87**:5-14.

Goldie, R. G., Fernandes, L. B., Rigby, P. J., and Paterson, J. W. (1988). Epithelial dysfunction and airway hyperreactivity in asthma. In *Mechanisms in Asthma: Pharmacology, Physiology, and Managment.* Alan R. Liss, New York, pp. 317-329.

Grandordy, B. M., Frossard, N., Rhoden, K. J., and Barnes, P. J. (1988). Tachykinin-induced phosphoinositide breakdown in airway smooth muscle and epithelium: relationship to contraction. *Mol. Pharmacol.* **33**:515-519.

Guc, M. O., Ilhan, M., and Kayaalp, S. O. (1988). The rat anococcygeus muscle is a convenient bioassay organ for airway epithelium-derived relaxing factor. *Eur. J. Pharmacol.* **148**:405-409.

Hay, D. W. P., Farmer, S. G., Raeburn, D., Robinson, V. A., Fleming, W. W., and Fedan, J. S. (1986a). Airway epithelium modulates the reactivity of guinea-pig respiratory smooth muscle. *Eur. J. Pharmacol.* **129**:11-18.

Hay, D. W. P., Raeburn, D., Farmer, S. G., Fleming, W. W., and Fedan, J. S. (1986b). Epithelium modulates the reactivity of ovalbumin-sensitized guinea-pig airway smooth muscle. *Life Sci.* **38**:2461-2468.

Hay, D. W. P., Farmer, S. G., Raeburn, D., Muccitelli, R. M., Wilson, K. A., and Fedan, J. S. (1987a). Differential effects of epithelium removal on the responsiveness of guinea-pig tracheal smooth muscle to bronchoconstrictors. *Br. J. Pharmacol.* **92**:381-388.

Hay, D. W. P., Muccitelli, R. M., Horstemeyer, D. L., Wilson, K. A., and Raeburn, D. (1987b). Demonstration of the release of an epithelium-derived inhibitory factor from a novel preparation of guinea-pig trachea. *Eur. J. Pharmacol.* **136**:247-250.

Hay, D. W. P., Raeburn, D., and Fedan, J. S. (1987c). Regional differences in reactivity and in the influence of the epithelium on canine intrapulmonary bronchial smooth muscle responsiveness. *Eur. J. Pharmacol.* **141**:363-370.

Hay, D. W. P., Muccitelli, R. M., and Raeburn, D. (1988). Does the epithelium-derived inhibitory factor (EpDIF) act via inhibition of phosphatidylinositol (PI) turnover in guinea-pig trachea (GPT)? *FASEB J.* **2**:A1057.

Hogg, J. C., Eggleston, P. A. (1984). Is asthma an epithelial disease? *Am. Rev. Respir. Dis.* **129**:207-208.

Holroyde, M. C. (1986). The influence of epithelium on the responsiveness of guinea-pig isolated trachea. *Br. J. Pharmacol.* **87**:501-507.

Holtzman, M. J., Aizawa, H., Nadel, J. A., and Goetzel, E. J. (1983a). Selective generation of leukotriene B$_4$ by tracheal epithelial cells from dogs. *Biochem. Biophys. Res. Commun.* **114**:1071-1076.

Holtzman, M. J., Fabbri, L. M., O'Byrne, P. M., Gold, B. D., and Aizawa, H., Walters, E. H., Alpert, S. E., Nadel, J. A. (1983b). Importance of airway inflammation for hyperresponsiveness induced by ozone. *Am. Rev. Respir. Dis.* **127**:686-690.

Hunter, J. A., Finkbeiner, W. E., Nadel, J. A., Goetzel, E. J., and Holtzman, M. J. (1985). Predominant generation of 15-lipoxygenase metabolites of arachidonic acid by epithelial cells from human trachea. *Proc. Natl. Acad. Sci.* **82**:4633-4637.

Ignarro, L. J., Byrms, R. E., Buga, G. M., Wood, K. S., and Chandhuri, G. (1988). Pharmacological evidence that endothelium-derived relaxing factor is nitric oxide: use of pyrogallol and superoxide dismutase to study endothelium-dependent and nitric oxide-elicited vascular smooth muscle relaxation. *J. Pharmacol. Exp. Ther.* **244**:181-189.

Ilhan, M., and Sahin, I. (1987). Tracheal epithelium releases a vascular smooth muscle relaxant factor: demonstration by bioassay. *Eur. J. Pharmacol.* **131**:293-296.

Laitinen, L. A., Elkin, R. B., Empey, D. W., et al. (1976). Changes in bronchial reactivity after administration of live attenuated influenza virus. *Am. Rev. Respir. Dis.* **113**:194.

Laitinen, L. A., Heino, M., Laitinen, A., Kava, T., and Haahtela, T. (1985). Damage of the airway epithelium and bronchial reactivity in patients with asthma. *Am. Rev. Respir. Dis.* **131**:599-606.

Lam, S., LeRiche, J., Phillips, D., and Chan-Yeung, M. (1987). Cellular and protein changes in bronchial lavage fluid after late asthmatic reaction in patients with red cedar asthma. *J. Allergy Clin. Immunol.* **80**:44-50.

Lamport, S. J., and Fedan, J. S. (1988). Temperature-dependent modulatory effect of epithelium on reactivity of guinea-pig isolated trachealis. *FASEB J.* **2**:A1057.

Leikauf, G. D., Ueki, I. F., Nadal, J., and Widdicombe, J. H. (1985). Release of cycloxygenase products from cultured epithelium derived from human and dog trachea. *Fed. Proc.* **44**:1920.

Leikauf, G. D., Ueki, I. F., Widdicombe, J. H., and Nadel, J. A. (1986). Alteration of chloride secretion across canine tracheal epithelium by lipoxygenase products of arachidonic acid. *Am. J. Physiol.* **250**:F47-F53.

Leikauf, G. D., Driscoll, K. E., and Wey, H. E. (1988). Ozone-induced augmentation of eicosanoid metabolism in epithelial cells from bovine trachea. *Am. Rev. Respir. Dis.* **137**:435-442.

Lewis, R. A., Austin, K. F., Drazen, J. M., Clark, D. A., Marfat, A., Corey, E. J. (1980). Slow-reacting substances of anaphylaxis: identification of leukotrienes C-1 and D from human rat sources. *Proc. Natl. Acad. Sci.* **77**:3710-3714.

Lev, A., Christensen, G. C., Ryan, J. P., Wang, M., Kelsen, S. G. (1988). Respiratory epithelial modulation of airway smooth muscle is calcium and temperature dependent. *Am. Rev. Respir. Dis.* **137**:A309.

Lorenz, R. R., Gao, Y., and Vanhoutte, P. M. (1988). The effects of epithelium-removal on airway contractility is not mediated by arachidonic acid metabolites or nitric oxide. *Physiologist* **31**:A124.

Lundblad, K. A. L., and Persson, C. G. A. (1988). The epithelium and the pharmacology of guinea-pig tracheal tone *in vitro*. *Br. J. Pharmacol.* **93**:909-917.

Manning, P. S., Jones, G. L., Lane, C. G., Daniel, E. E., O'Byrne, P. M. (1988). Decreased contractility occurs when epithelium is near, but not attached. *Am. Rev. Respir. Dis.* **137**:A309.

Morris, H. G. (1985). Physiology and pharmacology of prostaglandins and leukotrienes in bronchial asthma. In *Bronchial Asthma: Mechanisms and Therapeutics*. Edited by E. B. Weiss, M. S. Segal and M. Stein. Little Brown, Boston, p. 1650.

Munakata, M., Mitzner, W., and Menkes, H. (1988a). Osmotic stimuli induce epithelial-dependent relaxation in the guinea pig trachea. *J. Appl. Physiol.* **64**:466-471.

Munakata, M., Huang, I., Menkes, H., and Mitzner, W. (1988b). Protective role of epithelium on smooth muscle contractions. *Am. Rev. Respir. Dis.* **137**:A310.

Murlas, C. (1986). Effects of mucosal removal on guinea-pig airway smooth muscle responsiveness. *Clin. Sci.* **70**:571-575.

Murlas, C. G., and Roum, J. H. (1985). Sequence of pathologic changes in the airway mucosa of guinea pigs during ozone-induced bronchial hyperreactivity. *Am. Rev. Respir. Dis.* **131**:314-320.

Murphy, R. C., Hamarström, S., and Samuelson, B. (1979). Leukotriene C: A slow-reacting substance from murine mastocytoma cells. *Proc. Natl. Acad. Sci. USA* **76**:4275.

Nadel, J. A. (1983). Bronchial reactivity. *Adv. Intern. Med.* **28**:207-223.

Nijkamp, F. P., and Folkerts, G. (1987). Reversal of arachidonic acid-induced guinea-pig tracheal relaxation into contraction after epithelium removal. *Eur. J. Pharmacol.* **131**:315-316.

Orehek, J., Douglas, J. S., and Bouhuys, A. (1975). Contractile responses of the guinea-pig trachea *in vitro*: modification by prostaglandin synthesis-inhibiting drugs. *J. Pharmacol. Exp. Ther.* **194**:554-564.

Palmer, R. M. J., Ferrige, A. G., and Moncada, S. (1987). Nitric oxide release accounts for the biological activity of endothelium-derived relaxing factor. *Nature (Lond.)* **327**:524-527.

Persson, C. G. A. (1986). Role of plasma exudation in asthmatic airways. *Lancet* **2**:1126-1128.

Persson, C. G. A., and Karlsson, J. A. (1987). In vitro response to bronchodilator drugs. In *Drug Therapy for Asthma.* Lung Biology in Health and Disease. Edited by J. Jenne, T. Murphy, and C. Lenfant. New York, Marcel Dekker, pp. 129-176.

Raeburn, D., Hay, D. W. P., Robinson, V. A., Farmer, S. G., Fleming, W. W., and Fedan, J. S. (1986a). The effect of verapamil is reduced in isolated airway smooth muscle preparations lacking the epithelium. *Life Sci.* **38**:809-816.

Raeburn, D., Hay, D. W. P., Farmer, S. G., and Fedan, J. S. (1986b). Epithelium removal increases the reactivity of human isolated tracheal muscle to methacholine and reduces the effect of verapamil. *Eur. J. Pharmacol.* **123**:451-453.

Raeburn, D., Hay, D. W. P., and Fedan, J. S. (1987). Calcium uptake into guinea-pig trachealis: the effect of epithelium removal. *Cell Calcium* **8**:429-436.

Rubanyi, G. M., and Vanhoutte, P. M.)1985). Hypoxia releases a vasoconstrictor substance from the canine vascular endothelium. *J. Physiol.* **364**:45-56.

Ruff, F., Zander, J. F., Edoute, Y., Santais, M. C., Flavahan, N. A., Verbeuren, T. J., and Vanhoutte, P. M. (1987). Beta$_2$-adrenergic responses to tulobuterol in airway smooth muscle, vascular smooth muscle and adrenergic nerves. *J. Pharmacol. Exp. Ther.* **244**:173-180.

Russell, J. A. (1978). Responses of isolated canine airways to electric stimulation and acetylcholine. *J. Appl. Physiol.* **45**:690-698.

Russell, J. A. (1980). Noradrenergic inhibitory innervation of canine airways. *J. Appl. Physiol.* **48**:16-22.

Samhorn, M. N., and Piper, P. J. (1986). Actions of leukotrienes in nonhuman respiratory tissues. In *The Leukotrienes: Their Biological Significance.* Edited by P. J. Piper. Raven Press, New York, p. 151.

Shore, S. A., Powell, W. S., and Martin, J. G. (1985). Endogenous prostaglandins modulate histamine-induced contraction in canine tracheal smooth muscle. *J. Appl. Physiol.* **58**:859-868.

Smith, P. L., Welsh, M. J., Stoff, J. S., and Frizzell, R. A. (1982). Chloride secretion by canine tracheal epithelium: role of intracellular cAMP levels. *J. Membrane Biol.* **70**:217-226.

Stuart-Smith, K., and Vanhoutte, P. M. (1987). Heterogeneity in the effects of epithelium removal in the canine bronchial tree. *J. Appl. Physiol.* **63**:2510-2515.

Stuart-Smith, K., and Vanhoutte, P. M. (1988a). Arachidonic acid evokes epithelium-dependent relaxations of canine bronchi. *J. Appl. Physiol.* **65**:2170-2180.

Stuart-Smith, K., and Vanhoutte, P. M. (1988b). The airway epithelium modulates the responsiveness of porcine bronchial smooth muscle. *J. Appl. Physiol.* **65**:721-727.

Stuart-Smith, K., and Vanhoutte, P. M. (1990a). Epithelium-derived relaxing factor. In *Airway Smooth Muscle: Receptor Modulation and Response*. Edited by D. K. Argarwal. CRC Press, Boca Raton, Florida.

Stuart-Smith, K., and Vanhoutte, P. M. (1990b). Epithelium, Contractile Tone and Responses to Relaxing Agonists in Canine Bronchi. *J. Appl. Physiol.* In press.

Thompson, D. C., Stewart, A. B., and Fennessy, M. R. (1985). The effect of epithelium removal on the sensitivity of the guinea pig isolated trachea of contractile agonists. *Clin. Exp. Pharmacol. Physiol.* (Suppl. 9):21.

Thompson, D. C., Wells, J. L., Altiere, R. J., and Diamond, L. (1988). The effect of epithelium removal on non-adrenergic, non-cholinergic inhibitory responses in the isolated central airways of the cat and guinea pig. *Eur. J. Pharmacol.* **145**:231-237.

Torphy, T. J., Rinard, G. A., Rietow, M. G., and Mayer, S. E. (1983). Functional antagonism of canine tracheal smooth muscle: inhibition by methacholine of the mechanical and biochemical responses to isoproterenol. *J. Pharmacol. Exp. Ther.* **227**:694-698.

Torphy, T. J., Zheng, C., Peterson, S. M., Fiscus, R. R., Rinard, G. A., and Mayer, S. E. (1985). Inhibitory effect of methacholine and drug-induced relaxation, cyclic AMP accumulation, and cyclic AMP-dependent protein kinase, activation in canine tracheal smooth muscle. *J. Pharmacol. Exp. Ther.* **223**:409-417.

Tschirhart, E., and Landry, Y. (1986). Airway epithelium releases a relaxant factor: demonstration with substance P. *Eur. J. Pharmacol.* **132**:103-104.

Tschirhart, E., Frossard, N., Bertrand, C., and Landry, Y. (1987). Arachidonic acid metabolites and airway epithelium-dependent relaxant factor. *J. Pharmacol. Exp. Ther.* **243**:310-316.

Undem, B. J., Raible, D. G., Adkinson, Jr. N. F., and Adams G. K. III (1988). Effect of removal of epithelium on antigen-induced smooth muscle contraction and mediator release from guinea-pig isolated trachea. *J. Pharmacol. Exp. Ther.* **244**:659-665.

Vanhoutte, P. M. (1987a). Airway epithelium and bronchial reactivity. *Can. J. Physiol. Pharmacol.* **65**:448-450.

Vanhoutte, P. M. (1987b). Endothelium and the control of vascular tissue. *News in Physiol. Sci.* **2**:18-22.

Vanhoutte, P. M. (1987c). Endothelium-dependent contractions in arteries and veins. *Blood Vessels* **24**:141-144.

Vanhoutte, P. M. (1988a). Epithelium-derived relaxing factor(s) and bronchial reactivity. *Am. Rev. Respir. Dis.* **138**:S24-S30.

Vanhoutte, P. M. (1988b). Epithelium derived relaxing factor: myth or reality? *Thorax* **43**:665-668.

Vanhoutte, P. M., and Flavahan, N. A.)1987). Modulation of cholinergic neurotransmission in the airways. In: *The Airways: Neural Control in Health and Disease.* Edited by M. A. Kaliner and P. J. Barnes. New York, Marcel Dekker, pp. 203-216.

Vanhoutte, P. M., Rubanyi, G. M., Miller, V. M., and Houston, D. S. (1986). Modulation of vascular smooth muscle contraction by the endothelium. *Annu. Rev. Physiol.* **48**:307-320.

Vermeire, P. A., and Vanhoutte, P. M. (1979). Inhibitory effects of catecholamines in isolated canine bronchial smooth muscle. *J. Appl. Physiol.* **46**:787-791.

Weibel, E. R. (1985). Lung cell biology. In *Handbook of Physiology,* The Respiratory System, Circulatory and Nonrespiratory Functions, Section 3, Vol. I. Bethesda, MD, American Physiological Society, p. 47.

Welsh, M. J. (1987). Effect of phorbol ester and calcium ionophore on chloride secretion in canine tracheal epithelium. *Am. J. Physiol.* **253**(Cell Physiol. 22):C828-C834.

Xu, G. L., Sivarajah, K., Reen, W., Nettesheim, P., and Eling, T. (1986). Biosynthesis of prostaglandins by isolated and cultured airway epithelial cells. *Exp. Lung Res.* **10**:101-114.

Xue, Q.-F., Maurer, R., and Engel, G. (1983). Selective distribution of beta- and alpha$_1$-adrenoceptors in rat lung visualized by autoradiography. *Arch. Int. Pharmacodyn. Ther.* **266**:308-314.

6

Structure of Airway Smooth Muscle

EDWIN E. DANIEL, I. BEREZIN, and PAUL M. O'BYRNE

McMaster University
Hamilton, Ontario, Canada

I. Introduction

This review will focus on the ultrastructure of airway smooth muscle, especially the trachea and bronchi, and on structural elements that may affect muscle function: cell-to-cell junctions, innervation, and the presence of inflammatory cells and the changes they induce. Since our research has involved studies mostly of human and canine airways, the information presented is derived primarily from these species.

II. Methodological Considerations

We have studied human airway derived from autopsy material taken within 3 h after death and then exposed to oxygenated Krebs solution at 25 °C for several hours (Davis et al., 1982, 1983, 1986). This material therefore suffers from the possible presence of postmortem changes and from the absence of information about the status of the airways and especially the responsiveness of the airway in vivo.

We have also studied canine airways. The animals included as "normals" are those without any gross evidence of airway infection or inflammation in vivo. Also, in some cases, airway responsiveness to challenge (usually acetylcholine) has been studied prior to euthanasia (e.g., Daniel, 1988; Daniel et al., 1988; O'Byrne et al., 1988). To induce inflammation and hyperresponsiveness, ozone inhalation has been used (O'Byrne et al., 1988; Jones et al., 1988) and we have also studied genetically hyperresponsive Basenji-greyhound dogs (Hirshman and Downs, 1986; Daniel et al., 1989a), and compared them to normally responsive controls.

The animals were killed with an overdose of anesthetic, and the tissues rapidly dissected in Krebs-Ringer's solution. Human and animal airways were fixed by immersion in buffered glutaraldehyde (Daniel and Posey-Daniel, 1984; Daniel et al., 1987, 1988). Airway muscle was postfixed in osmium, the tissues were embedded, stained, en bloc with uranyl actate, sectioned, and stained with lead citrate. Sections were made so that muscle was cross-sectioned. When possible (with second or higher order bronchi), each section included muscle, epithelium, and the space between them. A standard protocol was used for examination of profiles of muscle and of nerves near (≤ 2.5 μm) muscle; the region between epithelium and muscle and the epithelium was examined for their normal cellular constituents and for changes after ozone administration (30 min, 2 h, and 6 h).

III. General Description

A. Muscle

Since the most complete systematic study has been made of canine airway, the general description will be based on this species. Canine airway muscles are arranged in bundles partly surrounded by fibroblasts. However, the profiles of cells in cross-section are not simple circles but are of complex configuration (Fig. 1). They often have long projections. The most unexpected observation is that they often have membrane-bounded lacunae within the cell profile. These are usually clearly connected to the extracellular space and they often contain collagen, elastin, or basement-membrane-like material. The cells have other structures common to smooth muscle: many membrane caveolae, thick myosin, thin actin and intermediate filaments, dense bodies in the cytoplasm and associated with the plasmalemma, typical nuclei, a limited Golgi apparatus near the nucleus, endoplasmic reticulum, often near the plasmalemma.

The cells are frequently connected by gap junctions usually located on cell processes (Fig. 2) and in the canine airway these are found in similar density from trachea down to sixth order bronchi. Gap junction profiles vary in

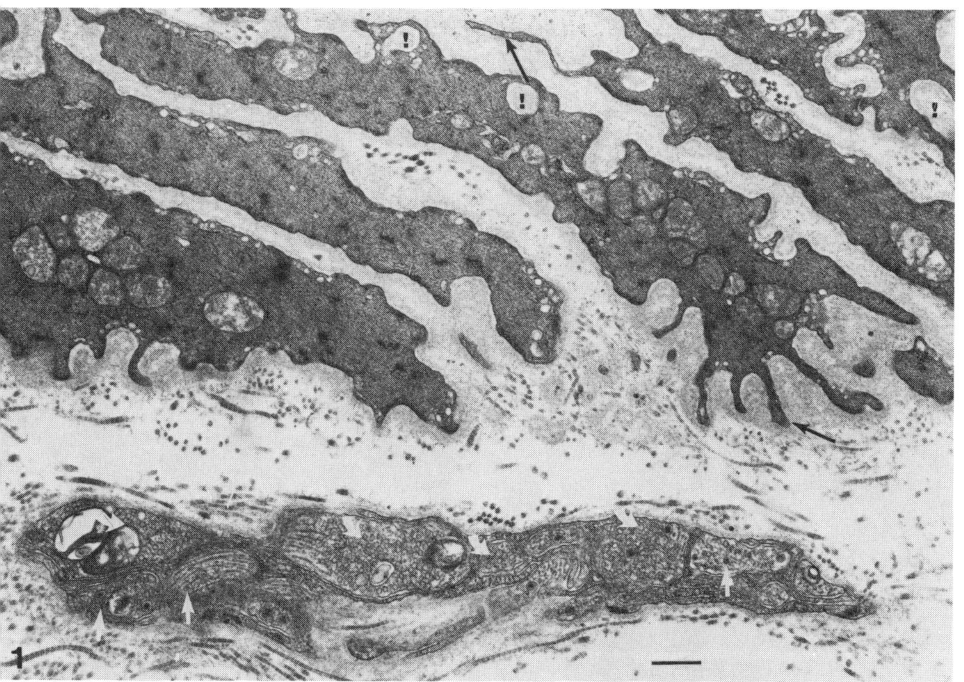

Figure 1 Profiles of muscle cells and nerves in a bundle from a fifth order bronchus fixed 6 h after ozone inhalation. Note the long projections of smooth muscle (dark arrows), the membrane-bounded lacunae (noted with !) containing basement membrane. Note also the absence of intermediate contacts, which is a common observation in canine airways. The nerve profiles are at the edge of the muscle bundle. Those containing small granular synaptic vesicles (adrenergic) are marked with a straight white arrow; those with small agranular vesicles (cholinergic) are marked with a curved white arrow. Note that adrenergic nerve profiles are closer to cholinergic profiles than to muscle profiles in this case (bar indicates approximately 487 nm).

size but average 200 nm and gap junction length is from 0.5 to 1 μm/1000 μm of cell membrane length. In human airway, they are present in trachea and first and second order bronchi, but in smaller bronchi typical gap junctions visible by electron microscopy are not present (Daniel et al., 1986). Other junctions normally present in airway smooth muscle include close appositions and intermediate contacts.

Intermediate contacts may be related in structure to desmosomes; they are regions in which the cell membranes run parallel, 200-600 nm apart, and with an electron-dense line or row of particles midway between the cell mem-

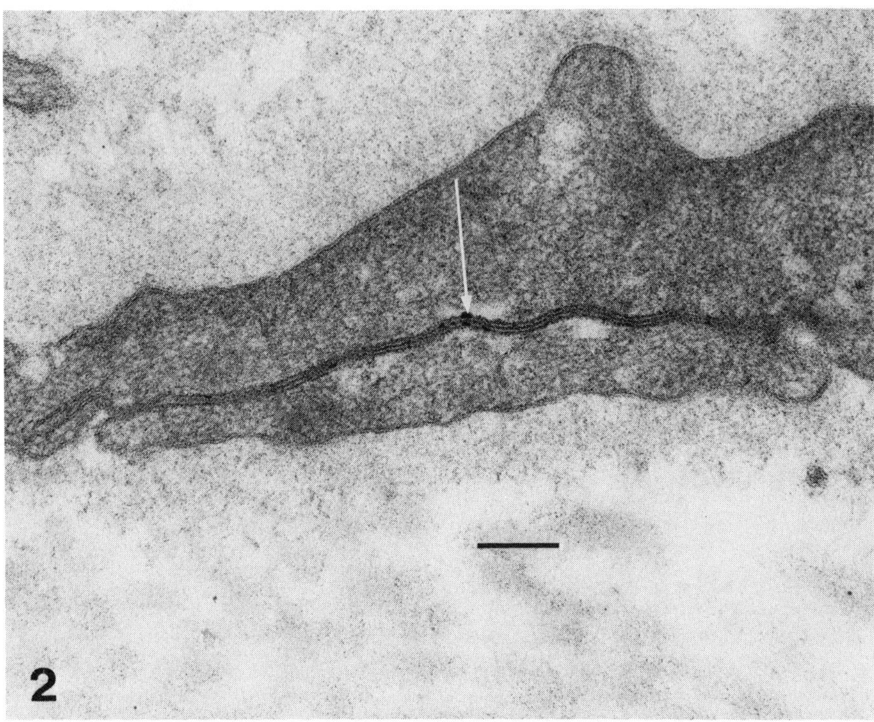

Figure 2 Profile of an unusually long gap junction (white arrow) between projections of two smooth muscle cells of a fifth order bronchus fixed 6 h after ozone inhalation. Gap junction profiles average 200 nm in length, but this is over 900 nm in length. The arrow also indicates some dense deposits occasionally found near gap junctions (bar indicates approximately 105 nm).

membranes in the region of the basement membrane and electron dense material (similar to the cytoplasmic dense bodies) in the cytoplasm subadjacent to the plasma membrane. They may provide sites of mechanical attachment between cells and for the contractile proteins within cells. The point of interest in airway muscle is that they are rare in the canine airway and probably in human airway as well. Whether this is generally true in the airway of other species requires further examination. The absence or rarity of intermediate contacts (e.g., Fig. 1) suggests that airway muscle cells may be mobile in relation to one another or may be anchored to one another by other means. The marked complexity of outlines of muscle cell profiles noted above (Fig. 1) may be related to the lack or the nature of the mechanical attachments of airway smooth muscle cells to one another. Consequences of this structural peculiarity need to be evaluated with respect to the elastic elements in the mechanical performance of airway muscle.

The other type of cell-to-cell junctions are the close appositions, which are short regions of close approximation (20-100 nm) between plasma membranes of two cells. In the airway they sometimes have electron-dense cytoplasmic regions subjacent to the junction but sometimes do not (Fig. 3). Their function is unknown.

B. Nerves

Nerves close enough to ($\leqslant$2-5 μm) smooth muscle to be assumed to provide neural control are present in markedly varied densities in different airways.

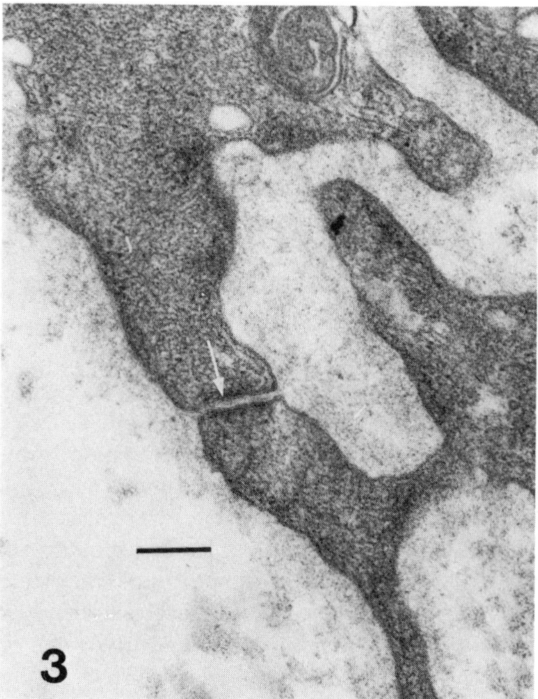

Figure 3 Profile of a close apposition (white arrow) between projections of two smooth muscle cells of a first order bronchus fixed 6 h after ozone inhalation. The gap between cell membranes is 15-20 nm in this type of junction, which has electron-dense material in the cytoplasm subadjacent to the apposition. Another type of close apposition (not shown) lacks this material (bar indicates approximately 144 nm).

In all species studied to date except guinea pig (Jones et al., 1980; Mansour and Daniel, 1987; Hoyes and Barber, 1980), the trachea is sparsely innervated by nerves that have their profiles at the periphery (Fig. 1) of muscle bundles (see Kannan and Daniel, 1980). The guinea pig trachea has a relatively dense innervation with nerves that are sometimes close to airway muscle (Jones et al., 1980). There seems to be some confusion among some who study airway regarding how many nerves supply the guinea pig trachea.

In the bronchi of humans (Daniel et al., 1986) and dogs (Daniel et al., 1988, 1989b; Daniel and O'Byrne, 1990, unpublished data), the density of nerves increases dramatically compared to trachea. Moreover the varicose nerve profiles found are within muscle bundles (Fig. 4) as well as at their periphery and sometimes are found quite close to smooth muscle cell profiles. In contrast to trachea, in which most varicose nerve profiles contain a preponderance of small agranular vesicles (SAV) or SAV along with a few large granular vesicles (LGV), a significant proportion of nerve profiles near bronchial muscle containing small granular vesicles (SGV). In most instances the SGV are known to contain adrenergic mediator (see Llewellyn-Smith et al., 1981; Gordon-Weeks, 1981, 1982; and Wilson et al., 1981 for exceptions in guinea pig intestine), while the SAV are presumed to contain acetylcholine. This last assumption is not generally true (Daniel et al., 1977; Gibbons, 1982) but may be correct in canine airway in which the major innervation is clearly either cholinergic or adrenergic (Daniel et al., 1988, 1981a,b; Janssen and Daniel, 1990, unpublished data). Of potential functional importance is the location of the nerve profiles containing SGV and lacking glial cell cover very near those with SAV (Fig. 1) as well as near smooth muscle cells (Fig. 4). This provides a structural arrangement for adrenergic nerves to influence airway function by both pre- and postsynaptic actions. We have recently obtained clear electrophysiological evidence that adrenergic nerves in bronchi can modulate the release of acetylcholine and affect smooth muscle function.

The structure of bronchial muscle, with many gap junctions between muscle cells and a dense close innervation, is inconsistent with classic descriptions of the control of smooth muscles: that they are either single-unit (few close nerves, many gap junctions), multiunit (many close nerves, few or no gap junctions) or in between. These muscles are endowed structurally with the means for both neural (multiunit) and myogenic (singleunit) control. Limitations to myogenic control could arise from the inability of those muscles to initiate action potentials, owing to rectification of depolarizing currents (Kannan et al., 1984). In the absence of action potentials, electrical events such as excitatory junction potentials can propagate only for limited distances that are determined by the passive membrane properties (primarily by the space constant). So far no critical examination has been made of the possibility that some pathophysiological conditions associated with airway

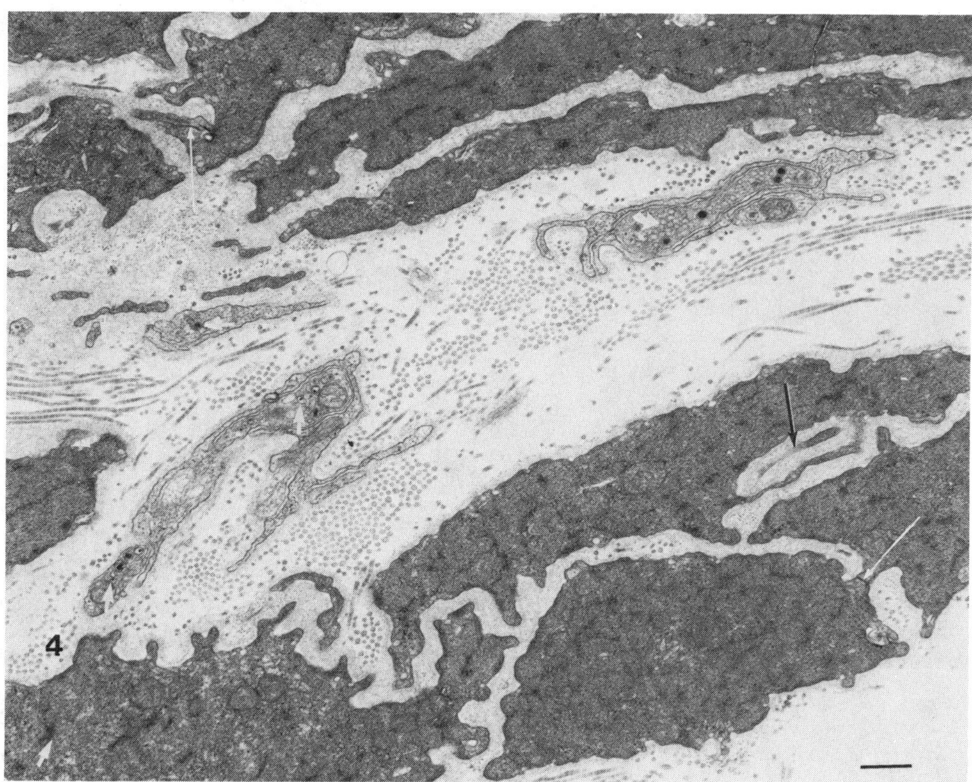

Figure 4 Profiles of nerves and muscles of a fifth order bronchus fixed 30 min after ozone inhalation. Note the gap junctions between muscle cells (long straight white arrows) and the membrane-bounded lacuna (straight black arrows) containing a profile that is probably a thin projection from another smooth muscle cell. Note the absence of intermediate contacts. The nerve profiles containing small granular synaptic vesicles (adrenergic) are marked by straight white arrows and are sometimes close to profiles of muscle cells, as are nerve profiles with small agranular vesicles (curved white arrow) (bar indicates approximately 454 nm).

hyperresponsiveness might result from loss of these rectifying properties or enhancement of cell-to-cell transmission.

C. Epithelium

In canine airway, there is a fairly typical arrangement of the cells of the epithelium (Fig. 5 shows the nearly normal epithelium present 6 h after ozone inhalation). Ciliated and mucous cells line the lumen and there are basal cells

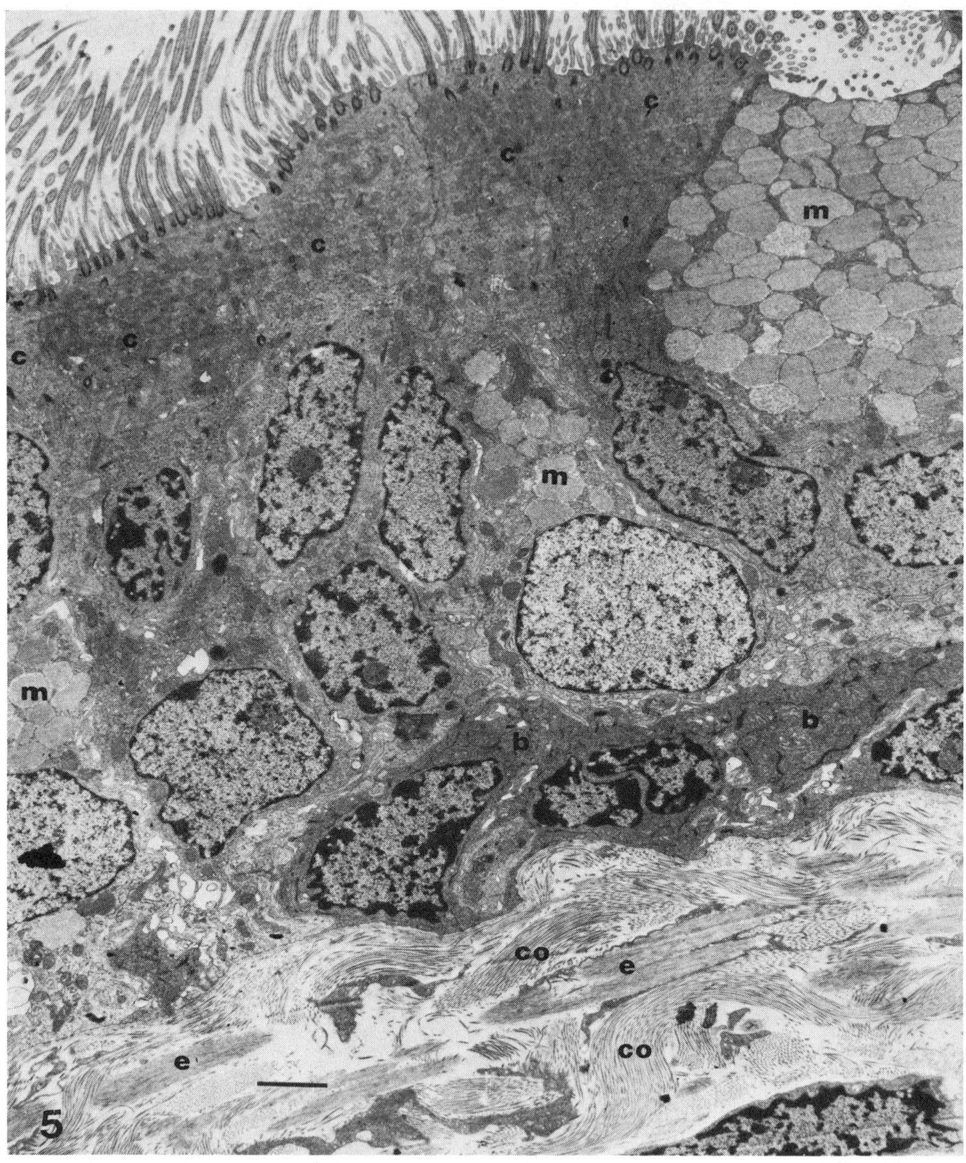

Figure 5 Epithelium and interstitial space from a fifth order bronchus fixed 6 h after ozone inhalation. Note the large number of ciliated cells (c) lining the lumen, goblet cells containing mucus (m), and basal cells (b) at the inner border of the epithelium. The interstitial space contains elastin bundles (e) and collagen (co) (bar indicates approximately 836 nm).

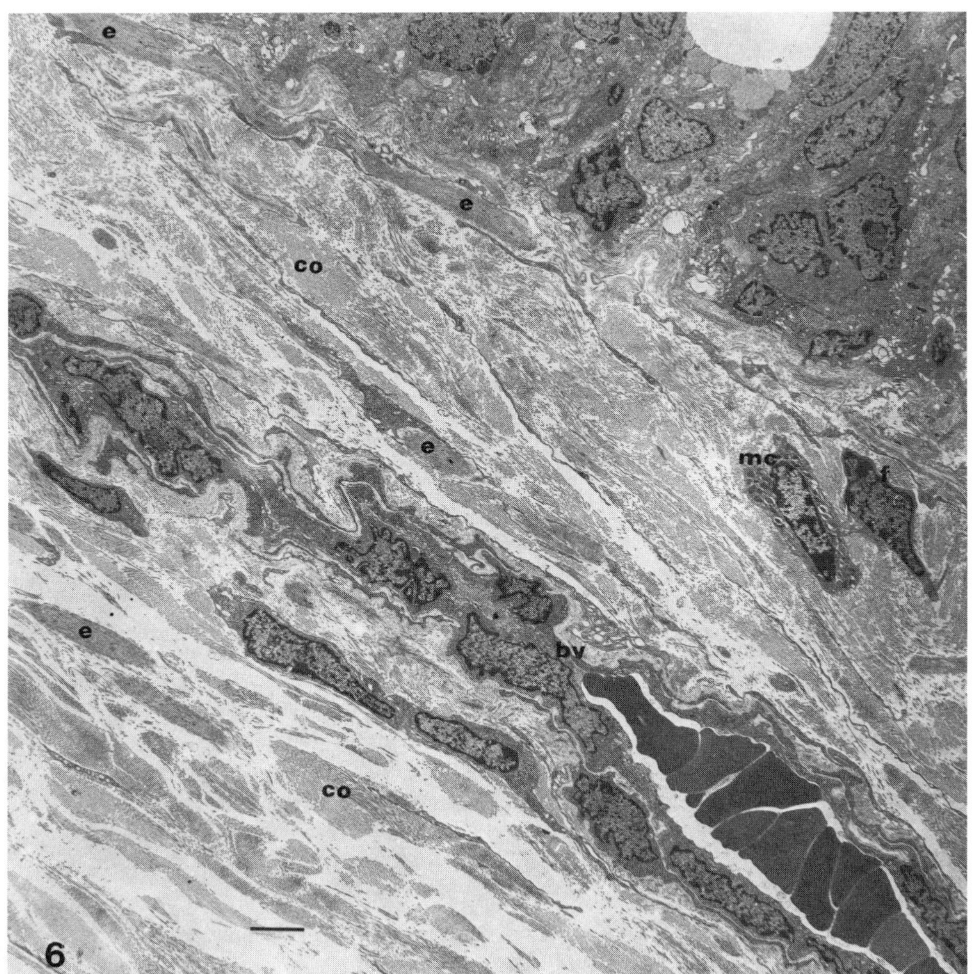

Figure 6 The interstitial space and inner part of the epithelial layer from a fifth order bronchus taken 6 h after ozone inhalation. Mast cells (mc), fibroblasts (f), and blood vessels (bv) are present as in control animals, as are elastin bundles (e) and collagen bundles (co) (bar indicates approximately 2184 nm).

along the inner border. In addition, there are profiles tentatively classified as neuroendocrine along that border that sometimes send projections toward the lumen. Nerve profiles, identified by the presence of neurotubules, neurofilaments, or synaptic vesicles, are rarely observed despite intensive searching and those found are near basal cells far from the lumen. Nerves approaching the inner border of the epithelium from the region of the muscle are almost nonexistent in the tissues we have studied, which is consistent with a sparse innervation in the canine epithelium. Since the same tubules, filaments, and vesicles are found in the neuroendocrine profiles, it seems possible that the profiles observed are really part of these cells. A full study of serial sections to reconstruct the neuroendocrine structures in three dimensions would be helpful.

The space between the inner border of the epithelium and the muscle is as wide or wider than the epithelium in canine airways (Daniel et al., 1988). For convenient reference, we call it the interstitial space. This space is much more narrow in rodents but in them as well as in dogs it contains blood vessels, connective tissue (elastin and collagen), and a few other cells. In the bronchi of dogs, these other cells and fibroblasts are both often closely associated with elastin or collagen, and occasional macrophages. Within 6 h after ozone inhalation the interstitial space, like the epithelium, is approaching normality (Fig. 6). In "normal" dogs, (see Daniel et al., 1988) the cells are exclusively fibroblasts and mast cells (Fig. 6). These are usually both closely associated with collagen and elastin.

IV. Structural Changes Associated with Airway Hyperresponsiveness

A. Basenji-Greyhound versus Greyhound Airways

There is essentially no qualitative difference between the airway structures considered in hyperresponsive Basenji greyhound (BG), normally responsive greyhound, and other normal dogs. The only quantitative difference appears to be a modest increase in the density of gap junctions in several orders of airway in the BG animals (Daniel et al., 1989a). Most surprising is the absence of inflammatory cells other than the normally occurring mast cells and the absence of epithelial damage.

B. Ozone Inhalation

Ozone inhalation (3.0 ppm for 30 min) caused enhanced responsiveness to inhaled acetylcholine and histamine (Holtzman et al., 1983, 1986; Fabbri et al., 1984; Jones et al., 1988) and also enhanced responsiveness of tracheal muscle to electrical field stimulation (Walters et al., 1986; O'Byrne et al.,

1988; Jones et al., 1988) and to acetylcholine (Jones et al., 1988; O'Byrne et al., 1988) of the trachea in vitro. The in vitro tracheal hyperresponsiveness is reported to be present at 2 h after and to disappear 6 h after ozone inhalation (Walters et al., 1986). Major roles for neutrophil influx (Fabbri et al., 1984; Holtzman et al., 1983; O'Byrne et al., 1984a,b) and the release of thromboxane A_2 in hyperresponsiveness after ozone have been suggested for both the in vivo (Aizawa et al., 1985) and the in vitro (Tamaoki et al., 1987; Daniel et al., 1988; Serio and Daniel, 1988) effects.

We have examined the structural effects of ozone inhalation 30 min, 2 h, and 6 h after the end of the exposure. The qualitative findings are summarized in Table 1. These results must be regarded as preliminary since quantitative analysis of the data is incomplete. Perhaps the most surprising observations have to do with the epithelium. Figures 7 and 8 illustrates the findings at 30

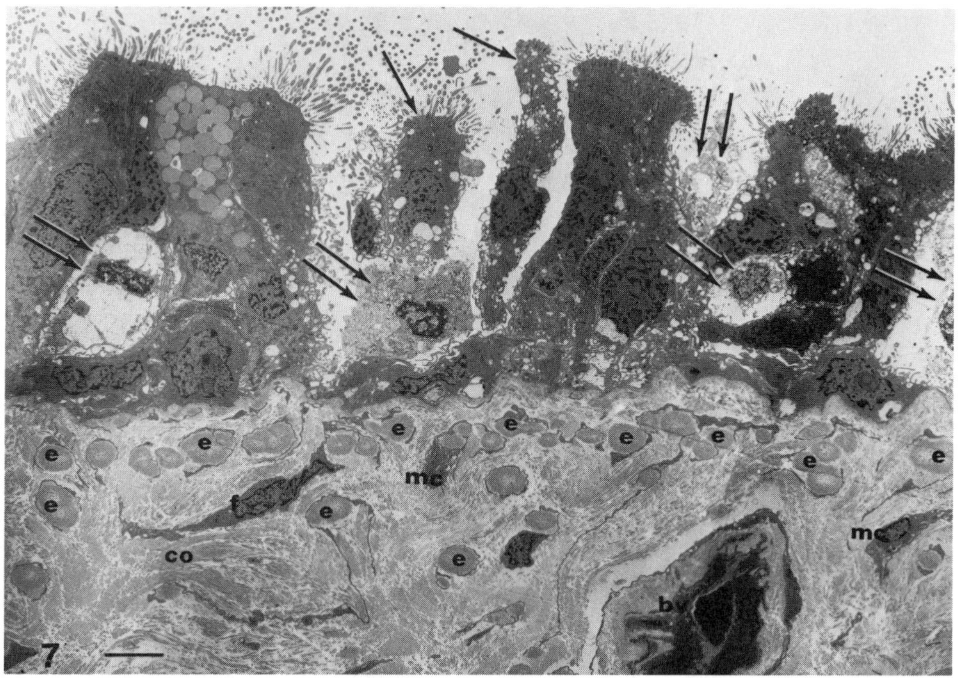

Figure 7 Damaged epithelium from a fifth order bronchus fixed 30 min after ozone inhalation. Note ciliated cells (single black arrow) in the process of desquamation from the epithelium. There are additional seriously damaged cells (double arrows) that cannot be identified with certainty. Some may be goblet cells and some may be ciliated cells. Note profiles of mast cells (mc) and fibroblast (f) in interstitial space, together with a blood vessel (bv), elastin (e), and collagen (co) (bar indicates approximately 2105 nm).

Table 1 Qualitative Major Effects of Ozone Inhalation on Structures of Canine Airway

Structure	Time After Ozone		
	30 min	2 h	6 h
Muscle bundles			
Muscles	No change	No change	No change
Nerves	No change	No change	No change
Other	Occasional macrophages, present	Occasional immune cells of various classes present	Occasional macrophages in some bronchi
Epithelium			
Ciliated cells	Severe damage (some lost); cilia matted	Focal damage	Rare focal damage
Mucous cells	Many discharging mucus	Many normal; others appear markedly depleted of mucus	Normal except for occasional depleted cells
Basal cells	Normal except in local regions of severe damage	Normal	Normal

"Neuroendocrine profiles"	Severe damage	Damage still present	Nearly normal
Immune cells	None or very rare	Occasional mast cells, neutrophils, macrophages present within epithelium	Occasional macrophages in some bronchi
Interstitial space			
Blood vessels	Platelets/neutrophils, etc. sequestered	Neutrophils etc. sequestered	Normal
Fibroblasts	Normal	Perhaps reduced in number	Nearly normal
Elastin	Structural changes	Structural changes	Structural changes
Collagen	Normal (mostly)	Normal	Normal
Mast cells	Activated	Perhaps reduced in number; activated	Present; still activated
Other immune cells	Macrophages present	Neutrophils and macrophages present	Neutrophils reduced in numbers and some phagocytized by macrophages, which are still present

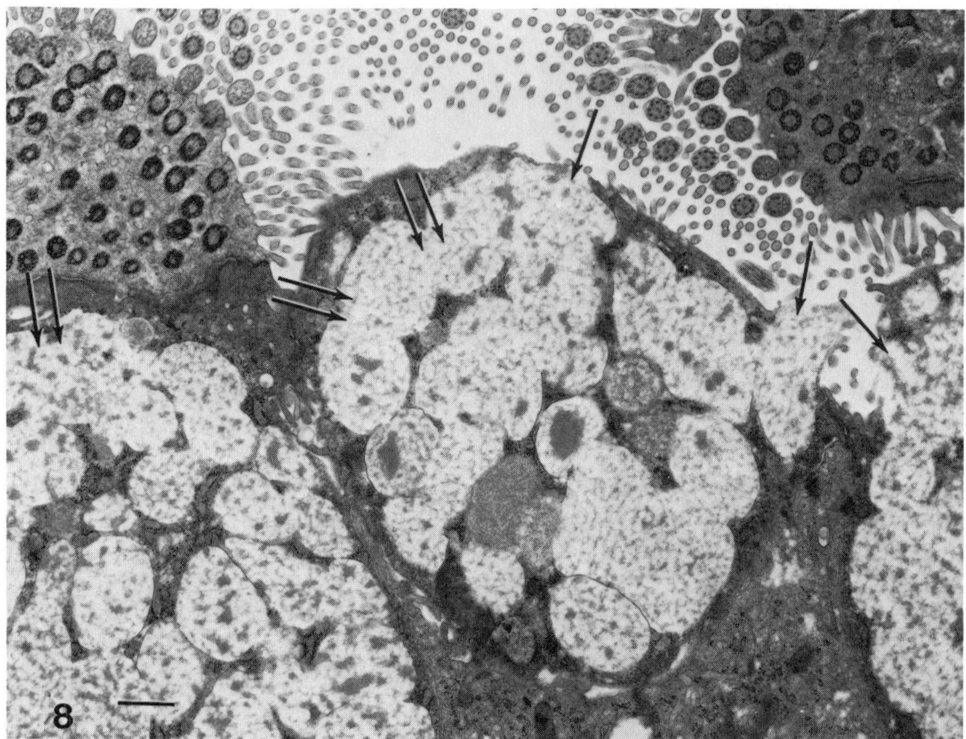

Figure 8 Higher-magnification micrograph of ciliated cells and goblet cells taken from a fifth order bronchus fixed 30 min after ozone inhalation. Note the appearance of mucous cell; some mucus globules (single arrow) are in the process of excreting mucus into the lumen; most show the loss of their boundary membranes (see double arrows) and all have an altered appearance of their mucus content (loss of electron density and segregation into a fibrous appearance) (bar indicates approximately 210 nm).

min and should be compared to those at 2 h (Daniel et al., 1988) and the similar (to results at 2 h) findings (Figs. 5, 6) at 6 h after administration of ozone. There was major damage, including desquamation of ciliated cells (Fig. 7) and matting of cilia at 30 min, but only focal damage was seen later, at 2 or 6 h. There was also extensive secretion from goblet cells and these were markedly depleted of mucus (Fig. 8). At 30 min also mast cells (Fig. 9) and other immune cells were occasionally present passing through the epithelium. These migrating cells were found frequently at 2 h and less frequently

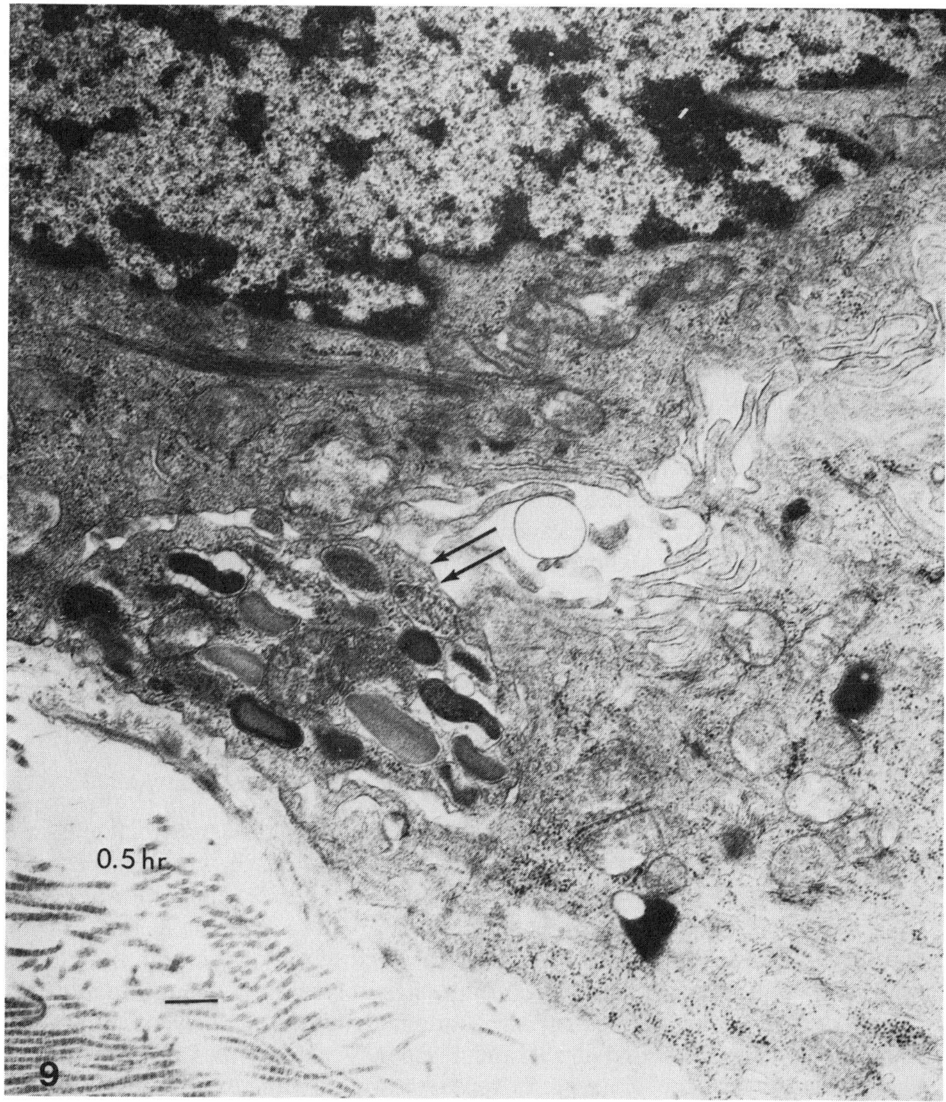

Figure 9 Micrograph of inner border of epithelium from a fifth order bronchus; part of a mast cell (double arrows) is apparently invading the epithelium. Note that the granules suggest that the cell is activated. One granule near the double arrows may be discharging its contents into the space, which has opened up between basal cells (bar indicates approximately 350 nm).

at 6 h. Consistent with the appearance of these immune cells in the interstitial space, we found neutrophils, platelets, and macrophage-like cells sequestered in blood vessels 0.5 and 2 h after administration of ozone. There was not, however, gross damage to endothelium. Occasionally immune cells, most frequently macrophages, were found within or very near muscle bundles after ozone at each time studied. Macrophages were also the most common immune cell at 30 min after ozone inhalation. Neutrophils were increased in the interstitial space 2 h after ozone and many fewer were present at 30 min or 6 h. Mast cells were found in reduced numbers at 2 h in the interstitial space but were noted at each study time usually to be activated. Eosinophils were not observed in blood vessels, interstitial space, or epithelium at any time. Overall, the summary in Table 1 points to a possible early role for macrophages (at 30 min) and the importance of neutrophils and macrophages in the interstitial space at the time (2 h) the muscle is hyperresponsive. This latter hypothesis is in contrast to the observations of Murlas and Roum (1985) in guinea pigs. These authors found that neutrophil infiltration followed after the onset of hyperresponsiveness present 2 h after ozone inhalation. They also found a marked depletion of mucosal goblet cells 2 h after ozone inhalation when the airway was hyperresponsive. This may correspond to our observation of the depletion of mucus in goblet cells (Fig. 8). Boatman and colleagues (1974) earlier exposed cats to ozone up to 1 ppm for 3 h and, as in our studies, found selective damage (vacuolization) to ciliated cells.

V. Conclusions

This study shows that in canine airways both the tracheal and bronchial muscle are well supplied with gap junctions and the bronchi of second to sixth order (but not trachea or first order bronchi) with a dense innervation. The nerve profiles include a significant proportion of adrenergic nerves. In bronchi, adrenergic nerve profiles are located close to both smooth muscle cells and other (cholinergic) nerves. These structures do not change qualitatively during ozone-induced inflammation and hyperresponsiveness. The epithelium, especially ciliated cells and neuroendocrine profiles, are severely damaged by ozone but have partly recovered by the time hyperresponsiveness is present in vitro and in vivo. The hyperresponsiveness seems to be associated with the presence of neutrophils and macrophages and the activation of mast cells in the space between epithelium and muscle and with occasional macrophages or other immune cells in or near muscle bundles.

Acknowledgments

This work was supported by the Medical Research Council of Canada. Dr. O'Byrne is the recipient of a Medical Research Council of Canada Scholarship.

Discussion

Leff: The ozone data you showed are in conflict with other published reports. Can you comment as to why?

Daniel: Yes, other authors have shown a correlation between neutrophil infiltration and ozone-induced hyperactivity in several other animal models. The data I reviewed apply only to the dog model.

Laitinen: Can you tell anything about the number of infiltrating cells?

Daniel: There were many more neutrophils at 2 h then at 6 h. Many were found in every grid square at 2 h but very few at 6 h.

Barnes: What is the source of the thromboxane you found?

Daniel: We cannot be sure.

O'Byrne: Do you see platelets as well?

Daniel: Very rarely.

Irvin: Do gap junctions increase with ozone exposure?

Daniel: Gap junctions are very labile and are regulated by inflammatory mediators. However, we did not detect increased numbers of internalized gap junctions after ozone exposure.

Drazen: We have just completed an analysis of complete dose-response curves in dogs before and after ozone exposure (Kerriya, J. Appl Physiol., 1988). There was no change in the plateau of the dose-response curve. In this respect, did you observe airway edema in your ozone exposed dogs?

Daniel: There is no ultrastructural evidence of endothelial damage. However, this method is not designed to measure vascular permeability.

Chung: In the rat, ozone exposure is not accompanied by microvascular permeability.

Fish: Do you have any idea what controls the migration of cells through the lamina propria after ozone exposure?

Daniel: We certainly observed reduced numbers of mast cells in the lamina propria at a time when epithelial mast cell numbers were increased. We cannot comment on the factors influencing these changes.

References

Aizawa, H., Chung, K. F., Leikauf, G. D., Ueki, I., Bethel, R. A., O'Byrne, P. M., Hirose, T., and Nadel, J. A. (1985). Significance of thromboxane generation in ozone-induced airway hyperresponsiveness in dogs. *J. Appl. Physiol.* **59**:1918-1923.

Boatman, E. S., Sato, S., and Frank, R. (1974). Acute effects of ozone on cat lungs. II. Structural. *Am. Rev. Respir. Dis.* **10**:157-169.

Daniel, E. E. (1988). Ultrastructure of airway smooth muscle. In *Mechanisms in Asthma: Pharmacology, Physiology and Management.* Edited by J. Wood. New York, Alan R. Liss, pp. 179-203.

Daniel, E. E., and Posey-Daniel, V. (1984). Neuromuscular structures in opossum esophagus: role of interstitial cells of Cajal. *Am. J. Physiol.* **246**(3):G305-G315.

Daniel, E. E., Taylor, G. S., Daniel, V. P., and Holman, M. E. (1977). Can non-adrenergic inhibitory varicosities be identified structurally? *Can. J. Physiol. Pharmacol.* **55**(2):243-250.

Daniel, E. E., Kannan, M., Davis, C., and Posey-Daniel, V. (1986). Ultrastructural studies on the neuromuscular control of human tracheal and bronchial smooth muscle. *Respir. Physiol.* **63**:109-128.

Daniel, E. E., Posey-Daniel, V., Jager, L. P., Berezin, I., and Jury, J. (1987). Structural effects of exposure in the sucrose gap apparatus. *Am. J. Physiol.* **21**(1):C77-C87.

Daniel, E. E., Serio, R., Jury, J., Pashley, M., and O'Byrne, P. (1988). Effects of inflammatory mediators on neuromuscular transmission in canine trachea *in vitro*. In *Mechanisms of Asthma: Pharmacology, Physiology and Management.* Edited by J. Wood. New York, Alan R. Liss, pp. 167-176.

Daniel, E. E., Berezin, I., and Hirshman, C. (1989a). Structures of airways from control (Greyhound) and hyperresponsive (Basenji-Greyhound) dogs. *J. Appl. Physiol.*

Daniel, E. E., Inoue, F., Jager, L. P., Jury, J., and Serio, R. (1989b). Excitatory junction potentials in canine trachealis smooth muscle cells mediated via an increased chloride conductance. *J. Physiol*

Davis, C., Kannan, M. S., Jones, T. R., and Daniel, E. E. (1982). The control of human airway smooth muscle (in vitro studies). *J. Appl. Physiol.* **53**(5):1080-1087.

Davis, C., Jones, T. R., and Daniel, E. E. (1983). Studies of the mechanism of passive anaphylaxis in human airway smooth muscle. *Can. J. Physiol. Pharmacol.* **61**:705-713.

Fabbri, L. M., Aizawa, H., Alpert, S. E., Walters, E. H., O'Byrne, P. M., Gold, B. D., Nadel, J. A., and Holtzman, M. J. (1984). Airway hyperresponsiveness and changes in cell counts in bronchoalveolar lavage after ozone exposure in dogs. *Am. Rev. Respir. Dis.* **129**:288-291.

Gibbons, I. L. (1982). Lack of correlation between ultrastructural and pharmacological types of non-adrenergic autonomic nerves. *Cell Tissue Res.* **221**:551-581.

Gordon-Weeks, P. R. (1981). Properties of nerve endings with small granular vesicles in the distal colon and rectum of the guinea-pig. *Neuroscience* **6**:1793-1811.

Gordon-Weeks, P. R. (1982). Noradrenergic and non-adrenergic nerves containing small granular vesicles in Auerbach's plexus of the guinea pig: evidence against the presence of noradrenergic synapses. *Neuroscience* **7**:2925-2946.

Hirshman, C. A., and Downes, H. (1986). Airway responses to methacholine and histamine in basenji greyhounds and other purebred dogs. *Respir. Physiol.* **63**:339-346.

Holtzman, M. J., Fabbri, L. M., O'Byrne, P. M., Gold, B. D., Aizawa, H., Walters, E. H., Alpert, S. E., and Nadel, J. A. (1983). Importance of airway inflammation for hyperresponsiveness induced by ozone. *Am. Rev. Respir. Dis.* **127**:686-690.

Holtzman, M. J., Fabbri, L. M., Skoogh, B. E., O'Byrne, P. M., Walters, E. H., Aizawa, H., and Nadel, J. A. (1986). Time course of airway hyperresponsiveness induced by ozone in dogs. *J. Appl. Physiol.* **55**:1232-1236.

Hoyes, A. D., and Barber, P. (1980). Innervation of trachealis muscle in the guinea-pig: a quantitative ultrastructural study. *J. Anat.* **130**:789-800.

Jones, T. R., Kannan, M. S., and Daniel, E. E. (1980). Ultrastructural study of guinea pig tracheal smooth muscle and its innervation. *Can. J. Physiol. Pharmacol.* **58**(8):74-983.

Jones, G. L., O'Byrne, P. M., Pashley, M., Serio, R., Jury, J., Lane, C. G., and Daniel, E. E. (1988). Airway smooth muscle responsiveness from dogs with airway hyperresponsiveness after O$_3$ inhalation. *J. Appl. Physiol.* **65**:57-74.

Kannan, M. S., and Daniel, E. E. (1980). Structural and functional study of control of canine tracheal smooth muscle. *Am. J. Physiol.* **238**:C27-C33.

Kannan, M. S., Jager, L. P., Daniel, E. E., and Garfield, R. E. (1984). Effects of 4-aminopyridine and tetraethylammonium chloride on the electrical activity and cable properties of canine tracheal smooth muscle. *J. Pharmacol. Exp. Ther.* **227**:706-715.

Llewellyn-Smith, I. J., Wilson, A. J., Furness, J. B., Costa, M., and Rush, R. A. (1981). Ultrastructural identification of noradrenergic axon and their distribution within the enteric plexuses of the guinea-pig small intestine. *J. Neurocytol.* **10**:331-352.

Mansour, S., and Daniel, E. E. (1987). Structural changes in tracheal nerves and muscle associated with *in vivo* sensitization of guinea pigs. *Respir. Physiol.* **72**:283-294.

Murlas, C. G., and Round, J. H. (1985). Sequence of pathologic changes in the airway mucosa of guinea pigs during ozone-induced bronchial hyperresponsiveness. *Am. Rev. Respir. Dis.* **131**:314-426.

O'Byrne, P. M., Walters, E. H., Aizawa, H., Fabbri, L. M., Holtzman, M. J., and Nadel, J. A. (1984a). Indomethacin inhibits the airway hyperresponsiveness but not the neutrophil influx induced by ozone in dogs. *Am. Rev. Respir. Dis.* **130**:220-224.

O'Byrne, P. M., Walters, E. H., Gold, B. D., Aizawa, H. A., Fabbri, L. M., Alpert, S. E., Nadel, J. A., and Holtzman, M. J. (1984b). Neutrophil depletion inhibits airway hyperresponsiveness induced by ozone exposure. *Am. Rev. Respir. Dis.* **130**:214-219.

O'Byrne, P. M., Jones, G. L., Lane, C. G., Pashley, M., and Daniel, E. E. (1988). Neural transmission during ozone-induced airway hyperresponsiveness. In *Mechanisms in Asthma: Pharmacology, Physiology and Management*. Edited by J. Wood. New York, Alan R. Liss, pp. 3-13.

Serio, R., and Daniel, E. E. (1988). Thromboxane effects on canine trachealis neuromuscular function. *J. Appl. Physiol.* **64**:1979-1988.

Tamaoki, J., Sekizawa, K., Osborne, M. L., Ueki, I. F., Graf, P. D., and Nadel, J. A. (1987). Platelet aggregation increases cholinergic neurotransmission in canine airway. *J. Appl. Physiol.* **62**:2246-2251.

Walters, E. H., O'Byrne, P. M., Graf, P. D., Fabbri, L. M., and Nadel, J. A. (1986). The responsiveness of airway smooth muscle *in vitro* from dogs with airway hyperresponsiveness *in vivo*. *Clin. Sci.* **71**:605-611.

Wilson, A. J., Furness, J. B., and Costa, M. (1981). The fine structure of the submucous plexus of the guinea-pig ileum II. Description and analysis of vesiculated nerve processes. *J. Neurocytol.* **10**:785-804.

7

Tracheobronchial Microcirculation in Asthma

CARL G. A. PERSSON

University Hospital of Lund and AB Draco
Lund, Sweden

Airway inflammation is generally considered to equal the presence of inflammatory cells on the mucosal surface and in the mucosal/submucosal tissue. However, this sign alone can be difficult to interpret. The cells may be present in the airways for no apparent reason, for tissue repair or to fuel an inflammatory process. To identify the latter inflammatory condition, measurements are needed to demonstrate whether the airway tissue itself is actively affected by the inflammation. Over 100 years ago, vascular leakage of plasma was proposed by Cohnheim (1882) to be a cardinal inflammatory event. Recent data suggest that the appearance of plasma macromolecules on the mucosal surface may demonstrate both the time course and the degree of airway inflammation (Erjefält and Persson, 1989). Determination of plasma tracers in mucosal fluids is also important because plasma exudation is a potentially important pathogenetic mechanism of asthma (Persson, 1986).

Just beneath the airway epithelium there is a rich network of microvessels (Sobin et al., 1963; Laitinen et al., 1987). Under the influence of inflammatory provocations, endothelial cells of postcapillary venules actively separate to produce transient gaps in the vessel wall. Through these gaps bulk leakage of proteinaceous plasma occurs. The extravasated plasma protein systems become activated to produce a large variety of peptides, many of which are significant inflammatory mediators. The increased amount of solutes in the proteinaceous exudate results in a subepithelial osmotic load. This load and the associated increase in interstitial hydrostatic pressure may separate epithelial cells, with subsequent luminal entry of plasma exudate/transudate. (Persson et al., 1990).

Whereas the epithelium is a tight barrier to material on the mucosal surface, it appears to be a poor barrier to exuded plasma solutes (Erjefält and Persson, 1989, 1990a; Persson, 1989a). Even at a threshold level of inflammatory insults, the plasma exudate will not stay within the wall tissue but is significantly exuded into the airway lumen. The concentration of plasma tracers in airway mucosal surface liquids thus reflects quantitatively the inflammatory exudation process in the airway mucosa/submucosa.

Perhaps the most significant component of hypersecretion in asthma is not a secretory product but a plasma exudate/transudate. The limited information available suggests that plasma proteins are abnormally abundant in asthmatic airways and that at symptom induction and prevention levels of plasma tracers increase and decrease, respectively (see Persson, 1988a).

The passage of macromolecules across the inflamed mucosa may be largely unidirectional into the lumen (Erjefält and Persson, 1989, 1990a). This selectivity seems highly desirable, particularly when plasma exudation operates in airway defense. Within a few minutes after a provocation, the potent plasma kinin, complement, fibrinolysis, coagulation, immunoglobulin, and other systems would be able to act on the mucosal surface without there being a concomitantly increased tissue penetration of inhaled factors such as allergens.

The plasma exudate is not merely a useful marker of airway inflammation in asthma. By its abundant content of mediators as well as other inflammatory factors, and by its physical effects including edema and increased mucus viscosity, the plasma exudate is a multipotential pathogenetic factor in asthmatic symptoms (Persson, 1986, 1988a). It cannot be excluded that a basic abnormality of asthma in part resides in exaggerated plasma exudation mechanisms.

I. Airway Microvessels

Leonardo da Vinci illustrated the distribution of the bronchial arteries as well distinguished from the pulmonary vascular system and discussed the fact that "Nature duplicated artery and vein in such an instrument" (Daly and Hebb, 1966). Laitinen et al. (1987), using light and electron microscopic examination of vascular casts, have recently demonstrated the organization of an impressive microvasculature in the tracheobronchial wall of dogs and humans, confirming and extending earlier work that used these species and guinea pigs (Sobin et al., 1963). Just beneath the epithelium there is a copious capillary-venular network (Fig. 1), which is continuous along the airways. There are also more deeply lying plexuses, including a peribronchial microvascular network.

The bronchial circulation receives 1-5% of the cardiac output and the mucosa/submucosa is particularly well perfused (Deffenbach et al., 1987; Parsons et al., 1985). In such species as the pig and the sheep, a single bronchial artery supplies almost the whole bronchial circulation but in humans, dog, and oxen, a number of bronchial arteries originate from the aorta, the intercostal, and other arteries. Bronchial arteries nurture not only bronchi but also nerves, pulmonary vessels, pleura, and some other tissues. Venous drainage of the extrapulmonary airways and the first few generations of bronchi goes to the right heart via the azygos and hemiazygos veins. A major part of the venous blood from the bronchial circulation goes to the pulmonary vein via tributaries along the airways and peripherally through anastomoses between bronchial capillaries and pulmonary capillaries or precapillaries.

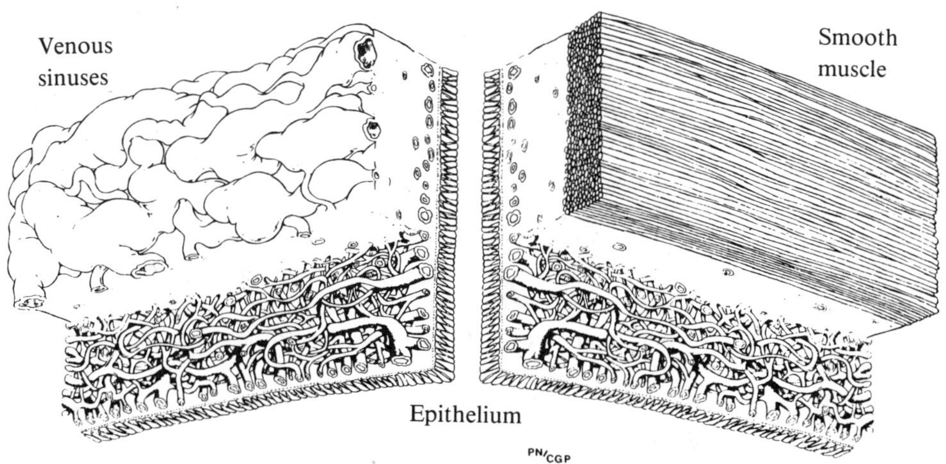

Figure 1 Differences and similarities between nasal and tracheobronchial airway tissues. A major obstruction mechanism of the nasal passages is filling of venous sinuses. A corresponding symptom-inducing event in the lower airways is tracheobronchial smooth muscle constriction. In mucosal/submucosal inflammation there is active involvement of the epithelium and the subepithelial plexus of microvessels. Plasma exudation across the vascular and mucosal barriers is an important process in inflammatory airway disease.

The distribution of tracheobronchial microvessels coincides with that of asthma, which is an airway and not a pulmonary disease. Also, the pharmacology of airway microcirculation is distinct from that of the pulmonary microcirculation. For example, proposed mediators of asthma produce plasma exudation in airways (Persson, 1988a) but not in pulmonary vascular beds (Persson et al., 1982; Hurley, 1983). The occurrence of exuded plasma in inflamed airways will not produce a wet lung. However, physical and physiological aspects of airway function may be severely affected.

II. Focus on Airway Vasculature Led to the Discovery of Major Antiasthma Drugs

Towards the end of the 19th century a number of German investigators considered that swelling of the bronchial mucus membrane was responsible for the asthmatic obstruction. This reasoning was based mainly on the assumption of similarities in this respect between the bronchi and the nasal airways (Persson, 1990). At the turn of the century, the vasodilator hypothesis of asthma had significant proponents in the United States. Encouraged by the information that adrenal extract produces vasoconstriction in various systems, Solis-Cohen (1900) gave large oral doses of desiccated adrenal glands to asthmatic subjects. The study was successful and Solis-Cohen furthered his view of asthma as a "vasomotor ataxia of the relaxing variety." This study has been quoted as the first evidence that epinephrine is an effective drug for the treatment of inasthma. However, this cannot be so. First, already by 1859 Salter had described the immediate "cure" of asthma in situations of either sudden alarm or violent pleasing excitements (Persson, 1985). Second, the epinephrine content of the adrenals could not have survived the oral route as an active drug. Indeed, Solis-Cohen (1900), in reporting a gradually increasing improvement, may have demonstrated the beneficial effect of repeated administrations of glucocorticoids in patients with asthma. This was 50 years before this remedy was definitely proven to be effective (Persson 1989b).

When epinephrine became available as a pure substance, Bullowa and Kaplan (1903) successfully gave injections of it to asthmatics. Like Solis-Cohen, they did the right thing for the wrong reason. They, too, set out to test the hypothesis that the "obstruction is caused by a turgidity of the bronchial mucosa." In fact, Bullowa and Kaplan (1903) concluded that the other, then prevailing, hypothesis of asthma ("spasm of the circular muscles of the bronchi") was not valid. In Prague in 1907, epinephrine was shown to relax airway muscle (Persson, 1985).

Although these findings were helpful for progress in drug research, it was incorrect to believe that the vascular mechanisms behind nasal blockage in rhinitis had an identical bronchial vascular correlate in asthma. Significant mechanisms of obstructive symptoms are clearly different between nasal and tracheobronchial passages. Thus filling of venous sinuses produces nasal blockage, whereas constriction of bronchial smooth muscle narrows the lower airways (Fig. 1).

On the other hand, complex mucosal inflammation is probably of primary pathogenetic importance in both rhinitis and asthma (Fig. 1; Persson and Pipkorn, 1990). The airway mucosal anti-inflammatory, antiexudative effects of glucocorticoids were first observed in human nasal passages (Persson, 1989b). The possibility that a cardinal vascular sign of inflammation, plasma exudation, is governed by similar mechanisms in nasal and tracheobronchial mucosa is important because in several respects the nasal mucosa is a superior locale to the bronchi for airway research in humans.

III. Blood Flow

It is of interest that a drug with potent α_2-receptor agonist properties, such as oximetazolin, inhibits nasal blockage and reduces blood flow but may not interfere with inflammatory stimulus-induced plasma exudation (Svensson et al., 1990). In theory, the inflammatory leakage of plasma is dependent on blood flow but since the airway mucosa/submucosa is so well perfused by a large fraction of the bronchial blood flow, changes in flow may not be critical to the exudation process. The fact that epinephrine, having vasoconstrictor as well as β_2-agonist properties, has not as yet demonstrated additional anti-asthma effects over those produced by β_2-agonists, which are vasodilators, further supports the view that drug-induced vasoconstriction may be of little consequence in asthmatic airways. Of course, locally applied large dosages of epinephrine produce a blanching effect on the tracheobronchial mucosa through α-receptor-mediated vasoconstriction, and this action will necessarily prevent inflammatory stimulus-induced plasma exudation (Persson et al., 1982).

In general, the neural, hormonal, and pharmacological regulation of bronchial and tracheal blood flow has many of the characteristics of a systemic vascular bed (Deffebach et al., 1987; Salonen et al., 1988). Through extensive anastomosis with the bronchial microcirculation, the pulmonary perfusion has a capacity to perfuse also the rich networks of airway microvessels should the bronchial arterial supply fail for some reason (Daly and Hebb, 1966; Deffebach et al., 1987; Kröll et al., 1987). Irrespective of where the blood comes from, the airway microcirculation has its particular role and reactivity in airway defense and in inflammatory airway disease.

IV. Plasma Exudation

Under physiological conditions, fluid equilibrium is maintained by a balance between the hydrostatic pressure in the capillary bed, which tends to drive fluid out of the vascular compartment, and the counteracting force of the transmural colloid osmotic pressure gradient upheld by plasma proteins. Inflammatory stimuli have dramatic effects on the postcapillary venule serving to open up gaps between endothelial cells. The ensuing leakage of protein-aceous plasma will practically abolish the colloid osmotic pressure gradient. The vascular leakage of large molecules, which is an active process under physiological and pharmacological control, is generally referred to as increased vascular permeability (Hurley, 1983).

The proposed bronchoconstrictory mediators of asthma (amines, peptides, lipid products, etc.) have, with few exceptions, the additional capacity of increasing airway microvascular permeability and hence inducing plasma exudation (Persson, 1988a). A neurogenic, possibly substance P- or other tachykinin-mediated, vascular-mucosal permeability of rodent airways, has attracted interest, but this mechanism may not operate in the airways of larger mammals including humans (Persson and Erjefält, 1988). Also, the cholinergic transmittor, acetylcholine, which is a potent bronchoconstrictor and secretagogue, seems to be without effect on vascular permeability. However, a large variety of nonneural mediators remain to account for plasma exudation in asthma.

The vascular target cells, which are responsible for increased permeability to macromolecules in inflammation, are the endothelial cells of postcapillary venules (8-30 μm in diameter). These cells harbor receptors for agents known to mediate and modulate vascular permeability (see Persson and Svensjö, 1985). They also have an intriguing organization of filaments and myoid proteins that could exert contractile activity. Majno and Palade (1961) therefore originally suggested that the mediator-induced deformation of endothelial cells resulting in the gaps was due to a contractile effect. Although direct proof of the validity of this hypothesis is lacking, it has been widely accepted. It is attractive because, as a corollary, relaxation of endothelial cells could explain the closure of the gaps that so readily takes place spontaneously after, or even during, an attack of an immediate-type inflammatory mediator such as histamine (Persson and Svensjö, 1985; Greiff et al., 1990).

Even if there is a degree of tachyphylaxis to inflammatory stimulus-induced plasma exudation, this can be overcome by introducing novel mediators, increasing the dosage of the mediator or allowing a small interval between provocations. Some recent human experiments illustrate that endothelial-epithelial plasma leakage can be induced frequently in a reproducible fashion. Svensson et al. (1989) examined effects of 3 repeated nasal challenges with histamine at 30 min intervals (in 12 normal subjects) and compared the result with the same procedure on a different day. Nasal lavages were performed every 10 min to recover the mucosal surface liquids. Histamine significantly increased the levels of plasma proteins and plasma-derived mediators in the lavage fluids. The plasma tracers returned to baseline, and the next dose of histamine produced the same responses. Histamine-induced sneezes decreased somewhat from the first to the second challenge but other symptoms (blockage, secretion) as well as the plasma exudate tracers were quite reproducible at the 3 challenges in the same session as well as between the 2 histamine challenge days. These findings support the view that noninjurious, reversible processes regulate the inflammatory flow of macromolecules across airway endothelial-epithelial barriers.

V. Epithelial Passage of Plasma Exudate/Transudate

It has been proposed and widely accepted as an attractive possibility that asthmatic bronchi absorb inhaled factors to an abnormally large extent. This hypothesis now remains unproven. It is more established that plasma macromolecules traverse the mucosa into the lumen of asthmatic airways. Passage of extravasated plasma macromolecules into the lumen does not necessarily mean that luminal macromolecules can freely enter airway tissues (Erjefält and Persson, 1989, 1990a; Persson, 1989a).

Some recent experimental data in animals may shed light on possible mechanisms of epithelial passage of exuded plasma. Paracellular routes must be considered because large volumes of plasma exudate/transudate may rapidly enter the airway lumen apparently without destroying the epithelium (Persson and Erjefält, 1986; Erjefält and Persson, 1989). It was further demonstrated that plasma tracers appear promptly on the mucosal surface of tracheobronchial airways after a large variety of mucosal provocations: mediators such as histamine, bradykinin, and PAF, a neurogenic stimulus, allergen (an IgE-driven reaction), and an occupational asthma agent (toluene diisocyanate). Such muscosal challenges produced immediate plasma leakage. Biphasic responses with a late-phase leakage, and quite sustained plasma leakage responses were also recorded (Erjefält and Persson, 1989) (Fig. 2).

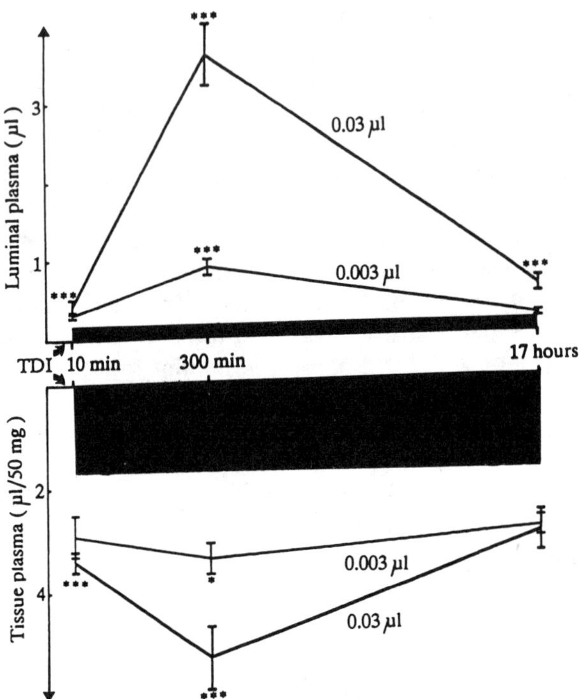

Figure 2 Toluene diisocyanate (TDI) applied in minimal amounts on guinea pig tracheobronchial mucosa produced prompt and sustained exudation of plasma into airway tissue (below) and lumen (above). A peak was reached 300 min after the single exposure. Shadowed areas show control vehicle data, which correspond to values obtained in untreated animals and are normal plasma pools.

All these agents produced concentration-dependent responses, and with all responses, even the threshold effects, there was an excellent correlation between plasma exuded into the interstitium of the airway wall and that appearing on the mucosal surface (Erjefält and Persson, 1989).

It is likely the closest microvessels, abundant just beneath the epithelium, that will be affected by the mucosal provocations and leak plasma. The subepithelial interstitium will then be endowed with exuded plasma. The negative surface charges and other factors in this milieu activate the exuded plasma protein systems. This activation will produce a large number of inflammatory peptides and the increased number of molecules will increase the osmotic load. Hence, the epithelium will be under attack from the basal side by the exudate and there will be some build up of interstitial hydrostatic pressure.

Even a small increase in pressure, perhaps together with mediator-induced destabilizaion of epithelium, will presumably cause the epithelial cells to separate transiently thus allowing passage of interstitial plasma along a gradient into the lumen. This possibility is supported by observations in vitro where tracheal luminal entry of serosal macromolecular solutes is reversibly induced by small increases (5 cmH$_2$O) in the serosal to luminal pressure ratio (Persson et al., 1990). Furthermore, both in vivo and in vitro the epithelium was intact promptly after the passage of the large solutes (Persson et al., 1987, 1990).

VI. Methods in Studies of Airway Plasma Exudation

So far there have been surprisingly few studies of airways plasma exudation. This is due in part to a scarcity of specific methods.

A. Particulate Tracers

Early observations on inflammatory vascular permeability (Pietra et al., 1971; Hurley, 1983) were made with particulate tracers such as carbon particles. If injected into the systemic circulation just before administration of an inflammatory mediator, the carbon particles will map out those microvessels that have become leaky. The particulate tracer will pass through the endothelial gaps but will then be trapped because they cannot pass the basement membrane. The particule tracer technique has been used to identify in airways that inflammatory permeability changes take place in postcapillary venules and, furthermore, that the tracheobronchial microvessels are reactive to proposed mediators of asthma whereas pulmonary microvessels are not.

The limitations of particulate tracers are many. They cannot estimate the extent of plasma exudation nor its distribution. Particulate tracers only provide a single point of measurement and cannot be given to humans. Most important is perhaps the fact that particle tracer measurement may show normal findings although plasma exudation is continuing to a significant degree. It was recently demonstrated that a late-phase airways plasma exudation phase induced by topical PAF on the guinea pig tracheal mucosa was not detectable with the carbon leakage method (O'Donnell et al., 1990).

B. Solute Tracers

The choice of solute tracers is not trivial. Albumin measurements are most commonly used but may not always provide specific information on the plasma exudation process. Albumin is a rather small plasma protein that is normally present in airway liquids. In fact, albumin may be actively secreted by the mucosa (Webber and Widdicombe, 1989) in addition to being a component of the exudate. The dye tags and the radiolabeling of albumin need more validation than usually is carried out. Evans blue dye may bind to other blood and tissue proteins than albumin and, although the binding between albumin and radioiodines may be firm, the corresponding attachment to technetium is not.

Larger solutes than albumin, such as α_2-macroglobulin and fibrinogen, have been measured and have provided the information that plasma exudation is a bulk extravasation of the various-sized plasma proteins. However, these proteins are metabolized after extravasation and their levels in the exudate may, therefore, not correctly reflect the exuded plasma volume. Another consideration is that fibrin formation may occur in the lamina propria. During late-phase plasma exudation after toluene-diisocyanate exposure, Erjefält and Persson (1989) observed that the airway wall to lumen ratio for amounts of exuded fibrinogen was much larger than that for albumin.

Fluorescein-labeled dextran macromolecules (FITC-D) (70,000 or 156,000 dalton) have been used successfully. FITC-D has less charge than the native proteins and charge may be one of the determinants of the ability of macromolecules to pass a variety of barriers in the airways (endothelial-epithelial and their basement membranes). Indeed, despite its greater size FITC-D 156,000 passed the mucosal barriers more readily than albumin (Erjefält and Persson, 1989). A possible drawback with the FITC-D tracers is that other fluorescent proteins will be comeasured in the inflammatory exudates sampled.

VII. Plasma Exudation or Changes in the Blood Pool?

By definition, the measurement of plasma exudation in tissue samples requires that the intravascular plasma content be known. The blood pool of tissue samples can be specifically quantitated and its amount of plasma be deducted from the total tissue plasma content (Persson et al., 1986b). Many authors (Sheppard et al., 1986; Lundberg et al., 1983; Boschetto et al., 1989) state that they do not need to measure the airway blood pool because by flushing saline through the vascular system they "eliminate" the airway tissue of blood. This claim is not well supported by actual data. It is, in fact, not possible to wash out more than about half of the blood pool of the airway microvessels (Erjefält and Persson, unpublished observations). Hence, "washout of blood pool" is not an acceptable technique unless validated by actual measurements of the remaining blood pool. This aspect would be particularly important under inflammatory conditions when more blood may be trapped in newly recruited and congested microvessels. What has been reported as "plasma leakage" may, to an unknown extent, have been a "noninflammatory" intravascular engorgement.

Recent observations of a good correlation between the content of plasma exudate in airway tissue and lumen, respectively (Erjefält and Persson, 1989) indicate that the problem of variations in the blood pool also can be circumvented by sampling and assaying mucosal surface material.

VIII. Sampling of Mucosal Surface Liquids

There have been several attempts to obtain proper samples of airway surface liquids, whether the purpose has been to assess plasma exudation or another event. In tracheobronchial airways, the techniques employed generally lack specificity. The so-called bronchial lavage retrieves, to an unknown extent, alveolar lining fluid. In ordinary bronchoalveolar lavage the latter may be 100 times as large as the airway fluid component (Reynolds, 1987). There are many other problems with bronchial lavages, including artefactual trauma, the necessity of using premedications, large and unknown variabilities in exposed and lavaged mucosal surface areas, ethical problems, and others. It is interesting to note that Lam et al. (1985) observed no difference between normal and asthmatic subjects in the plasma protein content of their bronchoalveolar lavage fluids, whereas the difference was 10-fold in material sampled by a small volume lavage of a main bronchus.

A. Specific Large Airway Lavages

In animals, a technique for specific and nontraumatic lavage of large tracheobronchial airways has been described (Erjefält and Persson, 1989). With use of this technique it has been possible to correlate the amount of exuded plasma in the airway lumen with that in the underlying tissue. The data suggest that just by sampling the surface liquids it is possible to determine the mucosal/submucosal inflammatory plasma exudation process, its intensity, and time course in great detail (Erjefält and Persson, 1989). This observation strongly supports the relevance of specific airway lavage procedures. Whereas specificity seems difficult to achieve in human bronchi it is quite feasible in human nasal airways.

Nasal provocations and washings can be performed safely in normal subjects and in patients with various rhinitic conditions. By repeated washings (which even can be carried out by patients themselves), the time course of plasma exudation and other events can be readily assessed. Indeed, a recently developed technique allows one to expose a defined area of the human nasal mucosa with known concentrations of mediators, tracers, or other agents for the desired length of time (Greiff et al., 1990). Moreover, the novel device gently lavages that same mucosal surface area. Thus actual concentration/response evaluations for effects of mediators on human airway mucosa and microvessels can now be assessed (Greiff et al., 1990).

B. Absorbing Disks: What Do They Sample?

The possibility of exposing a defined surface area as well as sampling its liquids has led to the use of absorbing disk techniques. A piece of filter paper containing known amounts of mediator or allergen has usually been applied on the airway mucosa (human nasal or animal tracheobronchial). However, the absorbing disk technique seems to destroy the barrier function of the epithelial lining. Thus, filter papers gently applied on the guinea pig tracheal mucosa sampled airway tissue fluid and its macromolecular solutes rather than or in addition to sampling the surface liquids (Erjefält and Persson, 1990b).

IX. Passage of White Cells

Sticking of white cells to endothelium and their subsequent migration across the vascular wall are characteristic of many inflammatory processes and are acknowledged events in asthmatic airways. As with protein leakage, the leukocyte-endothelium interactions occur mainly in postcapillary venules, and the diapedesis is through endothelial intercellular junctions. However, leukocytes can have a protein-tight seal suring migration and mediator-induced leakage of plasma macromolecules occurs without cellular escape, showing that different mechanisms are involved in the two types of exudative process (Hurley, 1983). It is likely that also the epithelial passage of white cells is distinct from the luminal entry of exuded plasma (Milks et al., 1983).

X. Plasma Exudation in the Pathogenesis of Asthma

An immediate result of tracheobronchial exudation, and a result that is generally thought of, is airway mucosal/submucosal edema. Edema is also consistently mentioned in discussions of airway pathology in asthma, but has, presumably due to technical difficulties, only scattered qualitative support from biopsies and postmortem examinations. Nevertheless, histological examination illustrating increased interstitial spaces seems to demonstrate convincingly the presence of edema in asthmatic airways (see chapter-Laitinen and Laitinen). Unlike luminal mucus material, the edema will not be moved away from critical sites of resistance. It can be deformed by constriction of more deeply lying airway smooth muscle but will not be compressed, and will therefore exaggerate the reduction in airway lumen that occurs during bronchoconstriction. As first calculated by Hutt and Wick (1956), this may have dramatic effects on the increase in airway resistance that is roughly dependent on the fourth power of the radius of free lumen. A peribronchial edema might reduce compliance and further facilitate bronchoconstriction by uncoupling bronchial muscle from the stabilizing forces of the parenchyma surrounding the pulmonary bronchi. Both mucosal and peribronchial edema might thus be important in bronchial hyperresponsiveness.

When plasma enters the airway lumen, many potential consequences relating to mucus viscosity and plug formation can occur (see Persson, 1988a). Mucociliary transport would be reduced by an increase in the periciliary fluid layer. The edema and the transepithelial passage of plasma may contribute to sloughing of epithelium. Plasma proteins may increase mucus production, prevent its normal hydration, and increase its viscosity by mucin-albumin complexes and by activation of the coagulation system with fibrin formation. Surfactant material may be destroyed by exuded plasma, leading to small airway narrowing.

In addition to the above-mentioned physical aspects, exuded plasma proteins, in particular in an inflamed airway, are not innocuous (Persson, 1986). The kinin, complement, clotting, fibrinolysis, and other systems would be activated to produce an immense variety of bronchoconstricting and inflammatory mediators, which also cause further recruitment of inflammatory cells. The presence of exuded plasma in the airways may also be necessary for conditioning and activation of inflammatory cells, which are abundant in patients with asthma.

XI. Inhibition of Plasma Exudation

On the basis of the potential importance of plasma exudation in asthma, it was suggested that its inhibition may be a major aspect of the pharmacological action of antiasthma drugs, especially glucocorticoids (Persson, 1986; Andersson and Persson, 1988). It is an intriguing observation that several antiasthma drugs may reduce inflammatory stimulus-induced airway leakage of plasma. Studies in animals and human subjects have shown that glucocorticoids reduce plasma exudation and its entry into the lumen of inflamed airways. Moreover, a close relationship between glucocorticoid-induced clinical improvement and reduction of plasma exudation has been observed in patients with rhinitis and asthma (Andersson and Persson, 1988). Although less effective than the glucocorticoids, the cromoglycates also reduce plasma exudation through a blend of actions including a stabilizing action on venular endothelial cells (Persson, 1987).

Studies carried out with a variety of xanthine derivatives demonstrated that antiasthma xanthines can be classified into adenosine blockers such as theophylline (and caffeine) and xanthines such as enprofylline, which does not antagonize effects of adenosine (Persson et al., 1986a). The xanthines may produce several airway anti-inflammatory effects, and in guinea pig airways enprofylline and theophylline reduced capsaicin-induced plasma exudation in a dose-dependent fashion. The antiexudative effect was shown to be a local airways action since superfusion with only a few μg/ml of enprofylline was active and the total topical dosage was more than 500 times less than that required by the intravenous route, while still a therapeutic dosage (1-5 mg/kg) (Persson et al., 1986b, 1988). Theophylline has been demonstrated to reduce both symptoms and plasma exudation in inflammatory stimulus-provoced human nasal mucosa (Naclerio et al., 1986). Symptom induction and pharmacological prevention correlated well with plasma proteins and plasma-derived mediators, whereas levels of cellular mediators such as histamine correlated less well (Persson, 1988b). It was interesting that enprofylline was as effective as a large dose of a PAF antagonist (WEB 2086) in inhibiting the late-phase plasma exudation occurring after application of PAF topically on guinea pig tracheal mucosa (O'Donnell et al., 1989). Failure by Boschetto et al. (1989) to find antiexudative effects of xanthines in guinea pig airways probably relates to the methodology used (see above), including the administration of near-shock dosages of PAF intravenously.

The postcapillary venular endothelium and mucosal epithelium seem to harbor anti-leakage-mediating β_2-receptors (Persson and Svensjö, 1985). β-receptor agonists such as terbutaline were among the first drugs demonstrated to exhibit antipermeability actions in a variety of systemic vascular beds (see Persson et al., 1982; Persson and Svensjö, 1985). Terbutaline given locally or systemically reduced an inflammatory stimulus-induced plasma exudation response in guinea-pig tracheobronchial airways in a dose-dependent fashion (Persson et al., 1986; Persson, 1988a; Erjefält and Persson, unpublished observations). If the stimulus was too strong, the β-agonist was not effective in this system. Lack of efficacy has also been reported by other workers. However, the techniques used to examine plasma exudation (Boschetto et al., 1989) have not differentiated between intravascular and extravascular plasma. Furthermore, both the inflammatory provocations and the drugs have been administered intravenously (Boschetto et al., 1989), which makes it difficult to interpret the data in terms of specific airway actions. Information is still scarce on the antiexudative effects of β-agonists in human airways.

Accepting that plasma exudation is a cardinal sign of inflammation (Cohnheim, 1882; Hurley, 1983) an antiexudative effect should be the result of almost any major anti-inflammatory action. For example, through inhibition of formation/release of vasoactive mediators, significant antiexudative effects can be achieved. It may also be possible to attenuate plasma exudation by constricting arterioles and thus reducing the delivery of plasma to the leaky microvessels. However, the most important vascular target cells are the endothelial cells of postcapillary venules. Through some stabilizing action drugs such as glucocorticoids, β-agonists, and xanthines variably reduce the ability of venular endothelial cells to separate and form the leaky gaps. Particular to the airways is the luminal entry of plasma exudates. Since the epithelial crossing may be brought about by the exudate itself (see above), it is through inhibition of the extravasation of plasma that luminal entry is also inhibited.

XII. Conclusion

Besides its role in nutrition, the tracheobronchial microcirculation is involved in the conditioning of incoming air, in clearing the airways of various factors, and other functions. It is possible that this circulation transports inhaled drugs to those parts of the lower airways that were not reached by the initially deposited dose. Such a mechanism would help to explain the clinical efficacy of inhaled drugs in the treatment of asthma.

It is now increasingly being understood that tracheobronchial plasma exudation may be an important pathogenetic mechanism of asthma. The abundant venular system beneath the epithelial lining may be seen as a giant inflammatory cell releasing its powerful mediator systems at a variety of provocations. The potential release is so great that physical changes in the airway wall and lumen would also result. These aspects may justify the focus in this chapter on plasma exudation mechanisms and studies thereof.

Discussion

O'Byrne: How quickly can exudation be reversed by drugs such as epinephrine or specific β_2 agonists?

Persson: The plasma exudation process can be stopped promptly. Even in the presence of inflammatory mediators, the endothelial gaps will close spontaneously after having been open for only a few minutes. It is another question whether exuded plasma can be cleared rapidly. Normally the lymphatic transport is very slow. Hence, the most efficient and rapid clearance route is probably the passage of plasma into the lumen. Whether this passage can be speeded up by drugs is not known.

Leff: How would β_2 agonists reverse exudation in vascular tissues?

Persson: Hypothetically, β-agonists can reduce ongoing vascular leakage by closing (relaxing) the separated (contracted) endothelial cells of postcapillary venules.

Chung: What is the mechanism of the prolonged and delayed protein leakage you find with PAF or isocyanates? Is this due to prolonged opening of the endothelial venular junctions?

Persson: Biphasic vascular leakage can occur in response to a variety of stimuli. PAF is the only single mediator for which we have observed both immediate and late-phase plasma leakage. Mechanisms involved in the late phase after toluene-diisocyanate have not been assessed. Particulate tracers such as carbon identify the immediate leak but not the late-phase airways plasma exudation occurring after topical PAF.

Hargreave: Has the degree of plasma exudation in sputum been compared between smokers with chronic bronchitis and nonsmokers with asthma? Is there any difference?

Persson: Such studies are highly warranted. By analyzing macromolecular plasma tracers in sputum, you should be able to determine the ongoing mucosal/submucosal inflammatory process. Its intensity and time course may preferably be studied by analyzing tagged macromolecules that you inject intravenously at specific time periods.

Kerrebijn: The fact that a high dosage of beta$_2$ agonist (1-2 mg inhaled) given *immediately* after histamine challenge, which results in a drop of FEV_1 of 20-25% of baseline, does produce an FEV_1 value that is significantly lower than that obtained without histamine whereas this is not the case *1 h* after histamine challenge may indicate that mucosal edema plays a significant role in the histamine reaction.

Persson: It is an interesting possibility. However, if you see similar phenomena with methacholine-β-agonist interactions, antiplasma leakage is not a likely mechanism mainly because muscarinic agonists do not produce leakage of plasma.

Widdicombe: After a histamine or methacholine challenge there would be more surface airway liquid because of either transudation or gland secretion. The subsequent β-agonist challenge would be into a larger absorptive volume of liquid and might be less effective.

Tattersfield: What is the effect of beta$_2$ agonists on the nasal response to inhaled histamine? In the skin beta agonists reduce the wheal response to histamine, but only with relatively high dosages.

Persson: No data are available as yet. β-agonists may only be effective against histamine-induced plasma leakage when threshold responses occur. β-agonists are not always active against large plasma leakage responses.

Paré: In the nose there is no smooth muscle and obstruction is largely due to engorgement of capacitance vessels in the nasal mucosa. We always mention hyperemia as a possible mechanism of bronchial narrowing, but how much does it really contribute? Do you and John Widdicombe have measurements that would allow calculation of the potential importance of bronchial vascular engorgement?

Persson: It is an interesting possibility that sinusoidal vascular pooling is contributing significantly to airway resistance in tracheobronchial airways. However, the failure of vasoconstrictors such as epinephrine and oximetazolin to reverse obstruction through vasoconstriction suggests that it may be of limited importance.

Widdicombe: Hyperemia in the dog trachea increases mucosal thickness by 10-20% at the most. But we do not know if changes in bronchial mucosal thickness may be proportionately larger than for the trachea; and the dog has a relatively less extensive airway vasculature than, for example, sheep and, probably, humans.

Barnes: Calcium antagonists (e.g., inhaled and oral nefedipine), which presumably cause airway hyperemia, do not obstruct airways as measured by FEV_1 of sGaw. This suggest that hyperemia by itself does not narrow airways, although whether an effect on *small* airways occurs is not known.

Sertl: Are there any experimental data that drugs (β-agonists, steroids) can clear edema formation more quickly than that occurring without any drugs?

Persson: Several drugs can reduce plasma leakage but they would have to act prophylactically because once plasma is exuded, you would have to increase its clearance and that may be more difficult to accomplish with drugs.

Schleimer: T. Williams, A. Issekutz, and others have demonstrated that vascular leak in the skin can occur: by both leukocyte-dependent and leukocyte-independent mechanisms. Have you studied the lung to determine whether this is also the case in the airways? If so, can PAF elicit both mechanisms?

Persson: I think there is a case for leukocyte involvement, in particular in the sustained plasma exudation responses that we see with occupational chemicals and allergen and PAF. Specific airway data on this point are scarce.

Paré: In addition to occupying space within the airway lumen and delivering plasma-derived mediators to the airway, plasma exudation could change the surface active properties of the liquid lining the airways and this could further narrow the airways.

Drazen: Airway edema, if it increased the external diameter of an airway, could result in airway narrowing by decreasing the elastic recoil forces that tend to keep the airway open. These forces are quite powerful.

Persson: The possibility that peribronchial edema in small airways unloads elastic recoil has been proposed by Peter Macklem. Also, small-airway narrowing secondary to plasma exudation-induced destruction of surfactant material has been discussed by Hogg and Macklem.

Platts-Mills: You talked about the poor transport of molecules from the lumen of the bronchi into the subepithelial space and stated correctly that little is known about the transport of allergens from the bronchial lumen inwards. However, inhaling a protein could produce a wheal and flare reaction at a Prausnitz-Kuestner site on the back, demonstrating that absorption of a protein (?) allergen would occur through the nasal mucosa into the bloodstream.

Persson: It is correct that allergens can penetrate airway mucosal barriers. The point I wanted to make is that plasma exudation into the lumen can occur without appreciably increasing the normal ability of large luminal molecules to penetrate the airway tissue.

References

Andersson, P., and Persson, C. G. A. (1988). Developments in antiasthma glucocorticoids. In *Directions for New Anti-Asthma Drugs*. Edited by S. R. O'Donnell and C. G. A. Persson. Basel, Birkhäuser, pp. 239-260.

Boschetto, P., Roberts, N. M., Rogers, D. F., and Barnes, P. J. (1989). Effect of anti-asthma drugs on microvascular leakage in guinea-pig airways. *Am. Rev. Respir. Dis.* **139**:416-421.

Bullowa, J. G. M., and Kaplan, D. M. (1903). On the hypodermatic use of adrenalin chloride in the treatment of asthmatic attacks. *Med. News* **83**:787-790.

Cohnheim, J. (1882). *Vorlesungen uber Allgemeine Pathologie I*. Berlin, August Hirschwald, pp. 232-367.

Daly, I. de B., and Hebb, C. (1966). *Pulmonary and Bronchial Vascular Systems*. London, Edward Arnold, pp. 42-88.

Deffebach, M. E., Charan, N. B., Lakshminarayan, S., and Butler, J. (1987). The bronchial circulation: small but a vital attribute of the lung. *Am. Rev. Respir. Dis.* **135**:463-481.

Erjefält, I., and Persson, C. G. A. (1986). Anti-asthma drugs attenuate inflammatory leakage of plasma into airway lumen. *Acta. Physiol. Scand.* **128**:653-654.

Erjefält, I., and Persson, C. G. A. (1989). Inflammatory passage of plasma macromolecules into airway tissue and lumen. *Pulmon. Pharmacol.* **2**: 93-102.

Erjefält, J., and Persson, C. G. A. (1990a). Plasma exudation into the airway lumen is a "one-way traffic". Effects of topical provocations on absorption and exudation across the mucosa in guinea-pig tracheobronchial airways. *Clin. Exp. Allergy,* submitted.

Erjefält, I., and Persson, C. G. A. (1990b). On the use of absorbing discs to sample airway mucosal surface liquids. *Clin. Exp. Allergy,* submitted.

Greiff, L., Pipkorn, U., Alkner, U., and Persson, C. G. A. (1989). The "Nasal Pool-device" applies controlled concentrations of solutes on human nasal airway mucosa and samples its surface exudations/secretions. *Clin. Exp. Allergy,* in press.

Hurley, J. V. (1983). *Acute Inflammation,* 2nd ed. Edinburgh, Churchill Livingstone.

Hutt, G., and Wick, H. (1956). Bronchial-luemn and Atemwiderstand. *Z. Aerosol Frosch. Ther.* **5**:131-140.

Kröll, F., Karlsson, J.-A., and Persson, C. G. A. (1987). Bronchial circulation perfused via the pulmonary artery in guinea-pig isolated lungs. *Acta Physiol. Scand.* **129**:437-440.

Laitinen, L. A., Laitinen, A., and Widdicombe, J. G. (1987). Effects of inflammatory and other mediators on airway vascular beds. *Am. Rev. Respir. Dis.* **135**:567-570.

Lam, S., Leriche, J. C., Kijek, K., and Phillips, R. T. (1985). Effect of bronchial lavage volume on cellular and protein recovery. *Chest* **88**:856-859.

Lundberg, J. M., Saria, A., Brodin, E., Rosell, S., and Folkers, K. (1983). A substance P antagonist inhibits vagally induced increase in vascular permeability and bronchial smooth muscle contraction in the guinea-pig. *Proc. Nat. Acad. Sci. U.S.A.* **80**:1120-1124.

Majno, G., and Palade, G. E. (1961). Studies on inflammation I. *J. Biophys. Biochem. Cytol.* **11**:571-605.

Milks, L., Uszler, J. M., Effros, R. M., and Reid, E. (1983). Transepithelial electrical resistance studies during in vitro neutrophil (PMN) migration. *Fed. Proc.* **43**(3):777.

Naclerio, R. M., Bartenfelder, D., Proud, D., Togias, A. G., Meyer, D. A., Kagey-Sobotka, A., Norman, P. S., and Lichtenstein, L. M. (1986). Theophylline reduces histamine release during pollen-induced rhinitis. *J. Allergy Clin. Immunol.* **78**:874-876.

O'Donnell, S. R., Erjefält, I., and Persson, C. G. A. (1990). Early and late tracheobronchial plasma exudation by PAF administered to the airway mucosal surface in guinea-pigs: effects of WEB 2086 and enprofylline. *J. Pharmacol. Exp. Ther.,* in press.

Persson, C. G. A. (1985). On the medical history of xanthines and other remedies for asthma: a tribute to H. H. Salter. *Thorax* **40**:881-886.

Persson, C. G. A. (1986). Role of plasma exudation in asthmatic airways. *Lancet* **2**:1126-1129.

Persson, C. G. A. (1987). Cromoglycate, plasma exudation and asthma. *Trends Pharmacol. Sci.* **8**:202-203.

Persson, C. G. A. (1988a). Plasma exudation and asthma. *Lung* **116**:1-23.

Persson, C. G. A. (1988b). Xanthines as airway antiinflammatory drugs. *J. Allergy Clin. Immunol.* **81**:615-617.

Persson, C. G. A. (1989a). Permeability changes in obstructive airway diseases. In *Bronchitis* IV. Edited by H. J. Sluiter and R. Van Der Lende. Assen, Van Gorcum, pp. 236-248.

Persson, C. G. A. (1989b). Glucocorticoids for asthma—early contributions. *Pulmon. Pharmacol.* **2**:163-166.

Persson, C. G. A. (1990). On the medical history of asthma and rhinitis. In *Rhinitis and Asthma. Similarities and Differences.* Edited by N. Mygind, U. Pipkorn and R. Dahl, Copenhagen, Munksgaard, pp. 9-20.

Persson, C. G. A., and Erjefält, I. (1986). Inflammatory leakage of macromolecules from the vascular compartment into the tracheal lumen. *Acta. Physiol. Scand.* **126**:615-616.

Persson, C. G. A., and Erjefält, I. (1987). Non-neural and neural regulation of airway microvascular leakage of macromolecules. *Neural Regulation of the Airways in Health and Disease.* Edited by M. A. Kaliner and P. Barnes. New York, Marcel Dekker, pp. 523-549.

Persson, C. G. A., and Pipkorn, U. (1990). On the pharmacology and pathophysiology of asthma and rhinitis. In *Rhinitis and Asthma. Similarities and Differences.* Edited by N. Mygind, U. Pipkorn, and R. Dahl. Copenhagen, Munksgaard. pp.

Persson, C. G. A., and Svensjö, E. (1985). Vascular responses and their suppression: drugs interfering with venular permeability. In *Handbook of Inflammation,* Volume 5: *The Pharmacology of Inflammation.* Edited by I. L. Bonta, M. A. Bray, and M. J. Parnhan. Amsterdam, Elsevier, pp. 61-81.

Persson, C. G. A., Erjefält, I., Grega, G. J., and Svensjö, E. (1982). The role of β-receptor agonists in the inhibition of pulmonary edema. *Ann. N.Y. Acad. Sci.* **384**:544-557.

Persson, C. G. A., Anderson, K.-E., and Kjellin, G. (1986a). Effects of emprofylline and theophylline may show the role of adenosine. *Life Sci.* **38**:1057-1072.

Persson, C. G. A., Erjefält, I., and Andersson, P. (1986b). Leakage of macromolecules from guinea pig tracheobronchial microcirculation. Effects of allergen, leukotriene, tachykinins, and anti-asthma drugs. *Acta. Physiol. Scand.* **127**:95-106.

Persson, C. G. A., Erjefält, J., Sundler, F. (1987). Airway microvascular and epithelial leakage of plasma induced by PAF-acether and capsaicin. *Am. Rev. Respir. Dis.* **135**:A401.

Persson, C. G. A., Erjefält, I., and Gustafsson, B. (1988). Xanthines—symptomatic or prophylactic in asthma? In *Directions for New Anti-Asthma Drugs*. Edited by S. R. O'Donnell and C. G. A. Persson. Basel, Birkhäuser, pp. 137-156.

Persson, C. G. A., Erjefält, J., Gustafsson, B., Luts, A. (1990). Subepithelial hydrostatic pressure may regulate plasma exudation across the mucosa. *Int. Arch. Allergy Appl. Immunol.* in press.

Pietra, C. G., Szidon, J. P., Leventhal, M. M., and Fishman, A. P. (1971). Histamine and interstitial pulmonary edema in the dog. *Circ. Res.* **29**: 323-337.

Reynolds, H. Y. (1987). State of art. Broncho-alveolar lavage. *Am. Rev. Respir. Dis.* **135**:250-263.

Salonen, R. O., Webber, S. E., and Widdicombe, J. G. (1988). Effects of neuropeptides and capsaicin on the canine tracheal vasculature in vivo. *Br. J. Pharmacol.* **95**:1262-1270.

Sheppard, D., Scypinski, L., Horn, J., Gordon, T., and Thompson, J. (1986). Granulocyte-mediated airway edema in guinea-pigs. *J. Appl. Physiol.* **60**:1213-1220.

Sobin, S. S., Frasher, W. G., Tremer, H. M., and Hadley, G. G. (1963). The microcirculation of the tracheal mucosa. *Angiology* **14**:165-170.

Solis-Cohen, S. (1900). The use of adrenal substance in the treatment of asthma. *JAMA* **34**:1164-1166.

Svensson, C., Baumgarten, C. R., Pipkorn, U., Alkener, U., and Persson, C. G. A. (1989). Reversibility and reproducibility of histamine-induced plasma leakage in nasal airways. *Thorax* **44**:13-18.

Svensson, C., Persson, C. G. A., Baumgarten, C. R., Alkner, U., and Pipkorn, U. (1990). Topical α-adrenoceptor stimulation may not reduce histamine-induced plasma leakage in human nasal airways. Thesis, Lund pp. 89-101.

Webber, S. E., and Widdicombe, J. G. (1989). The transport of albumin across the ferret in-vitro whole trachea. *J. Physiol.,* **408**:457-472.

8

Platelets in Asthma

ANDRÉ CAPRON, CLAUDE AURIAULT, JEAN-YVES CESBRON,
VÉRONIQUE PANCRÉ, JEAN-CLAUDE AMEISEN,
ANDRÉ-BERNARD TONNEL, MARTINE DAMONNEVILLE,
ANNE TSICOPOULOS, and MICHEL JOSEPH

Institut Pasteur
Lille, France

Asthma has long been viewed, similarly to other allergic diseases, as a conflict involving two partners: IgE antibody and mast cells. Extensive studies, initiated in parasitic diseases, have now unequivocally established that IgE antibodies can trigger mononuclear phagocytes, eosinophils, and platelets directly through specific surface IgE receptors now identified as $Fc_\epsilon RII$ (Capron et al., 1986a). Genes encoding for this class of receptors have been cloned and, although studies on molecular structure indicate a close homology between $Fc_\epsilon RII$ on inflammatory cells and on B cells, indications are now emerging of some degree of posttranscriptional heterogeneity among the second receptors for IgE. While the evidence for the direct participation of other inflammatory cells, such as eosinophils, in allergic reactions is now widely recognized, the role of platelets as effector cells remains a matter of controversy and the concept that platelets might be active cellular partners in allergy is still debatable.

In this chapter we discuss, in the light of recent information, the experimental evidence arguing for such an active participation of platelets, not only in allergic asthma but also in intrinsic asthma, such as aspirin-induced asthma.

I. Mechanisms of Platelet Activation: A Receptor for IgE on Platelets

In allergic disorders, platelet activation was long believed to occur indirectly through the effects of platelet-activating factor (PAF or PAF-acether). PAF is released by a variety of IgE-sensitized cells that express either $Fc_\epsilon RI$ (mast cells, basophils) or $Fc_\epsilon RII$ (macrophages, eosinophils). PAF is also released by stimulated endothelial cells and by activated platelets themselves (Barnes et al., 1988).

The concept that platelets can participate directly in some IgE-mediated processes has arisen from the demonstration of the involvement of this cell population in IgE-dependent killing of parasites (Joseph et al., 1983).

These studies, confirmed by others (Cines et al., 1986), indicated that human platelets can bind IgE in vitro and that cross-linking of surface-bound IgE with anti-IgE or antigen induced platelet activation and secretion. Further experiments led to the demonstration of a specific receptor for the Fc fragment of IgE on the platelet membrane. Scatchard analysis showed that there were between 600 and 1000 binding sites for IgE per platelet with an affinity constant of $3 \times 10^7 M^{-1}$ (Joseph et al., 1986).

Several lines of evidence pointed to similarities between the platelet IgE receptor and the $Fc_\epsilon R$ on monocytes, macrophages, and eosinophils. In particular, a unique monoclonal antibody BB10, raised against the eosinophil IgE receptor, inhibited IgE binding and IgE-dependent platelet activation. It should be stressed that the platelet IgE receptor clearly appears as distinct from the previously described IgG-binding sites and that cross-linking of surface-bound IgE can also be achieved with the so-called IgE-binding factors known as histamine-releasing factor (HRF), released by macrophages and platelets themselves.

Purification and subsequent gel analysis of the platelet IgE receptor have provided evidence of two subunits of 43kD and 30 kD, the latter differing from the smaller subunit in eosinophils and monocytes generally identified as a 23-25 kD molecule (Capron et al., 1986b). An interesting feature of the platelet $Fc_\epsilon RII$ is its association with a platelet membrane glycoprotein that plays an essential role in hemostatsis: the GPllb/llla complex. Platelets from patients with Glanzman's thrombasthenia selectively lacked both the GPllb/llla complex and the IgE receptor, and monoclonal antibodies to GPllb and llla inhibited the binding of IgE and the IgE-mediated cytotoxicity in normal platelets. This indicates that the binding of IgE to human platelets required the presence of the GPllb/llla complex (Ameisen et al., 1986). Recent studies performed in parallel on eosinophils and platelets indicated that $Fc_\epsilon RII$

and GPllb/llla share common characteristics of adhesiotopes and, more precisely, the RGD sequence commonly involved in the primary structure of adhesion proteins.

In the framework of allergic or inflammatory disorders, other biological mediators of platelet triggering have also been demonstrated. C-reactive protein, for instance, appeared as a potent inducer of platelet activation. Platelets collected during the acute phase of experimental infection of rodents by schistosomes were highly cytotoxic for schistosome larvae and normal platelets could be triggered into effector cells by highly purified C-reactive protein (Bout et al., 1986). More recently, it has been shown that the neuropeptide substance P could directly trigger platelet activation (Damonneville et al., 1988a). The amino acid sequence of substance P actively involved in platelet activation is confined to the N-terminal region of the molecule, as for stimulation of T lymphocyte proliferation, whereas amino acids of the C-terminal portion induce histamine release from peritoneal mast cells. The construction of various synthetic peptides derived from the sequence of substance P has allowed the demonstration that the AA sequence 5-11 correspond to the most active site of the molecule. In competition experiments it has been also demonstrated that platelet activation by substance P can be inhibited by IgE itself, and that the competitive inhibition observed might be related to the existence of limited but significant conformational homology between the primary structure of substance P and the domain of the ϵ chain.

Taken together, these examples, which do not represent an exhaustive list of the molecules potentially involved in platelet activation, provide evidence, in the framework of allergic disorders. that relevant stimuli such as IgE, IgE-binding factors, C-reactive protein, or substance P can directly participate in platelet activation and secretion of platelet-derived mediators.

II. Expression of Platelet Activation: A Scenario for Free Radicals in IgE-Mediated Platelet Activation

In both animals and humans, allergic challenge or asthmatic shock (but not the nonallergic bronchoconstriction mediated by methacholine) has been shown to induce the release into plasma of platelet-specific proteins, such as platelet factor 4 (PF4) (Knauer et al., 1981) and β-thromboglobulin (βTG) (Gresele et al., 1982). These increases, however, varied widely from patient to patient and were not observed by all investigators (Greer et al., 1984; Durham et al., 1985). In the bronchoalveolar lavage of asthmatic patients, significant elevations in levels of βTG and fibrinopeptide-A from fibrinogen were measured during early- and late-phase response to allergen challenge (Metzger et al., 1985).

In the framework of our studies, platelets isolated from patients with allergic asthma or with *Hymenoptera* venom hypersensitivity reacted *in vitro* to specific allergen or to anti-IgE by releasing cytotoxic mediators and oxygen-derived free radicals, evidenced respectively by the death of parasitic larvae and by chemiluminescence (Capron et al., 1987).

How can platelets affect cellular targets? Our challenging opinion sees the cytotoxicity of platelets as involving the participation of (OX)-type radical species. Four sets of arguments appear in support of this working hypothesis:

1. Free radical scavengers and oxidoreductases (superoxide dismutase, catalase, glutathione peroxidase) removing O_2^-, H_2O_2, and lipid peroxides strongly inhibit cytocidal effects of IgE-dependent platelet activation. The data obtained are consistent with a lipid peroxidation process in platelets (Cesbron et al., 1987).

2. Mobilized pools of metal ions, particularly iron, are important in accelerating damaging free radical reactions and, conversely, chelating agents can be used as protective compounds. We have, in this context, shown an increased IgE-dependent activation by Fe^{++} down to $10^{-11}M$. In addition, the presence of $10^{-6}M$ of the iron chelator *o*-phenanthroline abolished the action of Fe^{++} (Cesbron et al., 1987).

3. IgE-stimulated platelets induce significant catalase-inhibitable chemiluminescence, which reaches its maximum between 3 and 5 min after the stimulus and decays slowly

4. Spin trapping of hydroxyl radicals by reaction with stable nitroxyl radicals, and the generation of electron paramagnetic resonance (EPR) spectra have allowed the identification of OH$^\bullet$ radicals after IgE-dependent activation.

As a whole the data gathered render highly probable the participation of free radical reactions as a result of IgE-dependent platelet activation. The possibility that oxygen free radicals contribute directly to tissue damage seems unlikely considering the short life of these molecules. Whatever the primary radical event occurring within cells, it is reasonable to think that it sets off radical chain reactions, leading to lipoperoxidation of lipids in membranes. Lipid peroxides can fragment to give a wide range of more stable products, such as aldehydes, for example. No relationship between the arachidonic acid metabolism of platelets and their cytocidal properties after IgE-dependent activation has been evidenced in our research. We have, in particular, been unable to correlate significant changes in arachidonate products with platelet activation, although the cytotoxicity was abolished with various lipoxygenase and cycloxygenase inhibitors. Evidence that phospholipase A_2, which preferentially hydrolyzes peroxidized fatty acids rather than arachidonic acid, might play a crucial role in platelet cytotoxicity is consistent with the above observations. We are still left with working hypotheses in our understanding of molecular mechanisms governing cytocidal properties of platelets following IgE-dependent activation; much work in this area is still needed. It might be reassuring to remember that almost 20 years after the discovery of cytotoxic T cells and natural killer (NK) cells our understanding of their killing mechanism is still very fragmentary.

III. Regulatory Mechanisms: Lymphokines Modulate Platelet Functions

The demonstration of effector functions of platelets in parasitic diseases raised the question of their possible regulation by T cells. Normal human platelets treated with culture supernatants from mitogen- or antigen-stimulated $CD4^+/CD8^-$ T cells developed the capacity to kill the larvae of *S. mansoni* in the absence of IgE antibodies. The physicochemical properties of the factors involved strongly suggested that IFNγ was likely one of the lymphokines stimulating platelet cytotoxicity. The neutralization by monoclonal and polyclonal anti-IFNγ antibodies of the induction of the platelet killer effect, the presence of IFNγ in the $CD4^+/CD8^-$ lymphocyte supernatants, and the direct inducer effect of recombinant IFNγ clearly demonstrated that this lymphokine was one of the factors responsible for the induction of platelet cytotoxic functions (Pancré et al., 1987). The in vivo relevance of this effect was studied in the rat model: the passive transfer of normal rat platelets treated with rat recombinant IFNγ to normal syngeneic recipients on the day of challenge infection led to a high degree of protection. Moreover, IFNγ could also act on the IgE-dependent platelet cytotoxicity by enhancing the IgE receptor expression on the platelet membrane (Pancré et al., 1988).

The demonstration of an interrelationship between IFNγ and platelet function has to be related to the work of Molinas et al. (1987), who have demonstrated that human IFNγ was able to bind to an estimate 150-200 high-affinity specific receptors on human platelets with an apparent equilibrium dissociation constant (Kd) of 2×10^{-10}M.

A second inducing factor of platelet cytotoxicity exhibiting a neutral pI was also previously evidenced in $CD4^+/CD8^-$ stimulated T-lymphocyte supernatant. This factor was identified as tumor necrosis factor (TNF). Indeed, recombinant TNF β and, to a lesser extent TNFα induced normal platelets into cytotoxic effects for *S. mansoni* larvae (Damonneville et al., 1988b).

An additive effect of TNF and IFNγ has been also observed. The characterization of TNF receptor(s) onto the platelet membrane is presently underway.

We have demonstrated that concanavalin A (ConA) and antigen-stimulated CD4⁻/CD8⁺ T lymphocytes released a factor able to inhibit the IgE-, IFN-, and TNF β-dependent platelet cytotoxicity toward the parasitic larvae. The production of oxygen metabolites by platelets in an IgE-anti-IgE reaction was likewise strongly inhibited by the lymphokine (Pancré et al., 1986). This platelet-activity-suppressive lymphokine (PASL) was identified as an acid- and heat-stable polypeptide of 15-20 kD with a pI of 4.6. The factor was specifically absorbed by platelet membrane suggesting its actions through the binding to receptor. The in vivo relevance of PASL could be established by a complete abolition of the protection normally conferred toward a challenge infection by the intravenous passive transfer of platelets from immune to normal rats, after PASL-treatment of transferred platelets (Pancré et al., 1989). The molecular cloning of PASl is presently underway.

Taken together, these results demonstrated that, in addition to IgE antigen-specific CD4⁺/CD8⁻ T lymphocytes could activate platelets through IFN and TNF production, while a feedback regulation of the platelet immune functions should be under the control of CD4⁻/CD8⁺-stimulated T cells through the generation of PASL.

Of possible interest is the observation that wheras IL-4 has been shown to induce $Fc_\epsilon RII$ expression on B cells, monocytes, and eosinophils, IL-4 did not increase, in our hands, IgE-dependent platelet activation. Conversely, γ-IFN, which enhances the expression of $Fc_\epsilon RII$ on platelet membrane, does not exhibit such effect on eosinophils. These differences in the activity of this interleukin on $Fc_\epsilon RII$, together with the observation mentioned above of differences in the structure of one of the subunit of IgE platelet receptor, might be an indication of some heterogeneity among IgE receptors on inflammatory cells.

IV. Platelets and Asthma

While the participation of inflammatory cells expressing the low-afinity receptor for IgE, such as mononuclear phagocytes or eosinophils, is now largely accepted, the exact role of platelets in allergic diseases, and more particularly asthma, certainly remains to be more clearly established (Joseph, 1988).

A. Signs of Platelet Activation in Asthma

Platelets isolated from patients with allergic asthma (due to house dust, mites, or grass pollens) or platelets from patients with *Hymenoptera* venom hypersensitivity reacted in vitro to specific allergens or to IgE-specific ligands (such as anti-IgE antibody) by producing cytotoxic mediators, evidenced by the death of parasite larvae (Joseph et al., 1983) or oxygen-derived free radicals, evidenced by luminol-luciferin chemiluminescence (Joseph et al., 1986). Anti-IgG and nonspecific allergens were unable to induce such effects. Due to the presence of IgE receptors on at least 20% of the thrombocytic population, platelets isolated from healthy donors could be passively sensitized with IgE antibody by preincubation in the serum of allergic patients. The addition of specific allergens or anti-IgE-induced effector functions was demonstrated by the death of *Schistosoma mansoni* and by free radical-dependent chemiluminescence. Here again, anti-IgG was inactive on such platelets, whereas the role of bound IgE in the platelet reactivity was confirmed by isotype-specific adsorption of antibody from the serum of allergic donors: only the adsorption of IgE, and not that of IgG, could abrogate the ability of allergic patient serum to induce normal platelets into cytotoxic effectors. The participation of IgE in this activation process was further corroborated by the inhibitory role of polyclonal (Spiegelberg, 1984) and monoclonal antibodies (Capron et al., 1986b) against the $Fc_\epsilon RII$ on the passive senstization and activation of normal platelets by allergic patients' sera.

If platelets have a general role in asthma, the selective functional capacities of platelets linked to their IgE receptors might be triggered through IgE-independent mechanisms in asthmatic syndromes of nonimmunological origin. In this context, aspirin-sensitive asthma appeared as a good model for investigating such a hypothesis. This was the second situation explored in the perspective of platelet involvement in asthma.

Cases of common and severe aspirin-sensitive asthma have presented, until recently, no in vitro abnormality and no involvement of any cell population or humoral factor. In fact, platelets isolated from patients with aspirin-sensitive asthma exhibited in vitro an abnormal response to aspirin-generated oxygen metabolites and cytotoxic mediators in the presence of acetylsalicylic acid or nonsteroidal anti-inflammatory drugs (NSAID) such as indomethacin or flurbiprofen (Ameisen et al., 1985). Neither blood leukocytes nor purified leukocyte populations from the same patients could be triggered into cytotoxic effectors in the presence of aspirin or NSAID. Futhermore, the involvement of IgE in this abnormal response of platelets was ruled out by several lines of evidence, including the inability of serum from patients to sensitize in vitro platelets from healthy donors, and the absence of an inhibitory effect of polyclonal or monoclonal antibodies directed against the $Fc_\epsilon RII$.

Investigation of the mechanism of this platelet response showed it to be related to the inhibitory effect of NSAID on cyclooxygenase. The abnormal response of patients' platelets to NSAID might be caused by reduced binding of endogenous PGH_2 endoperoxides to their platelet receptor, which is an indirect consequence of the NSAID-induced inhibition of cyclooxygenase that reduces PGH_2 synthesis. Although the exact nature of the specific platelet abnormality remains to be defined, endoperoxides might play a crucial regulatory role in patients' platelets, which NSAID would disturb. One possibility is that PGH_2 might be involved in the control of the synthesis and/or of the biological effect of platelet lipoxygenase products (Ameisen, 1986; Fig. 1).

Since neither leukocytes nor any other cell population has yet been shown to respond abnormally to NSAID, and since drugs that prevent the platelet response (salicylate or salicylamide) appear to prevent the clinical symptoms (Ameisen, 1985), these observations strongly support the involvement of platelets in these asthmatic attacks. Whether the mediators released by the activated platelets have the capacity to induce bronchospasm, or to trigger other cell populations to release bronchoconstrictive factors, such as PAF or leukotrienes, is currently being investigated.

Another approach has recently been developed and has led to the identification of antiplatelet antibodies in some patients with nonallergic, so-called intrinsic asthma. Such antibodies can induce in vitro platelet activation and secretion, similar to what is observed after IgE-dependent activation.

B. Changes in the Behavior of Platelets from Allergic Patients

In aspirin-induced asthma, platelets lost their property to generate cytocidal factors after induction of a refractory period induced by daily ingestion of high dosages of aspirin. In this syndrome, platelets were deactivated at the very period when patients were insensitive to the drug, and they recovered full reactivity as soon as the aspirin treatment had been discontinued and patients were sensitive again (Ameisen, 1985).

Similarly, in *Hymenoptera* venom hypersensitivity, platelets from patients undergoing specific immunotherapy by rush desensitization lost their specific reactivity to allergens in vitro, becoming unable to generate free radicals and cytotoxic mediators, in contrast with the properties they exhibited before desensitization (Tsicopoulos et al., 1988). The in vitro sensitivity of platelets exactly correlated with the sensitivity of patients to venom. Recent experiments favor the possible intervention of lymphocytes in the observed modification of platelet reactivity. Indeed, lymphocyte supernatants obtained from patients after rush desensitization were able to downregulate platelet reactivity. In similar fashion, sera obtained from desensitized patients were able to suppress IgE-dependent platelet activation. Physicochemical character-

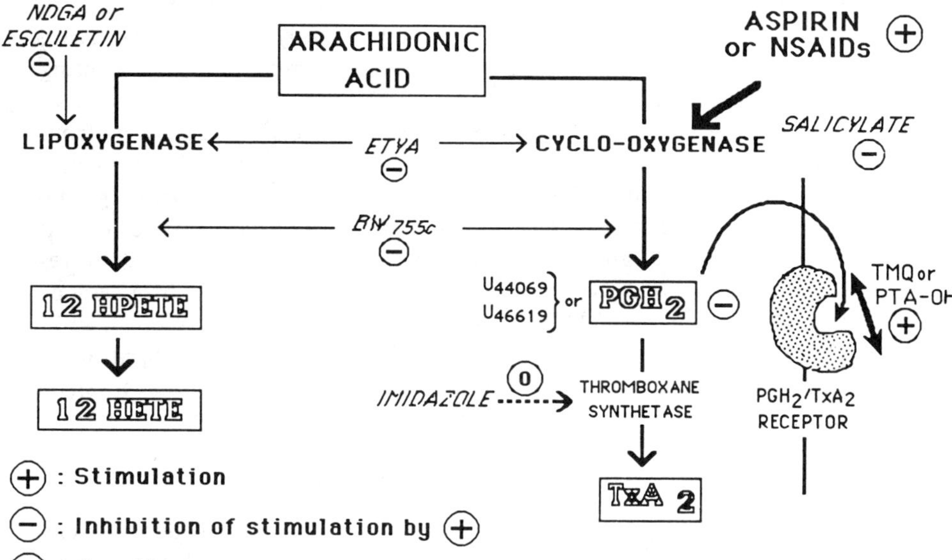

Figure 1 In vitro, platelets from patients with aspirin-induced asthma expressed antiparasite cytotoxicity and generated oxygen metabolites ⊕ in the presence of aspirin and nonsteroidal anti-inflammatory drugs (NSAIDs). The platelet anomaly seemed to be linked to a prostaglandin endoperoxide (PGH2) defect (and not to a thromboxane A2 (TxA$_2$) defect, since imidazole had no activity) induced by the cyclooxygenase (CO) inhibition by NSAIDs. In fact, the addition of PGH2 or one of its nonmetabolizable analogs (U44069 or U46619) impaired the activating effect of NSAIDs ⊖ Alternatively, the abnormal response could be associated with an impaired binding of PGH2 to its specific receptor on platelet membrane. This late hypothesis is supported by the induction of the abnormal response of aspirin-sensitive platelets by trimethoquinol (TMQ), or of a TxA$_2$ analog (PTA-OH), two antagonists of the PGH2/TxA$_2$ receptor, in the absence of NSAIDs. This TMQ or PTA-OH effect was abrogated by a preincubation with PGH2 or its stable analogs. However, the defect linked to PGH2 is not the only disorder in these platelets, since other metabolic inhibitors of CO, such as eicosatetranoic acid (ETYA), an analog of arachidonic acid, or BW755c, did not induce the abnormal response, and furthermore impaired the NSAID effect: these drugs are, simultaneously, lipoxygenase (LO) inhibitors. Nordihydroguaiaretic acid (NDGA) and esculetin, which are more specific inhibitors of LO, also impaired the abnormal response to NSAIDs. In conclusion, one metabolite of the LO pathway, yet unknown, is therefore crucial in the observed effect. Finally, sodium salicylate, by competing with aspirin at the CO level and/or by its scavenging properties, blocked the NSAID-dependent activation of platelets.

ization of the suppressive factor present in lymphocyte supernatants and in serum showed properties very similar to those previously described for PASL, indicating that this lymphocyte factor might be preferentially expressed during the course of desensitization.

Several authors have reported a reversible modification of platelets from atopic patients, which exhibit hypoaggregability (Solinger et al., 1973; Maccia et al., 1977; Rao and Walsh, 1983), associated with an increased bleeding time in patients (Szczeklik et al., 1986). The platelet turnover is also accelerated up to twice its normal value in asthmatic patients (Taytard et al., 1986), returning to control levels after treatment with an antiasthmatic drug such as ketotifen (Taytard et al., 1987).

These observations, even if not conclusive for a direct participation of platelets in asthma pathogenesis, bring evidence of their reactivity to environmental conditions.

C. Platelet Dependence of Bronchoconstriction

Beyond the events reported above, the exposure of airways to allergen challenge induces, in asthmatic patients or in sensitized rabbits and guinea pigs, bronchoconstriction as a primary effect. Platelet depletion in experimental animals suppressed the allergic respiratory syndrome (Pinckard et al., 1977). In this context, the role of PAF-acether in immediate response, although well documented (Barnes et al., 1988), is far from being fully understood. Nonetheless PAF-acether was shown to induce acute airway response after intravenous injection or intratracheal instillation (Denjean et al., 1983). Platelets seem to play a crucial role in this effect of PAF-acether. Thrombocytopenia has been associated with PAF-induced bronchoconstriction (Gateau et al., 1984). Platelet depletion, or platelet inhibition by prostacyclin, in rabbit or guinea pig, suppressed the effects induced by PAF-acether on the lungs (Vargaftig and Benveniste, 1983). In vitro PAF-acether strongly contracted surgical specimens of human bronchi, but only in the presence of platelets: neither PAF-acether nor platelets alone could induce bronchospasm (Schellenberg et al., 1983). Platelet activation mediated by PAF-acether is expressed by granule exocytosis. Compounds able to inhibit the platelet release also impaired the bronchoconstriction induced by antigen or PAF-acether (Vargaftig and Benveniste, 1983). In the rat, whose platelets have no PAF-acether receptors, the intravenous injection of this phospholipid was unable to provoke bronchoconstriction (Vargaftig and Benveniste, 1983).

V. Conclusion

In the light of the observations reported here, it appears that if the definitive demonstration of a platelet involvement in the immediate response of type I hypersensitive reactions and in their associated inflammatory effects is not acquired, the participation of these blood constituents in the cellular network leading to the physiopathological process of allergic reactions, and especially asthma, is largely documented and can be considered now as more than a hypothesis (Table 1). The suggestion that platelets could be generated mainly in the lung vasculature (Trowbridge et al., 1982) may strengthen the implication of thrombocytes in asthmatic pathological changes, and opens new possibilities of their involvement in various allergic and inflammatory disorders. Furthermore, as far as the cellular network is concerned, it should be unrealistic to stress only platelets as responsible for such pathological changes. Their reactivity must be reconsidered in the general concept of intercellular communications, with the recruitment of a large variety of active cell populations, especially eosinophils, perhaps endothelial cells, and, possibly, cells from the peripheral nervous system. In the context of eosinophils' participation in bronchial hyperreactivity and tissue damage, it has been reported that platelet depletion reduced PAF-acether- and allergen-mediated eosinophil infiltration into the lungs of normal and allergic animals, respectively (Lellouch-Tubiana et al., 1988). Such observations also add focus to

Table 1 Arguments Favoring Platelet Involvement in Allergy

In vitro
Allergen-induced IgE-dependent release of cytotoxic mediators from platelets
Abnormal selective response of platelets in aspirin-sensitive asthmatic patients (ASA)

In vivo
PF4 and β-TG in plasma and bronchoalveolar lavage of asthmatic patients
Pulmonary platelet aggregates after allergen challenge in asthmatic patients
Platelets in bronchoalveolar lavage of asthmatic patients

Platelet physiology
Reversible hypoaggregability and increased bleeding time in allergic patients
Accelerated turnover of blood platelets in asthmatic patients
Decrease of IgE-dependent stimulation after rush desensitization
Inhibition of aspirin-induced stimulation during refractory period of ASA

Bronchoconstriction
Allergen- or PAF-induced bronchoconstriction suppressed after platelet depletion or inhibition
No PAF-induced bronchoconstriction in the rat, platelets of which have no PAF receptors

Cell recruitment
Platelet-dependence of late-phase eosinophil infiltration into the lung

new therapeutic approaches to the control of allergic diseases and associated inflammatory disorders.

Discussion

Sertl: Did I understand right that substance P and IgE compete for the same receptor?

Capron: Experiments performed in our laboratory by M. Damonneville have established that IgE molecules significantly inhibit platelet activation induced by substance P. Experiments now in progress favor the existence of a specific and saturable binding site for substance P on the platelet membrane. IgE receptors ($Fc_\epsilon RII$) on platelets share a common sequence with a major membrane glycoprotein $GPIIb_\epsilon IIIa$. Antibodies to this GP, in particular the AP_2 monoclonal antibody, inhibit IgE-dependent platelet activation. This same antibody AP_2 inhibits SP-dependent platelet activation.

Kay: Does the IgE that binds to $Fc_\epsilon RII$ on platelets (or other cells) recognize the same major allergens as the IgE that binds to $Fc_\epsilon RI$? Also, on some cells there may be cooperation between cytophilic IgG and IgE in terms of certain components of a complex allergen mixture.

Capron: The question of a selective or even restricted isotype antibody response against defined epitopes is certainly a central issue. Extending from our previous experience with cloned proteins of various parasites, we have undertaken similar studies on allergens that have recently been cloned. The picture we have is that platelet activation by antibodies from allergic patients and, subsequently, specific antigen is clearly IgE restricted and IgG antibodies apparently have no role in the activation process.

Platts-Mills: Could you clarify the experiment in which platelet activation by venom protein is decreased following rush desensitization?

Capron: The main message is that in *Hymenoptera* venom sensitization, patients' platelets can be directly activated by the allergen. In contrast, the platelets of the same patients undergoing specific immunotherapy by rush desensitization lost their specific reactivity to allergens in vitro even at very high concentrations.

Church: Michel Joseph from your lab has reported that nedocromil sodium but not cromolyn sodium prevents aspirin-induced activation of platelets from aspirin-sensitive patients. Do you know why these drugs differ in their effects and what other drugs have this effect?

Capron: Michel Joseph has shown that cetirizine was also shown to inhibit platelet activation by IgE-dependent stimuli (Joseph, et al. (1989). *Int. Arch. Allergy Appl. Immunol.* in press).

Acknowledgments

This work was supported by the Unité Mixte INSERM U167-CNRS 624.

References

Ameisen, J. C. (1986). Aspirin sensitive asthma: a model for a role of platelets in hypersensitivity reactions. *Ann. Inst. Pasteur/Immunol.* **137D**:141-147.

Ameisen, J. C., Capron, A., Joseph, M., Maclouf, J., Vorng, H., Pancré, V., Fournier, E., Wallaert, B., and Tonnel, A. B. (1985). Aspirin-sensitive asthma: abnormal platelet response to drugs inducing asthmatic attacks. *Int. Arch. Allergy Appl. Immunol.* **78**:438-448.

Ameisen, J. C., Joseph, M., Caen, J. P., Kusnierz, J. P., Capson, M., Boizard, B., Wautier, J. L., Levy-Toledano, S., Vorng, H., and Capron, A. (1986). A role for glycoprotein IIb-IIIa complex in the binding of IgE to human platelets and platelet IgE-dependent cytotoxic functions. *Br. J. Haematol.* **64**:21-32.

Barnes, P. J., Chung, K. F., and Page, C. P. (1988). Platelet-activating factor as a mediator of allergic disease. *J. Allergy Clin. Immunol.* **81**:919-934.

Bout, D., Joseph, M., Pontet, M., Vorng, H., Deslée, D., and Capron, A. (1986). Rat resistance to schistosomiasis: platelet-mediated cytotoxicity induced by C-reactive protein. *Science* **231**:153-156.

Capron, A., Dessaint, J. P., Capron, M., Joseph, M., Ameisen, J. C., and Tonnel, A. B. (1986a). From parasites to allergy: a second receptor for IgE. *Immunol. Today*, **7**:15-18.

Capron, A., Joseph, M., Ameisen, J. C., Capron, M., Pancré, V., and Auriault, C. (1987). Platelets as effectors in immune and hypersensitivity reactions. *Int. Arch. Allergy Appl. Immunol.* **82**:307-312.

Capron, M., Jouault, T., Prin, L, Joseph, M., Ameisen, J. C., Butterworth, A. E., Papin, J. P., Kusnierz, J. P., and Capron, A. (1986b). Functional study of a monoclonal antibody to IgE Fc receptor (Fc_ER_2) of eosinophils, platelets, and macrophages. *J. Exp. Med.* **164**:72-89.

Cesbron, J. Y., Capron, A., Vargaftig, B. B., Lagarde, M., Pincemail, J., Braquet, P., Taelman, H., and Joseph, M. (1987). Platelets mediate the action of diethylcarbamazine on microfilariae. *Nature* **325**:533-536.

Cines, D. B., van der Keyl, H., and Levinson, A. I. (1986). In vitro binding of an IgE protein to human platelets. *J. Immunol.* **136**:3433-3440.

Damonneville, M., Joseph, M., Auriault, C., Gras-Masse, H., Tartar, A., Joseph, M., and Capron, A. (1988a). The neuropeptide substance P stimulates the effector functions of platelets. Ninth European Immunology Meeting, Roma, September 14-17, 1988.

Damonneville, M., Wietzerbin, J., Pancré, V., Joseph, M., Capron, A., and Auriault, C. (1988b). Recombinant tumor necrosis factors mediate platelet cytotoxicity to *Schistosoma mansoni* larvae. *J. Immunol.* **140**: 3962-3965.

Denjean, A., Arnoux, B., Masse, R., Lockart, A., and Benveniste, J. (1983). Acute effects of intratracheal administration of platelet-activating factor in baboons. *J. Appl. Physiol.* **55**:799-804.

Durham, S. R., Dawes, J., and Kay, A. B. (1985). Platelets in asthma. *Lancet* **2**:36.

Gateau, O., Arnoux, B., Deriaz, H., Viars, P., and Benveniste, J. (1984). Acute effects of intratracheal administration of PAF-acether in humans. *Am. Rev. Respir. Dis.* **129**:3A.

Greer, I. A., Winter, J. H., Gaffney, D., McLoughlin, K., Belch, J. J. F., Boyd, G., and Forbes, C. D. (1984). Platelets in asthma. *Lancet* **2**:1479.

Gresele, P., Todisco, T., Merante, F., and Nenci, G. G. (1982). Platelet activation and allergic asthma. *N. Engl. J. Med.* **306**:549.

Joseph, M. (1988). Platelets in allergy: assays and interpretation. *Clin. Rev. Allergy* **6**:191-210.

Joseph, M., Auriault, C., Capron, A., Vorng, H., and Viens, P. (1983). A new function for platelets: IgE-dependent killing of schistosomes. *Nature* **303**:810-812.

Joseph, M., Capron, A., Ameisen, J. C., Capron, M., Vorng, H., Pancré, V., Kusnierz, J. P., and Auriault, C. (1986). The receptor for IgE on blood platelets. *Eur. J. Immunol.* **16**:306-312.

Knauer, K. A., Lichtenstein, L. M., Adkinson, N. F., and Fish, J. E. (1981). Platelet activation during antigen-induced airway reactions in asthmatic subjects. *N. Engl. J. Med.* **304**:1404.

Lellouch-Tubiana, A., Lefort, J., Simon, M. T., Pfister, A., and Vargaftig, B. B. (1988). Eosinophil recruitment into guinea pig lungs after PAF-acether and allergen administration. Modulation by prostacyclin, platelet depletion, and selective antagonists. *Am. Rev. Respir. Dis.* **137**:948-954.

Maccia, C. A., Gallagher, J. S., Ataman, G., Glück, H. I., Brooks, S. M., and Bernstein, I. L. (1977). Platelet thrombopathy in asthmatic patients with elevated immunoglobulin E. *J. Allergy Clin. Immunol.* **59**:101-108.

Metzger, W. J., Hunninghake, G. W., and Richerson, H. B. (1985). Late asthmatic response: inquiry into mechanisms and significance. *Clin. Rev. Allergy* **3**:145-165.

Molinas, F. C., Wietzerbin, J., and Falcoff, E. (1987). Human platelets possess receptors for a lymphokine: demonstration of high specific receptors for Hu IFN. *J. Immunol.* **138**:802-806.

Pancré, V., Auriault, C., Joseph, M., Cesbron, J. Y., Kusnierz, J. P., and Capron, A. (1986). A suppressive lymphokine of platelet cytotoxic functions. *J. Immunol.* **137**:585-591.

Pancré, V., Joseph, M., Mazingue, C., Wietzerbin, J., Capron, A., and Auriault, C. (1987). Induction of platelet cytotoxic functions by lymphokine: role of gamma interferon. *J. Immunol.* **138**:4490-4495.

Pancré, V., Joseph, M., Capron, A., Wietzerbin, J., Kusnierz, J. P., Vorng, H., and Auriault, C. (1988). Recombinant human immune interferon induces increased IgE receptor expression on human platelets. *Eur. J. Immunol.* **18**:829-832.

Pancré, V., Joseph, M., Capron, A., Delanoye, A., Vorng, H., and Auriault, C. (1989). Characterization of a suppressive factor of platelet cytotoxic functions in human and rat *Schistosomiasis mansoni. Clin. Exp. Immunol.* **76**:417-421.

Pinckard, R. N., Halonen, M., Palmer, J. D., Butler, C., Shaw, J. O., and Henson, P. M. (1977). Intravascular aggregation and pulmonary sequestration of platelets during IgE-induced systemic anaphylaxis in the rabbit: abrogation of lethal anaphylactic shock by platelet depletion. *J. Immunol.* **119**:2185-2193.

Rao, A. K., and Walsh, P. N. (1983). Acquired qualitative platelet disorders. *Clin. Haematol.* **12**:201-238.

Schellenberg, R. R., Walker, B., and Snyder, F. (1983). Platelet-dependent contraction of human bronchi by platelet-activating factor. *J. Allergy Clin. Immunol.* **71**:145.

Solinger, A., Bernstein, J. S., Ataman, G., and Glück, H. I. (1973). The effect of epinephrine on platelet aggregation in normal and atopic subjects. *J. Allergy Clin. Immunol.* **51**:29-34.

Spiegelberg, H. L. (1984). Structure and function of Fc receptors for IgE on lymphocytes, monocytes and macrophages. *Adv. Immunol.* **35**:61-88.

Szczeklik, A., Milner, P. C., Birch, J., Watkins, J., and Martin, J. P. (1986). Prolonged bleeding time, reduced platelet aggregation, altered PAF-acether sensitivity, and increased platelet mass are a trait of asthma and hay fever. *Thromb. Haemost.* **56**:183-187.

Taytard, A., Guenard, H., Vuillemin, L., Bourot, J. L., Vergeret, J., Ducassou, D.,Piquet, Y., and Freour, P. (1986). Platelet kinetics in stable asthmatic subjects. *Am. Rev. Respir. Dis.* **134**:983-985.

Taytard, A., Vuillemin, L., Guenard, H., Rio, P., Vergeret, J., and Ducassou, D. (1987). Platelet kinetic in stable asthmatic patients: effect of ketotifen. *Am. Rev. Respir. Dis.* **135**:388A.

Trowbridge, E. A., Martin, J. F., and Slater, D. N. (1982). Evidence for a theory of physical fragmentation of megakaryocytes, implying that all platelets are produced in the pulmonary circulation. *Thromb. Res.* **28**:461-475.

Tsicopoulos, A., Tonnel, A. B., Wallaert, B., Joseph, M., Ameisen, J. C., Ramon, P. H., Dessaint, J. P., and Capron, A. (1988). Decrease of IgE-dependent platelet activation in *Hymenoptera* hypersensitivity after specific rush desensitization. *Clin. Exp. Immunol.* **71**:433-438.

Vargaftig, B. B., and Benveniste, J. (1983). Platelet-activating factor today. *Trends Pharmacol. Sci.* **4**:341-343.

A. BARRY KAY, C. J. CORRIGAN, and A. J. FREW

National Heart and Lung Institute
London, England

9

T Lymphocytes and Asthma

I. Introduction

An area of considerable current interest is the role of the T lymphocyte in the regulation and expression of the inflammation associated with allergy and asthma. The T-cell-derived lymphokines, interleukin (IL)-4, IL-5, and interferon (IFN)-gamma are intimately involved in the regulation of IgE production (Leung and Geha, 1987). Some lymphokines are active in the control of eosinophil production by the bone marrow (IL-5, granulocyte/ macrophage colony-stimulating factor [GM-CSF], IL-3) and in the regulation of mast cell differentiation. Others have chemotactic activity for neutrophils, eosinophils, and basophil granulocytes as well as monocytes and can activate or degranulate these effector cells. T lymphocytes also play a general role in the regulation of specific immune responses and might be one of the principal target cells for allergen injection immunotherapy.

Direct evidence for T-lymphocyte changes in asthma and allergy come from a variety of sources. Postmortem examination of the airways of asthmatic patients revealed large numbers of lymphocytes (Dunnill, 1960; Dunnill et al., 1969). Increased numbers of "atypical intraepithelial lymphocytes" have been found in an ultrastructural study of bronchial biopsies taken during life from subjects with mild asthma (Jeffery et al., 1987, 1989). These lymphocytes are probably activated T cells, but formal proof of this is not yet available. Increased natural killer (NK) activity has been described in the peripheral blood of asthmatic patients (Timonen and Stenius-Aarnala, 1985). NK activity is an inducible property of T cells and of non-T, non-B, lymphocytes and is thus a nonspecific indicator of lymphocyte activation. In recent years considerable progress has been made toward understanding the biology of the inflammation characteristic of asthma (particularly atopic allergic asthma). A picture is now emerging of a complex and ordered sequence of events, initiated by the recognition of allergen by IgE, and possibly also by T cells, leading to the selective recruitment of inflammatory effector cells. These processes seem to be regulated at several points by the coordinated release of intercellular mediators.

Of all the cells involved in the atopic allergic response, and indeed in any immune reaction, only the T and B lymphocytes are inherently antigen-specific. The actions of mast cells, neutrophils, eosinophils, and mononuclear phagocytes are only specific in so far as their activities are focused by interactions between surface receptors and specific immunoglobulin or complement molecules bound to target surfaces. In addition, their activation and efficiency appear to be regulated, at least in part, by soluble products released from T lymphocytes and other cells.

II. Atopic Allergic Asthma: The Need for a Model

Although useful information can be obtained from biopsies of affected sites in patients with chronic allergic asthma and rhinitis, most of our knowledge of the pathophysiology of allergic tissue responses comes from experimental models in which allergen is administered to the skin, nose, or lungs of sensitized individuals. The histopathological appearance of allergic inflammation in humans has been studied most often in the skin. In addition, a few key studies have used bronchial biopsy and lavage findings to supply corroborative evidence to support the extrapolation of skin study findings to the airways. However, allergen inhalation has mainly been used to obtain physiological and pharmacological data in patients with allergic asthma and rhinitis.

The introduction of allergen extracts into the skin of atopic subjects provokes an immediate reaction with itching, edema (wheal), and erythema (flare). This is accompanied histologically by mast cell degranulation, retraction of endothelial cell processes, and interstitial edema (Ting et al., 1980). Subsequently, some but not all subjects will experience a "late-phase reaction" (LPR) characterized macroscopically by edema and erythema; in addition, itching may occasionally be present. Biopsies from LPRs show cellular infiltration: initially neutrophils and eosinophils but by 24 h mononuclear cells, particularly lymphocytes, predominate.

Analogous immediate and LPR occur in the lungs (as airways obstruction), nose (as blockage and itching), and conjunctiva (as edema and itching) after exposure to relevant allergens. Pharmacologically and physiologically these LPRs resemble more closely the clinical disorders of allergic asthma, rhinitis, and conjunctivitis than do immediate responses to allergen. Thus antihistamine drugs, which are partially effective in preventing the immediate response to allergen exposure, are of limited use in treating clinical asthma. On the other hand, glucocorticoids are extremely effective in the treatment of asthma and ablate the LPR without affecting the immediate allergic response when given as single dose before allergen challenge.

The precise mode of action of corticosteroids in these situations remains unclear. Corticosteroids have a number of properties that might account, at least in part, for their anti-inflammatory effects and might be relevant to their efficacy in asthma. The more important of these can be summarized as follows: (1) inhibition of lymphocyte proliferation and lymphokine release, (2) inhibition of macrophage activation and mediator release, (3) inhibition of eosinophil colony formation (Butterfield et al., 1986) and eosinophil chemotaxis, (4) inhibition of human basophil (but not mast cell) mediator release (Lichtenstein and MacGlashan, 1986), (5) decrease in the number of mast cells (Otsuka et al., 1986) and eosinophils (Lichtenstein and MacGlashan, 1986) in the nasal mucosa after prolonged treatment, and (6) decreased bronchial hyperreactivity after prolonged treatment with inhaled corticosteroids (Kerrebijn et al., 1987).

In a recent immunohistological study of the human cutaneous LPR, monoclonal antibodies and immunocytochemistry were used to assess the cellular component of these reactions and to obtain evidence of eosinophil and T-lymphocyte activation (Frew and Kay, 1988).

Numerous eosinophils were present at allergen-challenged sites and persisted in the tissues for up to 48 h. The majority were activated as demonstrated by staining with the monoclonal antibody EG2 (Tai et al., 1984), which recognizes an epitope on the secreted form of the eosinophil cationic protein.

Increased numbers of T lymphocytes were also seen in and around small blood vessels at the site of cutaneous LPRs; this T-lymphocyte infiltrate persisted for at least 48 h. The majority of the infiltrating T lymphocytes were CD4 + (helper/inducer subset) and the infiltration appeared to be specific in that the CD4 + /CD8 + ratio of cells in the skin was substantially increased compared with peripheral blood. A small number of cells expressed the IL-2 receptor, providing evidence of T-cell activation. Supporting this observation, there was increased expression of HLA-DR by endothelial cells and of CD4 antigen by epidermal Langerhans cells. Both phenomena provide indirect evidence of interferon-gamma secretion from activated T cells (Miossec and Ziff, 1986; Walsh et al., 1987). There was no clear association between the numbers of infiltrating T cells and the size of the LPR, but there was a striking association of CD4+ T cell numbers with the number of activated eosinophils at 24 h and, to a lesser extent, 48 h (Frew and Kay, 1988).

III. Late Asthmatic Reactions

Allergic reactions are clearly important in episodes of acute extrinsic asthma, such as occur when sensitive individuals are exposed acutely to animals or grass pollen. It has also been proposed, although less widely accepted, that recurrent exposure to allergens may be important in the development and maintenance of airways inflammation in chronic asthma (Cockcroft, 1983). Various aspects of this hypothesis have been studied in the experimentally induced asthmatic reactions provoked by inhalation of relevant allergens. Late asthmatic reactions (LAR) are conventionally defined as 20% fall in forced expiratory volume in 1s (FEV_1) (or 50% fall in sGAW) 3-12 h after a standardized allergen inhalation challenge that evoked an early asthmatic response equivalent to a 20% fall in FEV_1. When this operational "definition" is used, LAR occurs in about 50% of atopic asthmatic subjects (Booij-Nord et al., 1971).

Several groups have used bronchoalveolar lavage (BAL) to study cellular infiltration in the human LAR. In a study of the LAR, Diaz et al. (1989) found no difference in total BAL cell counts in subjects with dual asthmatic responses (DAR) compared with single early responders (SER) after allergen inhalation. However, BAL eosinophils, lymphocytes, and neutrophils were increased in the DAR group. The majority of subjects in both the SER and DAR groups had elevated BAL concentrations of eosinophil basic proteins, which confirmed that eosinophil activation is a feature of the LAR.

Alterations in bronchoalveolar T-lymphocyte subsets after allergen challenge were found that support the concept that T cells are involved in the expression of the allergen-induced late-phase asthmatic reaction in humans. For instance, relative increases in CD8+ cells were found in bronchoalveolar lavage in SER, as compared with DAR (Gonzalez et al., 1987). In another study segmental bronchial allergen challenge was performed via the fiberoptic bronchoscope and a selective increase in CD4+ cells in lavage fluid was observed 48 hours after challenge in subjects who had previously been shown to experience DARs (Metzger et al., 1987). These findings are consistent with the decrease in CD4+ cells in the peripheral blood been reported after allergen inhalation (Gerblich et al., 1984). Taken together, these observations suggest that a process of selective recruitment and retention of CD4+ T lymphocytes is occurring in the lungs during the late asthmatic reaction.

We have studied allergen-induced accumulation of T cells in the bronchi, using a guinea pig model of the late asthmatic reaction (Frew et al., 1989). Following allergen inhalation, an elevation in T-lymphocyte numbers in the bronchial mucosa and adventitia was detected. The kinetics of this T-cell accumulation paralleled the changes in airways resistance. The numbers of T cells and eosinophils were significantly correlated preceding the peak of the late phase of the bronchoconstriction. Subset analysis showed that the majority of the infiltrating T cells were CD3+, CD8− (i.e., putative T-helper cells). In contrast to the striking changes observed in the tissues, analysis of BAL and blood T cell subsets did not show any significant changes in this model.

It is clearly of considerable importance to determine the mechanisms through which inflammatory cells are attracted and the extent to which cellular interactions modulate their activity after their arrival at the inflammatory site. A host of stimuli have been shown to activate eosinophils in vitro but to date it is less clear which of these actually operate in vivo. In vitro, the lipid mediators leukotriene (LT) B_4 and platelet-activating factor (PAF), the complement fragments C5a and C3a, the bacterial analog f-Met-Leu-Phe, opsonized zymosan, and calcium ionophore all result in impressive enhancement of eosinophil function (Gleich and Adolphson, 1986). Each of these stimuli is also an effective activator of neutrophil function and thus none can account for the apparently selective accumulation and activation of eosinophils seen in allergic inflammation. One of the few mediators that selectively activates eosinophil function is the T-cell product interleukin-5, which can enhance antibody-dependent cytotoxic capacity, superoxide generation, degranulation (Lopez et al., 1988), and adherence (Walsh et al., 1989). Interleukin-5 has also been reported to be weakly chemotactic for eosinophils, although this effect was weak and has not yet been confirmed (Yamaguchi et al., 1988; Kurihara et al., 1988).

In the absence of a clearly selective attractant for eosinophils, attention has turned to factors regulating the persistence of eosinophils at inflammatory sites. In vitro, eosinophils survive in culture for only a few days, but their survival can be prolonged by the addition of IL-3, IL-5, or GM-CSF, and especially if fibroblasts or endothelial cells are also present (Owen et al., 1987; Rothenburg et al., 1988). Such a mechanism might account for the persistence of activated eosinophils at late-phase skin reaction sites, and for the association of eosinophil persistence with the intensity of T-lymphocyte accumulation.

IV. T Lymphocytes as Effector Cells in Atopic Allergic Asthma

Until recently it was generally considered that the main role of T lympho-cytes in IgE-dependent hypersensitivity was the induction and regulation of IgE production by B lymphocytes. The intensive application of monoclonal antibodies and recombinant DNA technology has led to a reappraisal of the breadth of T lymphocyte function. It is clear that T cells are capable of operat-ing as proinflammatory cells in their own right, as well as orchestrating B-cell proliferation and differentiation. In addition, T lymphocytes have a clearly defined role in recruiting and activating other effector cells (Miyajima et al., 1988). Coordination of these various effector functions is achieved by the secretion of lymphokines by T cells in response to stimulation with specific antigen.

The cytokines interleukin-4 and interferon-gamma have important roles in the regulation of IgE production (Teale and Abraham, 1987), while IL-5 is also implicated in the mouse, but thus far apparently not in humans (Sander-son et al., 1988). These cytokines are also active on macrophages, eosino-phils, and endothelial cells and allergen-specific T lymphocytes attracted after allergen challenge will presumably release these various cytokines at the site of allergic inflammation. Thus there are a number of important and fundamental questions about the functional properties of T cells that recog-nize allergens.

It is of particular importance to determine the amount and proportions of cytokines secreted by T cells that recognize allergenic determinants. In the mouse it has been possible to classify CD4 + T lymphocytes into two distinct subsets on the basis of their profile of lymphokine production. Both subsets secrete IL-3 and GM-CSF; one subset of T lymphocytes (Th1 cells) produces IL-2 and IFN-gamma and mediates delayed-type hypersensitivity reactions. The other subset (Th2 cells) secretes IL-4 and IL-5 but not IL-2 or IFN-gamma, and supports IgE production (Mossmann et al., 1986).

It seems that atopic human subjects have an increased proportion of circulating T lymphocytes that elaborate IL-4 after activation (Maggi et al., 1988). This is consistent with their tendency to produce increased amounts of IgE, but it remains uncertain whether this increase in the numbers of IL-4-producing cells is confined to allergen-specific cells or whether IL-4-pro-ducing cells can recognize nonallergenic epitopes.

The functional repertoire of a limited number of allergen-specific human T-lymphocyte clones has been studied in detail. It has been shown that indi-vidual T-cell clones can provide support for IgE production that is at least partially mediated via interleukin-4 (O'Hehir et al., 1988). These same cells also elaborate substantial quantities of proinflammatory lymphokines, including lymphokines which attract and activate neutrophils (Tsai et al., 1988; Maestrelli et al., 1988).

The relative absence of monocyte infiltration in the human cutaneous LPR is also consistent with the hypothesis that a different subset of T lymphocytes is attracted in this model, compared with other forms of cell-mediated hypersensitivity.

V. Novel Lymphokines

The majority of the lymphokines that have thus far been characterized were first described in terms of their activity in T- or B-cell growth and differentiation assays. The two exceptions are tumor necrosis factor (TNF) and IFN-gamma, whose effects were initially thought to be specific for macrophages. As time has progressed, it has become clear that each lymphokine can have several different effects and that, broadly speaking, several lymphokines are active in any given assay system. Given the provenance of the currently available lymphokines, it is not really surprising that none of them is particularly active in the chemotaxis and activation of granulocytes. By focusing on the ability of T-cell products to modulate granulocyte function, two novel lymphokines have recently been characterized. One of these is a 12-15 kD protein that is chemotactic for neutrophils (Maestrelli et al., 1988). The other is a 35 kD protein that activates neutrophils and enhances neutrophil production of the lipid mediator LTB_4 (Tsai et al., 1988). Both these factors are released by lymphocytes specifically stimulated with antigen or nonspecifically with the lectin phytohemagglutinin or anti-CD3 monoclonal antibodies and are distinct from the lymphokines IL-1, IL-2, IL-3, IL-5, GM-CSF, and TNF.

Although both these lymphokines have greater effects on neutrophils than eosinophils, they illustrate the importance of using appropriate assay systems to study lymphokine effects on inflammatory cells. It seems likely that other cytokines will be described in the future whose primary effects are on granulocytes.

VI. T Cells and Acute Severe Asthma

Further evidence to support the view that T cells are involved in the pathogenesis of chronic asthma comes from studies of acute severe asthma (status asthmaticus). Corrigan et al. (1988) were able to demonstrate significant elevations of the expression of three surface proteins associated with T lymphocyte activation (interleukin-2 receptor [IL-2R], class II histocompatibility antigen [HLA-DR], and "very late activation" antigen [VLA-1] in patients with acute severe asthma compared with control subjects (those with mild asthma, chronic obstructive airways disease, and normal individuals). Phenotypic analysis of the IL-2R-positive T lymphocytes showed that these cells were exclusively of the CD4 "helper-inducer" phenotype. The percentages of IL-2R and HLA-DR-positive (but not VLA-1-positive) lymphocytes tended to decrease as the patients were treated and their condition improved clinically. In addition, the serum concentrations of interferon-gamma and soluble IL-2R were significantly elevated in patients with acute severe asthma compared with all the control groups (Corrigan and Kay, 1990). Concentrations decreased as the patients improved clinically during first 7 day period of hospital treatment. A significant correlation was observed between the degree of airways obstruction as measured by the peak expiratory flow rate and (1) the percentages of peripheral blood T lymphocytes expressing IL-2R and (2) the serum concentrations of soluble IL-2R.

Serum neutrophil chemotactic activity (NCA) was measured in patients with acute severe asthma and compared with than in control subjects (mild asthma, stable chronic irreversible airflow obstruction, allergic rhinitis, noninfective lung conditions, or asymptomatic) (Buchanan et al., 1987a,b). There were nine subjects in each group. Statistically significant elevations (p <0.002) in NCA were detected in patients with acute severe asthma compared with each control group. Serial measurements of NCA were subsequently undertaken in 12 patients with acute asthma, at the time of admission to hospital, after 3 days of treatment, and on discharge after approximately 7 days. A highly significant (p <0.001) reduction in serum NCA activity on day 7 compared with that on day 0 was observed, and this correlated inversely with the improvement in lung function (PEFR). Gel filtration by fast protein liquid chromatography (FPLC) using Superose 6 prep grade (6PG? indicated that NCA in patients with acute severe asthma was heterogeneous and consisted of at least four peaks of activity associated with proteins with molecular weights of approximately 800, 600, 150, and <20kD. The 800 and 150 kD peaks were also observed in control subjects, but to a lesser degree. The 600 and <20 kD activities were virtually confined to the patients with acute severe asthma. FPLC chromatofocusing of the 600 MW peak from the acute asthmatics, using a Mono-P column and a pH gradient from 8.3 to 5.0, revealed considerable activity in fractions eluting between pH 6.0 and 7.0, which was not observed in the normal control subjects. A second peak, associated with pI of >7.0, was observed in patients with acute asthma, mild asthma, and in normal subjects.

These observations indicate that (1) the asthma-associated high-molecular-weight neutrophil chemotactic activity (HMW-NCA) is present in serum in the acute form of the natural disease; (2) this activity significantly decreases with treatment; (3) HMW-NCA of severe asthma (and some control groups) is heterogeneous; and (4) the peak of chemotactic activity is associated with a molecular size of 600 kD and an isoelectric point between pH 6.0 and 7.0, and is therefore comparable in these respects with the activity previously described in association with allergen-and exercise-induced early- and late-phase asthmatic reactions.

We then investigated whether mononuclear cells (MNC) isolated from patients with acute severe asthma (ASA) generate NCA spontaneously in culture. Peripheral blood MNC (PBMNC) and serum were isolated from 14 patients on admission to hospital as an emergency with ASA, and in some cases 7 days later. PBMNC and serum were similarly isolated from control subjects (normals, those with mild asthma or chronic obstructive airways disease). PBMNC (2×10^6 cells/ml) were cultured for 24-72 h (37 °C, 5% CO_2) in RPMI 1640 medium buffered with 25 mM HEPES but in the absence of serum. Culture supernatants (SN) were assayed undiluted for NCA using a modified Boyden chamber technique. PBMNC from ASA patients elaborated significantly greater amounts of NCA into the culture SN after 24 h compared with all control groups (p <0.01). There was no further increase in SN NCA after 48 and 72 h. In all ASA patients a reduction was observed in the amount of this PBMNC-derived NCA after 1 week of therapy (p <0.001). SN from ASA and normal controls were pooled, concentrated by freeze drying, and subjected to 12 size fractionation and Mono P chromatofocusing using FPLC. A peak of NCA corresponding to a molecular size of 16-25 kD and a pI of 6.8 was detectable in the concentrated ASA SN but completely absent from the control SN. An activity with similar physicochemical characteristics was detectable in the serum of patients with ASA but not that of normal controls. This MNC-derived NCA may play a role in the genesis of asthmatic bronchial inflammation, and its presence is consistent with the hypothesis that lymphocyte activation is a feature of ASA.

VII. Asthma, T Cells, and Corticosteroids

Glucocorticoids, which are the mainstay for treatment of both day-to-day chronic asthma and acute severe asthma, have profound inhibitory effects on T-lymphocyte function. As well as inhibiting IL-2 elaboration (Bloemena et al., 1988), they can also inhibit the expression of low-affinity interleukin-2 receptors and rapidly reverse induced interleukin-2 receptor expression on cultured T lymphocytes in vitro (Horst and Flad, 1987). Methylxanthines exhibit a similar action (Mary et al., 1987). These observations further suggest that the T lymphocyte may be a primary target for such conventional antiasthma drugs. In a study by Poznansky et al. (1984), peripheral blood mononuclear cells from asthmatic patients were cultured in soft agar in the presence of phytohemagglutinin (PHA) and with and without methylprednisolone. Colony growth from patients whose asthma had responded satisfactorily to glucocorticoid medication was inhibited by methylprednisolone in vitro at concentrations as low as 10^{-9} M. In contrast, patients shown to be resistant to the therapeutic effects of glucocorticoids yielded colonies that differed little in number, size, or constituent phenotype when untreated or exposed to methylprednisolone at concentrations as high as 10^{-8} M. Higher concentrations of glucocorticoid inhibited colony growth from both types of patients. These observations led to the suggestion that in glucocorticoid-resistant asthma there might be a defect in the responsiveness of mononuclear cells to these drugs. The fact that colony formation was driven by PHA, a specific T-lymphocyte mitogen, suggests that these cells were the primary target for inhibition by methylprednisolone in this experiment, although an additional effect of this drug on the monocytic component of the colonies cannot be excluded.

Most asthmatic patients respond both symptomatically and objectively to regular inhaled glucocorticoids, a method that is both well tolerated and remarkably free of side effects. We have argued that the efficacy of glucocorticoids in treating asthma may be ascribable, at least in part, to their inhibitory effects on T-lymphocyte proliferation. Significant therapeutic problems arise, however, with those patients, with whom every chest physician is familiar, whose asthma is relatively (or even totally) refractory to treatment with inhaled or systemic glucocorticoids, even when given in very high dosages (Carmichael et al., 1981). By the same argument, this may be attributable to a relative refractoriness of the response of these patients' T lymphocytes to glucocorticoids (see above). There is no doubt that these patients are asthmatic since a pronounced reduction in airflow obstruction occurs after they inhale a bronchodilator aerosol. Nevertheless, because their asthma is resistant to glucocorticoids (and in many cases to other drugs including oral methylxanthines), their chronic symptoms can seldom be adequately controlled. The asthma in such patients is usually severe and they are seriously disabled for long periods; at any time they may develop acute exacerbations that require urgent hospitalization. Despite the lack of evidence that their disease is ameliorated by glucocorticoid therapy, they are often maintained on high oral dosages of these drugs, leading to the development of severe side effects. Although such patients are relatively few, they account for a high proportion of the total number of patients seen at most respiratory outpatient clinics.

VIII. Immunosuppressive Drugs and Asthma

How can patients with refractory, corticosteroid-resistant asthma be helped? In view of the hypothesis expounded in this chapter that activated T lymphocytes are important in the pathogenesis of asthma and form a primary target for glucocorticoid therapy, the question arises whether other "anti-inflammatory" or "immunosuppressive" drugs may be effective antiasthma drugs, particularly in those patients whose disease is relatively refractory to glucocorticoids.

A. Azathioprine, Methotrexate and Gold Salts

Previous attempts to treat asthma with immunosuppressive agents such as the purine antagonist azathioprine have been largely unsuccessful (Hodges et al., 1971; Asmundsson et al., 1971). Purine antagonists have relatively little effect on delayed-type hypersensitivity reactions in humans or on T lymphocyte proliferative responses in vitro. Their main mode of action seems to be directed at NK activity and antibody production (Rees and Lockwood, 1986). More success has been claimed with the antifolate drug methotrexate, which, in a double-blind crossover study in patients with chronic asthma, allowed a significant reduction in the use of oral glucocorticoids without deterioration in lung function (Mullarkey et al., 1988). Methotrexate does not, however, have a precise mode of action in the sense that it blocks DNA synthesis and so has an effect on all dividing cells. Experience with methotrexate therapy in other diseases, such as psoriasis (Roenigk et al., 1988), has shown that a number of hazards are associated with its use, including idiosyncratic pulmonary interstitial fibrosis and cumulative dose-dependent hepatotoxicity, necessitating repeated liver biopsies in some patients. Even when given in low dosages it often causes malaise, headaches, nausea, leukopenia, and other unpleasant side effects.

Gold salts, whether administered orally or parenterally, appeared in small studies to have a corticosteroid-sparing effect in patients with chronic asthma (Klaustermeyer et al., 1987; Bernstein et al., 1988). Proteinuria, necessitating cessation of therapy, is a significant side effect of such therapy, particularly with the use of parenteral formulations. Although these agents are undoubtedly effective in the treatment of inflammatory diseases such as rheumatoid arthritis, the mode(s) of action of gold salts remains obscure. Oral gold salt preparations have been shown to inhibit anti-IgE-induced release of histamine and leukotriene C_4 from human lung mast cells (Wotjecka-Lukasik et al., 1986) and to inhibit histamine-induced contraction of guinea pig tracheal smooth muscle rings (Malo et al., 1986). Whether these actions of gold salts are relevant to a corticosteroid-sparing effect in asthma therapy is unknown. Oral gold salts also inhibited mitogen-induced proliferation of T lymphocytes in vitro (Harth et al., 1977).

B. Cyclosporin A

Cyclosporin A (CyA) is a potent immunosuppressive agent that prolongs survival of allogeneic transplants (Cohen et al., 1984). It appears to arrest division of T lymphocytes in the G0 or early G1 phase of the cell cycle and inhibits, at a pretranslational level, the generation of interleukin-2 (Granelli-Piperno et al., 1984). There is some debate as to whether CyA inhibits expression of the high-affinity, physiologically relevant form of the interleukin-2 receptor on T lymphocytes (Lillehoj et al., 1984; Miyawaki et al., 1983), but the end result is a complete inhibition of the response of these cells to endogenous or exogenous interleukin-2 (Van Oers et al., 1985; Kay and Benzie, 1986). The available evidence suggests that CyA acts specifically on lymphocytes and that the effect is reversible: lymphocyte function returns to normal after use of the drug is discontinued.

Like other immunosuppressive drugs, CyA has many potential side effects including reversible increases in serum creatinine, potassium, and uric acid levels, hypertension, hepatotoxicity, tremor, paresthesia, hypertrichosis, gum hyperplasia, and nausea. Little is known of its effects, if any, on the developing fetus. Of foremost concern has been the possibility that CyA may cause irreversible renal damage. Renal transplant recipients have recently been described who developed interstitial renal fibrosis, tubular atrophy, and arteriolopathy while receiving CyA therapy (Farnsworth et al., 1983), although such changes are also seen when other immunosuppressive methods are employed (D'Ardenne et al., 1985). It seems, however, that the risk of such pathological changes is dose-related; in patients with renal allografts receiving CyA therapy, such changes have been seen to progress only in patients who received a high cumulative dosage of CyA during the first 6 months of treatment. Apparently a CyA dosage of up to 10.7 mg/kg/day was safe (Klintmalm et al., 1984) and there has certainly been no great deterioration of renal function in those patients who have taken CyA for a long time (Merion et al., 1984; Calne and Wood, 1985). If whole blood levels of CyA are kept to between 200 and 500 ng/ml, serious nephrotoxicity will be unusual, nor is there any good evidence that long-term CyA therapy at such low dosages causes serious harm to the kidneys, although patients will need to be followed up longer to be certain of this (Anon, 1986). It would seem reasonable therefore to appraise CyA for its possible benefits to the "hard core" of asthmatic patients who require or receive oral glucocorticoids in high dosages for prolonged periods of time. Unfortunately, because of the potential side effects of CyA, a large number of patients, such as those with existing renal disease or hypertension and all women of childbearing age, will have to be excluded from receiving CyA. There is an urgent need for alternative anti-inflammatory drugs with the potency of CyA but without its side effects. There is every reason to believe that such drugs would be of enormous benefit to those asthmatic patients whose disease is not satisfactorily controlled by regular inhaled glucocorticoid therapy.

IX. Conclusions

T lymphocytes act as effector cells in cell-mediated hypersensitivity reactions as well as collaborating with B cells in IgE production. Recent evidence suggests that the T lymphocyte may play a role in atopic allergic inflammation and asthma distinct from its participation in immunoglobulin production. Models of atopic allergic asthma in humans and guinea pigs support the hypothesis that T lymphocytes orchestrate eosinophil infiltration and activation and that eosinophil products lead directly to tissue damage. Activated T cells and their products have also been identified in the natural form of asthma in its acute severe form (status asthmaticus) and there is evidence that in patients whose disease fails to respond to corticosteroids T cells are "chronically activated." New approaches aimed at suppressing T cell function in the context of chronic asthma have been discussed.

Discussion

Hargreave: Could you define precisely what you mean by "steroid-resistant" asthma?

Kay: Patients with documented, reversible airflow obstruction who show no increase in FEV_1 or peak flow after 2 weeks of oral prednisolone (20 mg daily in first week, 40 mg daily in second week). These are nonsmokers and are not chronic bronchitics.

Dahl: Do these patients have eosinophilia in blood or BAL fluid?

Kay: Some do.

Kerrebijn: What is the role of T lymphocytes in "intrinsic" asthma?

Kay: I would speculate that both "intrinsic" and "extrinsic" asthma have a substantial T-cell component and that both may be disorders of local mucosal cell-mediated immunity.

Platts-Mills: You suggest that intrinsic asthma may be T-cell-mediated. We have looked at patients with "intrinsic" asthma who have a fungal infection (*Trichophyton*) of their toenails and have an immune response to *Trichophyton*. However, the association is with *immediate* hypersensitivity, not the delayed response. Thus, although IgE responses are accompanied by T-cell responses that may well play a role in asthma, it is not clear that T-cell responses alone are associated with asthma in this system or any other.

Hargreave: Could lymphokines from activated lymphocytes stimulate growth and activation of metochromatic cells (mast cells or basophils)?

Kay: T-cells produce histamine-releasing factors for basophils and mast cells (e.g., IL-3) and T cells can serve as precursors for mucosal mast cells.

Sybrecht: A recent report suggests that atopy can be transferred by bone marrow cells from allergic individuals.

Kay: This supports the view that T cells act as effector cells in allergic inflammation.

O'Byrne: In the guinea pig model, the appearance of T cells roughly corresponds to the physiological changes. What happens between the early, "late," and "late-late" response?

Kay: I am not sure why the T cell signal is not sustained, although the numbers of cells in the submucosa are always above control values.

Capron: Have you analyzed T cells into Mossman's TH1 and TH2 subtypes? Have you used phenotyping with CD4 +, CD45 +, and CD + BW29 + antibodies, which are said to be the functional equivalents in humans?

Kay: Mossman's classification does not hold up well in humans but we have some evidence that some of the CD4 + cell population in late-phase skin reactions are memory (primed) subsets (UCLHI + ve). We would need to study the cytokine profile of T cells in allergy to answer your question precisely.

References

Anon (1986). Cyclosporin for ever? *Lancet* 1:419-420.

Asmundsson, T., Kilburn Kaye, H., Lazzlo, J., and Krock, C. J. (1971). Immunosuppressive therapy of asthma. *J. Allergy* 47:136.

Bernstein, D. I., Bernstein, L., Bodenheimer, S. S., and Pietrusko, R. G. (1988). An open study of Auranofin in the treatment of steroid-dependent asthma. *J. Allergy Clin. Immunol.* 81:6-16.

Bloemena, E., Van Oers, M. H. J., Weinreich, S., Yong, S.-L., and Schellekens, P. T. A. (1988). Prednisolone and cyclosporin A exert differential inhibitory effects on T cell proliferation in vitro. *Clin. Immunol. Immunopathol.* 48:380-391.

Booij Nord, H., Orie, N. G. M., and DeVries, K. (1971). Immediate and late bronchial obstructive reactions to inhalation of house dust and protective effects of disodium cromoglycate and prednisolone. *J. Allergy Clin. Immunol.* 48:344-354.

Buchanan, D. R., Cromwell, O., and Kay, A. B. (1987a). Neutrophil chemotactic activity in acute severe asthma ("status asthmaticus"). *Am. Rev. Respir. Dis.* 136:1397-1402.

Buchanan, D. R., Fitzharris, P., Cromwell, O., and Kay, A. B. (1987b). Neutrophil chemotactic activity from cultured blood mononuclear cells in acute severe asthma. *Thorax* 42:749 (abs).

Butterfield, J. H., Ackerman, S. J., Weiler, D., Eisenberg, A. B., and Gleich, G. J. (1986). Effects of glucocorticoids on eosinophil colony growth. *J. Allergy Clin. Immunol.* **78**:450-457.

Calne, R. Y., and Wood, A. J. (1985). Cyclosporin in cadaveric renal transplantation: 3 year follow up of a European multicentre trial. *Lancet* **2**:549.

Carmichael, J., Paterson, I. C., Diaz, P., Crompton, G. K., Kay, A. B., and Grant, I. W. B. (1981). Corticosteroid-resistance in chronic asthma. *Br. Med. J.* **282**:1419-1422.

Cockcroft, D. W. (1983). Mechanisms of perennial allergic asthma. *Lancet* **2**:253-256.

Cohen, D. J., Loertscher, R., Rubin, M. F., Tilney, N. L., Carpenter, C. B., and Strom, T. B. (1984). Cyclosporine: a new immunosuppressive agent for organ transplantation. *Ann. Intern. Med.* **101**:667-682.

Corrigan, C. J., and Kay, A. B. (1990). CD4 T-lymphocyte activation in acute severe asthma. Relationship to disease severity and atopic status. *Am. Rev. Respir. Dis.* **141** (in press).

Corrigan, C. J., Hartnell, A., and Kay, A. B. (1988). T lymphocyte activation in acute severe asthma. *Lancet* **1**:1129-1132.

D'Ardenne, A. J., Dunnill, M. S., Wood, R. F. M., Thompson, J. F., and Morns, P. J. (1985). Cyclosporin treatment does not cause specific histologic changes in human renal allografts. *Transplant Proc.* **17**:1166-1167.

Diaz, P., Gonzalez, M. C., Galleguillos, F. R., Ancic, P., Cromwell, O., Shepherd, D., Durham, S. R., Gleich, G. J., and Kay, A. B. (1989). Leukocytes and mediators in bronchoalveolar lavage during allergen-induced late-phase asthmatic reactions. *Am. Rev. Respir. Dis.* **139**:1383-13.

Dunnill, M. S. (1960). The pathology of asthma with special reference to changes in the bronchial mucosa. *J. Clin. Pathol.* **13**:27-33.

Dunnill, M. S., Massarella, G. R., and Anderson, J. A. (1969). A comparison of the quantitative anatomy of the bronchi in normal subjects, in status asthmaticus, in chronic bronchitis and in emphysema. *Thorax* **24**:176-179.

Farnsworth, A., Hall, B. M., Kirwan, P., Bishop, G. A., Duggin, G. C., Goodman, B., Horrath, J., Johnson, J., Ng, A., Sheil, A. G. R., and Tiller, D. J. (1983). Pathology in renal transport patients treated with cyclosporin. *Transplant. Proc.* **15**:2852-2854.

Frew, A. J., and Kay, A. B. (1988). The relationship between infiltrating CD4+ lymphocytes, activated eosinophils and the magnitude of the allergen-induced late phase cutaneous reaction. *J. Immunol.* **141**:4158-4164.

Frew, A. J., Moqbel, R., Varley, J., Azzawi, M., Hartnell, A., Barkans, J., Scheper, R. J., Church, M. K., Holgate, S. T., and Kay, A. B. (1990).

T lymphocytes and eosinophils in allergen-induced late phase asthmatic reactions in the guinea pig. *Am. Rev. Respir. Dis.* **141**:407-413.

Gerblich, A. A., Campbell, A. E., and Schuyler, M. R. (1984). Changes in T lymphocyte subpopulations after antigenic bronchial provocation in asthmatics. *N. Engl. J. Med.* **310**:1349-1352.

Gleich, G. J., and Adolphson, C. R. (1986). The eosinophil leukocyte: structure and function. *Adv. Immunol.* **39**:177-253.

Gonzalez, M. C., Diaz, P., Galleguillos, F. R., Ancic, P., Cromwell, O., and Kay, A. B. (1987). Allergen-induced recruitment of bronchoalveolar (OKT4) and suppressor (OKT8) cells in asthma. Relative increases in OKT8 cells in single early responders compared with those in late-phase responders. *Am. Rev. Respir. Dis.* **136**:600-604.

Granelli-Piperno, A., Inaba, K., and Steinman, R. M. (1984). Stimulation of lymphokine release from T lymphoblasts. Requirement for mRNA synthesis and inhibition by cyclosporin A. *J. Exp. Med.* **160**:1792-1802.

Harth, M., Stiller, C. R., Sinclair, St. C., Evans, J., McGirr, D., and Zuberi, R. (1977). Effects of a gold salt on lymphocyte responses. *Clin. Exp. Immunol.* **27**:357-364.

Hodges, N. G., Brewis, R. A. L., and Howell, J. B. L. (1971). An evaluation of azathioprine in severe chronic asthma. *Thorax* **26**:734.

Horst, H. J., and Flad, H. D. (1987). Corticosteroid/interleukin-2 interactions: inhibition of binding of interleukin-2 to interleukin-2 receptors. *Clin. Exp. Immunol.* **68**:156-162.

Jeffery, P. K., Nelson, F. C., Wardlaw, A. J., and Kay, A. B. (1987). Quantitative analysis of bronchial biopsies in asthma. *Am. Rev. Respir. Dis.* **135**:A316.

Jeffery, P. K., Wardlaw, A. J., Nelson, F. C., Collins, J. V., and Kay, A. B. (1989). Bronchial biopsies in asthma: an ultrastructural quantitative study and correlation with hyperreactivity. *Am. Rev. Respir. Dis.* **140**: 1745-1753.

Kay, J. E., and Benzie, C. R. (1986). Lymphocyte activation by OKT3: cyclosporine sensitivity and synergism with phorbol ester. *Immunology* **57**: 195-199.

Kerrebijn, K. F., van Essen-Zandvliet, E. E. M., and Neijens, H. J. (1987). Effect of long term treatment with inhaled corticosteroids and beta-agonists on the bronchial responsiveness in children with asthma. *J. Allergy Clin. Immunol.* **79**:653-659.

Klaustermeyer, W. B., Noritake, D. T., and Kwong, F. K. (1987). Chrysotherapy in the treatment of corticosteroid-dependent asthma. *J. Allergy Clin. Immunol.* **79**:720-725.

Klintmalm, G., Bohman, S. O., Sundelin, B., and Wilczek, H. (1984). Interstitial fibrosis in renal allografts after 12-16 months of cyclosporin treatment: beneficial effect of low doses in early post-transplantation period. *Lancet* **2**:950-955.

Kurihara, K., Wardlaw, A. J., Maestrelli, P., Tsai, J.-J., and Kay, A. B., (1988). IL-1, IL-2, TNF, INF-gamma, GM-CSF and PHA-stimulated leukocyte supernatants have negligible eosinophil chemotactic activity compared with platelet activating factor (PAF). *FASEB J.* **2**: A1449.

Leung, D. Y. M., and Geha, R. S. (1987). Regulation of the human IgE antibody response. *Int. Rev. Immunol.* **2**:75-91.

Lichtenstein, L. M., and MacGlashan, D. W., Jr. (1986). The concept of basophil releasibility. *J. Allergy Clin. Immunol.* **77**:291-294.

Lillehoj, H. S., Malek, T. R., and Shevach, E. M. (1984). Differential effect of cyclosporin A on the expression of T and B lymphocyte activation antigens. *J. Immunol.* **133**:244-250.

Lopez, A. F., Sanderson, C. J., Gamble, J. R., Campbell, H. D., Young, I. G., and Vadas, M. A. (1988). Recombinant human interleukin-5 is a selective activator of human eosinophil function. *J. Exp. Med.* **167**: 219-224.

Maestrelli, P., Tsai, J.-J., Cromwell, O., and Kay, A. B. (1988). The identification and partial characterization of a human mononuclear cell-derived neutrophil chemotactic factor apparently distinct from IL-1, IL-2, GM-CSF, TNF and IFN-gamma. *Immunology* **64**:219-225.

Maggi, E., Del Prete, G., Mucchia, D., Parronchi, P., Tiri, A., Chretien, I., Ricci, M., and Romagnani, S. (1988). Profiles of lymphokine activities and helper function for IgE in human T cell clones. *Eur. J. Immunol.* **18**(7):1045-1050.

Malo, P. E., Wasserman, M., Parris, D., and Pfeiffer, D. (1986). Inhibition by Auranofin of pharmacologic and antigen-induced contractions of the isolated guinea pig trachea. *J. Allergy Clin. Immunol.* **77**:371-376.

Mary, D., Aussel, C., Ferrua, B., and Fehlmann, M. (1987). Regulation of interleukin-2 synthesis by cAMP in human T cells. *J. Immunol.* **139**:1179-1184.

Merion, R. M., White, D. J. G., Thiru, S., Evans, D. B., and Calne, R. Y. (1984). Cyclosporine: five years experience in cadaveric renal transplantation. *N. Engl. J. Med.* **310**:148-154.

Metzger, W. J., Zavala, D., Richerson, H. B., Moseley, P., Iwamota, P., Monick, M., Sjoerdsma, K., and Hunninghake, G. W. (1987). Local allergen challenge and bronchoalveolar lavage of allergic asthmatic lungs. Description of the model and local airway inflammation. *Am. Rev. Respir. Dis.* **135**:433-440.

Miossec, P., and Ziff, M. (1986). Immune interferon enhances the production of interleukin 1 by human endothelial cells stimulated with lipopolysaccharide. *J. Immunol.* **137**:2848-2852.

Miyajima, A., Miyatake, S., Schreurs, J., DeVries, J., Arai, N., Yokota, T., and Arai, K. (1988). Coordinate regulation of immune and inflammatory responses by T cell-derived lymphokines. *FASEB J.* **2**:2462-2473.

Miyawaki, T., Yachie, A., Ohzeki, S., Nagaoki, T., and Taniguchi, N. (1983). Cyclosporin A does not prevent expression of Tac antigen, a probably TCGF receptor molecule, on mitogen-stimulated human T cells. *J. Immunol.* **130**:2737-2742.

Mossmann, T. R., Cherwinski, H., Bond, M. W., Giedlin, M. A., and Coffman, R. L. (1986). Two types of murine helper T cell clone. 1. Definition according to profiles of lymphokine activities and secreted proteins. *J. Immunol.* **136**:2348-2357.

Mullarkey, M. F., Blumenstein, B. A., Andrade, W. P., Bailey, G. A., Olason, I., and Wetzel, C. E. (1988). Methotrexate in the treatment of corticosteroid-dependent asthma. A double-blind crossover study. *N. Engl. J. Med.* **318**:603-607.

O'Hehir, R. E., Bal, V., Quint, D., Moqbel, R., Kay, A. B., Zanders, E., and Lamb, J. R. (1988). IgE induction by human cloned T lymphocytes specific for house dust mite is IL-4 dependent. *FASEB J.* **2**:A1442.

Otsuka, H., Denburg, J. A., Befus, A. D., Hitch, D., Lapp, P., Rajan, R. S., Bienenstock, J., and Dolovich, J. (1986). Effect of beclomethasone dipropionate on nasal metachromatic cell subpopulations. *Clin. Allergy* **16**:589-595.

Owen, W. F., Rothenburg, M. E., Silberstein, D. S., Gasson, J. C., Stevens, R. L., Austen, K. F., and Soberman, R. J. (1987). Regulation of human eosinophil viability, density and function by granulocyte/macrophage colony stimulating factor in the presence of 3T3 fibroblasts. *J. Exp. Med.* **166**:129-141.

Poznansky, M. C., Gordon, A. C. H., Douglas, J. G., Krajewski, A. S., Wyllie, A. H., and Grant, I. W. B. (1984). Resistance to methylprednisolone in cultures of blood mononuclear cells from glucocorticoid-resistant asthmatic patients. *Clin. Sci.* **67**:639-645.

Rees, A. J., and Lockwood, C. M. (1986). Immunosuppressive drugs in clinical practice. In: *Clinical Aspects of Immunology*, 4th ed. Edited by P. J. Cochmans and D. K. Peters. London, Blackwell Scientific, pp. 507-564.

Roenigk, H. H., Auerbach, R., Maibach, H. I., and Weinstein, G. D. (1988). Methotrexate in psoriasis: revised guidelines. *J. Am. Acad. Dermatol.* **19**:145-156.

Rothenburg, M. E., Owen, W. F., Silberstein, D. S., Woods, J., Soberman, R. J., Austen, K. F., Stevens, R. L. (1988). Human eosinophils have prolonged survival, enhances functional properties, and become hypodense when exposed to human interleukin-3. *J. Clin. Invest.* **81**:1986-1992.

Sanderson, C. J., Campbell, H. D., and Young, I. G. (1988). Molecular and cellular biology of eostinophil differentiation factor (Interleukin-2) and its effects on human and mouse B cells. *Immunol. Rev.* **102**:29.

Tai, P. C., Spry, C. J. F., Peterson, C., Venge, P., and Olsson, I. (1984). Monoclonal antibodies distinguish between storage and secreted forms of eosinophil cationic peptide. *Nature* **309**:182-184.

Teale, J. M., and Abraham, K. M. (1987). The regulation of antibody class expression. *Immunol. Today* **8**:122-126.

Timonen, T., and Stenius-Aarnala, B. (1985). Natural killer cell activity in asthma. *Clin. Exp. Immunol.* **59**:85-90.

Ting, S., Dunsky, E. H., Lavker, R. M., and Zweiman, B. (1980). Patterns of mast cell alterations and *in vivo* mediator release in human allergic skin reactions. *J. Allergy Clin. Immunol.* **66**:417-423.

Tsai, J.-J., Maestrelli, P., Cromwell, O., Moqbel, R., Fitzharris, P., and Kay, A. B. (1988). A T lymphocyte-derived factor which enhances IgG-dependent release of leukotriene B_4 (LTB_4) from human neutrophils *Immunology* **65**:449-456.

Van Oers, M. H. J., Yong, S.-L., Schellekens, P. T. A., and Aarden, L. A. (1985). The mechanism of action of cyclosporine is not primarily at the level of the interleukin-2 system. *Transplant. Proc.* **17**:2700-2705.

Walsh, G. M., Kurihara, K., and Kay, A. B. (1989). Effect of platelet activating factor (PAF) and interleukin-5 (IL-5) on eosinophil adherence reactions. *FASEB J.* **3**:A1330.

Walsh, L. J., Parry, A., Scholes, A., and Seymour, G. J. (1987). Modulation of CD4 antigen on human gingival Langerhans cells by gamma interferon. *Clin. Exp. Immunol.* **70**:379-385.

Wojtecka-Lukasik, E. W., Sopata, I., and Maslinski, S. (1986). Auranofin modulates mast cell histamine and polymorphonuclear leucocyte collagenase release. *Agents Actions* **18**:68-70.

Yamaguchi, Y., Hayashi, Y., Sugama, Y., Miura, Y., Kasahara, T., Kitamura, S., Torisu, M., Mita, S., Tominaga, A., Takatsu, K., and Suda, T. (1988). Highly purified murine interleukin-5 stimulates eosinophil function and prolongs in vitro survival. *J. Exp. Med.* **167**:1737-1742.

10

Platelet-Activating Factor and Asthma

K. F. CHUNG and PETER J. BARNES

National Heart and Lung Institute
London, England

I. Introduction

In 1972, Benveniste and colleagues coined the term "platelet-activating factor" (PAF) to describe a substance released from rabbit basophils after IgE stimulation, which was capable of causing platelet aggregation (Benveniste et al., 1972). In 1979, three separate groups announced the semisynthesis of 1-alkyl-2-acetyl-sn-glycero-3-phosphocholine (AAGPC), which had biological and chemical properties identical to natural PAF (Benveniste et al., 1979; Demopoulos et al., 1979; Blank et al., 1979). Subsequently, PAF isolated from IgE-stimulated rabbit basophils was shown to be AAGPC by gas-liquid chromatography and mass spectrometry (Hanahan et al., 1980).

In this chapter, we review current knowledge concerning PAF, particularly its effects on the airways, and the evidence for a possible role in asthma. Over the past 10 years there has been increasing evidence that inflammatory responses within the airways may play a crucial role in causing bronchial hyperresponsiveness and the clinical symptoms characteristic of asthma (Chung, 1986). PAF is a potent inflammatory mediator that appears to be capable of mimicking many of the features of asthma, such as airway edema, bronchial hyperresponsiveness, and eosinophil recruitment and activation (Barnes et al., 1988). The availability of specific antagonists of PAF receptors may provide more direct evidence for a role of PAF in asthma (Chung and Barnes, 1988) and such studies are now underway.

II. Metabolism of PAF

A. Synthesis

PAF is synthesized de novo as a two-step process involving the activation of phospholipase A2 to generate lyso-PAF from 1-alkyl-2-acyl-glycerophosphocholine in membrane phospholipids, followed by acetylation of lyso-PAF by an acetyltransferase enzyme (Fig. 1) (Wykle et al., 1980). This process has been demonstrated in a number of inflammatory cell types in vitro, including macrophages, neutrophils, eosinophils, and platelets. Activity of acetyltransferase is markedly increased by the calcium ionophore A23187 or by the phagocytosis of zymosan-activated particles (Ninio et al., 1983). However, the regulatory processes governing acetyltransferase activity during normal physiology are not well understood.

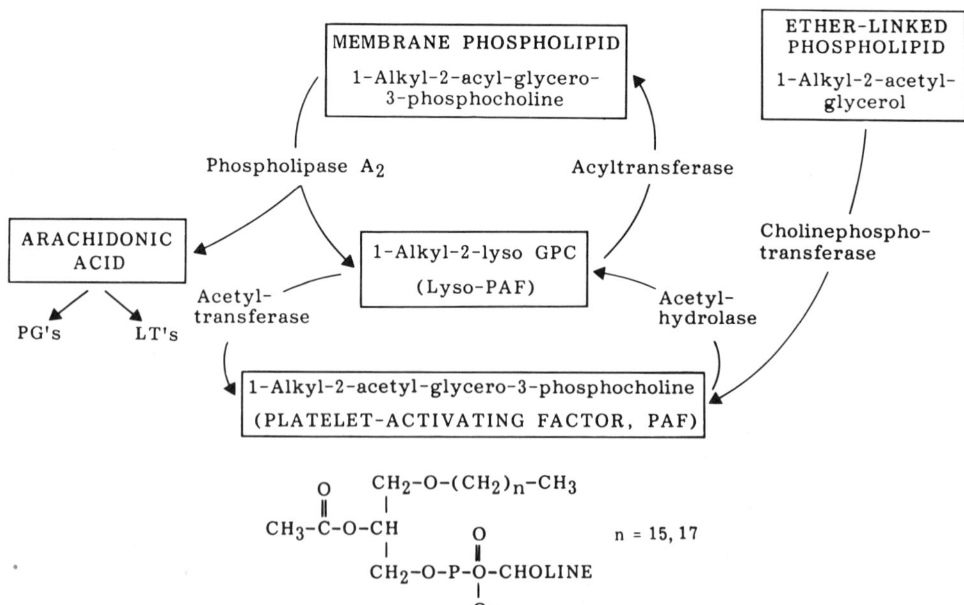

Figure 1   Synthesis and catabolism of platelet-activating factor (PAF). GPC, glycero-3-phosphocholine; PG, prostaglandins; LT, leukotrienes.

An alternative synthetic pathway involves the generation of PAF directly from ether-linked phospholipids such as alkyl-acetyl-glycerols, under the action of a highly specific phosphocholinetransferase present in several tissues, including the lungs of rats and human neutrophils (Renooij and Synder, 1981). Although the role of this enzyme in PAF metabolism remains to be elucidated, it is thought that this pathway may operate under physiological conditions, perhaps for the maintenance of normal cellular function. The acetyltransferase pathway may, on the other hand, be preferentially activated by inflammatory signals such phagocytosis and chemotaxis (Snyder, 1987).

B. Catabolism

PAF is rapidly metabolized by an acetylhydrolase that hydrolyzes the acetate moiety to yield lyso-PAF and acetate (Fig. 1). This enzyme is found intracellularly in the cytosolic fraction of a wide variety of tissues and human blood cells (Lee et al., 1982; Blank et al., 1981). In addition, an extracellular form exists in plasma and serum obtained from several species including humans and is associated with the lipoprotein fraction (Farr et al., 1980). Its activity may be important in regulating the potent biological effects of PAF. Serum, but not platelet, PAF acetylhydrolase activity is reduced in asthmatic children, leading to the hypothesis that this may underlie the severity of asthma in these patients (Miwa et al., 1988). In the rat, PAF administered by the intratracheal route is rapidly taken up by bronchiolar and alveolar epithelial cells and is metabolized to lyso-PAF and phosphatidylcholine (Haroldsen et al., 1987). Inflammatory cells, such as neutrophils, also rapidly incorporate PAF into its fatty acyl derivative (Chilton et al., 1983). Finally, Lyso-PAF is degraded to a fatty alcohol and 3-phosphatidylcholine glycerol. Thus, PAF synthesis and catabolism appear to be regulated primarily by phospholipase A_2, acetyltransferase, and acetylhydrolase.

C. Cellular Sources

A wide range of cell types produce PAF in vitro. Within a few minutes of activation of neutrophils by opsonized zymosan or calcium ionophore, PAF is synthesized, although only 3-4% is released (Lynch and Henson, 1986). Normal human eosinophils exhibit no detectable acetyltransferase activity, in contrast to eosinophils from patients with eosinophilia, which show high activity (Lee et al., 1984). Thus, these latter eosinophils release PAF after stimulation with various chemotactic factors including eosinophilic chemotactic factor of anaphylaxis (ECF-A) and f-met-leu-phe (FMLP) (Lee et al., 1984). Human eosinophils also have the most abundant PAF precursor, alkylacyl-glycerophosphocholine of all types of circulating cells (Ojima-Uchiyama et al., 1988). Purified human hypodense eosinophils release PAF after IgE- (but not IgG-) mediated activation (Capron et al., 1988). Human alveolar macrophages obtained by bronchoalveolar lavage of allergic asthmatic subjects also release PAF following stimulation with the appropriate antigen in vitro but not with zymosan (Arnoux et al., 1987). Cultured human endothelial cells release a small percentage of synthetized PAF after activation by calcium ionophore, bradykinin, thrombin, and interleukin-1 (McIntyre et al., 1985; Prescott et al., 1984). Purified human lung mast cells also generate PAF when stimulated with anti-IgE but most of the PAF is also retained intracellularly (Schleimer et al., 1986). The role of intracellular PAF is not known, but one possibility is that it may regulate surface receptors to increase the attachment of inflammatory cells to endothelial cells (Lynch and Henson, 1986).

III. Cellular Activation by PAF

A. Effects on Cells

PAF has potent effects on a wide variety of cells. At picomolar concentrations, PAF causes aggregation of washed rabbit and human platelets, with the release of serotonin (O'Donnell et al., 1979). The stimulation of neutrophils by PAF results in the release of lysosomal enzymes and superoxide anions, the generation of leukotriene B_4, and chemotaxis (O'Flaherty, 1985; Lin et al., 1982; Wardlaw et al., 1986). PAF is extremely potent in causing the release of the granule-associated enzyme eosinophil peroxidase from human and guinea pig eosinophils (Kroegel et al., 1988) (Fig. 2). In addition, it induces a dose-dependent enhancement of eosinophil cytotoxicity as measured by the killing of *Schistosoma mansoni* schistosomula coated with C3b and IgG antibodies (Macdonald et al., 1986). PAF is the most potent chemotactic and chemokinetic mediator for eosinophils in vitro (Wardlaw et al., 1986) and promotes the adhesion of neutrophils and eosinophils to vascular endothelial cells, primarily through an effect on the endothelial cell (Garcia et al., 1988; Kimani et al., 1988). PAF has a priming effect on the respiratory burst response of stimulated neutrophils (Dewald and Baggiolini, 1988).

B. Interactions with Arachidonic Acid Metabolism

Because PAF and arachidonic acid are released from a common precursor (alkyl-acyl-GPC) when cells are stimulated in vitro (Fig. 1), interactions of PAF with arachidonic metabolites should be considered. Responses of human neutrophils to PAF, such as the release of granule-associated enzymes, may be mediated by products of the lipoxygenase pathway (Smith and Bowman, 1982). Another interaction between arachidonate metabolites and PAF is illustrated by the potentiating effect of 5-HETE on the degranulation of human

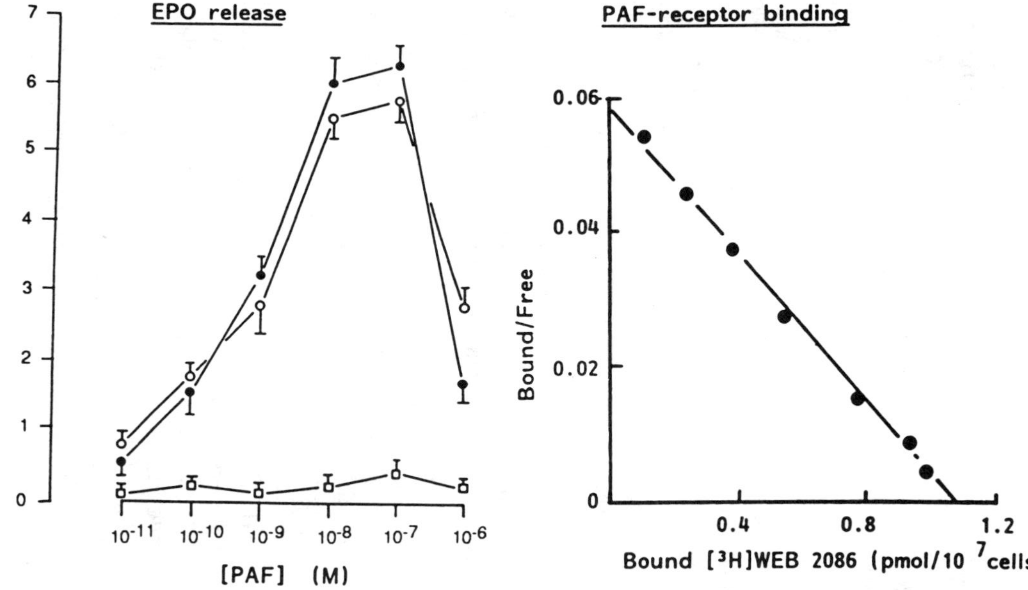

Figure 2 Left panel: Effect of platelet-activating factor on eosinophil peroxidase (EPO) release from purified human eosinophils. EPO activity was measured by luminol-enhanced chemiluminescence ($\bullet$) and by colorimetry using o-phenyleneclamine ($\bigcirc$). The results referred to a standard using horseradish peroxidase. EPO activity was inhibited by the specific EPO inhibitor, 3-amino-1,2,4-triazole ($\square$; data from Kroegel et al., 1988). Right panel: Scatchard plot of the specific binding of the PAF antagonist ligand, [³H]WEB 2086, to intact human eosinophils obtained from a patient with hypereosinophilia syndrome. The derived linear Scatchard plot indicates a homogeneous population of noninteracting binding sites with a binding capacity (Bmax) of 64,000 sites/cell and a binding affinity (k_D) of 18.5 nM.

neutrophils by PAF (O'Flaherty et al., 1983); thus the rapid synthesis of both mediators in activated neutrophils may be the cause of rapid degranulation. PAF also stimulated the release of LTB_4 from human neutrophils and eosinophils (Lin et al., 1982; Bruynzeel et al., 1986). Other effects of PAF, such as the aggregation of human platelets, may be mediated through thromboxane A_2 generation (Miller et al., 1982).

C. PAF Receptors

The stereoselectivity of PAF effects, its high biological potency, and the development of specific tachyphylaxis suggest that the surface membrane receptors are involved in mediating these effects. With the use of [³H]PAF as a radioligand, high-affinity binding sites on human and rabbit platelets (Valone et al., 1982), human neutrophils (O'Flaherty et al., 1986; Valone and Goetzl, 1983), and human lung membranes (Hwang et al., 1985a) have been demonstrated. This binding appears to be specific and can be inhibited by PAF antagonists. However, there is generally a high level of nonspecific binding. In addition, PAF is rapidly metabolized. For example, in the neutrophil, [³H]PAF is rapidly converted into its acyl derivative at 37 °C and transferred into specific granules, but this metabolism was not present at 4 °C (O'Flaherty et al., 1986). Labeled PAF antagonists have been used more recently and proven to be more suitable as radioligands. Thus, [³H]dihydrokadsurenone has been shown to bind specifically to rabbit platelet membranes with saturation and to be displaced by PAF and other PAF antagonists (Hwang et al., 1986). Similar results were obtained with the binding of [³H] WEB 2086 to intact human platelets, although [³H]52770 RP binding was not displaced by labeled PAF or WEB 2086, which suggest that [³H] 52770 RP binding sites were not identical to those of PAF (Ukena et al., 1988). Specific binding on isolated human neutrophils and eosinophils has also been described with [³H]WEB 2086 (Dent et al., 1988; Fig. 2). PAF-receptor binding to human and guinea pig lung has also been described with [³H] WEB 2086, and preliminary autoradiographic studies suggest that these receptors are widely distributed (Dent et al., 1989).

D. Intracellular Mechanisms

The intracellular mechanisms are not fully elucidated. PAF induces calcium uptake in rabbit platelets, an effect that is dependent on extracellular concentration of calcium and blocked by the calcium channel blocker verapamil (Lee et al., 1983). Calmodulin antagonists inhibit PAF-induced aggregation of human platelets (Levy, 1983), which may therefore be mediated by a calmodulin-dependent mechanism. Degranulation of human neutrophils and eosinophils is greatly reduced by the absence of extracellular calcium (O'Flaherty et al., 1981; Kroegel et al., 1988). PAF-activated platelets, eosinophils, and macrophages show an early rapid rise in intracellular calcium levels (Conrad and Rink, 1986; Kroegel et al., 1989; Hallam et al., 1984). PAF also stimulates the metabolism of phosphatidylinositides in platelets (Shukla and Hanahan, 1982), which may be related to intracellular calcium mobilization.

IV. Effect of PAF on Airways

A. Airway Microvascular Leakage and Edema

When administered intravenously, PAF is one of the most potent inducers of airway microvascular leakage in the guinea pig, being approximately 10,000 times more potent than histamine and 10 times more potent than LTD_4 (Evans et al., 1987, 1989; O'Donnell and Barnett, 1987). PAF is active throughout the respiratory tract, in contrast to the effects of histamine, which are limited to central airways. This effect is independent of circulating platelets or of eicosanoid generation (Evans et al., 1987). Both an immediate and a delayed increase (at 5 h) in airway microvascular leakage of radiolabeled albumin have been observed with the intratracheal administration of PAF; there was also a concomitant exudation of plasma proteins across the airway epithelium (Persson et al., 1987), which may underlie the slowing of mucociliary clearance induced by PAF (Aursudkij et al., 1987). When infused into the bronchial circulation of sheep, PAF induces a significant decrease in bronchial blood flow associated with a fall in cardiac output (Long et al., 1988).

Whether PAF-induced airway microvascular leakage and edema result in airway narrowing is more difficult to establish directly. In the guinea pig made hyperresponsive after intravenous PAF administration, there is a reduced bronchodilator response to isoproterenol despite a normal relaxation response of tracheal smooth muscle in vitro and a normal density and affinity of tracheal and pulmonary β-receptors (Barnes et al., 1987). This imparied bronchodilator response to a β-agonist in vivo may result from the presence of airway edema induced by PAF, which would not be easily reversed by a β-agonist (Boschetto et al., 1988). In humans, PAF-induced bronchoconstriction is only partially inhibited by a dose of a β-agonist (albuterol) that completely blocks a similar degree of bronchoconstriction induced by smooth muscle constrictor, methacholine (Chung et al., 1989). It is also possible that the bronchoconstrictor response resistant to the β-agonist may represent the effect of edema.

B. Airway Narrowing

PAF is a potent bronchoconstrictor agent in vivo but has negligible direct contractile effects on airway smooth preparations in vitro (Cuss et al., 1986;

Denjean et al., 1983; Mazzoni et al., 1985; Halonen et al., 1985; Chung et al., 1986; Schellenberg, 1987; Popovich et al., 1988). Thus, PAF causes airway narrowing by indirect mechanisms in vivo such as the release of smooth muscle constrictor mediators or the induction of airway edema. Human and canine airway smooth muscle contracts to PAF in the presence of platelets in vitro (Schellenberg, 1987; Popovich et al., 1988). In the canine airway, serotonin released from PAF-activated platelets was implicated as the constrictor mediator (Popovich et al., 1988). However, the secondary cells involved in PAF-induced bronchoconstriction in vivo are not known and may depend on the route of administration of PAF and the species studied. In the guinea pig, PAF-induced bronchoconstriction by the intravenous route is dependent on circulating platelets, but the nature of platelet-derived mediators is uncertain; neither antihistamines, serotonin antagonists, nor indomethacin inhibits the bronchoconstrictor response (Vargaftig et al., 1982). When PAF is administered by aerosol, this effect is not dependent on platelets but is reduced by cyclooxygenase inhibitors (Lefort et al., 1984); it may involve the activation of alveolar macrophages (Maridonneau-Parini et al., 1985). In the dog, aerosolized-PAF-induced bronchoconstriction is dependent on thromboxane A2 generation (Chung et al., 1986), but when PAF is administered intravenously PAF-induced tracheal smooth muscle contraction in vivo is only slightly attenuated by cyclooxygenase inhibition with indomethacin (Leff et al., 1987). In the sheep, depletion of circulating platelets or granulocytes does not interfere with PAF-induced changes in lung mechanics (Christman et al., 1988). PAF has been shown to cause the release of neuropeptides such as substance P from guinea pig lungs (Rodrique et al., 1988), which could explain the activation of efferent postganglionic parasympathetic nerves underlying PAF-induced contraction of tracheal smooth muscle in the dog (Leff et al., 1987; Tanaka and Grunstein, 1986).

The effects of PAF aerosol have now been documented in humans (Cuss et al., 1986; Rubin et al., 1987). PAF aerosol induces bronchoconstriction within 2-3 min of inhalation, with an onset slower than that observed with histamine or methacholine (Cuss et al., 1986). However, the duration of effect is no longer than that induced by the other constrictors and there is no evidence of a delayed bronchoconstrictor response. A transient episode of facial flushing maximal at 5 min, with little change in systemic blood pressure and a significant increase in pulse rate, occurs concomitantly (Cuss et al., 1986). Rapid tachyphylaxis develops to the bronchoconstrictor effect of PAF, which probably underlies the small responses obtained by Rubin and colleagues with administration of increasing concentrations of PAF (Rubin et al., 1987). In normal subjects, airway responsiveness to PAF aerosol is approximately 100 times less than that to methacholine, and there is no significant linear relationship between the responsiveness to either stimulus

(Cuss et al., 1986; Fig. 3). Subjects with mild asthma who are hyperresponsive to methacholine do not appear to be more sensitive to PAF than normal subjects (Chung and Barnes, 1989). It is possible that this may reflect an equal propensity of PAF to induce airway narrowing by causing edema in these two groups rather than by a direct effect on airway smooth muscle. Alternatively, if PAF were released endogenously in patients with mild asthma, this may represent a tachyphylactic response.

The role of cells and mediators in PAF-induced bronchoconstriction in man remains unclear. Prostacyclin infused at a concentration needed to inhibit PAF-induced platelet aggregation ex vivo does not inhibit PAF-induced bronchoconstriction, which suggests that platelets do not contribute to this response (Lammers et al., 1988). A thromboxane receptor antagonist is also ineffective (Stenton et al., 1989). Whether release of sulfidopeptide leukotrienes is involved is not known. Although histamine may mediate PAF-induced wheal formation in the skin, it is not likely to do so in the airways (Chung et al., 1988), contrary to the inhibitory effect of chlorpheniramine against intravenously administered PAF in the rabbit (Halonen et al., 1985).

C. Effect on Circulating and Bronchoalveolar Cells

PAF causes a rapid fall in circulating neutrophils and platelets when administered either intravenously or intratracheally (Chung et al., 1988; Gateau et al., 1984; Halonen et al., 1985). When inhaled by both normal and asthmatic subjects, PAF induces profound neutropenia at 5 min, with a rebound neutrophilia at 15 min and the development of tachyphylaxis to subsequent inhalations (Chung et al., 1988, 1989). No significant fall in platelet count was

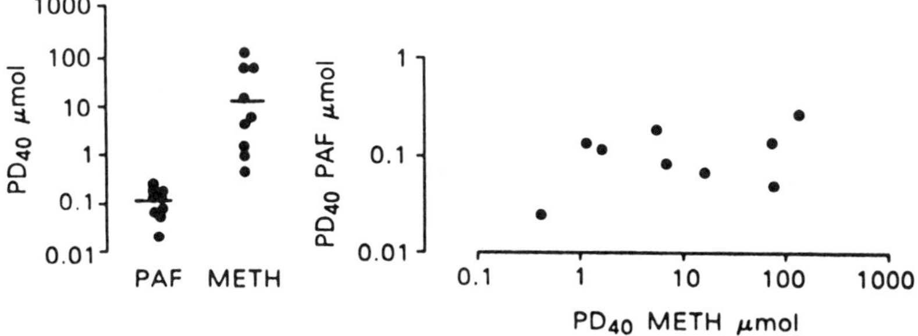

Figure 3 Provocative dose of methacholine or platelet-activating factor (PAF) needed to cause a 40% fall in partial expiratory flow rates (PD$_{40}$) in normal subjects. There is no significant linear correlation between PD$_{40}$-methacholine and PD$_{40}$-PAF (reproduced from Cuss et al., 1986).

observed, probably due to the lower dosage of PAF administered than is used in animal studies.

These falls in circulating blood cell levels could be the result of a combination of hemodynamic factors, such as slowing of pulmonary blood flow and increased adhesiveness of cells to the pulmonary vascular endothelium, both of which result from a direct effect of PAF. Radiolabeled platelets transiently accumulate within the pulmonary vasculature following intravenous administration of PAF in guinea pigs or endotracheal instillation in baboons (Robertson and Page, 1987; Arnoux et al., 1988). In humans, circulating neutrophils become hypodense within 15 min of inhalation of PAF, as a result of an increase in cell volume, probably indicating neutrophil activation that would predispose towards an increased adherence to the endothelium (Wardlaw et al., 1988).

Following PAF inhalation, circulating platelets do not show desensitization of PAF-induced aggregation ex vivo; however, circulating neutrophils are less responsive in their chemiluminescent response to PAF activation at 90 min (Kioumis et al., 1988). Thus, it is not possible to use ex vivo platelet desensitization to PAF as evidence for endogenous release of PAF. Improved techniques for the study of PAF receptors on intact cells may help to clarify the mechanisms of tachyphylactic response to PAF.

In the baboon and guinea pig, PAF induces a significant increase in eosinophil counts in bronchoalveolar lavage fluid, occurring within 1 h of challenge by the endotracheal routes (Arnoux et al., 1988; Coyle et al., 1988). In the guinea pig given intravenous PAF, histological examination reveals infiltration in the bronchial walls, together with mucous plugs containing eosinophils in the bronchial lumen (Lellouch-Tubiana et al., 1988). This eosinophil infiltration is suppressed by prostacyclin and by platelet depletion with antiplatelet serum. Thus, in the guinea pig, platelets may be involved in mediating PAF-induced eosinophil accumulation. In nonasthmatic human subjects, 4 h after inhalation there is an approximate doubling of neutrophil recovery in bronchoalveolar lavage fluid, without any significant increase in eosinophil counts (Wardlaw et al., 1988); this study has not been performed in asthmatic subjects. Of great interest is the selective accumulation of eosinophils as measured by the skin window technique, when PAF is injected intradermally in allergic subjects (Henocq and Vargaftig, 1988). The mechanism by which this occurs is intriguing because PAF has chemotactic activity for both eosinophils and neutrophils in vitro (Wardlaw et al., 1986). It is possible that under certain conditions the response of eosinophils is selectively enhanced by cytokines such as interleukin so as to respond specifically to PAF.

D. Bronchial Hyperresponsiveness

PAF induces an increase, sometimes prolonged, in bronchial responsiveness to methacholine and histamine in several species including humans (Table 1) (Barnes et al., 1987; Cuss et al., 1986; Chung et al., 1986; Fitzgerald et al., 1987; Christman et al., 1987; Mazzoni et al., 1985; Rubin et al., 1987). In normal subjects, a single exposure to PAF aerosol resulted in a mean tripling of bronchial responsiveness at 3 days, with a continuing effect up to 1-3 weeks: five of the six subjects showing such a response (Cuss et al., 1986; Fig. 4). By constrast, asthmatic subjects do not show an overall increase in airway responsiveness; there is also no significant effect of PAF on the bronchodilator response to isoproterenol (Chung and Barnes, 1989). These observations are similar to those reported by Rubin and colleagues (1987), who showed a 2.5-fold increase in methacholine responsiveness at 1 h after recovery from PAF-induced bronchoconstriction in normal but not in asthmatic subjects. The lack of response observed in asthmatic subjects is difficult to explain but may reflect the difficulty in further enhancing inflammatory mech-

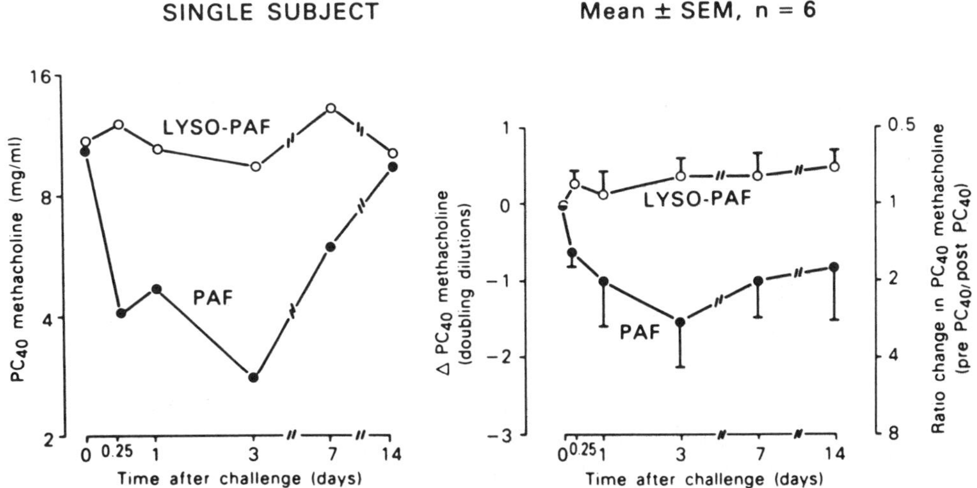

Figure 4   Changes in mean PC_{40}- methacholine in six normal subjects after inhalation of platelet-activating factor. There is a significant increase in airway responsiveness within 6 h, an effect lasting up to 2 weeks. Changes in PC_{40} in a single subject are also shown in the left-hand panel (data reproduced from Cuss et al., 1986).

Table 1 Platelet-Activating Factor and Bronchial Hyperresponsiveness

Species	Dose of PAF	Effect on responsiveness	Reference
Human			
Normal	Aerosol (0.11 μmol)	Threefold increase in PC_{40}-methacholine detectable at 6 h and lasting 1-2 weeks	Cuss et al. (1986)
	Aerosol (1,000 μg/ml)	2.5-fold increase in PC_{35}-methacholine at 1 h	Rubin et al. (1987)
Asthmatic			
	Aerosol (1,000 μg/ml)	No increase	Rubin et al. (1987)
	Aerosol (132 μg delivered)	No overall change in responsiveness to methacholine or isoprenaline at 3 days	Chung et al. (1989)
Guinea pig			
	Stepwise intravenous (iv) infusion (600 ng/kg)	Increase in responsiveness to iv histamine, substance P and acetylcholine within 1-2 h	Mazzoni et al. (1985)
	Aerosol (10 μg/ml)	Increased response to serotonin aerosol at 15 min (fourfold increase in pulmonary inflation pressure)	Fitzgerald et al. (1987)
	Aerosol (250-1000 μg/ml)	Increased response to iv acetylcholine and histamine at 24 h (doubling of pulmonary inflation pressure)	Coyle et al. (1988)
Dog			
	Aerosol (total 1000 μg delivered)	Fourfold increase in responsiveness to acetylcholine aerosol maximal at 3 h, lasting less than 6 h	Chung et al. (1986)
Sheep			
	IV (0.5 μg/kg)	Doubled increase in responsiveness measured at $ED_{65}C_{dyn}$ to aerosol histamine	Christman et al. (1987)

anisms that are maintaining bronchial hyperresponsiveness in the asthmatic subject and that would not be present in the normal subject.

The mechanisms underlying PAF-induced bronchial hyperresponsiveness are of interest. Induction of airways edema by PAF may account in part for the acute component of the increase in bronchial responsiveness (Moreno et al., 1986), but the more sustained component may result from an inflammatory response initiated by PAF, such as the recruitment of inflammatory cells to the airway wall. Although there is an increase in neutrophil count in bronchoalveolar lavage fluid in humans after PAF administration, this correlated inversely with the degree of bronchial hyperresponsiveness, suggesting a protective effect of the neutrophil (Wardlaw et al., 1988). Whether the eosinophil appears later in lavage fluid or would have been observed in biopsies of the airway wall is not known. However, the eosinophil remains the most attractive candidate (Fig. 5). In the guinea pig, platelet depletion inhibits PAF-induced eosinophil accumulation in the airways (Lellouch-Tubiana et al., 1988) and bronchial hyperresponsiveness (Coyle et al., 1988), which suggests that these events may be linked. Release of granule-associated enzymes such as eosinophil peroxidase and major basic protein from the eosinophil by PAF may result in damage to the airway epithelium (Frigas and Gleich, 1986), which is another pathological hallmark of asthma. Thus, incubation of guinea pig tracheal segments with eosinophils causes extensive epithelial damage in the presence of PAF (Read et al., 1989). Epithelial damage may in turn contribute to bronchial hyperresponsiveness through several distinct pathways (Cuss and Barnes, 1987). A summary of these putative mechanisms is shown in Figure 5.

E. Mucus Secretion

PAF stimulates secretion of mucin from explants of trachea from the guinea pig, rat, rabbit, and ferret in organ culture; however, this effect is small and only significant at high concentrations (10^{-4}M). Enhanced secretion by PAF was not the result of a cytotoxic effect of PAF or due to the secondary release of histamine, but this could occur through activation of leukotriene biosynthesis (Adler et al., 1987).

V. Antagonists of PAF

Over the past 5-6 years, there has been a great interest among pharmaceutical companies in the development of specific antagonists of PAF. Such compounds would be useful tools for defining the role of PAF under both

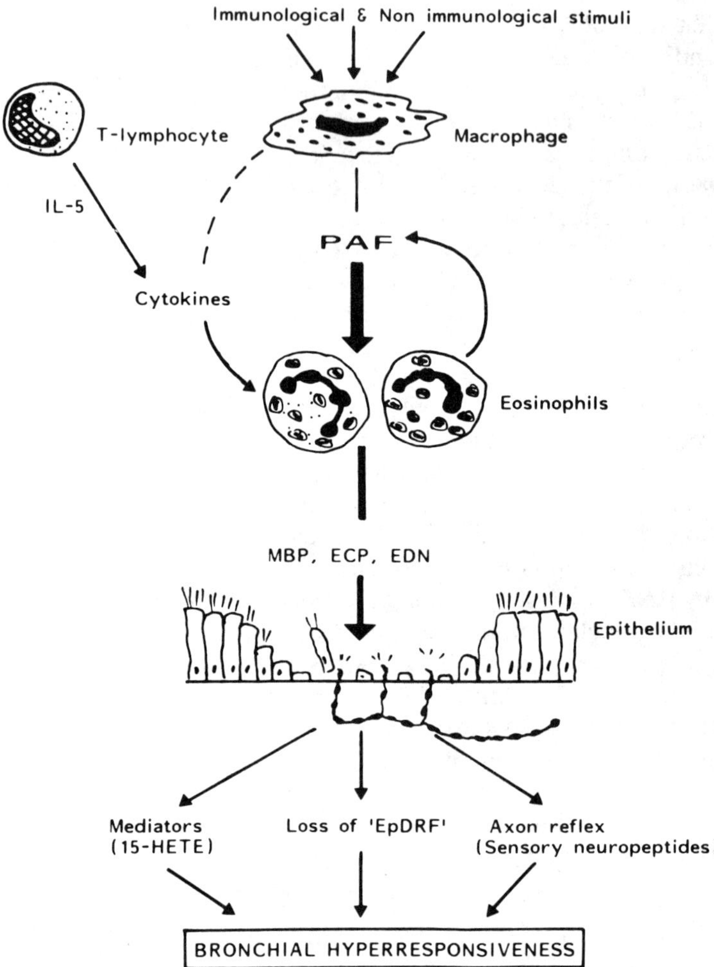

Figure 5 Putative mechanisms for PAF-induced bronchial hyperresponsiveness. MBP, major basic protein; ECP, eosinophil cationic protein; EDN, eosinophil-derived neurotoxin; EpDRF, epithelial-derived relaxant factor; 15-HETE, 15-hydroxy-eicosatetraenoic acid.

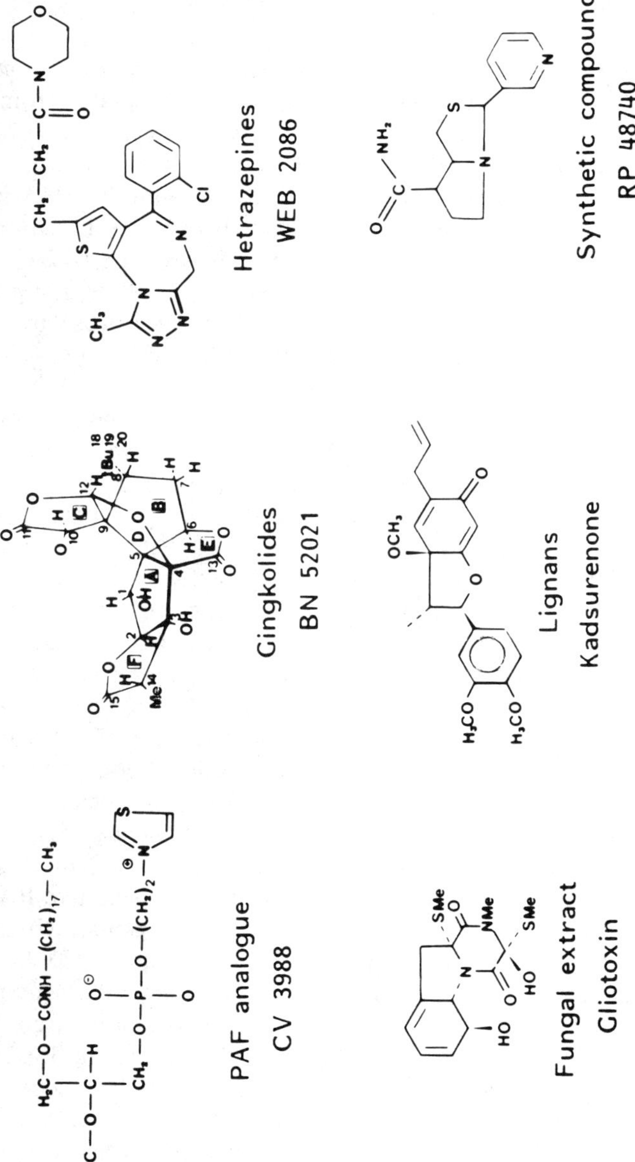

Figure 6 Chemical structures of antagonists of platelet-activating factor. Major classes with an example from each are shown.

normal and pathological conditions; in addition, these compounds may represent a novel class of agents for the treatment of some inflammatory conditions such as asthma.

Antagonists of PAF have either been developed by modification of the PAF molecule or discovered from natural compounds isolated from plants (Fig. 6). Structural analogues of PAF such as CV3988 were the first compounds with PAF antagonistic activities described (Terashita et al., 1983). Although CV3988 was first reported specifically to inhibit PAF-induced platelet aggregation, it has now been shown to also possess antagonistic activity against arachidonic acid and adenosine diphosphate (ADP) at high concentrations (Nunez et al., 1986). Another analog, CV6209, is reported to be 80 times more potent than CV3988 but is poorly absorbed by the oral route. Other related antagonists such as SRI 63-119 and Ro 19-3704 have been described.

Extensive screening tests of a number of natural compounds have shown them to antagonize the actions of PAF. Kadsurenone was obtained from the Chinese medicinal herb, haifenteng (*Piper futokadsurae*) and is a natural benzofuranoid neolignan (Shen et al., 1985). More potent analogs such as L-652,731 have also been developed (Hwang et al., 1985b). Kadsurenone is a specific and potent inhibitor of PAF-induced platelet aggregation and inhibits the binding of [³H]PAF to receptors on platelets and lung membranes. It is also active in vivo in blocking PAF-induced cutaneous wheal responses in the guinea pig (Hwang et al., 1985c). Another group of naturally occurring antagonists of PAF, the ginkgolides, are extracted from the leaves of the *Ginkgo biloba* tree; they have been used since ancient times as a remedy for chest complaints including cough and wheeze (Braquet et al., 1985). Ginkgolide B (BN 52021) is the most potent of this family and has recently been synthesized. These compounds inhibit the binding of labeled PAF from its receptor in both human platelets and lung tissue. BN 52021 inhibits PAF-induced platelet aggregation; this effect appears to be specific to PAF since it demonstrated no antagonism of other aggregating agents such as ADP, collagen, arachidonic acid, thrombin, or calcium ionophore A23187 (Nunez et al., 1986; Braquet et al., 1985). BN 52021 also inhibits PAF-induced degranulation of human neutrophils and chemotaxis of human eosinophils (Braquet et al., 1985; Kurihara et al., 1988). In the guinea pig, BN 52063 (a mixture of ginkgolides with 40% of BN 52021) caused a dose-dependent inhibition of airway microvascular leakage induced by PAF (Evans et al., 1987). Another class of natural PAF antagonist gliotoxins has been extracted from a wood fungus (Okamoto et al., 1986).

One well-defined pharmacological class of compound, the triazolobenzodiazepines, such as alprazolam and triazolam, has recently been shown to possess PAF antagonist activity (Kornecki et al., 1985). More recently, compounds now termed hetrazepines have been developed with more potent antagonistic effects but devoid of sedative effects (Casals-Stenzel and Weber, 1987). WEB 2086, for example, was found to be more potent than the BN 52063 compound in inhibiting PAF-induced human platelet aggregation in vitro (Evans et al., 1988a). More potent hetrazepines such as WEB 2170 and STY 2108 have been shown to be effective at dosages of 1-100 mg/kg in the guinea pig (Heuer et al., 1988).

Evaluation of these PAF antagonists in humans is at an early stage. The ginkgolide mixture, BN 52063, administered orally at single doses of 80 mg or 120 mg, is well tolerated by normal volunteers and potently inhibits PAF-induced wheal and flare responses in the skin in a dose-dependent fashion within an hour of ingestion (Chung et al., 1987; Fig. 7). This is associated with an inhibition of PAF-induced platelet aggregation ex vivo. The PAF analog, CV3988, has been infused in normal volunteers and results in a dosage-dependent inhibition of PAF-induced platelet aggregation ex vivo at dosages that resulted in small degrees of hemolysis (Arnout et al., 1988). WEB 2086 has been administered intravenously (0.5-50 mg), orally (1-400 mg), or by aerosol (0.05-1.0 mg) and found to be extremely potent in inhibiting PAF-induced platelet aggregation with no side effects (Adamus et al., 1988a,b). However, only a small inhibitory effect of BN 52063 (120 mg orally) against PAF-induced bronchoconstriction was observed (Fig. 8), with no effect on the accompanying neutropenia (Roberts et al., 1988a), which suggests that the bioavailability of the BN compound within the airways is small, and that more potent antagonists, preferably administered by the inhaled route, will be necessary for the treatment of asthma.

VI. Evidence for a Role of PAF in Asthma

A. Measurement of PAF Release

Measurement of PAF in biological fluids such as plasma and bronchoalveolar lavage fluid remains difficult. PAF is rapidly hydrolyzed to lyso-PAF by acetylhydrolase in plasma and is degraded rapidly by inflammatory cells such as neutrophils and by bronchiolar and alveolar epithelial cells (Chilton et al., 1983; Haroldsen et al., 1987). In addition, synthetized PAF may be preferentially stored within the activated cell rather than released outside the cell (Lynch and Henson, 1986). Loss of PAF during extraction procedures prior to bioassay using aggregation of washed platelets can be variable and considerable. Confirmation of the presence of PAF using mass spectrometry is necessary. Despite these difficulties, recovery of PAF in plasma and bronchoalveolar lavage fluid has been reported in asthmatic subjects, but without confirmation by mass spectrometry (Nakamura et al., 1987;

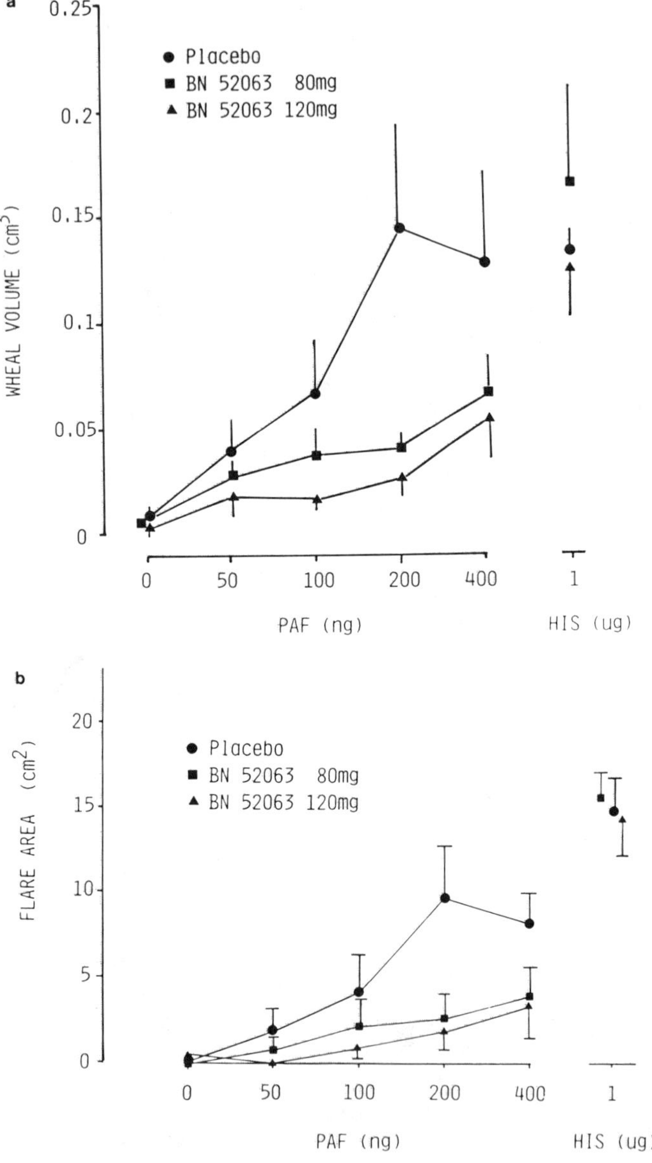

Figure 7 Effect of the ginkgolide mixture (80 mg ■ or 120 mg ▲ orally) or placebo (●) on flare areas and wheal volumes induced by intradermal platelet-activating factor (PAF) and histamine (HIS) in six normal subjects. There was significant inhibition of both wheal and flare responses particularly at the 200 and 400 ng dosage of PAF, with no effect on the histamine response. Values are means and SEM (reproduced from Chung et al., 1986).

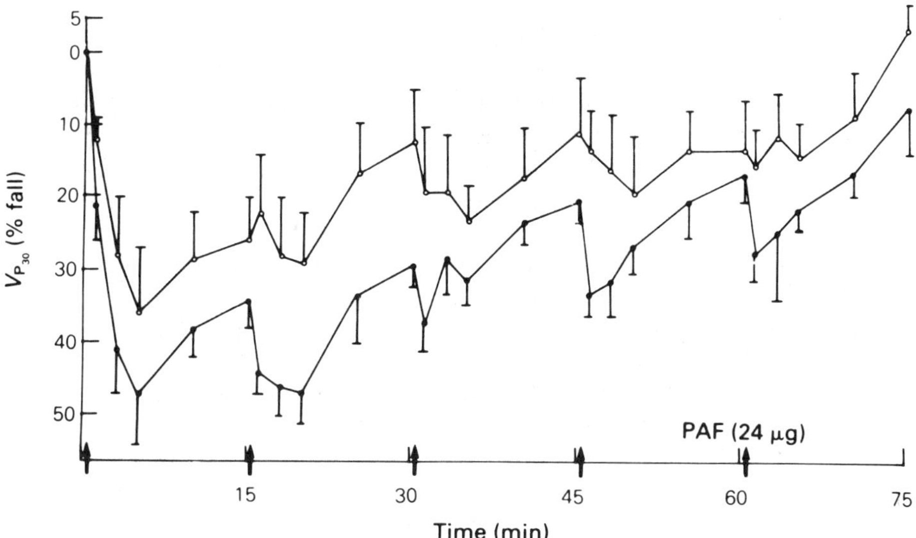

Figure 8 Time course of PAF-induced bronchoconstriction, indicated by changes in flow at 30% vital capacity (Vp30) after pretreatment with placebo (●) and the ginkgolide mixture, BN 52063, 120 mg orally (○) given 2 h prior to PAF challenge. Arrows indicate repeated inhalations of 25 µg PAF; mean values ± SEM for eight normal subjects. The response was significantly inhibited after BN 52063 after the first and second but not after subsequent inhalations of PAF ($p < 0.05$, t-test of differences between means; data from Roberts et al., 1988a).

Court et al., 1987). Nakamura et al. (1987) measured PAF activity in the plasma of asthmatic subjects following allergen challenge by acetylation of circulating lyso-PAF into the biologicaly active form of PAF. An increase in PAF activity, using a platelet-aggregating assay, was observed in subjects during the late asthmatic response but not in those with a single immediate response at 6 h after antigen challenge. There is no detectable PAF activity prior to acetylation in plasma. It is difficult to interpret this study because lyso-PAF can be both a precursor and a metabolite of PAF. Detectable amounts of PAF-like activity have been demonstrated in the plasma of patients with cold-induced urticaria within minutes after cold challenge (Grandel et al., 1985). PAF and lyso-PAF release has been shown in lung perfusates of sensitized lungs from guinea pigs challenged with ovalbumin aerosol (Fitzgerald et al., 1986). There are no data on whether PAF is released during IgE-mediated bronchoconstriction in subjects with allergic asthma.

B. Use of PAF Antagonists

In view of the difficulties in measuring PAF in biological fluids, specific and potent PAF antagonists are the best probes available for studying the role of PAF in asthma. The effects of PAF antagonists on the airway responses to ovalbumin in sensitized guinea pigs have been studied. BN 52021 antagonizes both heterologous and homologous passive bronchoconstriction in response to intravenous allergen challenge (Touvay et al., 1985). The histamine- and leukotriene-independent contraction induced by ovalbumin of sensitized lung parenchymal strips in vitro and of intact lungs in vivo was also suppressed by kadsurenone (Darius et al., 1986). However, both BN 52063 and WEB 2086 at dosages that were effective in blocking the effects of PAF of up to 100 mg/kg did not affect ovalbumin-induced airway microvascular leakage in the guinea pig (Evans et al., 1988a,b). Of greater interest is the effect of PAF antagonists on the late-phase airway response after antigen challenge, which is associated with an influx of eosinophils into the airways (DeMonchy et al., 1985). Preliminary reports show that a continuous infusion of WEB 2086 in the *Ascaris*-sensitive sheep inhibits the late-phase response after challenge with *Ascaris* antigen, without affecting the early response (Stevenson et al., 1987). Because sulfidopeptide leukotriene antagonists also produce similar results (Abraham et al., 1986), interactions between leukotrienes and PAF in this model of late-phase response must be considered. BN 52021 has been reported to blunt the late response and the associated increase in bronchial responsiveness after allergen challenge in ragweed-sensitized rabbits, but this is achieved at a rather high dosage of BN 52021 (100 mg/kg) (Coyle et al., 1987). BN 52021 (20 mg/kg) also inhibits both ovalbumin-induced bronchial hyperresponsiveness and eosinophil recovery into bronchoalveolar lavage fluid in the ovalbumin-sensitized guinea-pig (Coyle et al., 1988). Both BN 52021 (3 mg/kg) and WEB 2086 (3 mg/kg) inhibit the influx of eosinophils into the airway wall in a similar model (Lellouch-Tubiana, 1988). These observations suggest that PAF may induce bronchial hyperresponsiveness by recruitment and activation of circulating eosinophils. In vitro studies also suggest that PAF may be involved in some models of eosinophil activation. Thus, BN 52021 dosage-dependently decreased the cytotoxicity of purified human hypodense eosinophils for *Schistosoma* larvae in the presence of specific IgE antibodies (Capron et al., 1988).

There are virtually no studies of PAF antagonists to review, particularly their effects on the late-phase response or the bronchial hyperresponsiveness after allergen challenge in humans. The effects of the ginkgolide mixture BN 52063 on the skin response to allergen in atopic subjects have recently been reported (Roberts et al., 1988). BN52063 (at a dosage of 120 mg orally)

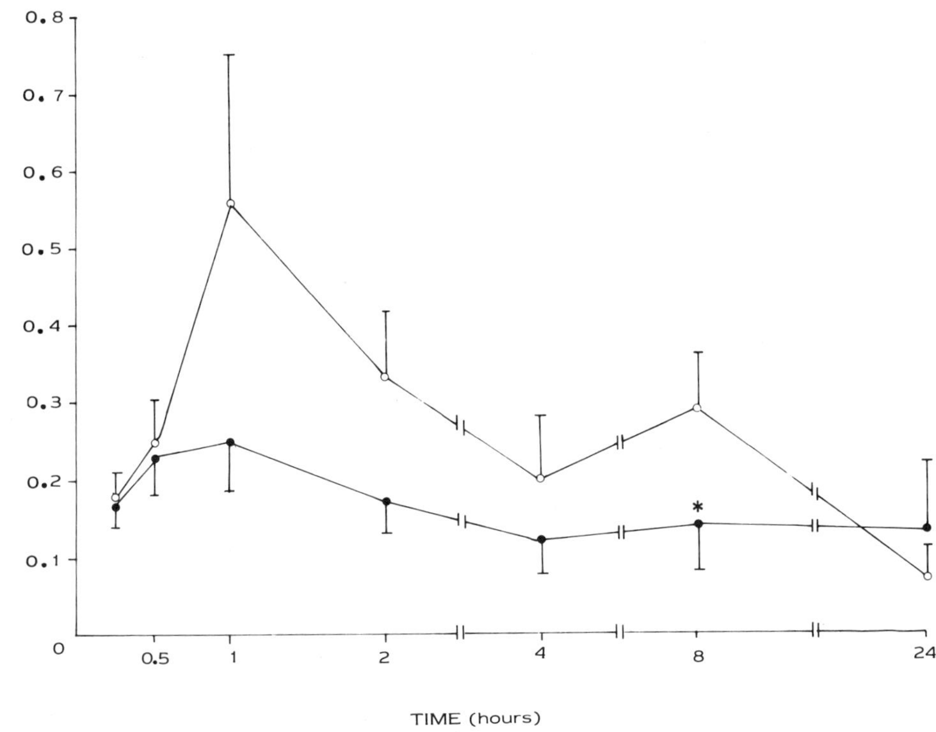

Figure 9 Effect of the ginkgolide mixture BN 52063 (120 mg orally) (●) 2 h before intradermal injection of antigen on inflammatory swelling volume compared to responses after placebo (diluent; ○) in 10 atopic subjects. Note the significant inhibition of late-phase induration (* $p < 0.05$, Wilcoxon as signed rank test). Data are shown as mean ± SEM (reproduced from Roberts et al., 1988b).

inhibits PAF-induced wheal and flare responses and significantly attenuated the late-phase induration without significant alteration in the early wheal response (Fig. 9). This probably indicates an inhibitory effect of BN 52063 on eosinophil infiltration into the skin. There are no data on the effects of chronic dosing with PAF antagonists on the airways.

VII. Conclusions

Much remains to be discovered about the biology of PAF and its possible role in the inflammatory process in asthma. Regulation of the metabolism of

PAF in normal and inflamed tissues has to be elucidated, and the localization of receptors of PAF within the airways of normal and asthmatic subjects may help us to understand the mechanisms of action of PAF. The interactions of PAF with other mediators, particularly of the lipoxygenase and cyclooxygenase pathway, need to be clarified further. The special relationship between PAF and the eosinophil could be crucial in the pathogenesis of bronchial hyperresponsiveness of asthma. Such information will be necessary for the interpretation of results of PAF antagonist treatment in patients with asthma and in planning their best use. Whether PAF antagonists will be of use in the treatment of asthma and their place in our antiasthma armamentarium remain to be determined.

Discussion

Kaliner: How can a molecule as short-lived as PAF cause such long-lasting effects in tissues?

Chung: PAF may interact with eosinophils, which may be stimulated to release more PAF, with consequent amplification of the response.

Barnes: In primates, PAF can stimulate eosinophil accumulation in lungs for up to 2 weeks after a single inhalation, which suggests that it can initiate a sequence of events.

Fuller: Why are asthmatic subjects not responsive to PAF?

Chung: PAF did not significantly increase airway responses to methacholine in a group of 8 patients with mild asthma, although some showed an increase. Perhaps it is more difficult to measure the small increase in responsiveness in patients with asthma, or perhaps it is more difficult to increase further responsiveness in airways that are already hyperresponsive.

Irwin: Can you comment on "priming" of inflammatory cells by PAF?

Chung: PAF has been shown by Braquet et al. to prime inflammatory cells such as neutrophils in very low concentrations. In patients with asthma we find eosinophils to be more responsive to PAF, perhaps because these cells have been primed by cytokines such as GM-CSF or IL-5.

Fabbri: Studies in dogs suggest that PAF-induced hyperresponsiveness is related to neutrophils. Is this true for humans?

Chung: In normal subjects we have shown that there is a significant increase in neutrophils in BAL fluid 3 h after a PAF inhalation; this increase is *inversely* related to the increase in responsiveness, however.

Leff: In dog the *acute* effects of PAF are mediated via release of serotonin from platelets. In humans serotonin is not a constrictor, so do you know the mechanism of acute bronchoconstriction?

Chung: We believe that the acute airway narrowing after PAF may be partly due to airway edema and partly due to release of a secondary bronchoconstrictor. This does *not* seem to be either histamine or thromboxane, and we cannot inhibit it with infused prostacyclin, so we have no evidence that platelet activation is involved.

Fish: The fact that asthmatic patients are not more responsive to PAF than normal subjects may be due to a lack of smooth muscle constrictor effect.

Chung: We agree that it could reflect edema. After administration of albuterol 200 μg, which completely blocked methacholine-induced bronchoconstriction, there was only about a 50% reduction in the PAF response.

Laitinen: Is there any evidence that PAF-induced increased BHR is related to epithelial damage, as with viral infection?

Chung: This may be so. There is certainly histological evidence in animals demonstrating epithelial shedding after intravenous or inhaled PAF.

O'Byrne: Does PAF cause a late-phase response?

Chung: We have not seen one in airways or skin, but perhaps this may be possible with higher local dosages of PAF.

Pipkorn: PAF at high dosages in the nose never gives a late-response.

Karlsson: Platelet supernatants, after stimulation with PAF, are reported to increase airway responsiveness in guinea pigs. Is there any evidence of this in humans.

Chung: Not in humans. In guinea pigs there is also evidence that platelets may mediate PAF- and allergen-induced eosinophil recruitment into the lungs.

Acknowledgments

Part of the work quoted in this chapter was supported by the Asthma Research Council and Medical Research Council (UK). We are grateful to Margaret Sherrington for her help during the preparation of this chapter.

References

Abraham, W. M., Wanner, A., Stevenson, J. S., and Chapman, G. A. (1986). The effect of an orally active leukotriene D4/E4 antagonist, LY 171883, an antigen-induced airway responses in allergic sheep. *Prostaglandins* **31**:457-467.

Adamus, W. S., Heuer, H., Meade, C. J., and Brecht, H. M. (1988a). Effect of peroral WEB 2086 on *ex-vivo* platelet- activating factor induced platelet aggregation in man (Abstract). *Prostaglandins* **35**:836.

Adamus, W. S., Heuer, H., Meade, C. J., Kempe, E. R., and Brecht, H. M. (1988b). Effect of intravenous or inhalative WEB 2086 on *ex-vivo* platelet-activating factor induced platelet aggregation in man. *Prostaglandins* **35**:797.

Adler, K. B., Schwartz, J. E., Anderson, W. H., and Welton, A. F. (1987). Platelet activating factor stimulates secretion of mucin by explants of rodent airways in organ culture. *Exp. Lung Res.* **13**:25-43.

Arnout, J., Hecken, A. V., Delpeleire, I., Miyamoto, Y., Holmes, I., De Schepper, and Vermylen, J. (1988). Effectiveness and tolerability of CV3988, a selective PAF antagonist, after intravenous administration in man. *Br. J. Clin. Pharmacol.* **25**:445-452.

Arnoux, B., Joseph, M., Simoes, A. H., Tonnel, A. B., Duroux, P., Capron, A., and Benveniste, J. (1987). Antigenic release of PAF-acether and beta-glucuronidase from alveolar macrophages of asthmatics. *Bull. Eur. Physiopathol. Respir.* **23**:119-124.

Arnoux, B., Denjean, A., Page, C. P., Nolibe, D., Morley, J., and Benveniste, J. (1988). Accumulation of platelets and eosinophils in baboon lung after PAF-acether challenge: inhibition by ketotifen. *Am. Rev. Respir. Dis.* **137**:855-860.

Aursudkij, B., Rogers, D. F., Evans, T. W., Alton, E. W. F. W., Chung, K. F., and Barnes, P. J. (1987). Reduced tracheal mucus velocity in guinea pig *in-vivo* by platelet activating factor (abstract). *Am. Rev. Respir. Dis.* **35**:160.

Barnes, P. J., Grandordy, B. M., Page, C. P., Rhoden, K. J., and Robertson, D. N. (1987). The effect of platelet activating factor on pulmonary beta-adrenoceptors. *Br. J. Pharmacol.* **90**:709-715.

Barnes, P. J., Chung, K. F., and Page, C. P. (1988). Platelet-activating factor as a mediator of allergic disease. *J. Allergy Clin. Immunol.* **81**:919-934.

Benveniste, J., Henson, P. M., and Cochrane, C. G. (1972). Leucocyte dependent histamine release from rabbit platelets: the role of IgE, basophils and a platelet activating factor. *J. Exp. Med.* **136**:1356-1377.

Benveniste, J., Tence, M., Varenne, P., Bidault, J., Boullet, C., and Polonsky, J. (1979). Semi-synthese et structure proposée du facteur activant les plaquettes (PAF): PAF-acether, un alkyl ether analogue de la lysophosphotidylcholine. *C. R. Acad. Sci.* **289**:1037-1040.

Blank, M. L., Snyder, F., Byers, W. L., Brooks, B., and Muirhead, E. E. (1979). Antihypertensive activity of an alkyl ether analog of phosphatidylcholine. *Biochem. Biophys. Res. Commun.* **90**:523-534.

Blank, M. L., Lee, T. C., Fitzgerald, V., and Snyder, F. (1981). A specific acetylhydrolase for 1-alkyl-2-acetyl-sn-glycero-3-phosphocholine (a hypotensive and platelet-activating lipid). *J. Biochem.* **256**:175-178.

Boschetto, P., Roberts, N. M., Rogers, D. F., and Barnes, P. J. (1988). Effect of anti-asthma drugs on microvascular leakage in guinea-pig airways (abstract). *Am. Rev. Respir. Dis.* **137**:179.

Braquet, P., Spinnewyn, B., Braquet, M., Bourgain, R. H., Taylor, J. E., Etienne, A., and Drieu, K. (1985). BN 52021 and related compounds: a new series of highly specific PAF-receptor antagonists isolated from *Ginkgo biloba. Blood Vessels* **16**:559-572.

Bruynzeel, P. L. B., Koenderman, L., Kok, P. T. M., Hameling, M. L., and Verhagen, J. (1986). Platelet-activating factor (Paf-acether)-induced leukotriene C4 formation and luminol-dependent chemiluminescence by human eosinophils. *Pharmacol. Res. Commun.* **18**:61-70.

Capron, M., Benveniste, J., Braquet, P., and Capron, A. (1988). Role of PAF-acether in IgE-dependent activation of eosinophils. In *New Trends in Lipid Mediators Research: The Role of Platelet-Activating Factor in Immune Disorders.* Edited by P. Braquet. Basel, Karger, pp. 10-17.

Casals-Stenzel, J., and Weber, K. H. (1987). Triazolobenzodiazepines: dissociation of their Paf (platelet-activating factor) anatagonistic and CNS activity. *Br. J. Pharmacol.* **90**:139-146.

Chilton, F. H., O'Flaherty, J. T., Ellis, J. M., Swendsen, C. L., and Wykle, R. L. (1983). Metabolic fate of platelet-activating factor in neutrophils. *J. Biol. Chem.* **258**:6357-6361.

Christman, B. W., Lefferts, P. L., and Snopper, J. R. (1987). Effect of platelet activating factor on aerosol histamine responses in awake sheep. *Am. Rev. Respir. Dis.* **135**:1267-1270.

Christman, B. W., Lefferts, P. L., King, G. A., and Snapper, J. R. (1988). Role of circulating platelets and granulocytes in PAF-induced pulmonary dysfunction in awake sheep. *J. Appl. Physiol.* **64**:2033-2041.

Chung, K. F. (1986). Role of inflammation in the hyperreactivity of the airways in asthma. *Thorax* **41**:657-662.

Chung, K. F., and Barnes, P. J. (1988). PAF antagonists: their potential therapeutic role in asthma. *Drugs* **35**:93-103.

Chung, K. F., and Barnes, P. J. (1989). Effects of platelet-activating factor on airway calibre, airway responsiveness and circulating cells in asthmatic subjects. *Thorax* **44**:108-115.

Chung, K. F., Aizawa, H., Leikauf, G. D., Ueki, I. F., Evans, T. W., and Nadel, J. A. (1986). Airway hyperresponsiveness induced by platelet-activating factor: role of thromboxane generation. *J. Pharmacol. Exp. Ther.* **236**:580-584.

Chung, K. F., Dent, G., McCusker, M., Guinot, Ph., Page, C. P., and Barnes P. J. (1987). Effect of a ginkgolide mixture (BN 52063) in antagonising skin and platelet responses to platelet activating factor in man. *Lancet* **1**:248-251.

Chung, K. F., Minette, P., McCusker, M., and Barnes, P. J. (1988). Ketotifen inhibits the cutaneous but not the airway responses to platelet-
activating factor in man. *J. Allergy Clin. Immunol.* **81**:1192-1197.

Chung, K. F., Dent, G., and Barnes, P. J. (1989). Effects of salbutamol on
bronchoconstriction, bronchial hyperresponsiveness and leucocyte responses induced by platelet activating factor in man. *Thorax* **44**:102-107.

Conrad, G. W., and Rink, T. J. (1986). Platelet activating factor raises intracellular calcium ion concentration in macrophages. *J. Cell Biol.* **103**:
439-450.

Court, E. N., Goadby, P., Hendrick, D. J., Kelly, C. A., Kingston, W.,
Stenton, S. C., and Walters, E. H. (1987). Platelet-activating factor in
bronchoalveolar lavage fluid from asthmatic patients (abstract). *Br. J.
Clin. Pharmacol.* **24**:258.

Coyle, A., Sjoerdsma, K., Page, C. P., Brown, L., and Metzger, W. J. (1987).
Modification of the late asthmatic response and bronchial hyperreac-
tivity by BN 52021, a platelet-activating factor antagonist (abstract).
Clin. Res. **35**:254.

Coyle, A. J., Unwin, S. C., Page, C. P., Touvay, C., Villain, B., and Braquet,
P. (1988). The effect of the selective antagonist Bn 52021 on PAF and
antigen-induced bronchial hyperreactivity and eosinophil accumulation.
Eur. J. Pharmacol. **148**:51-58.

Cuss, F. M., and Barnes, P. J. (1987). Epithelial mediators. *Am. Rev. Respir.
Dis.* **136**:32S-35S.

Cuss, F. M., Dixon, C. M. S., and Barnes, P. J. (1986). Effects of inhaled
platelet activating factor on pulmonary function and bronchial responsiveness in man. *Lancet* **2**:189-192.

Darius, H., Lefer, D. J., Smith, B., and Lefer, A. M. (1986). Role of platelet-
activating factor-acether in mediating guinea pig anaphylaxis. *Science*
232:58-60.

De Monchy, J. G. R., Kauffman, H. F., Venge, P., Koeter, G. H., Jansen,
H. M., Sluiter, H. J., and de Vries, K. (1985). Bronchoalveolar eosino-
phils during allergen-induced late asthmatic reactions. *Am. Rev. Respir.
Dis.* **131**:373-376.

Demopoulos, C. A., Pinckard, R. N., and Hanahan, D. J. (1979). Platelet-
activating factor. Evidence for 1-0-alkyl-2-acetyl-sn-glyceryl-3-phos-
phorylcholine as the active component (a new class of lipid chemical
mediators). *J. Biol. Chem.* **254**:9355-9358.

Denjean, A., Arnoux, B., Masse, R., Lockhart, A., and Benveniste, J. (1983).
Acute effects of intratracheal administration of platelet-activating factor
in baboons. *J. Appl. Physiol.* **55**:799-804.

Dent, G., Ukena, D., Chanez, P., Sybrecht, G. W., and Barnes, P. J. (1988). Characterization of platelet-activating factor (PAF) receptors in human neutrophils and eosinophils using the new competitive PAF antagonist WEB 2086 (Abstract). *Am. Rev. Respir. Dis.* **137**:236.

Dent, G., Ukena, D., Mak, J. C. W., Sybrecht, G. W., and Barnes, P. J. (1989). Platelet-activating factor receptors in human and guinea-pig lung: demonstration using the novel antagonist ligand [3H] WEB 2086 (Abstract). *Am. Rev. Respir. Dis.* **139**:A94.

Dewald, B., and Baggiolini, M. (1985). Activation of NADPH oxidase in human neutrophils. Synergism between fMLP and the neutrophil products PAF and LTB4. *Biochem. Biophys. Res. Commun.* **128**:297-304.

Evans, T. W., Chung, K. F., Rogers, D. F., and Barnes, P. J. (1987). Effect of platelet-activating factor on airway vascular permeability: possible mechanisms. *J. Appl. Physiol.* **63**:479-484.

Evans, T. W., Dent, G., Rogers, D. F., Aursudkij, B., Chung, K. F., and Barnes, P. J. (1988a). Effect of a PAF antagonist, WEB 2086, on airway microvascular leakage in the guinea pig and platelet aggregation in man. *Br. J. Pharmacol.* **94**:164-168.

Evans, T. W., Rogers, D. F., Aursudkij, B., Chung, K. F., and Barnes, P. J. (1988b). Inflammatory mediators involved in antigen-induced airway microvascular leakage in guinea-pigs. *Am. Rev. Respir. Dis.* **138**:395-399.

Evans, T. W., Rogers, D. F., Aursudkij, B., Chung, K. F., and Barnes, P. J. (1989). Regional and time-dependent effects of inflammatory mediators on airway microvascular permeability in guinea pigs. *Clin. Sci.* **76**:479-485.

Farr, R. S., Cox, C. P., Wardlow, M. L., and Jorenson, R. (1980). Preliminary studies of an acid labile factor (ALF) in human sera that inactivates platelet-activating factor (PAF). *Clin. Immunol. Immunopathol.* **15**:318-330.

Fitzgerald, M. F., Moncada, S., and Parente, L. (1986). The anaphylactic release of platelet-activating factor from perfused guinea-pig lungs. *Br. J. Pharmacol.* **88**:149-153.

Fitzgerald, M. F., Lees, I. W., Parente, L., and Payne, A. N. (1987). Exposure to Paf-acether aerosol induced airway hyperresponsiveness to 5-HT in guinea-pigs (abstract). *Br. J. Pharmacol.* **90**:112.

Frigas, E., and Gleich, G. J. (1986). The eosinophil and the pathology of asthma. *J. Allergy Clin. Immunol.* **77**:527-537.

Garcia, J. G. N., Azghani, A., Callahan, K. S., and Johnson, A. R. (1988). Effect of platelet-activating factor on leukocyte-endothelial cell interactions. *Thromb. Res.* **51**:83-96.

Gateau, O., Arnoux, B., Deriaz, H., Viars, P., and Benveniste, J. (1984). Acute effects of intratracheal administration of PAF-acether (platelet-activating factor) in humans (Abstract). *Am. Rev. Respir. Dis.* **129**:A3.

Grandel, K. E., Farr, R. S., Wanderer, A. A., Eisenstadt, D. T., and Wasserman, S. I. (1985). Association of platelet-activating factor in primary acquired cold urticaria. *N. Engl. J. Med.* **313**:405-409.

Hallam, J. T., Sanchez, A., and Rink, T. J. (1984). Stimulus-response coupling in human platelet: changes evoked by platelet-activating factor in cytoplasmic free calcium monitored with the fluorescent calcium indicator Quin 2. *Biochem. J.* **218**:819.

Halonen, M., Lohman, I. C., Dunn, A. M., McManus, L. M., and Palmer, J. D. (1985). Participation of platelets in the physiologic alterations of the AGEPC response and of IgE anaphylaxis in the rabbit. *Am. Rev. Respir. Dis.* **131**:11-17.

Hanahan, D. J., Demopoulos, C. A., Liehr, J., and Pinkard, R. N. (1980). Identification of platelet-activating factor isolated from rabbit basophils as acetylglyceryl ether phosphorlcholine. *J. Biol. Chem.* **255**:5514-5516.

Haroldsen, P. E., Voelkel, N. F., Henson, J. E., Henson, P. M., and Murphy, R. C. (1987). Metabolism of platelet-activating factor in isolated perfused rat lung. *J. Clin. Invest.* **79**:1860-1867.

Henocq, E., and Vargaftig, B. B. (1988). Skin eosinophilia in atopic patients. *J. Allergy Clin. Immunol.* **81**:691-695.

Heuer, H., Casals-Stenzel, J., Maucevig, G., Stransky, W., and Weber, K. H. (1988). Activity of the new and specific PAF-antagonists WEB 2170 and STY 2108 on PAF-induced bronchoconstriction and intrathoracic accumulation of platelets in the guinea-pig (Abstract). *Prostaglandins* **35**:798.

Hwang, S.-B., Lam, M.-H., and Shen, T. Y. (1985a). Specific binding sites for platelet'activating factor in human lung tissues. *Biochem. Biophys. Res. Commun.* **128**:972-979.

Hwang, S. B., Lam, M. H., Biftu, T., Beattie, T. R., and Shen, T. Y. (1985b). Trans-2, 5-Bis- (3,4,5,-trimethotyphenyl) tetrahydrofuran: an orally active specific and competitive receptor antagonist of platelet activating factor. *J. Biol. Chem.* **260**:15639-15645.

Hwang, S. B., Li, C. L., Lam, M. H., and Shen, T. Y. (1985c). Characterization of cutaneous vascular permeability induced by platelet-activating factor in guinea-pigs and rats and its inhibition by a platelet-activating factor antagonist. *Lab. Invest.* **52**:617-630.

Hwang, S. B., Lam, M. H., and Chang, M. N. (1986). Specific binding of [3H]dihydrokadsurenone to rabbit platelet membranes and its inhibition by the receptor agonists and antagonists of platelet-activating factor. *J. Biol. Chem.* **261**:13720-13726.

Kimani, G., Tonnesen, M. G., and Henson, P. G. (1988). Stimulation of eosinophil adherence to human vascular endothelial cells *in vitro by* platelet activating factor. *J. Immunol.* **140**:3161-3166.

Kioumis, I., Lammers, J. W., Dent, G., Chung, K. F., and Barnes, P. J. (1988). Effect of inhaled platelet-activating factor on circulating neutrophils and platelets in vivo and ex vivo in man. *Prostaglandins* **36**:343-354.

Kornecki, E., Garlich, Y. H., and Lenox, R. H. (1985). Platelet-activating factor-induced aggregation of human platelets specifically inhibited by triazolobenzodiazepines. *Science* **226**:1954-1956.

Kroegel, C., Yukawa, T., Dent, G., Chanez, P., Chung, K. F., and Barnes, P. J. (1988). Platelet activating factor induces eosinophil peroxidase release from purified human eosinophils. *Immunology* **64**:559-562.

Kroegel, C., Pleass, R., Yukawa, T., Chung, K. F., Westwick, J., and Barnes, P. J. (1989). Characterization of platelet-activating factor-induced elevation of cytosolic free calcium concentrations in eosinophils. *FEBS Letts.* **243**:41-46.

Kurihara, K., Wardlaw, A. J., Moqbel, R., and Kay, A. B. (1988). The ginkgolide (BN52021) inhibits PAF-induced chemotaxis and specific finding to human eosinophils and neutrophils (abstract). *J. Allergy Clin. Immunol.* **81**:159.

Lammers, J. W., Kioumis, I., McCusker, M. N., Nichol, G. M., Barnes, P. J., Chung, K. F. (1990). Effect of prostaglandin against bronchoconstriction induced by platelet-activating factor. *J. Allergy Clin. Immunol.* In Press.

Lee, T. C., Malone, E., Wasserman, S. I., Fitzgerald, V., and Snyder, F. (1982). Activities of enzymes that metabolises PAF in neutrophils and eosinophils from humans and the effect of calcium ionophore. *Biochem. Biophys. Res. Commun.* **105**:1301-1308.

Lee, T. C., Malone, B., and Snyder, F. (1983). Stimulation of calcium uptake by 1-alkyl-2-actetyl-sn-glycero-3-phosphocholine (platelet-activating factor) in rabbit platelets: possible involvement of the lipoxygenase pathway. *Arch. Biochem. Biophys.* **223**:33-39.

Lee, T. C., Lenihan, D. J., Malone, B., Roddy, L. L., and Wasserman, S. I. (1984). Increased biosynthesis of platelet activating factor in activated human eosinophils. *J. Biol. Chem.* **259**:5526-5530.

Leff, A. R., White, S. R., Munoz, N. M., Popovich, K. J., Shioya, T., and Stimler-Gerard, N. P. (1987). Parasympathetic involvement in PAF-induced contraction in canine trachealis in-vivo. *J. Appl. Physiol.* **62**:599-605.

Lefort, J., Rotilio, D., and Vargaftig, B. B. (1984). The platelet-independent release of thromboxane A2 by PAF-acether for guinea-pig lungs involves mechanisms distinct from those for leukotriene C4 and bradykinin. *Br. J. Pharmacol.* **82**:525-531.

Lellouch-Tubiana, A., Lefort, J., Simon, M. T., Pfister, A., and Vargaftig, B. B. (1988). Eosinophil recruitment into guinea-pig lungs after PAF-acether and allergen administration: modulation by prostacyclin, platelet depletion and selective antagonists. *Am. Rev. Respir. Dis.* **137**:948-954.

Levy, J. V. (1983). Calmodulin antagonists inhibit aggregation of human, guinea-pig, and rabbit platelets induced with platelet-activating factor. *FEBS Letts.* **154**:262-264.

Lin, A. H., Morton, D. R., and Gorman, R. R. (1982). Acetylglyceryl ether phosphorylcholine stimulates leukotriene B4 synthesis in human polymorphonuclear leukocytes. *J. Clin. Invest.* **70**:1058-1065.

Long, W. M., Jackowski, J. T., and Cortes, A. (1988). Reversal of PAF-induced changes in bronchial blood flow (Qbr) and airflow resistance (R1) by prostaglandin (PG)E1 (abstract). *Am. Rev. Respir. Dis.* **137**:532.

Lynch, J. M., and Henson, P. M. (1986). The intracellular retention of newly synthetized platelet-activating factor. *J. Immunol.* **137**:2653-2661.

Macdonald, A. J., Moqbel, R., Wardlaw, A. J., and Kay, A. B. (1986). Platelet-activating factor (PAF-acether) enhances eosinophil cytotoxicity in-vitro (abstract). *J. Allergy Clin. Immunol.* **77**:227.

McIntyre, T. M., Zimmerman, G. A., Satoh, K., and Prescott, S. M. (1985). Cultured endothelial cells synthesize both platelet-activating factor and prostacyclin in response to histamine, bradykinin, and adenosine triphosphate. *J. Clin. Invest.* **76**:271-280.

Maridonneau-Parini, I., Lagente, V., Lefort, J., Randon, J., Russo-Marie, F., and Vargaftig, B. B. (1985). Desensitization of PAF-induced bronchoconstriction and to activation of alveolar macrophages by repeated inhalation of PAF in the guinea-pig. *Biochem. Biophys. Res. Commun.* **131**:42-49.

Mazzoni, L., Morley, J., Page, C. P., and Sanjar, S. (1985). Induction of airway hyper-reactivity by platelet activating factor in the guinea-pig (abstract). *J. Physiol.* **365**:107.

Miller, O. V., Ayer, D. E., and Gorman, R. R. (1982). Acetyl glyceryl phosphorylcholine inhibition of prostaglandin I2-stimulated adenosine 3, 5-cyclic monophosphate levels in human platelets. Evidence for thromboxane A2 dependence. *Biochem. Biophys. Acta* **711**:445-451.

Miwa, M., Miyake, T., Yamanaka, T., Sugatani, J., Suzuki, Y., Sakata, S., Araki, Y., and Matsumoto, M. (1988). Characterization of serum platelet-activating factor (PAF) acetylhydrolase: correlation between deficiency of serum PAF acetylhydrolase and respiratory symptoms in asthmatic children. *J. Clin. Invest.* **82**:1983-1991.

Moreno, R. H., Hogg, J. C., and Pare, P. D. (1986). Mechanics of airway narrowing. *Am. Rev. Respir. Dis.* **133**:1171-1180.

Nakamura, T., Morita, Y., Kuriyama, M., Ishihara, K., Ito, K., and Miyamoto, T. (1987). Platelet-activating factor in late asthmatic response. *Int. Arch. Allergy Appl. Immunol.* **82**:57-61.

Ninio, E., Mencia-Huerta, J. M., and Benveniste, J. (1983). Biosynthesis of platelet-activating factor (paf-acether). V. Enhancement of acetyltransferase activity in murine peritoneal cells by the calcium ionophere A 23187. *Biochim. Biophys. Acta* **751**:298-304.

Nunez, D., Chignard, M., Korth, R., Le-Couedic, J.-P., Norel, X., Spinnewyn, B., Braquet, P., and Benveniste, J. (1986). Specific inhibition of PAF-acether-induced platelet activation by BN 52021 and comparison with the PAF-acether inhibitors kadsurenone and CV 3988. *Eur. J. Pharmacol.* **123**:197-205.

O'Donnell, M. C., Henson, P. M., and Fiedel, B. A. (1979). Activation of human platelets by platelet-activating factor (PAF) derived from sensitized rabbit basophils. *Immunology* **35**:953-958.

O'Donnell, S. R., and Barnett, C. J. K. (1987). Microvascular leakage to platelet activating factor in guinea-pig trachea and bronchi. *Eur. J. Pharmacol.* **138**:385-396.

O'Flaherty, J. (1985). Neutrophil degranulation: evidence pertaining to its mediation by the combined effects of leukotriene B4, platelet-activating factor, and 5-HETE. *J. Cell Phys.* **122**:229-239.

O'Flaherty, J. T., Wykle, R. L., Miller, C. H., Lewis, J. C., Waite, M., Bass, D. A., McCall, C. E., and DeChatelet, L. R. (1981). 1-0-alkyl-sn-glyceryl-3-phosphorylcholines: a novel class of neutrophil stimulants. *Am. J. Pathol.* **103**:70-79.

O'Flaherty, J. T., Thomas, M. J., Hammett, M. J., Carroll, C., McCall, C. E., and Wykle, R. L. (1983). 5-L-hydroxy-6,8,11,14-eicosatetraenuate potentiates the human neutrophil degranulating action of platelet-activating factor. *Biochem. Biophys. Res. Commun.* **111**:1-7.

O'Flaherty, J. T., Surles, J. R., Redman, J., Jacobson, D., Piantadosi, C., and Wykle, R. L. (1986). Binding and metabolism of platelet-activating factor by human neutrophils. *J. Clin. Invest.* **78**:381-388.

Ojima-Uchiyama, A., Masazawa, Y., Sugiura, T., Waku, K., Saito, H., Yui, Y., and Tomioka, H. (1988). Phospholipid analysis of human eosinophils: high levels of alkylacylglycerophosphocholine (PAF precursor). *Lipids* **23**:815-817.

Okamoto, M., Yoshida, K., Uchida, I., Kohsaka, M., and Aoki, H. (1986). Studies of platelet activating factor (PAF) antagonists from microbial products. II. Pharmacological studies of FR-49175 in animal models. *Chem. Pharm. Bull. (Tokyo)* **34**:345-348.

Persson, C. G. A., Erjefalt, I., and Sundler, F. (1987). Airway microvascular and epithelial leakage of plasma induced by PAF-acether (PAF) and capsaicin (CAP). *Am. Rev. Respir. Dis.* **135**:A401.

Popovich, K. J., Sheldon, G., Mack, M., Munoz, N. M., Denberg, P., Blake, J., White, S. R., and Leff, A. R. (1988). Role of platelets in contraction of canine tracheal muscle elicited by PAF *in vitro*. *J. Appl. Physiol.* **65**:914-920.

Prescott, S. M., Zimmerman, G. A., and McIntyre, T. M. (1984). Human endothelial cells in culture produce platelet-activating factor (1-alkyl-2-acetyl-sn-glycero-3-phosphocholine) when stimulated with thrombin. *Proc. Natl. Acad. Sci. USA.* **81**:3534-3538.

Renooij, W., and Snyder, F. F., (1981). Biosynthesis of 1-alkyl-2-acetyl-sn-glycero-3-phosphocholine (platelet activating factor and a hypotensive lipid) by cholinephosphotransferase in various rat tissues. *Biochim. Biophys. Acta* **663**:545-556.

Roberts, N. M., McCusker, M., Chung, K. F., and Barnes, P. J. (1988a). The effect of PAF antagonist, BN 52063, on PAF-induced bronchoconstriction and neutropenia in man. *Br. J. Clin. Pharmacol.* **26**:65-72.

Roberts, N. M., Page, C. P., Chung, K. F., and Barnes, P. J. (1988b). The effect of a specific PAF antagonist, BN 52063, on antigen-induced cutaneous responses in man. *J. Allergy Clin. Immunol.* **82**:236-241.

Robertson, D. N., and Page, C. P. (1987). Effect of platelet agonists on airway reactivity and intrathoracic platelet accumulation. *Br. J. Pharmacol.* **92**:105-111.

Rodrique, F., Hoff, P., Touvay, C., Vilain, B., Carre. C., Mencia-Huerta, J. M., and Braquet, P. (1988). Platelet-activating factor induces the release of substance P and vasoactive intestinal peptide from guinea-pig lung tissues. In Braquet P. (ed): *The Role of Platelet-Activating Factor in Immune Disorders. New Trends in Lipid Mediators Research.* Edited by P. Braquet. Basel, Karger, pp. 93-98.

Rubin, A.-H., Smith, L. J., and Patterson, R. (1987). The bronchoconstrictor properties of platelet-activating factor in humans. *Am. Rev. Respir. Dis.* **136**:1145-1151.

Schellenberg, R. R. (1987). Airway responses to platelet-activating factor. *Am. Rev. Respir. Dis.* **136**:28-31.

Schleimer, R. P., MacGlashan, D. W., Peters, S. P., Pinckard, R. N., Adkinson, N. F., and Lichtenstein, L. M. (1986). Characterization of inflammatory mediator release from purified human lung mast cells. *Am. Rev. Respir. Dis.* **133**:614-617.

Shen, T. Y., Huang, S.-B., Chang, M. N., Doebber, T. W., Lam, M.-H., Wu, M. S., Wang, X., Han, G. Q., and Li, R. Z. (1985). Characterization of platelet-activating factor receptor antagonist isolated for haifenteng (Piper futokadsura): specific inhibition of in vitro and in vivo platelet-activating factor-induced effects. *Proc. Natl. Acad. Sci.* **82**:672-676.

Shukla, S. D., and Hanahan, D. J. (1982). AGEPC (platelet activating factor) induced stimulation of rabbit platelets: effects on phosphatidylinositol, di and triphosphoinositides. *Biochem. Biophys. Res. Commun.* **106**: 697-703.

Smith, R. J., and Bowman, B. J. (1982). Stimulation of human neutrophil degranulation with 1-0-octadecyl-2-0-acetyl-sn-glyceryl-3-phosphorylcholine: modulation by inhibitors of arachidonic acid metabolism. *Biochem. Biophys. Res. Commun.* **104**:1495-1501.

Snyder, F. (1987). The significance of dual pathways for the biosynthesis of platelet activating factor: 1-alkyl-2-lyso-sn-glycero-3-phosphate as a branchpoint. In *New Horizons in Platelet Activating Factor Research.* Edited by C. M. Winslow and M. L. Lee. London, John Wiley, pp. 13-25.

Stenton, S. C., Harris, A. H., Palmer, J. B., Hendrick, D. J., and Walters, E. H. (1989). The effects of a thromboxane receptor antagonist (GR32191) on PAF-induced bronchoconstriction and bronchial hyperresponsiveness (abstract). *Thorax* **44**:337P.

Stevenson, J. S., Tallet, M., Blinder, B., and Abraham, W. M. (1987). Modification of antigen-induced late responses with an antagonist of platelet-activating factor (WEB 2086) (abstract). *Fed. Proc.* **46**:1454.

Tanaka, D. T., and Grunstein, M. M. (1986). Effect of substance P on neurally mediated contraction of rabbit airway smooth muscle. *J. Appl. Physiol.* **60**:458-463.

Terashita, Z., Tsushima, S., Yoshioka, Y., Nomura, H., Inada, Y., and Nishikawa, K. (1983). CV-3988, a specific antagonist of platelet activating factor (PAF). *Life Sci.* **32**:1975-1982.

Touvay, C., Etienne, A., and Braquet, P. (1985). Inhibition of antigen-induced lung anaphylaxis in the guinea-pig by BN 52021 a new specific PAF-acether receptor antagonist isolated from Ginkgo biloba. *Agents Actions* **17**:371-372.

Ukena, D., Dent, G., Birke, F. W., Robaut, C., Sybrecht, G. W., and Barnes, P. J. (1988). Radioligand binding of antagonists of platelet-activating factor to intact human platelets. *FEBS Letts.* **2**:285-289.

Valone, F. H., and Goetzl, E. J. (1983). Specific binding by human polymorphonuclear leucocytes of the immunological mediator 1-0-hexadecyl/octadecyl-2-acetyl-sn-glycero-3-phosphorylcholine. *Immunology* **48**: 141-149.

Valone, F. H., Coles, E., Reinhold, V. R., and Goetzl, E. J. (1982). Specific binding of phospholipid platelet-activating factor by human platelets. *J. Immunol.* **129**:1637-1641.

Vargaftig, B. B., Lefort, J., Wal, F., Chignard, M., and Medeiros, M. C. (1982). Interference of non-steroidal anti-inflammatory drugs associated to anti-histamine and anti-serotonin agents with the bronchial and platelet effects of "platelet-activating factor" (PAF-acether). *Eur. J. Pharmacol.* **82**:121-130.

Wardlaw, A. J., Moqbel, R., Cromwell, O., and Kay, A. B. (1986). Platelet activating factor. A potent chemotactic and chemokinetic factor for human eosinophils. *J. Clin. Invest.* **78**:1701-1706.

Wardlaw, A. J., Chung, K. F., Moqbel, R., Hartnell, A., McCusker, M., Barnes, P. J., Collins, J. V., and Kay, A. B. (1990). Effect of inhaled platelet-activating factor on lung cells and circulating neutrophils in vivo: Relationship to changes in lung function. *Am. Rev. Respir. Dis.* In press.

Wykle, R. L., Malone, B., and Snyder, F. (1980). Enzymatic synthesis of 1-alkyl-2-acetyl-sn-glycero-3-phosphocholine, a hypotensive and platelet-aggregating lipid. *J. Biochem.* **255**:10256-10260.

Yukawa, T., Read, R., Kroegel, C., Rutman, R., Churg, K. F., Wilson, R., Cole, P., and Barnes, P. J. (1990). The effects of activated eosinophils and neutrophils on guinea-pig airway epithelium in vitro. *Am. J. Cell. Respir. Biol.* In press.

11

Arachnoids and Asthma
The Role of Receptors for Leukotrienes

JEFFREY M. DRAZEN

Beth Israel Hospital
Brigham and Womens' Hospital
Children's Hospital
and Harvard Medical School
Boston, Massachusetts

WILLIAM MAGUIRE and ELLIOT ISRAEL

Beth Israel Hospital and
Harvard Medical School
Boston, Massachusetts

BOHDAN PICHURKO

Brigham and Womens' Hospital
and Harvard Medical School
Boston, Massachusetts

I. Introduction

Arachidonic acid is a ubiquitous 20 carbon fatty acid containing 4 unsaturated *cis* double bonds (at the 5, 8, 11, and 14 positions); it is found esterified to phospholipids in numerous plasma membranes. Free arachidonic acid is liberated into the microenvironment on activation of certain enzymes, namely phospholipase A_2 or phospholipase C followed by diglyceride lipase, and by a variety of biological events including antigen-antibody interaction or receptor ligand coupling (Abdel-Latif, 1986; Vades and Pruzanski, 1986; Chang et al., 1987). Once free arachidonic acid becomes available, it can be enzymatically transformed into a number of biomolecules some of which possess the ability to mediate a wide variety of biological effects. This family of biomolecules is referred to by the term *eicosanoids* or, more specifically, *arachnoids*. There are two major pathways leading to the formation of arachnoids from arachidonic acid: the cyclooxygenase pathway and the lipoxygenase pathway. In general the bioactive products of the former pathway are the prostaglandins and thromboxanes while the bioactive products of the latter pathway are the leukotrienes, hydroxyeicosatetraenoic acids (HETEs), and the lipoxins.

The formation, metabolism, and biological actions relative to the lung of this family of compounds constitutes an extensive body of knowledge and have been recently reviewed in this series (Shore et al., 1989) and elsewhere (Hedqvist et al., 1982; Dahlen et al., 1987; Samuelsson et al., 1987; Oates et al., 1988; O'Byrne, 1988). This general topic will *not* be the focus of this chapter; in this chapter we will consider the evidence for sulfidopeptide leukotrienes in mediating airway constriction and hyperresponsiveness in asthma.

II. Brief Historical Perspective

The possible importance of leukotrienes in asthma has been postulated for almost half a century. Kelleway and Trethewie (1940) originally observed that the supernatant of isolated perfused guinea pig lungs, when placed on certain tissues, resulted in a slow-onset but sustained contractile response. Brocklehurst (1962) conclusively proved that this "slow-reacting substance" (SRS) was not histamine and further demonstrated that SRS derived from anaphylactic sources (so called SRS-A) was an extremely potent constrictor of human airway smooth muscle. The identification of SRS-A as an admixture of the sulfidopeptide* leukotrienes, LTC$_4$, LTD$_4$, and LTE$_4$ (Murphy et al., 1979; Hammarstrom et al., 1979; Corey et al., 1980; Lewis et al., 1980a,b; Orning et al., 1980; Parker et al., 1980) represented a major step in understanding the role of SRS-A in the pathobiology of asthma.

In the 10 years since the identification of the sulfidopeptide leukotrienes as the constituents of SRS-A, five lines of evidence have emerged regarding the role of the sulfidopeptide leukotrienes in asthma. These are the potential of various cells implicated in the asthmatic response to produce the leukotrienes; the identification of leukotrienes in biological fluids from patients during asthma attacks; the possible role that leukotrienes may play in the induction of a hyperresponsive state; the effects of leukotriene receptor antagonists in asthma; and the similarity of the pulmonary mechanical response to inhaled leukotrienes and acute airway obstruction in asthma. An in-depth review of each of these lines of evidence implicating leukotrienes in asthma could easily fill an entire volume of this series. Thus we have chosen to review briefly some of the points while considering others in depth.

---

*The term *sulfidopeptide* leukotrienes is used to identify those leukotrienes with a peptide chain bound via a thio-ether link to the fatty acid backbone at the C-6 position. This differentiates LTC$_4$, LTD$_4$, and LTE$_4$ from LTB$_4$ which is *not* a sulfidopeptide leukotriene.

III. Cells Capable of Synthesizing Sulfidopeptide Leukotrienes

A number of cells, which are normally resident in the lung or found in the lung in asthmatic conditions, have been shown to possess the ability to synthesize the sulfidopeptide leukotrienes. These cells include mast cells (McGlashan et al., 1982), eosinophils (Weller et al., 1983), macrophages (Rankin et al., 1984), platelets (Maclouf and Murphy, 1988), and vascular endothelial cells (Feinmark and Cannon, 1986). Mast cells, eosinophils, and macrophages have the ability to synthesize leukotrienes directly from arachidonic acid, while vascular endothelial cells and platelets require a source of LTA_4, such as neutrophils, to produce these products. Since there is a chapter in this volume devoted to each of these cell types and their possible role in asthma, the reader is referred to these for a discussion of the synthetic capabilities of each cell type.

IV. Recovery of Leukotrienes from Biological Fluids of Patients with Asthma

If leukotrienes are released in an acute asthmatic response, it seems reasonable to try to recover leukotrienes, or their metabolites, from biological fluids of individuals who are undergoing attacks of asthma. The first report in this regard was from Isono et al. (1985). These investigators demonstrated immunoreactive LTC_4 (i-LTC_4) in the plasma of children presenting to the emergency room with an acute attack of asthma. They were unable to detect i-LTC_4 in the plasma of normal children or the plasma of children with asthma in remission. Furthermore, they noted that the more severe the attack of asthma, the higher the level of i-LTC_4 in the plasma. Okubo et al. (1987) extended these observations to adults with asthma. In addition this latter report provided more substantive evidence for the identity of the materials isolated from the lung as LTC_4. They performed radioimmunoassay on material isolated from samples that had been subjected to reverse-phase high-performance liquid chromatography and assayed the fractions that had the retention time of authentic leukotriene standards. These investigators were thus able to separate LTC_4 and LTD_4 and were able to demonstrate that either or both were detectable in the plasma during acute asthma attacks. The mean levels during an asthma attack of LTC_4 and LTD_4 were 410 and 540 pg/ml, respectively. As in the findings of Isono et al., neither leukotriene was detectable in the plasma of normal subjects.

Ferrari and co-workers (1988) were able to detect i-LTC_4 in the nasal lavage fluid of three of four aspirin-sensitive asthmatic subjects who developed wheezing after aspirin ingestion. The FEV_1 fell in these subjects at the time that LTC_4 was detectable in the lavage fluid, but, because of the small number of subjects, a relationship between leukotriene levels and the severity of the asthma could not be established. Lam and co-workers (1988) were able to detect LTE_4 in the bronchoalveolar lavage fluid of 15 of 17 subjects with mild to moderate asthma; there was not a significant relationship between the amount of leukotriene detected and the severity of the asthma. Leukotrienes were not detectable in the lavage fluid from normal subjects. The identity of the LTE_4 was established by both RP-HPLC and positive ion fast atom-bombardment mass spectrometry, thus providing an unequivocal demonstration of the authenticity of the LTE_4.

These data demonstrate that leukotrienes can be identified in biological fluids from individuals during asthmatic responses. However the extreme bronchoconstrictor potency of the sulfidopeptide leukotrienes raises the need to detect accurately small quantities of these materials while demonstrating their authenticity. In addition, detection of intact leukotrienes probably underestimates the amount of total leukotriene released in any circumstance. For example, we now appreciate that leukotrienes may undergo n-acetylation, beta-oxidation, omega terminus hydroxylation and carboxylation, or conversion to their respective sulfoxide forms after their release at their putative site of response (Lee et al., 1984; Orning et al., 1985; Denzlinger et al., 1986; Foster et al., 1987; Stene and Murphy, 1988). Thus it seems likely that accurate quantitation of the amount of leukotriene released in a given circumstance will require a complete understanding of their metabolish and development of sensitive and specific assays for the more stable metabolites.

V. Leukotrienes and Airway Hyperresponsiveness

There are data to suggest that leukotrienes have the capacity to alter the responsiveness of airway contractile tissues to the actions of other mediators. In general this effect is small (a 1.5 to 3-fold shift of the dose-response curve to unrelated agonists) compared to the differences in responsiveness in normal and asthmatic human subjects (estimated to be on the order of 10-100 fold). The ability of the leukotrienes to alter airway responsiveness has been recently reviewed in this series (Shore et al., 1989) and will not be considered further here.

VI. Leukotriene Receptor Antagonists in Asthma

To understand the effects of leukotriene receptor antagonists in asthma, it is necessary to understand the biology of leukotriene receptors. Since this subject has not been reviewed in depth recently, it will be covered in detail in this chapter.

It has been shown that there are distinct receptors for at least two and possibly three of the known sulfidopeptide leukotrienes found in humans and that activation of such receptors results in the biological effects attributed to the leukotrienes. The presence of more than one type of functional leukotriene receptor has important implications for the understanding of asthma and related airway diseases. In this section we consider the role possibly played by distinct receptors for LTC_4 and LTD_4 in the asthmatic response. To do so it is necessary to consider studies performed in both animals and humans and to consider functional studies of antagonists, studies of receptor binding, and the mechanisms linking receptor occupation to functional responses.

A. Evidence for Multiple Leukotriene Receptors from Contractile Studies in Isolated Tissues

Guinea Pigs

Shortly after the definition of the structure of LTC_4 and LTD_4, analysis of Schild plots of the effects of the prototypical leukotriene receptor antagonist FPL55712 on contractile responses of guinea pig pulmonary tissues stimulated with either LTC_4 or LTD_4 suggested that these two sulfidopeptide leukotrienes had distinct receptors (Drazen et al., 1980; Snyder and Krell, 1984). The LTD_4 receptor differed from the LTC_4 receptor in that FPL55712, and subsequently other LTD_4 receptor antagonists, were shown to be more effective at inhibiting responses resulting from LTD_4 action than from LTC_4 (Fleisch et al., 1985; Jones et al., 1986; Snyder et al., 1987; Weichman et al., 1984). On this basis it was suggested that there were distinct receptors for LTC_4 and LTD_4 in both pulmonary parenchymal and tracheal tissues.

Although more than 10 molecules capable of inhibiting contractile responses mediated by LTD_4 have been identified (Fleisch et al., 1985; Jones et al., 1986; Snyder et al., 1987; Weichman et al., 1984; Gapinski et al., 1988; Chang et al., 1988; Tomioka et al., 1988; Young, 1988; Snyder and Bernstein, 1988; Abraham et al., 1988), in general these molecules have little effect on contractile responses mediated by LTC_4 if steps are taken to prevent metabolic interconversion to LTD_4. The potency of these LTD_4 antagonists varies substantively, but many of them will ''shift the LTD_4 dose-responsive curve'' by a factor of 2 at nanomolar concentrations. Thus these new LTD_4 receptor antagonists are on the order of 1000 times more potent than FPL-55712. Although many LTD_4 receptor antagonists have been developed, specific and selective LTC_4 receptor antagonists have not been identified. The LTC_4 receptor antagonists that have been defined also share activity LTD_4-induced muscle contraction, and thus lack specificity.

When appropriate precautions are taken to prevent metabolic interconversion, (Krillis et al., 1983) the distinction between LTC_4 and LTD_4 administration and subsequent contractile responses is more clearly evident. For example, in the presence of serine-borate complex, contractions induced by LTC_4 are not antagonized effectively by beta-$_2$ adrenergic agonists, while similar magnitude contractions induced by LTD_4 are antagonized (Charette and Jones, 1987; Hay et al., 1986; 1988). The use of serine-borate complex as a tool to prevent the metabolic interconversion of LTC_4 to LTD_4 is limited by the fact that treatment with this complex changes the baseline contractile state of the tissues and thus tissue tensions must be adjusted mechanically or studied at altered baseline tensions.

Use of an alternative gamma-glutamyl transpeptidase inhibitor known as AT-125 (Capraro and Hughey, 1985; Hill et al., 1985) offers distinct advantages over serine-borate complex. We have shown that this agent prevents the metabolic interconversion of $[^3H]LTC_4$ to $[^3H]LTD_4$ by isolated tracheal spirals from guinea pigs (Maguire et al., 1988; Fig. 1). Concentrations of AT-125 capable of greater than a 95% inhibition of the conversion of LTC_4 to LTD_4 are not associated with changes in either baseline tissue tension or contractile responses to histamine.

Although these data suggest that LTC_4 and LTD_4 act at distinct receptors, another line of evidence, in which the effects of altering the stereochemistry of the ligand molecule at or near the critical chiral centers were investigated, has not shown a clear distinction between LTC_4 and LTD_4 contractile receptors (Drazen et al., 1981; Lewis et al., 1981). However, this is likely due to the fact that such studies have been conducted without inhibiting the metabolic interconversion of LTC_4 to LTD_4. Since gamma-glutamyl transpeptidase, which catalyzes the interconversion of LTC_4 to LTD_4, likely only requires the glutathione moiety for recognition and catalysis it seems likely that molecular analogs structured to explore the LTC_4 receptor were converted to their LTD_4 counterparts by endogenous contractile tissue gamma glutamyl transpeptidase. Thus the data gathered in such studies cannot be used to address the question of distinct receptors for LTC_4 and LTD_4.

Humans

Systematic studies of in vitro human airway responses to leukotrienes in the presence of appropriate receptor antagonists and inhibitors of metabolic interconversion of LTC_4 to LTD_4 have not been completed until recently (Hay et al., 1988; Buckner et al., 1986, 1988). In these studies the responses elicited by LTC_4 and LTD_4 were both inhibited to a similar degree by FPL55712, LY171883, or SKF104353 (each of these molecules is a relatively selective LTD_4 receptor antagonist in the guinea pig) under conditions when metabolic

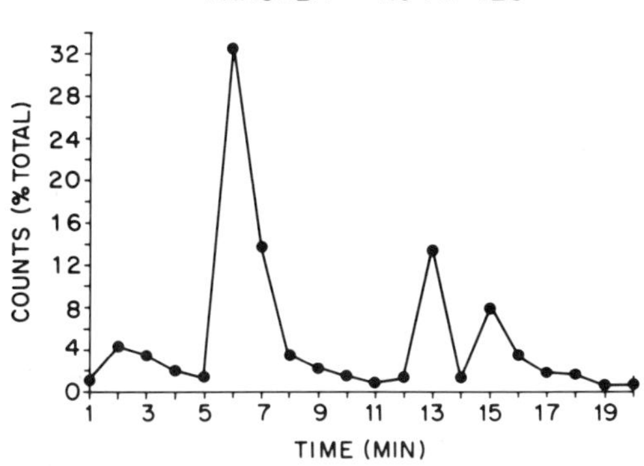

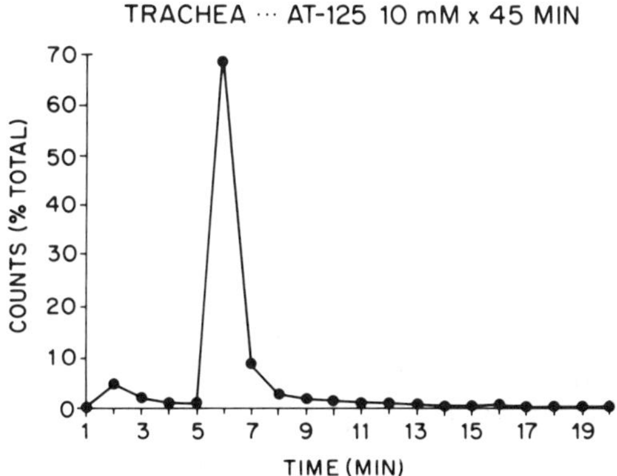

Figure 1 HPLC chromatograms of the supernatant obtained from guinea pig tracheas incubated with $[^3H]LTC_4$ added to cold LTC_4 to achieve a final bath concentration of 0.01 μM LTC_4; incubations were carried out at 37 °C for 45 min with or without 10mM AT-125. In the trachea not treated with this gamma-glutamyl transpeptidase inhibitor, there was conversion of about 30% of the added LTC_4 to LTD_4 and LTE_4 (as reflected in the peaks at 13 and 15 min), while in the trachea treated with AT-125 there was less than 1% conversion of the added material (note the single peak at 6 min).

interconversion of LTC_4 to LTD_4 was prevented. These data have been interpreted to suggest that human airways contain only a single leukotriene receptor subtype, similar to the guinea pig LTD_4 receptor, and that this receptor can be cross-activated by LTC_4. These data are flawed: although metabolic interconversion between LTC_4 and LTD_4 was *thought* to be prevented by the addition of serine-borate complex this point was not established experimentally. If the interconversion was in fact prevented, the conclusion is probably valid, if the interconversion was not prevented then this conclusion cannot be safely drawn. Furthermore, it is important to note that these studies were performed only on 2-4 airways from normal subjects, thus site-specificity and possible alterations in disease have not been explored. It is possible that had airways of a different size class been used, such as 0.5-1.0 mm airways, which are thought to be the airway predominantly involved in an asthmatic response, or had airways from individuals with asthma been used, different results may have been obtained. The effects of leukotriene receptor antagonists on the response to leukotriene inhalation are considered later in this chapter.

B. Evidence for Distinct LTC_4 and LTD_4 Binding Sites in Airway Tissues and Isolated Cells

LTD_4 Binding

A number of investigative groups have demonstrated the presence of specific, saturable, and inhibitable binding sites for LTD_4 in lung tissues (Cheng et al., 1984a, 1985; Mong et al., 1984b, 1985; Lewis et al., 1985); such sites have not been identified at similar densities in tissues without a defined pharmacological response to LTD_4. The k_d values for the binding of LTD_4 to guinea pig lung membranes, between 0.15 and 8 nM, are similar to the concentrations required for one-half maximal contractions of isolated guinea pig or human airway tissues. LTE_4 is an effective ligand for displacement of LTD_4 from its binding sites on lung membrane preparations, whereas a much greater concentration (approximately 100-fold) of LTC_4 is required for this effect, which suggests that the binding site is the LTD_4/LTE_4 receptor (Cheng et al., 1984b). The LTD_4-binding unit complex has been characterized as a heat-, trypsin-, and chymotrypsin-labile moiety with an apparent molecular weight of 240-500 kD (Mong et al., 1986a). GTP gamma S and Gpp[NH]p inhibit LTD_4 binding to its putative receptor protein, while ATP and GDP have little effect on binding (Mong et al., 1984b; Bruns et al., 1983). This suggests that LTD_4 binding is regulated by a G-type coupling protein.

LTC_4 Binding

In contrast to the tissue selectivity of LTD_4 binding sites, LTC_4 binding sites have been demonstrated in lung, brain, liver, and kidney as well as circulating polymorphonuclear leukocytes (Mong et al., 1985; Bruns et al., 1983; Lewis et al., 1984; Rovati et al., 1985; Pong et al., 1983; Baud et al., 1987). The binding of LTC_4 to pulmonary sites occurs with k_d values from 15 to 70 nM and Bmax values of 31,000-136,000 fmol/mg protein, compared to Bmax values of 70-1,100 fmol/mg protein for LTD_4. Although these findings are consistent with the existence of a specific LTC_4 receptor that transduces functional responses, a poor correlation between specific agonist binding and pharmacological effects raises the possibility that LTC_4 binding sites may not be receptors. One explanation for this effect is that LTC_4 binds to the ubiquitous human enzyme glutathione-S-transferase via the Ya subunit (Sun et al., 1986, 1987) with characteristics that mimic receptor binding. Thus LTC_4 binding could involve high-affinity variable-density enzymatic sites that, under certain experimental conditions, could prevent a putative spasmogenic receptor from being recognized as a distinct entity.

Civelli et al. (1987) examined binding of [^{3}H]LTC$_4$ in preparations of excised human bronchi obtained at the time of thoracic surgery requiring resection of airway tissues. No asthmatic subjects were included in their sample. They demonstrated specific binding of LTC$_4$ to membrane fractions prepared from these bronchi; the data obtained were best fit with a two-site model. The high-affinity site had a k$_d$ of 70 nM and a Bmax of 136,000 fmol/mg protein, while the low-affinity site had a k$_d$ of 580 nM and a Bmax of 38,300 fmol/mg protein. They demonstrated that these binding characteristics were not changed in the presence of hematin, a glutathione-S-transferase inhibitor, at concentrations between 10^{-8} and 10^{-5} M. This latter experiment was interpreted to indicate that binding was not occurring to glutathione-S-transferase, but they failed to use an optimal unspecified ligand such as hexylglutathione to demonstrate the specificity of the binding site. Furthermore, the k$_d$ that they observed is 20-50 times greater than the EC$_{50}$ that others have observed for LTC$_4$ contractile activity in human airways of similar size (Hay et al., 1987). Thus, although the binding units identified by Civelli et al. (1987) in human airways are clearly specific and saturable LTC$_4$ binding units, the functional role of these units has yet to be determined.

C. Mechanisms Linking Receptor Occupation to Functional Responses

LTD$_4$

The transmembrane signal associated with activation of LTD$_4$ receptors has been studied extensively in a variety of cell and tissue types. In BC3H$_1$ cells activation of LTD$_4$ receptors with LTD$_4$ is accompanied by synthesis and release of thromboxane (Tx) A$_2$ as indicated by the presence of its stable metabolite TxB$_2$. Coupling of activation to TxA$_2$ synthesis requires protein synthesis, as indicated by the inhibitory effects of cycloheximide and actinomycin D. Addition of free arachidonic acid to the cell cultures results in the formation of TxB$_2$, indicating that the availability of arachidonic acid was the limiting step (Clark et al., 1985). In BC3H$_1$ cells the limiting step appears to be de novo synthesis of phospholipase A$_2$ (Clark et al., 1986a). LTD$_4$-receptor-stimulation-coupled mobilization of arachidonic acid occurs not only in isolated cell systems but also in minced guinea pig lung preparations (Mong et al., 1986b).

In minced guinea pig lung, *Bordetella pertussis* treatment (1 μg/ml for 40 min), which ADP-ribosylates Gi and thus should inhibit many of the biological effects attributed to Gi, results in a 76% inhibition of TxB$_2$ synthesis and release in response to LTD$_4$ stimulation. These data have been interpreted to suggest that Gi regulates the coupling of LTD_4 receptor activation to downstream processes. In bovine endothelial cells (Clark et al., 1986b) *Bordetella pertussis* treatment likewise blocked LTD_4-induced arachidonic acid release and metabolism and also resulted in ADP- ribosylation of a 41 kD membrane protein. In contrast, in RBL-1 cells (Sarau et al., 1987) treatment with *Bordetella pertussis* had a similar effect on the 41 kD membrane protein, but did not have an effect on LTD_4-induced phosphatidyl-inositol (PI) turnover. These data demonstrate heterogeneity of Gi-coupled responses among tissues stimulated with LTD_4.

Activation of LTD_4 receptors results in dose-related PI hydrolysis in RBL-1 cells. The effects of LTD_4 on PI turnover are inhibitable with LTD_4 receptor antagonists, thus demonstrating the specific nature of the effect (Mong et al., 1987). The effects of LTD_4 receptor stimulation on arachidonic acid metabolism occur downstream from the effects of LTD_4 stimulation on PI metabolism, suggesting that activation of phospholipase C in the process of receptor occupancy precedes secondary activation of phospholipase A_2.

LTC_4

In contrast to the extensive data available on the coupling of LTD_4 receptors to intracellular events, there are very few data on the transduction of LTC_4-mediated effects. There are data from isolated guinea pig pulmonary parenchymal strips that LTC_4 and LTD_4 coupling mechanisms are distinct. When the effects of the calcium channel blockers diltiazem (0.67 mM), verapamil (0.61 mM), and nifedipine (0.29 mM) were compared on the contractile responses initiated by LTC_4 or LTD_4 (Israel et al., 1987) in guinea pig parenchymal strips, the contractile effects of LTC_4 but not LTD_4 were inhibited by these calcium channel blockers (Fig. 2). They also found that in the presence of diltiazem K_b values derived for the effects of FPL55712 on LTC_4- or LTD_4-induced contractions became similar, 0.32 and 0.47 μM respectively. This suggests that in this tissue LTC_4 can directly activate the LTD_4 receptor without bioconversion to LTD_4. This may explain the difficulties encountered in the functional characterization of LTC_4-mediated airway constriction.

D. Effects of Leukotriene Receptor Antagonists in Asthma

Antagonists with activity at the LTD_4 receptor have been studied in two forms of laboratory-induced asthma: antigen inhalation (Britton et al., 1987) and cold air inhalation (Israel et al., 1988). In the former case an oral dose of L-649,923 sufficient to shift the dose-response curve to inhaled LTD_4 3.8-fold (see above, Section VII) in normal subjects was administered to asthmatic subjects 2 h before inhalation of a dose of antigen known to result in an acute decrease of the FEV_1 by 20%. Compared to placebo, L-649,923 had no effect on baseline pulmonary function and resulted in a smaller response to

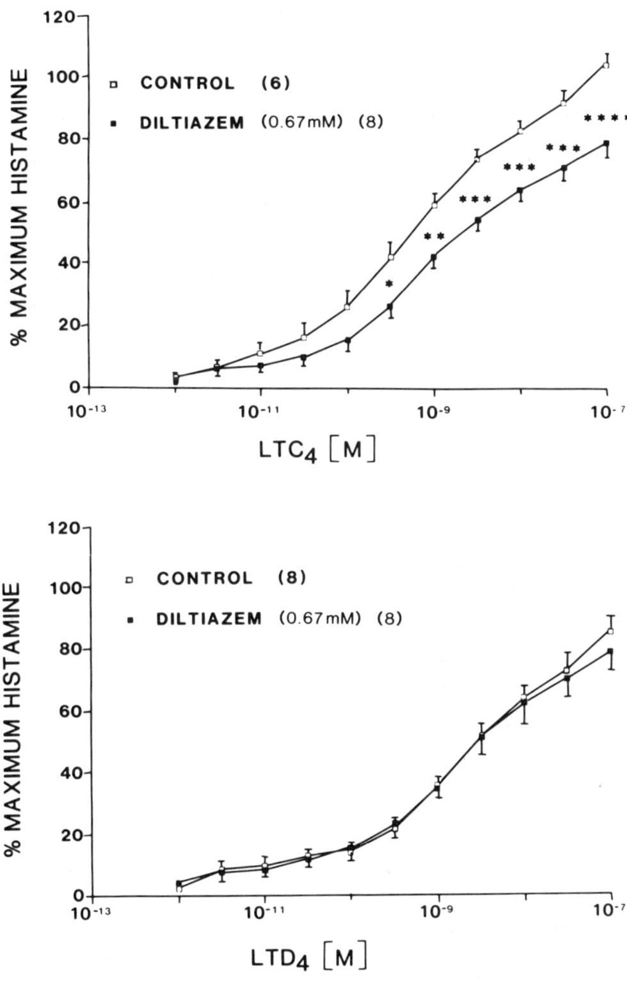

Figure 2 Effects of diltiazem (0.67 mM) on the contractile response of isolated guinea pig pulmonary parenchymal strips. In the upper panel LTC_4 was the agonist; in the lower panel LTD_4 was the agonist. Note that diltiazem treatment only inhibited the response to LTC_4 not LTD_4 (reprinted from Israel et al. (1987), with permission from the *Journal of Pharmacology and Experimental Therapeutics*).

inhaled antigen. However the magnitude of the effect was small; for example, the mean maximal fall in the FEV_1 during placebo treatment was 1.78 L and during L-649,923 treatment was 1.35 L; no effect was observed when specific conductance was used as the outcome index. In addition these investigators found no effect of treatment on the late response to inhaled antigen, that is, a late response of similar magnitude was observed after both active agent and placebo treatment. Israel and co-workers (1988) examined the effects of LY171883 on the acute bronchoconstrictor response to cold air inhalation in appropriate asthmatic subjects. An oral dose of LY171883, sufficient to shift the dose-response curve to inhaled LTD_4 about four fold, had a small, but significant protective effect on cold air-induced bronchospasm. Compared to placebo, there was no effect of LY171883 on baseline pulmonary function. Thus in these two forms of laboratory-induced asthma, relatively weak (i.e., less than fivefold shift of the dose-response curve) LTD_4 receptor antagonists had only minimal effects. However, because of the weakness of the antagonists used, one cannot determine if the failure to observe an effect results from the lack of involvement of LTD_4 in the response to inhaled antigen.

Cloud and co-workers (1987) examined the effects of LY171883 on lung function and symptoms in a group of over 100 subjects with mild asthma in a 6 week double-blind placebo-controlled trial. To enroll in the trial, subjects had to have asthma that could be controlled by the use of a beta-inhaler alone. They found that the group that took the LTD_4 antagonist had improved pulmonary function (an FEV_1 that had improved by about 0.3 L over the 6 weeks of the trial) compared to the placebo group, and at the same time required lower dosages of beta-agonist to control their asthma. These findings represent the first report of a salutary effect of a LTD_4 receptor antagonist in spontaneous asthma. Although the effect observed was small, the LTD_4 antagonist used was not very potent; studies are now underway with more potent LTD_4 receptor antagonists. The results of such studies should provide important new information on the role of the LTD_4 receptor in patients with asthma.

VII. Response of Human Airways In Vivo to Inhaled Leukotrienes

A. Normal Subjects

Potency and Site of Response

When aerosols of leukotrienes are inhaled by normal subjects, airway obstruction, as manifested by a decrease in flow rates during a forced exhalation, occurs (Holroyde et al., 1981; Weiss et al., 1982; Barnes et al., 1984; Smith et al., 1985, 1987; Bisgaard et al., 1983, 1985, 1987; Roberts et al., 1986a,b; Adelroth et al., 1986). Both LTC_4 and LTD_4 are potent bronchoconstrictor agonists, each being approximately 3000 times more potent than histamine in normal subjects. None of the studies reported thus far have been conducted with an agent capable of inhibiting the action of gamma-glutamyl transpeptidase administered to the subjects; thus, the actions observed after inhalation of LTC_4 could be due either to the native molecule or to LTD_4 derived from the administered LTC_4. The mechanism of response appears to be direct bronchoconstriction rather than bronchoconstriction resulting from secondarily generated prostaglandins (Smith et al., 1987).

The specific airways involved in the bronchoconstrictor response to inhaled leukotrienes are not clear at this time. In studies in which both the S_{Gaw} and flow rates from partial flow-volume curves were used as outcome indicators there was no difference in the dosage of inhaled leukotriene required to result in a change in either index of lung mechanics (Smith et al., 1985; Bisgaard et al., 1985). In contrast, when the FEV_1 and the flow rate at 30% of vital capacity measured from partial flow-volume curves ($\dot{V}30$) are used as outcome indicators, there is a clear distinction in the concentration of inhaled leukotriene required to achieve a decrease in the measured effect. Higher concentrations of inhaled leukotrienes are required to decrease the FEV_1 than the V30 (Davidson et al., 1987). These data are compatible with the hypothesis that in normal subjects the central airways are less responsive to inhaled leukotrienes than the peripheral airways. This conclusion rests on somewhat shaky grounds: more sophisticated tests of the sites of airway response, other than the differential response of the FEV_1 and $\dot{V}30$, are available but have not been applied to the problem. Furthermore, these data do not address the specific receptor (i.e., an LTC_4 versus and LTD_4 receptor) involved in mediating the contractile response observed.

Effects of Receptor Antagonists

The LTD_4 receptor in human airways in vivo has been identified as similar to the LTD_4 in the guinea pig airways, based on functional antagonism studies in which it has been shown that agents capable of inhibiting the LTD_4 response in the guinea pig also have similar effect in normal humans. FPL55712, L619,923, and LY171883 are each capable of inhibiting the response to inhaled LTD_4 (Holroyde et al., 1981; Bruns et al., 1983; Phillips et al., 1988). In the first report of the effects of an inhaled leukotriene on lung function in normal humans, Holroyde and co-workers (1981) demonstrated that the SRS-A antagonist FPL55712 inhibited the bronchoconstrictor response to inhaled LTD_4. This compound was not developed further because of its short in vivo duration of effect. Barnes et al. (1987) examined the effects of L-649,923 on airway constriction induced by inhalation of histamine or LTD_4 in normal subjects. They used a double-blind placebo-controlled protocol and demonstrated no effect on baseline pulmonary function and a geometric mean 3.8-fold shift in the LTD_4 dose-response curve. There was no effect on the histamine dose-response curve. Phillips and co-workers (1988) demonstrated that oral ingestion of a single dose of 400 mg of LY171883 resulted in a significant ($p \leqslant 0.01$) increase in the average concentration of LTD_4 that had to be inhaled to decrease the FEV_1 by 12% (from 5.5 to 25.3 nmol). These data establish that human airways in vivo have a receptor that mediates constriction similar to the guinea pig LTD_4 receptor; whether there is a receptor similar to the guinea pig LTC_4 receptor has yet to be established.

B. Asthmatic Subjects

Potency

When asthmatic subjects breath aerosols of LTC_4 or LTD_4 there is a decrement in the S_{Gaw}, FEV_1, or $\dot{V}30$, depending on the outcome indicator used by the study group (Griffin et al., 1983; Smith et al., 1985, 1987; Bisgaard et al., 1983, 1985, 1987; Roberts et al., 1986; Adelroth et al., 1986). When the $\dot{V}30$ is the outcome index, the asthmatic group is 3-10 times more sensitive to the bronchoconstrictor effects of inhaled leukotrienes than are normal subjects. Although there have been a relatively large number of studies in which the effects of inhaled LTD_4 have been examined in subjects with asthma, there are relatively few data on the effects of inhaled LTC_4 in asthmatic subjects (Adelroth et al., 1986; Pichurko et al., 1989). Regardless of the specific leukotriene inhaled, the overall effects on pulmonary mechanics appear to be quite similar. When the FEV_1 is used as the outcome index there is an approximately 100-fold difference in the sensitivity to these agonists between the two groups. In addition, the degree of hyperresponsiveness exhibited by the asthmatic subjects to LTD_4 is less than the degree of hyperresponsiveness exhibited to a reference agonist such as histamine or methacholine (Griffin et al., 1983; O'Byrne et al., 1988).

Physiological Implications

The possible physiological implications of this relative lack of hyperresponsiveness to inhaled leukotrienes in asthmatic individuals have been recently reviewed by O'Byrne et al. (1988) and include induction of tachyphylaxis to leukotrienes in patients with asthma, a site specificity of effect for leukotrienes, or an endogenous leukotriene antagonist in subjects with asthma. In regard to the site specificity of response, to the extent that the FEV_1 and the $\dot{V}30$ reflect differences in the predominant locus of airway responses (as outlined above), asthmatic central airways may be more sensitive to the effects of inhaled leukotrienes than the airways of normal subjects. Pichurko and co-workers (1989) have recently provided some evidence for the issue of site-specific responses to inhaled leukotrienes. They examined the effects of inhalation of aerosols of LTC_4 in seven patients with mild asthmatic symptoms by measuring maximal expiratory flow rates with patients breathing either air or a mixture of helium and oxygen (He/O_2). They found that prior to induction of airway obstruction by LTC_4 inhalation, the ratio of maximal expiratory flow at 30% of vital capacity while breathing He/O_2 to that measured while breathing air (the so-called density dependence), was 1.13 ± 0.16 (mean $\pm$ SEM). This ratio increased in proportion to the degree of induced obstruction when LTC_4 was the contractile agonist, but stayed the same or decreased in proportion to induced obstruction when histamine was the inhaled agonist. In a separate study of four normal subjects, using a slightly different protocol, they found that there was not a significant change in the density dependence after LTC_4 inhalation. Figure 3 shows the data obtained before induced obstruction and after an approximate 30% reduction in maximal expiratory flow rate (while the subjects or patients were breathing air). The observation that density dependence increased only after LTC_4 inhalation and only in asthmatic subjects is consistent with the hypothesis that there is selective expression of a leukotriene receptor in the central airways of asthmatic subjects. Although these data suggest a site predominance of leukotriene receptors in asthmatic subjects, no studies have been specifically designed to address the question of functional expression of specific receptors for LTC_4 or LTD_4 in asthmatic persons.

Selective Expression of an LTC_4 Receptor in Asthma?

Additional evidence is consistent with a difference in receptor expression between the two groups, but it is only suggestive at best. In particular, when

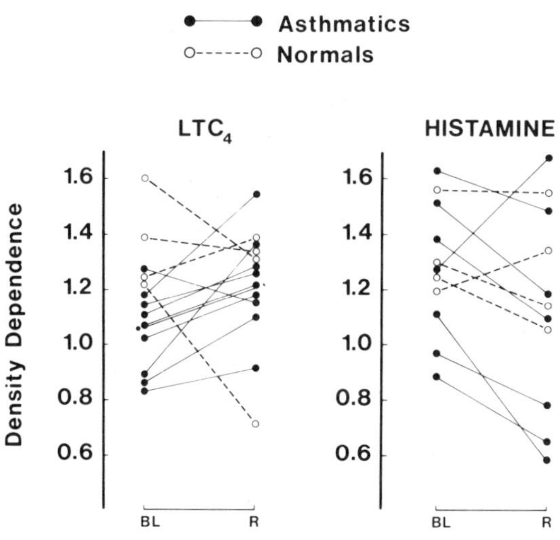

Figure 3 Change in density dependence (see text) of maximal expiratory airflow from baseline (BL) to response (R) following inhalation of LTC_4 or histamine in asthmatic (solid circles) or normal (open circles) subjects. The concentration of LTC_4 or histamine in the nebulizer was adjusted for each subject to achieve a 25-35% decrement in the maximal expiratory flow rate measured from partial flow volume curves at 30% of vital capacity (asthmatic data from Pichurko et al., 1989).

normal subjects inhale LTC_4 the onset of effect is slow compared to that resulting from inhalation of LTD_4 (Barnes et al., 1984; Drazen, 1986). This observation is consistent with a requirement for metabolic interconversion from LTC_4 to LTD_4 to be completed before normal subjects manifest a contractile response that is likely mediated by an LTD_4 receptor. In asthmatic subjects the response to inhaled LTC_4 is rapid in onset and sustained in duration compared with that achieved in normal subjects (Adelroth et al., 1966; Pichurko et al., 1989). In contrast, the time course of response to inhaled LTD_4 is similar in both groups. Among the possible explanations of the differences in time course is the possibility that the airways of asthmatic subjects have a specific receptor for LTC_4. Thus the rapid onset of contractile effects in this subject group may reflect action at an LTC_4 receptor that may not be present in normal subjects. The data are also compatible with other explanations, such as a difference in the permeability of the normal and the asthmatic airway to the less lipophilic LTC_4 compared to the more lipophilic LTD_4. It is also possible that the asthmatic airway expresses more accessible or greater quantities of gamma-glutamyl transpeptidase than normal airways, resulting in a more rapid interconversion of LTC_4 to LTD_4. Specific experiments designed to probe the functional expression of an LTC_4 receptor in asthmatic airways have not been performed. If asthmatic subjects selectively express an LTC_4 receptor, the functional consequences of inhalation of LTC_4 should not be blocked by an LTD_4 receptor antagonist, while in normal subjects LTC_4 effects would be blocked by an LTD_4 receptor antagonist.

Discussion

Fuller: Buckner's studies used airways from normal, not asthmatic subjects. It may be that normal subjects express only an LTD receptor while asthmatics express receptors for both LTC and LTD. What is the role of leukotrienes in the early and late phase asthmatic responses?

Drazen: I agree that Buckner's group did show that normal subjects do not express the LTC receptor. The data available suggest that leukotrienes are only important in the acute phase of asthma in humans, since leukotriene antagonists only affect the acute phase.

Fuller: I find that the data suggesting that leukotrienes are *not* important in the late phase of asthma are not compelling. The failure to demonstrate LTE in the urine of asthmatic patients may have multiple explanations. The clinical data with LT antagonists have largely employed very weak antagonists, and more potent antagonists are currently under study. We will have to wait for the results of these studies before we can make conclusions about the importance of leukotrienes in chronic asthma.

Drazen: In chronic asthma there are probably many activated cell types capable of producing substantial quantities of leukotrienes and other mediators.

Fuller: We have also studied a thromboxane A2 inhibitor, which reduced thromboxane generation but had no effect on antigen-driven responses.

References

Abraham, W, M., Stevenson, J. S., and Garrido, R. (1988). A leukotriene and thromboxane inhibitor (Sch 37224) blocks antigen-induced immediate and late responses and airway hyperresponsiveness in allergic sheep. *J. Pharmacol. Exp. Ther.* **247(3)**:1004-1011.

Abdel-Latif, A. A. (1986). Calcium-mobilizing receptors, polyphosphoinositides, and the generation of second messengers. *Pharmacol. Rev.* **38**: 227-272.

Adelroth, E., Morris, M. M., Hargreave, F. E., and O'Byrne, P. M. (1986). Airway responsiveness to leukotrienes C_4 and D_4 to methacholine in patients with asthma and normal controls. *N. Engl. J. Med.* **315**:480-484.

Barnes, N. C., Piper, P. J., and Costello, J. F. (1984). Comparative effects of inhaled leukotriene C_4, leukotriene D_4 and histamine in normal human subjects. *Thorax* **39**:500-504.

Barnes, N., Piper, P. J., and Costello, J. (1987). The effect of an oral leukotriene antagonist L-649,923 on histamine and leukotriene D4-induced bronchoconstriction in normal man. *J. Allergy Clin. Immunol.* **79**:816-821.

Baud, L., Koo, C. H., and Goetzl, E. J. (1987). Specificity and cellular distribution of human polymorphonuclear leucocyte receptors for leukotriene C_4. *Immunology* **62**:53-59.

Bisgaard, H., Groth, S., and Dirksen, H. (1983). Leukotriene D_4 induces bronchoconstriction in man. *Allergy* **38**:441-443.

Bisgaard, H., Groth, S., and Masden, F. (1985). Bronchial hyperreactivity to leukotriene D_4 in exogenous asthma. *Br. Med. J.* **290**:1468-1471.

Bisgaard, H., Poulsen, L., and Sondergaard, I. (1987). Nebulization and selective deposition of LTD_4 in human lungs. *Allergy* **42**:336-342.

Britton, J. R., Hanley, S. P., and Tattersfield, A. E. (1987). The effect of an oral leukotriene D_4 antagonist L-649,923 on the response of inhaled antigen in asthma. *J. Allergy Clin. Immunol.* **79**:811-816.

Brocklehurst, W. E. (1962). Slow-reacting substance and related compounds. *Progr. Allergy* **6**:539-558.

Bruns, R. F., Thomsen, W. J., and Pugsley, T. A. (1983). Binding of leukotrienes C_4 and D_4 to membranes from guinea pig lung: regulation by ions and guanine nucleotides. *Life Sci.* **33**:645-653.

Buckner, C. K., Krell, R. D., Laravuso, R. B., Coursin, D. B., Bernstein, P. R., and Will, J. A. (1986). Pharmacological evidence that human intralobar airways do not contain different receptors that mediate contractions to leukotriene C_4 and leukotriene D_4. *J. Pharmacol. Exp. Ther.* **237**:558-562.

Buckner, C. K., et al. (1988). Pharmacological evidence for leukotriene receptors in human intralobar airways. *Ann. N. Y. Acad. Sci.* **524**:181-186.

Capraro, M. A., and Hughey, R. P. (1985). Use of acivicin in the determination of rate constants for turnover of rat renal gamma-glutemyltranspeptidase. *J. Biol. Chem.* **260**:3408-3412.

Chang, J., Borgeat, P., Schleimer, R. P., Musser, J. H., Marshall, L. A., and Hand, J. M. (1988). Wy-48, 252 (1,1,1-trifluoro-N-[3-(2-quinolinylmethoxy)phenyl]membrane sulfonamide), an orally active leukotriene antagonist: effects on arachidonic acid metabolism in various inflammatory cells. *Eur. J. Pharmacol.* **148**:131-141.

Chang, M., Rao, M. K., Reddanna, P., Li, C. H., Tu, C. P., Corey, E. J., Reddy, C. C. (1987). Specificity of the glutathione S-transferases in the conversion of leukotriene A4 to leukotriene C4. *Arch. Biochem. Biophys.* **259(2)**:536-547.

Charette, L., and Jones, T. R. (1987). Effects of L-series borate on antagonism of leukotriene C_4-induced contractions of guinea pig trachea. *Br. J. Pharmacol.* **91**:179-188.

Cheng, J. B., and Townley, R. G. (1984a). Evidence for a similar receptor site for binding of [3H] leukotriene E_4 and [3H] leukotriene D_4 to the guinea pig crude lung membrane. *Biochem. Biophys. Res. Commun.* **122**:949-954.

Cheng, J. B., and Townley, R. G. (1984b). Identification of leukotriene D_4 receptor binding sites in guinea pig lung homogenates using [3H] leukotriene D_4. *Biochem. Biophys. Res. Commun.* **118**:20-26.

Cheng, J. B., Lang, D., Bewta, A., and Townley, R. G. (1985). Tissue distribution and functional correlation of [3H]leukotrine C_4 and [3H] leukotriene D_4 binding sites in guinea-pig uterus and lung preparations. *J. Pharmacol. Exp. Ther.* **232**:80-87.

Civelli, M., Oliva, D., Mezzetti, M., and Nicosia, S. (1987). Characteristics and distribution of specific binding sites for leukotriene C_4 in human bronchi. *J. Pharmacol. Exp. Ther.* **242(3)**:1019-1024.

Clark, M. A., Cook, M., Mong, S., and Crooke, S. T. (1985). The binding of leukotriene C_4 and leukotriene D_4 to membranes of a smooth muscle cell line (BC3H$_1$) and evidence that leukotriene induced contraction in these cells is mediated by thromboxane, protein and RNA syntheses. *Eur. J. Pharmacol.* **116**:207-220.

Clark, M. A., Conway, T. M., Bennett, C. F., Crooke, S. T., and Stadel, J. M. (1986a). Islet-activating protein inhibits leukotriene D_4- and leukotriene C_4- but not bradykinin- or calcium ionophore-induced prostacyclin synthesis in bovine endothelial cells. *Proc. Natl. Acad. Sci. USA* **83**:7320-7324.

Clark, M. A., Littlejohn, D., Conway, T. M., Mong, S., Steiner, S., and Crooke, S. T. (1986b). Leukotriene D_4 treatment of bovine aortic endothelial cells and bovine smooth muscle cells in culture results in an increase in phospholipase A_2 activity. *J. Biol. Chem.* **261**:10713-10718.

Cloud, M., Enas, G., Kemp, J., Platts-Mills, T., Altman, L., Townley, R., Tinkleman, D., King, T., Middleton, E., Sheffer, A., and McFadden, E. (1989). A specific LTD_4/LTE_4 receptor antagonist improves pulmonary function in patients with mild, chronic asthma. *Am. Rev. Resp. Dis.* **140**:1336-1339.

Corey, E. J., Clark, D. A., Goto, G., Marfat, A., Mioskowski, C., Samuelsson, B., and Hammarstrom, S. (1980). Stereospecific total synthesis of a "slow reacting substance" of anaphylaxis, Leukotriene C-1. *J. Am. Chem. Soc.* **102**:1436-1439.

Creese, B. R., and Bach, M. K. (1983). Hyperreactivity of airways smooth muscle produced *in vitro* by leukotrienes. *Prostaglandins Leukotrienes Med.* **11**:161-169.

Dahlen, S. E., Bjorck, T., and Hedqvist, P. (1987). Bioassay of leukotrienes. *Adv. Prostagland. Thrombox. Leukotriene Res. 1987.* **17B**:615-621.

Davidson, A. B., Lee, T. H., Scanlon, P. D., Solway, J., McFadden, E. R., Jr., Ingram, R. H., Jr., Corey, E. J., Austen, K. F., and Drazen, J. M. (1987). Bronchoconstrictor effects of leukotriene E4 in normal and asthmatic subjects. *Am. Rev. Respir. Dis.* **135(2)**:333-337.

Denzlinger, C., Gutiemann, A., Scheuber, P. H., Wilker, D., Hammer, D. K., and Keppler, D. (1986). Metabolish and analysis of cysteinyl leukotrienes in the monkey. *J. Biol. Chem.* **261**:15601-15606.

Drazen, J. M. (1986). Inhalation challenge with sulfidopeptide leukotrienes in human subjects. *Chest* **89**:414-419.

Drazen, J. M., Austen, K. F., Lewis, R. A., Clark, D. A., Goto, G., Marfat, A., and Corey, E. J. (1980). Comparative airway and vascular activities of leukotrienes C_1 and D *in vivo* and *in vitro*. *Proc. Natl. Acad. Sci. USA* **77**:4354-4358.

Drazen, J. M., Lewis, R. A., Austen, K. F., Toda, M., Brion, F., Marfat, A., and Corey, E. J. (1981). Contractile activities of structural analogs of leukotrienes C and D: necessity of a hydrophobic region. *Proc. Natl. Acad. Sci. USA* **78**:3195-3198.

Feinmark, S. J., and Cannon, P. J. (1986). Endothelial cell leukotriene C_4 synthesis results from intercellular transfer of leukotriene A_4 synthesized by polymorphonuclear leukocytes. *J. Biol. Chem.* **261**:16466-16472.

Ferreri, N. R., Howland, W. C., Stevenson, D. D., and Spiegelberg, H. L. (1988). Release of leukotrienes, prostaglandins, and histamine into nasal secretions of aspirin-sensitive asthmatics during reaction to aspirin. *Am. Rev. Respir. Dis.* **137**:847-854.

Fleisch, J. H., Rinkema, L. E., Haisch, K. D., Swanson-Bean, D., Goodson, T., Ho, P. P., and Marshall, W. S. (1985). LY171883, 1-less than 2-hydroxy-3-propyl-4-less than 4-(1H-tetrazol-5-yl) butoxy greater than phenyl greater than ethanone, an orally active leukotriene D_4 antagonist. *J. Pharmacol. Exp. Ther.* **233**:148-157.

Foster, A., Fitzsimmons, B., Rokcach, J., and Letts, S. (1987). Metabolism and excretion of peptide leukotrienes in the anesthetized rat. *Biochem. Biophys. Acta* **921**:486-493.

Gapinski, D. M., Roman, C. R., Rinkema, L. E., and Fleisch, J. H. (1988). Leukotriene receptor antagonists, 4, Syntheses and leukotriene D4/E4 receptor antagonist activity of 4-(alkyl)acetophenone derivatives. *J. Med. Chem.* **31**:172-175.

Griffin, M. Weiss, J. W., Leitch, A. G., McFadden, E. R. Jr., Corey, E. J., Austen, K. F., and Drazen, J. M. (1983). Effects of leukotriene D on the airways in asthma. *N. Engl. J. Med.* **308**:436-439.

Hammarstrom, S., Murphy, R. C., Samuelsson, B., Clark, D. A., Mioskowski, C., and Corey, E. J. (1979). Structure of leukotriene C: identification of the amino acid part. *Biochem. Biophys. Res. Commun.* **91**:1266-1272.

Hay, D. W., Muccitelli, R. M., Wilson, K. A., Wasserman, M. A., and Torphy, T. J. (1986). Differences in the ability of salbutamol to prevent and reverse LTC_4 induced contractions of the guinea-pig isolated trachea: influence of 1-serine borate. *Eur. J. Pharmacol.* **126**:323-327.

Hay, D. W., Muccitelli, R. M., Tucker, S. S., Vickery-Clark, L. M., Wilson, K. A., Gleason, J. G., Hall, R. F., Wasserman, M. A., and Torphy, T. J. (1987). Pharmacologic profile of SK&F 104353: a novel, potent, and selective peptiodoleukotriene receptor antagonist in guinea pig and human airways. *J. Pharmacol. Exp. Ther.* **243**:474-481.

Hay, D. W., Muccitelli, R. M., Wilson, K. A., Wasserman, M. A., and Torphy, T. J. (1988). Functional antagonism by salbutamol suggests differences in the relative efficacies and dissociation constants of the peptidoleukotrienes in guinea pig trachea. *J. Pharmacol. Exp. Ther.* **244**:71-78.

Hedqvist, P., Dahlen, S. E., and Bjork, J. (1982). Pulmonary and vascular actions of leukotrienes In *Leukotrienes and Other Lipoxoygenase*

Products. Edited by B. Samuelsson and R. Paoletti. New York, Raven Press, pp. 187-200.

Hill, K. E., Von Hoff, D. D., and Burk, R. F. (1985). Effect of inhibition of gamma-glutamyltranspeptidase by AT-125 (acivicin) on glutathione and cysteine levels in rat brain and plasma. *Invest. New Drugs.* 3:31-34.

Holroyde, M. C., Altounyan, R. E. C., Cole, M., Dixon, M., and Elliott, E. V. (1981). Bronchoconstriction produced in man by leukotrienes C & D. Lancet 2:17-18.

Isono, T., Koshihara, Y., Murota, S., Fukada, Y., and Furukawa, S. (1985). Measurement of immunoreactive leukotriene C4 in blood of asthmatic children. *Biochem. Biophys. Res. Commun.* 130:486-492.

Israel, E., Robin, J. L., and Drazen, J. M. (1987). Differential effects of calcium channel blockers on leukotriene C_4 and D_4 induced contractions in guinea pig pulmonary parenchymal strips. *J. Pharmacol. Exp. Ther.* 243:424-429.

Israel, E., Juniper, E. F., Morris, M. M., Dowell, A. R., Hargreave, F. E., and Drazen, J. M. (1988). Leukotriene D (LTD) receptor antagonist, LY171883, reduces the bronchoconstriction induced by cold air challenge in asthmatics: a randomized, double-blind, placebo controlled trial. *Am. Rev. Respir. Dis.* 137(4):27.

Jones, T. R., Young, R., Champion, E., Charette, L., Denis, D., Ford-Hutchinson, A. W., Frenette, R., Gauthier, J. Y., Guindon, Y., Kakushima, M., et al. (1986). L-649,923, sodium (beta S*, gamma R*)-4-(3-(4-acetyl-3-hydroxy-2-propylphenoxy)-propylthio)-gamma-hydroxy-beta-methyl-benzenebutanoate, a selective, orally active leukotriene receptor antagonist. *Can. J. Physiol. Pharmacol.* 64:1068-1075.

Kellaway, C. H., and Trethewie, E. R. (1940). The liberation of a slow-reacting smooth muscle-stimulating substance in anaphylaxis. *Q. J. Exp. Physiol.* 30:121-145.

Krilis, S., Lewis, R. A., Corey, E. J., and Austen, K. F. (1983). Bioconversion of C-6 sulfidopeptide leukotrienes by the responding guinea pig ileum determines the time course of its contraction. *J. Clin. Invest.* 71:909-915.

Lam, S., Chan, H., LeRiche, J. C., Chan Yeung, M., and Salari, H. (1988). Release of leukotrienes in patients with bronchial asthma. *J. Allergy Clin. Immunol.* 81(4):711-717.

Lee, H. K., and Murlas, C. (1985). Ozone-induced hyperreactivity in guinea pig is abolished by BW755C or FPL55712 but not by indomethacin. *Am. Rev. Respir. Dis.* 132:1005-1009.

Lee, T. H., Austen, K. F., Corey, E. J., and Drazen, J. M. (1984). LTE_4 induced airway hyperresponsiveness of guinea pig tracheal smooth muscle to histamine and evidence of three sulfidopeptide leukotriene receptors. *Proc. Natl. Acad. Sci. USA* **81**:4922-4961.

Lewis, R. A., Austen, K. F., Drazen, J. M., Clark, D. A., Marfat, A., and Corey, E. J. (1980a). Slow reacting substances of anaphylaxis: identification of leukotrienes C-1 and D from human and rat sources. *Proc. Natl. Acad. Sci. USA* **77**:3710-3714.

Lewis, R. A., Drazen, J. M., Austen, K. F., Clark, D. A., and Corey, E. J. (1980b). Identification of the C(6)-S-conjugate of leukotriene A with cysteine as a naturally occurring substance of anaphylaxis. Importance of the 11-*cis* geometry for biological activity. *Biochem. Biophys. Res. Commun.* **96**:271-277.

Lewis, R. A., Drazen, J. M., Austen, K. F., Toda, M., Brion, F., Marfat, A., and Corey, E. J. (1981). Contractile activities of structural analogs of leukotrienes C and D: role of the polar substituents. *Proc. Natl. Acad. Sci. USA* **78**:4579-4583.

Lewis, M. A., Mong, S., Vessilla, R. L., Hogaboom, G. K., Wu, H. L., and Crooke, S. T. (1984). Identification of specific binding sites for leukotriene C_4 in human fetal lung. *Prostaglandins* **27**:961-974.

Lewis, M. A., Mong, S., Vessilla, R. L., and Crooke, S. T. (1985). Identification and characterization of leukotriene D_4 receptors in adult and fetal human lung. *Biochem. Pharmacol.* **34**:4311-4317.

MacGlashan, D. W., Jr., Schleimer, R. P., Peters, S. P., Schulman, E. S., Adams, G. K., III, Newball, H. H., and Lichtenstein, L. M. Generation of leukotrienes by purified human lung mast cells. *J. Clin. Invest.* **70**:747-751.

Maclouf, J. A., and Murphy, R. C. (1988). Transcellular metabolism of neutrophil-derived leukotriene A_4 by human platelets. A potential cellular source of leukotriene C_4. *J. Biol. Chem.* **263**:174-181.

Maguire, W., Gerard, N., Israel, E., and Drazen, J. (1988). Acivicin (AT-125) prevents biotransformation of leukotriene (LT)C_4 to LTD_4 by guinea pig trachea. *Pharmacologist* **30**(3):A92.

Mong, S., Wu, H. L., Hogaboom, G. K., Clark, M. A., Stadel, J. M., and Crooke, S. T. (1984a). Regulation of ligand binding to leukotriene D_4 receptors: effects of medications and guanine nucleotides. *Eur. J. Pharmacol.* **106**:241-253.

Mong, S., Wu, H. L., Clark, M. A., Stadel, J. M., Gleason, J. G., and Crooke, S. T. (1984b). Identification of leukotriene D_4 specific binding sites in the membrane preparation isolated from guinea pig lung. *Prostaglandins* **28**:805-822.

Mong, S., Wu, H. L., Scott, M. O., Lewis, M. A., Clark, M. A., Weichman, B. M., Kinzig, C. M., Gleason, J. G., Crooke, S. T. (1985). Molecular heterogeneity of leukotriene receptors: correlation of smooth muscle contraction and radioligand binding in guinea-pig lung. *J. Pharmacol. Exp. Ther.* **234**:316-325.

Mong, S., Wu, H. L., Clark, M. A., Gleason, J. G., and Crooke, S. T. (1986a). Leukotrienes D_4 receptor-mediated synthesis and release of arachidonic acid metabolites in guinea pig lung: induction of thromboxane and prostacyclin biosynthesis by leukotriene D_4. *J. Pharmacol. Exp. Ther.* **239**: 63-70.

Mong, S., Wu, H. L., Stadel, J. M., Clark, M. A., and Crooke, S. T. (1986b). Solubilization of [3H] leukotriene D_4 receptor complex from guinea pig lung membranes. *Mol. Pharmacol.* **29**:235-243.

Mong, S., Wu, H. L., Miller, J., Hall, R. F., Gleason, J. G., and Crooke, S. T. (1987). SKF 104353, a high affinity antagonist for human and guinea pig lung leukotriene D4 receptor, blocked phosphatidylinositol metabolism and thromboxane synthesis induced by leukotriene D4. *Mol. Pharmacol.* **32**:223-229.

Murphy, R. C., Hammarström, S., and Samuelsson, B. (1979). Leukotriene C: a slow reacting substance from murine mastocytoma cells. *Proc. Natl. Acad. Sci. USA* **76**:4275-4279.

Oates, J. A., Fitzgerald, G. A., Branch, R. A., Jackson, E. K., Knapp, H. R., and Roberts, L. J., II. (1988). Clinical implications of prostaglandin and thromboxamne A_2 formation. *N. Engl. J. Med.* **319**:689-698.

O'Byrne, P. M. (1988). Leukotrienes, airway hyperresponsiveness, and asthma. *Ann. N.Y. Acad. Sci.* **524**:282-288.

Okubo, T., Takahashi, H., Sumitomo, M., Shindoh, K., and Suzuki, S. (1987). Plasma levels of leukotrienes C_4 and D_4 during wheezing attack in asthmatic patients. *Int. Arch. Allergy Appl. Immunol.* **84**:149-155.

Örning, L., Hammarström, S., and Samuelsson, B. (1980). Leukotriene D: a slow-reacting substance from rat basophilic leukemia cells. *Proc. Natl. Acad. Sci. USA* **7**:2014-2017.

Orning, L., Kaijser, L., and Hammarström, S. (1985). In vivo metabolism of LTC_4 in Man. *Biochem. Biophys. Res. Comm.* **130**:214-220.

Parker, C. W., Del Koch, D., Huber, M. M., and Falkenhein, S. F. (1980). Formation of the cysteinyl form of slow reacting substance (leukotriene E_4) in human plasma. *Biochem. Biophys. Res. Commun.* **97**:1038-1046.

Phillips, G. D., Rafferty, P., Robinson, C., and Holgate, S. T. (1988). Dose-related antagonism of leukotriene D_4-induced bronchoconstriction by p.o. administration of LY-171883 in nonasthmatic subjects. *J. Pharmacol. Exp. Ther.* **246**(2):732-738.

Pichurko, B. M., Scanlon, P. D., Sperling, R., Austen, K. F., Corey, E. J., Lafleur, J., and Drazen, J. M. (1989). Site of bronchoconstrictor activity of LTC_4 and histamine in normal and asthmatic subjects. *Am. Rev. Respir. Dis.* **140**:334-339.

Pong, S. S., DeHaven, R. N., Kuehl, F. A., Jr., and Egan, R. W. (1983). Leukotriene C_4 binding to rat lung membranes. *J. Biol. Chem.* **258**: 9616-9619.

Rankin, J. A., Hitchcock, M., Merrill, W. W., Huang, S. S., Brashler, J. R., Bach, M. K., and Askenase, P. W. (1984). IgE immune complexes induce immediate and prolonged release of leukotriene $C_4(LTC_4)$ from rat alveolar macrophages. *J. Immunol.* **132**:1993-1999.

Roberts, J. A., Rodger, I. W., and Thomson, N. C. (1986a). Effect of verapamil and sodium cromoglycate on leukotriene D_4 induced bronchoconstriction in patients with asthma. *Thorax* **41**:753-758.

Roberts, S. A., Giembycz, M. A., Raeburn, D., Rodger, I. W., and Thomson, N. C. (1986b). *In vitro* and *in vivo* effect of verapamil on human airway responsiveness to leukotriene D_4. *Thorax* **41**:12-16.

Rovati, G. E., Oliva, D., Sautebin, L., Folco, G. C., Welton, A. F., and Nicosia, S. (1985). Identification of specific binding sites for leukotriene C_4 in membranes from human lung. *Biochem. Pharmacol.* **34**:2831-2837.

Samuelsson, B., Dahlen, S. E., Lindgren, J. A., Rouzer, C. A., and Serhan, C. N. (1987). Leukotrienes and lipoxins: structures, biosynthesis, and biological effects. *Science* **237**(4819):1171-1176.

Sarau, H. M., Mong, S., Foley, J. J., Wu, H. L., and Crooke, S. T. (1987). Identification and characterization of leukotriene D_4 receptors and signal transduction processes in rat basophilic leukemia cells. *J. Biol. Chem.* **262**:4034-4041.

Shore, S. A., Austen, K. R., and Drazen, J. M. (1989). Eicosanoids and the lung. In *Cell Biology of the Lung*. Edited by D. Massaro. New York, Marcel Dekker.

Smith, L. J., Greenberger, P. A., Patterson, R., Krell, R. D., and Bernstein, P. R. (1985). The effect of inhaled leukotriene D_4 in humans. *Am. Rev. Respir. Dis.* **131**:368-372.

Smith, L. J., Kern, R., Patterson, R., Krell, R. D., and Bernstein, P. R. (1987). Mechanism of leukotriene D_4-induced bronchoconstriction in normal subject. *J. Allergy Clin. Immunol.* **80**:340-347.

Snyder, D. W., and Bernstein, P. R. (1988). U19052 (ICIAm): a novel leukotriene analog which antagonizes LTC_4, LTD_4, and LTE_4. *Prostaglandins* **35**:903-915.

Snyder, D. W., and Krell, R. D. (1984). Pharmacological evidence for a distinct leukotriene C_4 receptor in guinea-pig trachea. *J. Pharmacol. Exp. Ther.* **231**:616-622.

Snyder, D. W., Giles, R. E., Keith, R. A., Yee, Y. K., and Krell, R. D. (1981). *In vitro* pharmacology of ICI 198,615: a novel, potent, and selective peptide leukotriene antagonist. *J. Pharmacol. Exp. Ther.* **243**:548-556.

Stene, D. O., and Murphy, R. C. (1988). Metabolism of leukotriene E_4 in isolated rat hepatocytes. Identification of beta-oxidation products of sulfidopeptide leukotrienes. *J. Biol. Chem.* **263**:2773-2778.

Sun, F. F., Chau, L. Y., Spur, B., Corey, E. J., Lewis, R. A., and Austen, K. F. (1986). Identification of a high affinity leukotriene C4-binding protein in rat liver cytosol as glutathione S-transferase. *J. Biol. Chem.* **261**:8540-8546.

Sun, F. F., Chau, L. Y., and Austen, K. F. (1987). Binding of leukotriene C4 by glutathione transferase: a reassessment of biochemical and functional criteria for leukotriene receptors. *Fed. Proc.* **46**:204-207.

Tomioka, K., Yamada, T., Mase, T., Hara, H., and Murase, K. (1988). Pharmacological properties of the orally active leukotriene antagonist [C5-CC3-(4-acetyl-3-hydroxy-2-propylphenoxy)-propyl]thio]-1,3,4-thiadiazol-2-yl]thio]acetic acid. *Arzneimittelforsch.* **38**:682-685.

Vadas, P., and Pruzanski, W. (1986). Role of secretory phospholipases A2 in the pathobiology of disease. *Lab. Invest.* **55**:391-404.

Weichman, B. M., Wasserman, M. A., and Gleason, J. G. (1984). SK and F 88046: a unique pharmacologic antagonist of bronchoconstriction induced by leukotriene D_4, thromboxane and prostaglandins F2 alpha and D_2 *in vitro*. J. Pharmacol. Exp. Ther. **228**:128-132.

Weiss, J. W., Drazen, J. M., Coles, N., McFadden, E. R., Jr., Lewis, R., Weller, P., Corey, E. J., and Austen, K. F. (1982). Bronchoconstrictor effects of leukotriene C in humans. *Science* **216**:196-198.

Weller, P. F., Lee, C. W., Foster, D. W., Corey, E. J., Austen, K. F., and Lewis, R. A. Generation and metabolism of 5-lipoxygenase pathway leukotrienes by human eosinophils: predominant production of leukotriene C_4. *Proc. Natl. Acad. Sci. USA* **80**:7626-7630.

Young, R. N. (1988). L-648.051, a potent and specific aerosol active leukotriene D4 antagonist. *Agents Actions* (Suppl.) **23**:113-119.

12

Cholinergic Mechanisms in Bronchial Hyperresponsiveness and Asthma

JOHN G. WIDDICOMBE

St. George's Hospital Medical School
London, England

PETER J. BARNES

National Heart and Lung Institute
London, England

J.-A. KARLSSON

AB Draco
Lund, Sweden

I. Introduction

The three main motor systems of the airways, smooth muscle, submucosal glands, and vascular beds, are all influenced by cholinergic mechanisms, but to different degrees. Acetylcholine released from airway nerves may also have actions on epithelium and migratory cells such as mast cells, although these have been less frequently studied. It must also be remembered that the neurotransmitter to laryngeal and upper airways striated muscle is acetylcholine, the transmission being nicotinic and not affected by atropine.

The classic view of the neural control of airway tissues is that the adrenergic (sympathetic) and cholinergic (parasympathetic) systems act as a seesaw, with opposing actions on each target organ. For different tissues one neural system is thought to be dominant: the parasympathetic for smooth muscle and glands, and the sympathetic for blood vessels. This view has had to be modified in recent years for four reasons. First, the actions of sympathetic and parasympathetic systems are not always opposing. For example, both acetylcholine and catecholamines enhance the secretion of submucosal glands (Richardson and Somerville, 1988), and the action of the sympathetic nervous system on airway smooth muscle in some species is difficult to establish and may be absent in humans (Barnes, 1986). Second, the existence of cotransmission in airway motor nerves, both sympathetic and parasympathetic, with release of neuropeptides and possibly purines means that we can no longer consider cholinergic control in isolation from the actions of other transmitters (Lundberg et al., 1987; Barnes, 1988). A third complication is that airway and pulmonary sensory nerves, which activate central cholinergic reflexes to the respiratory tract, also cause local effects via axon reflexes with the release of sensory neuropeptides (McDonald, 1987; Barnes, 1988). Finally, these same afferent nerves may connect to intramural ganglia in the airways and modulate transmission from central nervous system to the periphery (Burnstock et al., 1987).

Airway nervous tone can be reflexly altered by sensory input from within and outside the respiratory tract. The cholinergic reflexes consist of afferent pathways in and outside the vagal nerves, a central integrating component, and vagal efferent motor nerves to the lung. Efferent vagal activity is transmitted through cholinergic (nicotinic) ganglia located within the airway wall. It is conceivable that cholinergic motor effects can originate also in higher centers in the central nervous system (CNS) since, for example, antimuscarinic drugs can be effective in patients with psychogenic asthma (McFadden et al., 1969; Rebuck and Marcus, 1979; Neild and Cameron, 1985).

This chapter will concentrate on cholinergic mechanisms, but some discussion of their interaction with other neurotransmitter systems is inevitable.

II. Cholinergic Control of Airways

A. Nerve Pathways

All the cholinergic nerves to the lower airways are in the parasympathetic system, and therefore are in the vagus nerve and its branches. The superior laryngeal nerve, part of this system, arises from the vagus high in the neck and, as well as supplying the larynx, gives sensory and motor innervation to much of the cervical trachea. Since this nerve contains few or no sympathetic motor fibers, it is mainly parasympathetic and gives the experimental advantage of being useful for studying control of cervical tracheal function without sympathetic involvement. This does not apply to the lower cervical vagus, which, at least in dogs, has sympathetic nerves looping up from the stellate ganglion and then passing caudally to the lungs (Daly and Mount, 1951); thus stimulation of the cervical vagus gives mixed sympathetic and parasympathetic actions. In similar fashion, the pulmonary branches of the sympathetic trunk in the chest join the vagus high in the thorax and run with the parasympathetic fibers down into the lower trachea and lungs.

In the neck some species have separate recurrent and pararecurrent laryngeal nerves. The former supply all the striated muscles of the larynx apart from cricothyroid, and have some afferent fibers from the larynx and cervical trachea passing caudally to join the vagus (Vidruk, 1983). The pararecurrent laryngeal nerve connects with the external branch of the superior laryngeal nerve and conducts cranially many of the afferent fibers from the cervical trachea. The relative importance of recurrent and pararecurrent laryngeal nerves in supplying the motor tissues of the trachea has not been clearly determined.

B. Ganglia

Preganglionic parasympathetic nerves to the airways and lungs synapse in the intramural ganglia found mainly in the adventitia of the posterior trachea and around the hili and bronchi of the lungs. Transmission at these ganglia is cholinergic and nicotinic. It is blocked by classic ganglion-blocking drugs such as hexamethonium. It is becoming increasingly clear that these intramural ganglia are a source of complex integration and modulation of activity (Baker, 1986; Baker et al., 1986; Burnstock et al., 1987). The ganglia contain neurons of different sizes and histochemical make-up, indicating more than one type of neuron (Chiang and Gabella, 1986). There are also differences in cell population between the main paratracheal ganglia in the posterior wall of the trachea and the smaller ganglia found in the submucosa. Baker et al. (1986) describe type I neurons mainly in the former ganglia, with large diameters, and type II neurons located mainly in the submucosa with smaller diameters. The type I neurons have been studied electrophysiologically by recording action potentials, and seem to have two subgroups (Cameron and Coburn, 1984). The A-cells have a strong afterhyperpolarization probably due to activation of calcium-dependent potassium currents. The B-cells have slow excitatory postsynaptic potentials and possibly some of the features characteristic of glial cells. Burnstock et al. (1987) have studied rat tracheal neurons in culture and also observed two cell types, although these differ in properties from those described by Cameron and Coburn (1984) for the ferret. For the tracheal neurons in culture, direct application of acetylcholine causes excitation.

The existence of at least two types of ganglionic neuron suggests that ganglionic transmission may be complex functionally. A number of studies show that cholinergic transmission can be modulated by other mediators and nervous inputs. For example, α_2- and possibly α_1-adrenoceptor agonists inhibit transmission (Fig. 1) (Baker et al., 1983; Grundstrom and Andersson, 1985), raising the possibility of sympathetic inhibition of cholinergic con-

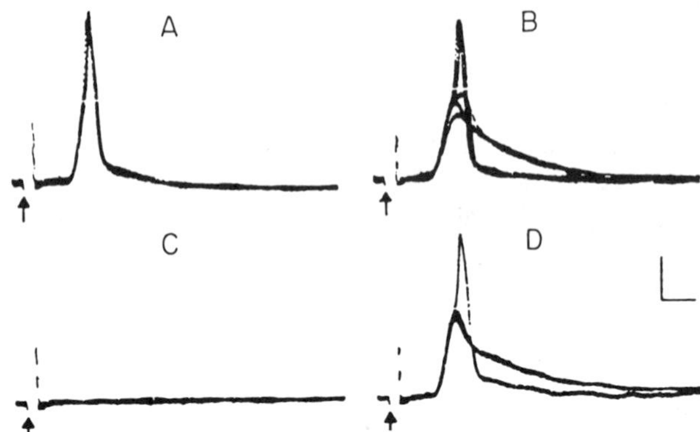

Figure 1   Inhibition of nicotinic transmission by norepinephrine and the reversal of this inhibition by phentolamine in ferret airway parasympathetic ganglion. Before (A) and 5 (B) and 6 (C) min after addition of epinephrine (10^{-5} M) to the reservoir perfusing the recording dish. D. 5 min after addition of phentolamine (5×10^{-5}M) to the same reservoir. In panels A-D, five consecutive traces are superimposed. In B, traces were recorded just as the response fell below the threshold for a spike; in D, traces were recorded just as the response rose above threshold. Horizontal and vertical bars equal 10 ms and 15 mV, respectively (from Baker et al., 1983).

traction of airway smooth muscle acting at a ganglionic site. β_2-Adrenoceptors, possibly activated by bloodborne catecholamines, can also inhibit ganglionic transmission (Skoogh and Svedmyr, 1989). Neurotransmitters such as vasoactive intestinal polypeptide (VIP) are found in the tracheal ganglia (Dey et al., 1981), and in rat tracheal neuronal cultures neuropeptide Y (NPY) and other neuropeptides have been identified (Burnstock et al., 1987). Sensory fibers connect to intramural ganglia and activate cholinergic postganglionic cells. The ganglionic synapse also has M_1-cholinoceptors, which, when excited, augment transmission and therefore lead to more powerful cholinergic motor actions (Lammers et al., 1989; see also below).

It is clear that cholinergic ganglionic transmission is highly complex in terms of both structure and neurotransmitters involved, and much work needs to be done to clarify the relevant anatomy and pharmacology. There seems to be a concentration of mast cells close to the tracheal intramural ganglia (Baker et al., 1986), somewhat reminiscent of the close association between mast cells and nerves in the gut. The result of this close relationship is not understood, but inflammatory mediators may influence ganglionic neurotransmission. Thus histamine has an inhibitory action on parasympathetic ganglia in guinea pig trachea. This effect is mediated by H_3-receptors, which operate at low concentrations of histamine (Ichinose et al., 1989).

C. Airway Smooth Muscle

Acetylcholine and cholinergic drugs contract airway smooth muscle at all levels of the tracheobronchial tree. Stimulation of the caudal end of the vagus nerves causes a tracheo- and bronchoconstriction, predominantly by contraction of smooth muscle (Fig. 2) (Nadel, 1980; Barnes, 1986; Nadel et al., 1985; Gross, 1988a). Field stimulation of airway smooth muscle preparations, including from humans, causes a contraction (Daniel et al., 1980). All of these effects are blocked by atropinic drugs. In some experimental preparations they are complicated by the fact that antidromic activation of sensory nerves can release neuropeptides such as substance P that cause smooth muscle contraction, although these responses are not sensitive to atropine (Barnes, 1986, 1988). With regard to neural control, most experimental results indicate that this is far stronger on the trachea and cartilaginous bronchi than on the distal noncartilaginous airways. The last have cholinoceptors present, but seem to be minimally activated by motor nerves. This general conclusion is supported by histological studies mapping the distribution of acetylcholinesterase-containing nerve fibers in the airways; few of these fibers are seen in the bronchioles (Laitinen and Laitinen, 1988).

The existence of cotransmission in parasympathetic motor cholinergic nerves (Lundberg et al., 1987; Barnes, 1988; see Chap. 15) (Fig. 2) complicates the story considerably. The unanswered question is whether all motor nerves to the airways contain equal proportions of acetylcholine and of neuropeptides such as VIP. There are at least two indications that some motor nerves to airway smooth muscle release only acetylcholine. Ichinose et al. (1987) showed that pulmonary C-fiber activation caused consecutively reflex

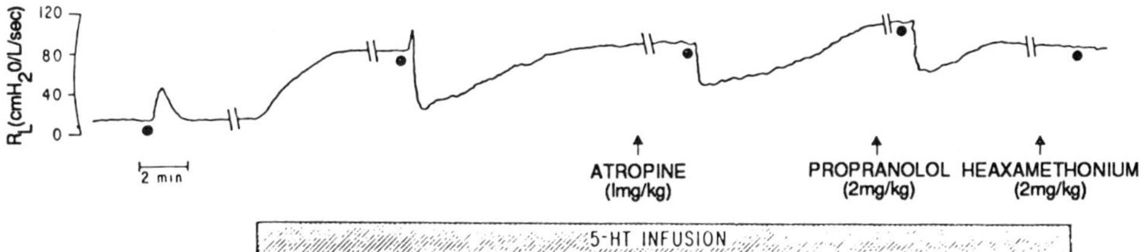

Figure 2 Changes in lung resistance (R_L) caused by mechanical stimulation of the larynx (shown by the closed circles) in an anesthetized, artificially ventilated cat. Initially the larynx was stimulated under basal conditions (far left). Thereafter baseline airway tone was enhanced by a continuous infusion of 5-hydroxytryptamine (5-HT) to allow observation of bronchodilatory responses. Note that the bronchoconstriction is blocked by atropine, leaving a bronchodilation blocked by hexamethonium (from Baker et al., 1983).

bronchoconstriction and dilatation due to release of acetylcholine and neuropeptides, respectively; however, when bronchomotor tone was changed reflexly by chemoreceptor activation, the response was entirely a cholinergic constriction without peptidergic dilatation. Don et al. (1988) have likewise shown that in the cat vagal nerve stimulation causes consecutive and separable bronchoconstriction and dilatation in the lungs, but that the tracheal response exhibits only smooth muscle contraction. They suggest that in this species the motor nerves to tracheal smooth muscle are cholinergic and not peptidergic. However many other studies, in particular with field stimulation, have shown that tracheal muscle from various species including cat contains nerves that release acetylcholine and relaxant transmitters, presumably neuropeptides (Daniel et al., 1980; Ito and Takeda, 1982; Leff, 1988). If there are two (or more) types of nerve to airway smooth muscle, cholinergic and cholinergic plus peptidergic, this raises the question whether the two groups can be separately controlled reflexly or centrally, and whether neuromodulation of transmission in intramural ganglia acts on the two systems in the same or different ways.

D. Submucosal Glands

Classic studies show that the main control of submucosal gland secretion is parasympathetic and cholinergic, being blocked by atropine (Richardson and Somerville, 1988). More recent work has indicated that catecholamines and sympathetic nerves also excite gland secretion, although the relative importance of this control has not been established (Phipps et al., 1980; Basbaum et al., 1981; Peatfield and Richardson, 1982). Peatfield and Richardson (1983) measured glycoprotein output from the trachea of cats, during repeated stimulation of the vagus nerves. They found that even very high dosages of atropine systemically and into the tracheal lumen did not completely inhibit the stimulated output (Fig. 3). The conclusion must be that other transmitters, presumably neuropeptides, are stimulating the output. Studies on the effect of neuropeptides on submucosal gland secretion indicate a complex modulatory action (Webber and Widdicombe, 1987; Webber, 1989; Widdicombe and Webber, 1990). Depending on the mechanism of mucus secretion (cholinergic or adrenergic), a neuropeptide such as VIP may enhance or inhibit gland secretion. If there is cholinergic and peptidergic cotransmission to submucosal glands, acetylcholine probably is the primary stimulus to secretion and any release of neuropeptides has a modulatory action on the volume and chemical composition of output.

E. Tracheobronchial Vasculature

Early studies on the vagal cholinergic control of the bronchial vasculature indicated that there was a cholinergic vasodilator system, which might modify

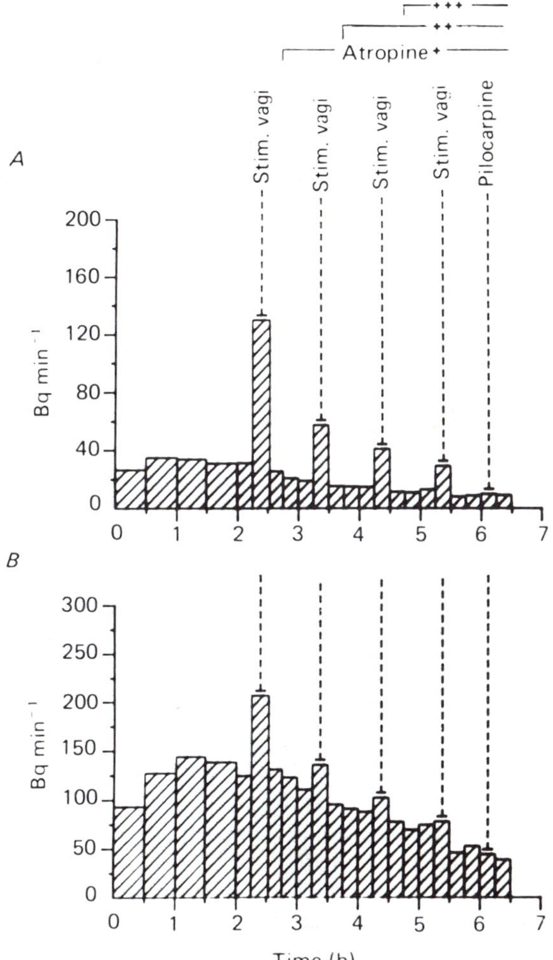

Figure 3 Rate of output of mucin-bound radioactivity from the cat trachea (A = ^{35}S, B = ^{3}H) against time. Electrical stimulation of the vagus nerve stimulated mucin release both in the presence and absence of increasing dosages of atropine. The normally potent effect of pilocarpine (0.5 mg/ml intraluminally) was not observed when atropine was present. Atropine +, 0.3 mg/kg intravenously and 0.6 μg/ml intraluminally. Atropine + +, 1.0 mg/kg intravenously and 20 μg/ml intraluminally. Apropine + + +, 3.0 mg/kg intravenously and 60 μg/ml intraluminally (from Peatfield and Richardson, 1983).

the dominant sympathetic adrenergic constrictor control (Daly and Hebb, 1966; Deffebach et al., 1987). However experiments with the bronchial vasculature were somewhat difficult to interpret because the results might be affected by the pronounced bronchoconstriction seen with vagal stimulation and by alterations in the pulmonary vascular bed into which most of the bronchial circulation drains. More recently the subject has been reopened by observing the effects of vagal stimulation (superior laryngeal nerve) on the tracheal vasculature of the dog (Laitinen et al., 1987a), pig (Matran et al., 1989), and cat (Martling et al., 1985). The response to such stimulation is a clear vasodilation (Fig. 4). Administration of atropine approximately halved the vasodilator effect of nerve stimulation, the residual response pre-

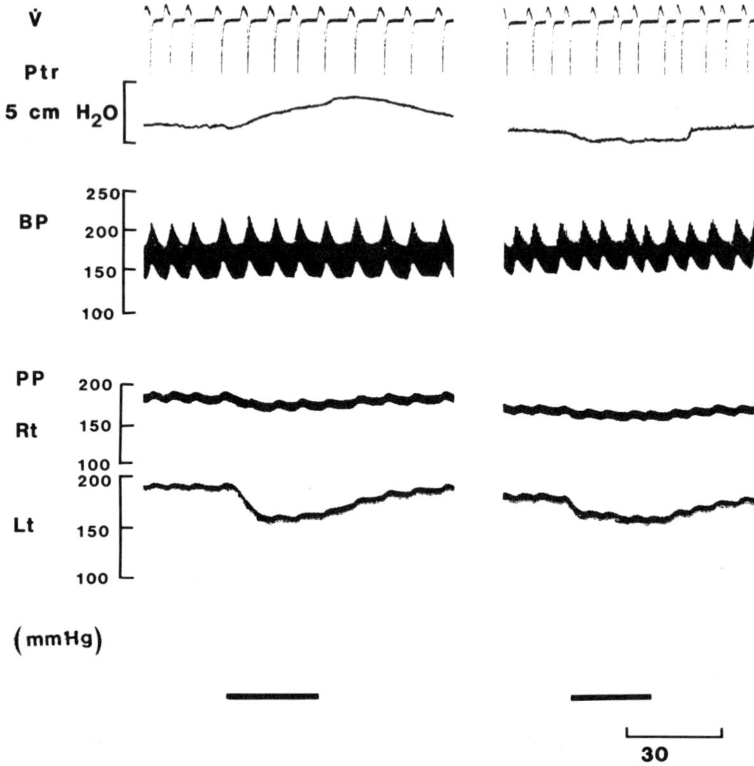

Figure 4   Electrical stimulation (5 V, 1 ms, 10 Hz) of the peripheral end of the cut left superior laryngeal nerve in a spontaneously breathing dog before (left) and after (right) administration of atropine (1 mg/kg intravenously). $\dot{V}$, airflow; P_{tr}, tracheal pressure; BP, blood pressure; RPP, right, and LPP, left perfusion pressures. Before atropine, stimulation causes falls in both perfusion pressures greater on the ipsilateral side, an increase in tracheal pressure, and no change in blood pressure. After atropine, the falls in perfusion pressures are smaller and there is a decrease in tracheal pressure (from Laitinen et al., 1987a).

sumably being due to release of neuropeptides from motor nerves and from antidromic activation of sensory nerves. The atropine-sensitive response indicates that there is a cholinergic dilator supply to tracheal blood vessels, consistent with the earlier studies on bronchial vascular control. The response can be mimicked by injections of methacholine, which are powerfully vasodilating, confirming the presence of dilator cholinoceptors on the vascular smooth muscle (Laitinen et al., 1987b). The fact that atropine itself did little to change vasomotor tone indicates that in the particular preparation used there is probably not much cholinergic vasodilator tonic activity in the vagal nerves.

F. Other Cholinergic Actions in Airways

Acetylcholine released into the airway mucosa can potentially affect cells there, such as those in the epithelium and migratory cells, including mast cells. For example, vagal nerve stimulation can enhance histamine release from mast cells due to antigen challenge, an effect that is blocked by atropine (Leff et al., 1986). In similar fashion, cholinergic agonists promote release of mediators such as histamine and leukotrienes from lung tissue in vitro, an effect that is also blocked by atropine (Kaliner et al., 1972). In the gut, mast cells are found anatomically very close to cholinergic nerves (Stanisz et al., 1987), and such a relationship could also apply to the airways or lungs (Bienenstock et al., 1988).

Ciliary beat activity in the epithelium can be increased by drugs such as methacholine, an effect that is blocked by atropine (Gross, 1988a). Lung C-fiber receptor stimulation can increase mucociliary activity, an effect that is blocked by atropine, suggesting a reflex cholinergic mechanism (Anggard et al., 1983). Thus there are indicators of the possibility that cholinergic mechanisms modify the secretion of migratory cells and the activity of epithelial cells. However, the role of vagal cholinergic nerves in these processes has not been established.

III. Muscarinic Receptors

A. Airway Muscarinic Receptors

Acetylcholine released from postganglionic cholinergic nerve fibers activates muscarinic receptors on target cells in airways (Barnes, 1989). These receptors are localized to several cell types, and their distribution has been studied by autoradiographic mapping techniques (Barnes et al., 1982, 1983).

In ferret lung, muscarinic receptors localized by [^{3}H] quinuclidinyl benzilate (QNB) binding are found on airway smooth muscle of cartilaginous airways, but there are few receptors in peripheral airways (Barnes et al., 1983), which suggests that cholinergic effects predominate in large airways in this species. In human trachea and bronchi, muscarinic receptors are also localized to airway smooth muscle (van Koppen et al., 1987) as well as in smooth muscle of peripheral airways (Mak and Barnes, 1989a,b). Muscarinic receptors are also found in submucosal glands in both animal and human airways (Barnes et al., 1983; van Koppen et al., 1987), consistent with the potent effect of cholinergic agonists on airway mucus secretion. Muscarinic receptors are also present on airway nerves and intramural ganglia (van Koppen et al., 1987; Mak and Barnes, 1989a,b), where they may have a neuromodulatory role.

B. Signal Transduction Mechanisms

The biochemical pathways by which occupation of muscarinic receptors leads to cell activation have now been extensively studied. Contraction of airway smooth muscle depends on release of calcium ions from intracellular stores. This involves hydrolysis of phosphoinositides (PI) with formation of inositol trisphosphate (IP3), which directly releases intracellular calcium (Grandordy and Barnes, 1987; Hall and Chilvers, 1989). There is a close relationship between occupation of muscarinic receptors and stimulation of PI turnover in airway smooth muscle, but the contractile response is considerably more sensitive than the PI response to cholinergic agonists, indicating the existence of "spare" receptors in this tissue (Grandordy et al., 1986). Muscarinic receptor stimulation of airway smooth muscle results in the rapid formation of IP3 and also of IP4, which may be important in refilling the intracellular calcium stores (Hall and Chilvers, 1989; Chilvers et al., 1988).

Muscarinic receptor stimulation inhibits adenylate cyclase, resulting in reduction of intracellular cyclic AMP formation (Jones et al., 1987), but how this relates to stimulation of PI hydrolysis is not yet certain.

C. Muscarinic Receptor Subtypes

Several subtypes of muscarinic receptor have now been identified pharmacologically (Mitchelson, 1988) and at least five subtypes have now been cloned and expressed (Bonner et al., 1987). Three muscarinic receptor subtypes have been demonstrated in lung and their functional significance is emerging (Barnes et al., 1988; Minette and Barnes, 1990) (Fig. 5).

M1-muscarinic receptors are differentiated by their high affinity for pirenzipine. The remaining muscarinic receptors are termed M2-receptors, but it is now clear that M2-receptors are heterogeneous. Antagonists such as gallamine, AF-DX 116, and methoctramine are potent on cardiac muscarinic (still called M2) receptors, which are clearly different from muscarinic receptors in smooth muscle and glands (called M3-receptors). These last are selectively inhibited by antagonists such as 4-DAMP and hexahydro-siladifenidol (Mitchelson, 1988).

M2-Receptors (Autoreceptors)

Muscarinic receptors, which inhibit the release of acetylcholine (autoreceptors), have been demonstrated on cholinergic nerves of airways in several

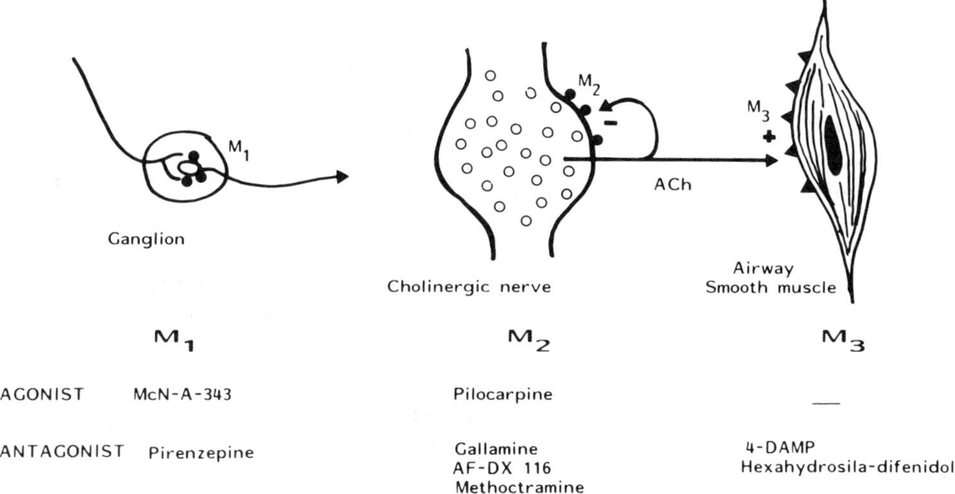

Figure 5 Muscarinic receptor subtypes in airways (from Barnes et al., 1988).

animal species, both in vivo and in vitro (Fryer and Maclagan, 1984; Blaber et al., 1985; Faulkner et al., 1986; Ito and Yoshitomi, 1988). Muscarinic receptors have also been demonstrated on human bronchial nerves in vitro (Minette and Barnes, 1990). These receptors inhibit acetylcholine release and therefore serve to limit vagal bronchoconstriction; they are of the M2-subtype and are clearly different pharmacologically from M3-receptors on airway smooth muscle (Fig. 5). Drugs such as atropine, which block pre-junctional receptors and those on smooth muscle with equal affinity, therefore increase acetylcholine release, which may then overcome the postjunctional blockade. This means that such drugs will not be as effective against vagal bronchoconstriction as against cholinergic agonists; it may be necessary to reevaluate the contribution of cholinergic nerves when drugs selective for the muscarinic receptors on airway smooth muscle (M3-antagonists) are developed. Indeed, low dosages of the nonselective antagonist ipratropium bromide potentiate vagal bronchoconstriction in the guinea-pig (Fryer and Maclagan, 1987), and this might contribute to the paradoxical bronchoconstriction that has been reported with anticholinergics.

Evidence has recently been obtained for muscarinic autoreceptors in human subjects in vivo. A cholinergic agonist, pilocarpine, which selectively activates M2-receptors, inhibits cholinergic reflex bronchoconstriction induced by sulfur dioxide in normal subjects, but such an effect does not appear to operate in asthmatic subjects, suggesting that there may be dysfunction of these autoreceptors (Minette et al., 1988).

M1-Receptors

M1-receptors, which are excitatory, are present in airway ganglia of animals and may be inhibited by pirenzepine (Bloom et al., 1987,1988). The function of these M1-receptors in regulation of airway tone is not yet certain. They may play an active role in "setting" vagal tone, since they appear to be important in the chronic control of ganglionic transmission, whereas the classic nicotinic receptors may be more important in rapid neurotransmission, as in reflexes. Similar receptors are also probably present in human parasympathetic ganglia, since pirenzipine inhibits reflex bronchoconstriction (induced by sulfur dioxide) at dosages that do not inhibit the direct effect of cholinergic agonists in airway tone (Lammers et al., 1989).

Receptor binding studies have demonstrated a surprisingly high proportion of M1-receptors in human lung (Casale and Ecklund, 1988; Mak and Barnes, 1989a). Autoradiographic studies have shown that while airway smooth muscle has only M3-receptors, submucosal glands have a mixture of M1- and M3-receptors (30% M1: 70% M3) and alveolar cells have only M1-receptors. The function of these alveolar M1-receptors is unknown.

IV. Cholinergic Reflexes

A. Upper Airways

The striated muscles of the larynx have a cholinergic innervation through the recurrent and, to a smaller extent, the superior laryngeal nerves. Here cholinergic effects are mediated via nicotinic receptors on the striated fiber, and cholinergic control of the laryngeal structures can therefore not be assessed by the use of antimuscarinic drugs. Laryngeal tone can be affected by mediators acting directly or indirectly through reflexes from the upper and lower airways (Higenbottam, 1980; Widdicombe, 1986). Weak nasal irritation may cause laryngeal narrowing in the expiratory phase (Szereda-Przestaszewska and Widdicombe, 1973). Irritation of the lower airways also produces laryngeal constriction (Stransky et al., 1973; Higenbottam, 1980). The larynx is narrowed in asthma, presumably by reflex mechanisms (Higenbottam, 1980).

The larynx can be assumed to be an important reflexogenic area due to its central position in the airways. It seems to be particularly sensitive to mechanical and chemical stimuli, which can cause laryngeal narrowing, bronchoconstriction (Fig. 2), airway mucus secretion, and tracheal vasodilation (Nadel and Widdicombe, 1962a; Tomori and Widdicombe, 1969; Boushey et al., 1972; Schultz et al., 1982). A laryngeal bronchodilator reflex has recently been demonstrated in cats (Szarek et al., 1986) (Fig. 2) and humans (Michoud et al., 1987, 1988; Lammers et al., 1989). This reflex seems to be mediated by neuropeptides such as VIP or a congener released from noncholinergic nonadrenergic nerves. Its physiological significance remains to be elucidated since it was only demonstrable when reflex bronchoconstriction was blocked by a cholinergic antagonist and airway smooth muscle tone was raised by an exogenous bronchoconstrictor agent.

Irritation of the nose usually causes a decrease in lower airways resistance, as well as sneezes and local nasal reflexes, but airways obstruction is sometimes also produced (Widdicombe, 1986). In asthmatic subjects, nasal irritation consistently increases airways resistance (Konno and Togawa, 1979; Nolte and Berger, 1983; Yan and Salome, 1983). The various results may be explained by differences in strength of the stimuli and by differences in the deposition of the irritant, possibly reaching the larynx, from which potent bronchoconstrictor reflexes can be triggered. Another possibility is that bronchodilation is produced from the nose but that total airways resistance is increased due to laryngeal narrowing. A final possibility is that there may be opposing effects of acetylcholine and of dilator neuropeptides on airway smooth muscle.

B. Tracheobronchial Tree

It is generally believed that reflex bronchoconstriction can be activated from the whole of the tracheobronchial tree, but little is known about the precise sites in the airways from which it can be evoked. No particularly sensitive sites seem to have been identified.

The involvement of a reflex is convincingly demonstrated when the site of stimulation is anatomically separated from the site of measurement and when it is sensitive to neuronal interruption. Gold et al. (1972) showed that histamine and allergen administered to one side of the lungs increased airways resistance also in the other side and that this effect could be abolished by ipsilateral vagotomy or by atropine. Administration of mediators or irritants such as histamine, capsaicin, bradykinin, and prostaglandins to the lower airways of dogs increases tracheal smooth muscle tone via a neural mechanism (Coleridge et al., 1965; Russell and Lai-Fook, 1979; Coleridge and Coleridge, 1986). Sensory input from the airways in the motor cholinergic reflex is carried in the vagus nerves and includes activity from rapidly adapting (irritant) receptors (RAR) with myelinated afferent nerves and bronchial and pulmonary C-fiber endings with nonmyelinated afferents.

The involvement of RAR is supported by the observation that the activity in this type of fiber is stimulated by agents causing an atropine-sensitive bronchoconstriction (Sellick and Widdicombe, 1971). Thus, for example, the histamine-induced increase in airways resistance in rabbits is inhibited by vagal cooling to 7 °C, which blocks conduction in myelinated afferents but leaves intact that in nonmyelinated nerves (Karczewski and Widdicombe, 1969).

In dogs, the response to histamine that is inhibited by antimuscarinic drugs (Gold et al., 1972) is likewise accompanied by enhanced activity in RAR (Vidruk et al., 1977). The mechanosensitive RAR are stimulated also by smooth muscle contraction and by a decrease in dynamic compliance (Sellick and Widdicombe, 1970; Jonzon et al., 1986) and it could therefore be argued that the increase in afferent neural activity is secondary to smooth muscle contraction. Arguing against this view is the observation that iso-proteranol abolishes the tracheal contraction but does not affect RAR receptor discharge to histamine (Vidruk et al., 1977). In rabbits (Mills et al., 1969) and guinea pigs (Bergren and Sampson, 1982), data remain inconclusive. Nevertheless, stimulation of RAR by muscle contraction may augment the bronchoconstrictor response (Sellick and Widdicombe, 1971).

RAR are more concentrated in the proximal parts of the airways (Sant'-Ambrogio, 1987), particularly at branching points of the tracheobronchial tree (Fillenz and Widdicombe, 1972). This is also the major site of constriction to cholinergic stimulation.

A variety of reflexes including bronchoconstriction, airway mucus secretion, vasodilatation, and possibly plasma protein extravasation are mediated by vagal C-fiber afferents (Coleridge and Coleridge, 1984; Karlsson et al., 1988). Evidence for the involvement of C-fibers in bronchoconstriction includes observations that stimuli such as capsaicin and bradykinin that may excite C-fiber endings selectively cause a constrictor response. This bronchoconstriction, at least in part, is sensitive to antimuscarinics (Simonssen et al., 1973; Fuller et al., 1985,1987). Various mediators and drugs applied to the lower airways of dogs increase tracheal smooth muscle tension including when the vagi are cooled to 7 °C but not when they are cooled to 0 °C (see Coleridge and Coleridge, 1986), which would block nonmyelinated fibers.

Activation of pulmonary C-fiber receptors can cause a reflex bronchodilatation when the usual constrictor response is prevented by atropine and bronchomotor tone is restored by a drug such as 5-hydroxytryptamine (Ichinose et al, 1987; Don et al., 1988). This response is thought to be due to the release of neuropeptides from vagal motor fibers. The mechanism is said not to apply to the cat trachea, unlike the bronchi.

In the guinea pig, neurogenic bronchoconstriction involves not only a cholinergic reflex (Clay and Thompson, 1985; Allott et al., 1980; Karlsson and Forsberg, unpublished data) but also a tachykinin peptide-mediated constrictor reflex (Lundberg and Saria, 1982; Karlsson and Persson, 1983; Szolcsanyi, 1983). RAR and capsaicin-sensitive sensory neurons constitute afferent pathways in these reflexes (see Karlsson et al., 1988). It has recently been established by the use of tetrodotoxin that the tachykinin-mediated bronchoconstriction is a local axon reflex within the airway wall (Kroll et al., 1990). Bronchoconstrictor reflexes have been examined in conscious animals but even with agents such as anticholinergic drugs and tachykinin antagonists it is not possible to determine from which site the reflex is evoked. In a group of conscious guinea pigs with sectioned superior laryngeal nerves, the bronchoconstrictor response to inhaled citric acid and histamine was unchanged, whereas the cough response was increased compared to sham-operated controls (Karlsson, Forsberg, and Lundberg, unpublished results). These reflexes seem thus to be evoked from the tracheobronchial tree rather than from the larynx in awake guinea pigs.

Sympathetic afferents through cervical ganglia seem to play a minor role in bronchoconstriction evoked from middle and upper parts of the airways (Tomori et al., 1957), but those passing through the stellate ganglia may be involved in bronchoconstriction from the lower airways (Cromer et al., 1933).

In contrast to the reflex responses to RAR and C-fiber receptors, slowly adapting pulmonary stretch receptors (SAR) reduce efferent vagal excitatory activity to the smooth muscle and mediate bronchodilation (Widdicombe and Nadel, 1963). The intense activity in SAR during tracheal constriction (Bartlett et al., 1976) may therefore serve to limit the bronchoconstrictor response.

We have considered the cholinergic reflexes acting on airway smooth muscle. Similar patterns have been seen for the control of secretion from airway submucosal glands (Richardson and Somerville, 1988; Nadel et al., 1985). Thus secretion is promoted by irritation of the nose and larynx, and by activation of pulmonary C-fiber receptors. Where transmitter mechanisms have been tested, they seem to be cholinergic, in that the secretions are prevented by atropinic drugs.

Stimulation of pulmonary C-fiber receptors also causes vasodilatation in the nose and trachea (Lung and Widdicombe, 1987; Sahin et al., 1987); however these responses are mainly due to the decrease in sympathetic adrenergic tone, and cholinergic mechanisms may not be involved.

C. Other Reflexes

In experimental animals, stimulation of arterial baroreceptors (Nadel and Widdicombe, 1962b), as well as of sensory receptors in skeletal muscle (Rybicki et al., 1983) and the diaphragm (McCallister et al., 1986), causes reflex bronchodilatation, whereas irritation of the tympanic membrane may cause bronchoconstriction (Todisco, 1982). Chemoreceptor stimulation causes a reflex bronchoconstriction (Nadel and Widdicombe, 1962b).

V. Cholinergic Control in Asthma

Since cholinergic nerves are the dominant bronchoconstrictor neural pathway, it has long been suggested that cholinergic mechanisms may be exaggerated in patients with asthma and may contribute to bronchial hyperresponsiveness. The imbalance between cholinergic and adrenergic control was first suggested by Alexander and Paddock (1921), who demonstrated an excessive bronchoconstrictor response to the cholinomimetic drug pilocarpine that could be reversed by epinephrine. There are several sites at which cholinergic control of the airways could be enhanced in asthma, from central control to receptors in target tissues. Enhanced responses to cholinomimetic drugs have even been demonstrated in extrapulmonary tissues (Kaliner et al., 1982), which suggests that there may be a more generalized abnormality in cholinergic control.

A. Increased Central Vagal Control

Since psychological factors may lead to bronchoconstriction, the cerebral cortex may influence cholinergic control of airways, but there is no evidence to support a fundamental psychological abnormality in asthma. Vagal tone is generated from a brainstem center and, although direct recording of vagal tone in human subjects has not been possible, there is some evidence for an increase in vagal tone in asthma since the sinus arrhythmia that reflects cardiac vagal tone is increased in asthmatic patients (Kallenbach et al., 1985). There is also evidence for an increase in vagal tone at night, which may underlie nocturnal asthma (Postma et al., 1985).

B. Enhanced Cholinergic Reflexes

Cholinergic reflex bronchoconstriction may be present in asthma in a number of ways, such as activation of afferent nerves in the respiratory tract (including larynx) and extrapulmonary receptors (e.g., esophagus stimulated by acid reflux; Barnes, 1987a). Several triggers to bronchoconstriction are mediated via cholinergic reflexes, as revealed by the inhibitory action of anticholinergic drugs. Inflammatory mediators, such as histamine or prostaglandins, may "sensitize" afferent nerve endings in the airway, making them more likely to be excited. In asthmatic patients, inhaled PGD_2 increases the bronchoconstrictor response to histamine (Fuller et al., 1986). This result can be explained by such a sensitizing action since histamine stimulates RARs in airways (and its bronchoconstrictor action can be reduced, albeit to a variable extent, by anticholinergic drugs).

C. Facilitation of Cholinergic Neurotransmission

There are several possible reasons why increased release of acetylcholine from postganglionic nerves in airways, or facilitated neurotransmission through parasympathetic ganglia, may occur. Some inflammatory mediators may facilitate release of acetylcholine from airway postganglionic nerves by acting at peripheral receptors. Thus a thromboxane mimetic U46619 and serotonin have this effect in canine airways (Chung et al., 1985; Sheller et al., 1982). Tachykinins also increase cholinergic neurotransmission at postganglionic nerves in rabbit and guinea pig airways (Tanaka and Grunstein, 1984; Hall et al., 1989), suggesting possible interactions between peptidergic and cholinergic nerves. Thus, if axon reflex mechanisms are activated, this may lead to an enhancement of cholinergic reflexes. Whether sensory input to parasympathetic ganglia in airways can also facilitate neurotransmission or lead to a "ganglionic reflex" has not yet been established. It is possible that M1-receptors in airway ganglia may increase neurotransmission and that such receptors may be upregulated in airways of asthmatic patients.

By contrast, activation of other receptors inhibits cholinergic neurotransmission. β-Agonists inhibit cholinergic neurotransmission in canine airways (via a β_1-receptor) and in human airways (via a β_2-receptor; Danser et al., 1987; Rhoden et al., 1988). Thus any dysfunction of β-receptors that might occur in asthma would lead to enhanced acetylcholine release. Indeed, blockade of the effect of circulating epinephrine on β_2-receptors on airway cholinergic nerves may underlie β-blocker-induced asthma, which may be prevented by anticholinergic treatment (Ind et al., 1989). Both neuropeptides and α_2-agonists inhibit cholinergic neurotransmission in guinea pig trachea (Stretton and Barnes, 1988; Grundstrom et al., 1981), and thus any defect in sympathetic nerve function might be reflected by an increase in vagal tone.

As discussed above, muscarinic autoreceptors are a powerful inhibitory mechanism in animal and human airway cholinergic nerves. A recent study has suggested that these receptors may be dysfunctional in asthmatic patients (Minette et al., 1988) and this would lead to exaggerated cholinergic reflex bronchoconstriction. This may also help to explain why β-blockers may precipitate strong bronchocontriction, even in patients with mild asthma, since the increased acetylcholine release due to blockade of prejunctional β-receptors would not be switched off in asthmatic patients (Barnes, 1989).

VIP may be a cotransmitter of acetylcholine in airway cholinergic nerves and, as a functional antagonist of airway smooth muscle contraction, may serve to limit excess reflex bronchoconstriction. If VIP is broken down more rapidly by enzymes released from inflammatory cells in airways of asthmatic patients, this would lead to an enhancement of cholinergic nerve effects

(Barnes, 1987b). Indeed, mast cell tryptase is remarkably effective in degrading VIP and this enzyme is probably released in asthmatic airways.

D. Enhanced Muscarinic Receptor Function

The bronchoconstrictor response to cholinergic agonists is exaggerated in asthmatic subjects, which raises the possibility that muscarinic receptors in airway smooth muscle may be increased or more efficiently coupled. However, the increased responsiveness is not specific for cholinergic agonists, and enhanced responses of a similar magnitude are also seen with other spasmogens such as histamine, leukotrienes, and prostaglandins (which contract smooth muscle directly through specific receptors; Boushey et al., 1980). There are conflicting reports about the responses of asthmatic airways in vitro to cholinergic agonists, but there is no convincing evidence for increased responsiveness (Thomson, 1987). In guinea pigs that become hyperresponsive to acetylcholine after intravenous or inhaled administration of platelet activating factor (PAF), there is no parallel increase in response of airways in vitro to acetylcholine, no increase in muscarinic receptor density or affinity (measured by direct binding), and no change in coupling or biochemical consequences of receptor activation (measured by PI turnover) (Robertson et al., 1988). This indicates that increased cholinergic responsiveness in vivo cannot be accounted for by enhanced muscarinic receptor function and is perhaps more likely to be due to mechanical factors such as airway edema induced by PAF.

VI. Implications for Treatment

Considerable evidence indicates that cholinergic mechanisms contribute to bronchoconstriction and increased mucus secretion in patients with asthma, although the role of cholinergic pathways was perhaps exaggerated in the past.

Anticholinergic drugs have been used widely in the treatment of asthma, and it is now possible to evaluate their effectiveness (Gross and Skorodin, 1984; Mann and George, 1985; Gross, 1988b). These drugs are surprisingly useful when given by nebulizer to patients with acute severe asthma, and may produce bronchodilation similar to that seen with nebulized β_2-agonists (Ward et al., 1981; Rebuck et al., 1987), which suggests that cholinergic mechanisms are predominant in the acute asthma attack. In patients with chronic asthma, anticholinergic drugs are considerably less effective as bronchodilators (Barnes, 1987c) than 5β-agonists. This is not surprising since airway smooth muscle is probably constricted directly by inflammatory mediators such as histamine and leukotrienes and this constriction can be reversed by β-agonists but not by anticholinergic agents. Anticholinergic drugs have no documented anti-inflammatory action in asthma; by contrast, they are as effective as β-agonists in chronic obstructive lung disease in which vagal tone is the only reversible component of airway obstruction (Gross, 1988b).

Perhaps the currently available anticholinergic drugs are not the most effective drugs at blocking cholinergic nerve effects. Both atropine and ipratropium bromide are nonselective and block both M2-receptors localized to cholinergic nerves and M3-receptors on muscle and glands. Thus, in theory, they may increase acetylcholine release, which may increase postjunctional blockade. This suggests that M3-selective blockers would be far more effective in blocking cholinergic nerve-induced effects in airways (Barnes, 1989), and such drugs are now being actively developed.

Discussion

Kaliner: Atropine is relatively ineffective in asthma: does this suggest that cholinergic mechanisms are not as important as once believed?

Widdicombe: Atropine-resistant bronchoconstriction is partly due to the direct action of local mediators, but some of the airway narrowing may be due to vascular congestion from vagal neurotransmitters (acetylcholine and VIP).

Irvin: We studied various irritants in cat larynx without evidence of a bronchodilator response.

Widdicombe: There may be different reflex responses depending on which afferent pathways are activated. There are at least five different sensory receptors in the laryngeal mucosa and so different irritants may excite different populations of receptor. In addition, the afferent pathway may interact in the CNS in gating airway reflexes.

Daniel: In dog airways the muscarinic receptors on cholinergic nerves are of the M1 subtype (blocked by pirenzepine and stimulated by McN A343).

Barnes: In human, guinea pig, and cat airways the muscarinic receptors on postganglionic cholinergic nerves are of the M2-subtype: sensitive to gallamine, AF-DX 116, and methoctramine, but not to pirenzepine. This may suggest species differences.

Fuller: What is the site of increased reflex responsiveness in asthma: nerves or muscle?

Widdicombe: In experimentally induced asthma, afferent receptors may be sensitized by airway inflammation. In humans the evidence is indirect. Many asthmatic patients have a hyperreactive cough reflex and the sensation of "tightness" in the chest, which suggest that sensory endings are being stimulated in asthma.

References

Alexander, H. L., and Paddock, R. (1921). Bronchial asthma: response to pilocarpine and epinephrine. *Arch. Intern. Med.* **27**:184-191.

Allott, C. P., Evans, D. P., and Marshall, P. W. (1980). A model of irritant-induced bronchoconstriction in the spontaneously breathing guinea-pig. *Br. J. Pharmacol.* **71**:165-168.

Anggard, A., Lundberg, J. M., and Lundblad, L. (1983). Nasal autonomic innervation with special reference to peptidergic nerves. *Eur. J. Respir. Dis.* **64**(Suppl):143-148.

Baker, D. G. (1986). Parasympathetic motor pathways to the trachea: recent morphologic and electrophysiologic studies. *Clin. Chest Med.* **7**:223-229.

Baker, D. G., Basbaum, C. B., Herbert, D. A., and Mitchell, R. A. (1983). Transmission in airway ganglia of ferrets: inhibition by norepinephrine. *Neurosci. Lett.* **41**:139-143.

Baker, D. G., McDonald, D. M., Basbaum, C. B., and Mitchell, R. A. (1986). The architecture of nerves and ganglia of the ferret trachea as revealed by acetylcholinesterase histochemistry. *J. Comp. Neurol.* **246**:513-526.

Barnes, P. J. (1986). Neural control of human airways in health and disease. *Am. Rev. Respir. Dis.* **134**:1289-1314.

Barnes, P. J. (1987a). Cholinergic control of airway smooth muscle. *Am. Rev. Respir. Dis.* **136**(Suppl):S42-S45.

Barnes, P. J. (1987b). Airway neuropeptides and asthma. *Trends Pharm. Sci.* **8**:24-27.

Barnes, P. J. (1987c). Using anticholinergics to best advantage. *J. Respir. Dis.* **8**:84-95.

Barnes, P. J. (1988). Airway neuropeptides. In *Asthma: Basic Mechanisms and Clinical Management*. Edited by P. J. Barnes, I. W. Rodger and N. C. Thomson. London, Academic Press, pp. 395-413.

Barnes, P. J. (1989). Muscarinic receptor subtypes: implications for lung disease. *Thorax* **44**:161-167.

Barnes, P. J., Nadel, J. A., Roberts, J. M., and Basbaum, C. B. (1982). Muscarinic receptors in lung and trachea: autoradiographic localization using [^{3}H]quinuclidinyl benzilate. *Eur. J. Pharmacol.* **86**:103-106.

Barnes, P. J., Basbaum, C. B., and Nadel, J. A. (1983). Autoradiographic localization of autonomic receptors in airway smooth muscle: marked differences between large and small airways. *Am. Rev. Respir. Dis.* **127**:758-762.

Barnes, P. J., Minette, P. A., and Maclagan, J. (1988). Muscarinic receptor subtypes in lung. *Trends Pharm. Sci.* **9**:412-416.

Bartlett, D., Jr., Jeffery, P., Sant'Ambrogio, G., and Wise, J. C. M. (1976). Location of stretch receptors in the trachea and bronchi of the dog. *J. Physiol Lond.* **258**:409-420.

Basbaum, C. B., Ueki, I., Brezina, L., and Nadel, J. A. (1981). Tracheal submucosal gland serous cells stimulated in vitro with adrenergic and cholinergic agonists. A morphometric study. *Cell Tissue Res.* **220**:481-498.

Begren, D. R., and Sampson, S. R. (1982). Characterization of intrapulmonary, rapidly adapting receptors of guinea pigs. *Respir. Physiol.* **47**:83-95.

Bienenstock, J., Perdue, M., Blennerhassett, M., Stead, R., Katuha, N., Sestini, P., Vancheri, C., and Marshall, J. (1988). Inflammatory cells and the epithelium. *Am. Rev. Respir. Dis.* **138**(Suppl):S31-S34.

Blaber, L. C., Fryer, A. D., and Maclagan, J. (1985). Neuronal muscarinic receptors attenuate vagally-induced contraction of feline bronchial smooth muscle. *Br. J. Pharmacol.* **86**:723-728.

Bloom, J. W., Yamamura, H. I., Baumgartner, C., and Halonen, M. (1987). A muscarinic receptor with high affinity for pirenzepine mediates vagally-induced bronchoconstriction. *Eur. J. Pharmacol.* **133**:21-27.

Bloom, J. W., Baumgartner-Folkerts, C., Palmer, J. D., Yamamura, H. I., and Halonen, M. (1988). A muscarinic receptor subtype modulates vagally-stimulated bronchial contraction. *J. Appl. Physiol.* **85**:2144-2150.

Bonner, T. I., Buckley, N. J., Young, A. C., and Brann, M. R. (1987). Identification of a family of muscarinic acetylcholine receptor genes. *Science* **237**:5.

Boushey, H. A., Richardson, P. S., and Widdicombe, J. G. (1972). Reflex effects of laryngeal irritation on the pattern of breathing and total lung resistance. *J. Physiol. Lond.* **224**:501-513.

Boushey, H. A., Holtzman, M. J., Sheller, J. R., and Nadel, J. A. (1980). Bronchial hyperreactivity. *Am. Rev. Respir. Dis.* **121**:389-413.

Burnstock, G., Allen, T. G. J., and Hassall, C. J. S. (1987). The electrophysiologic and neurochemical properties of paratracheal neurones in situ and in dissociated cell culture. *Am. Rev. Respir. Dis.* **136**(Suppl):S23-S26.

Cameron, A. R., and Coburn, R. F. (1984). Electrical and anatomical characteristics of the cells of the ferret paratracheal ganglion. *Am. J. Physiol.* **224**:1072-1080.

Casale, T. B., and Ecklund, P. (1988). Characterization of muscarinic receptor subtypes in human peripheral lung. *J. Appl. Physiol.* **65**:594-600.

Chiang, C.-H., and Gabella, G. (1986). Quantitative study of the ganglion neurones of the mouse trachea. *Cell Tissue Res.* **246**:243-252.

Chilvers, E. R., Barnes, P. J., and Nahorski, S. R. (1988). Muscarinic receptor stimulated turnover of polyphosphoinositides and inositol polyphosphates in bovine tracheal smooth muscle. *Br. J. Pharmacol.* **95**:778P.

Chung, K. F., Evans, T. W., Graf, P. D., and Nadel, J. A. (1985). Modulation of cholinergic neurotransmission in canine airways by thromboxane-mimetic U46619. *Eur. J. Pharmacol.* **117**:373-375.

Clay, T. P., and Thompson, M. A. (1985). Irritant induced cough as a model of intrapulmonary airway reactivity. *Lung* **163**:183-191.

Coleridge, H. M., Coleridge, J. C. G., and Luck, J. C. (1965). Pulmonary afferent fibres of small diameter stimulated by capsaicin and hyperinflation of the lungs. *J. Physiol. Lond.* **179**:248-262.

Coleridge, J. C. G., and Coleridge, H. M. (1984). Afferent vagal C-fiber innervation of the lungs and airways and its functional significance. *Rev. Physiol. Biochem. Pharmacol.* **99**:1-110.

Coleridge, J. C. G., and Coleridge, H. M. (1986). Reflexes evoked from tracheobronchial tree and lungs. In *Handbook of Physiology, 3. The Respiratory System, vol. II.* Edited by N. S. Cherniack and J. G. Widdicombe. Bethesda, MD, American Physiological Society, pp. 395-430.

Cromer, S. P., Young, R. H., and Ivy, A. C. (1933). On the existence of afferent respiratory impulses mediated by the stellate ganglia. *Am. J. Physiol.* **104**:468-475.

Daly, I. de B., and Hebb, C. (1966). *Pulmonary and Bronchial Vascular System.* London, Edward Arnold.

Daly, M. de B., and Mount, L. E. (1951). The origin, course and nature of bronchomotor fibres in the cervical sympathetic nerve of the cat. *J. Physiol. Lond.* **113**:43-62.

Daniel, E. E., Davis, C., Jones, T., and Kannan, M. S. (1980). Control of airway smooth muscle. In *Airway Reactivity.* Edited by F. E. Hargreave. Missisauga, Ontario, Astra Pharmaceuticals Canada Ltd, pp. 80-107.

Danser, A. H. J., van den Ende, R., Lorenz, R. R., Flavahan, N. A., and Vanhoutte, P. M. (1987). Prejunctional beta$_1$-adrenoceptors inhibit cholinergic neurotransmission in canine bronchi. *J. Appl. Physiol.* **62**:785-790.

Deffebach, M. E., Charan, N. B., Lakshminarayan, S., and Butler, J. (1987). The bronchial circulation. Small, but a vital attribute of the lung. *Am. Rev. Respir. Dis.* **135**:463-481.

Dey, R. D., Shannon, W. R., and Said, S. I. (1981). Localization of VIP-immunoreactive nerves in airways and pulmonary vessels of dogs, cats and human subjects. *Cell Tissue Res.* **220**:231-238.

Don, H., Baker, D. G., and Richardson, C. A. (1988). Absence of nonadrenergic noncholinergic relaxation in the cat cervical trachea. *J. Appl. Physiol.* **65**:2514-2530.

Faulkner, D., Fryer, A. D., and Maclagan, J. (1986). Postganglionic muscarinic inhibitory receptors in pulmonary parasympathetic nerves in guinea-pig. *Br. J. Pharmacol.* **88**:181-187.

Fillenz, M., and Widdicombe, J. G. (1972). Receptors of the lungs and airways. In *Handbook of Sensory Physiology*. Edited by E. Neil. Berlin, Springer-Verlag, pp. 81-112.

Fryer, A. D., and Maclagan, J. (1984). Muscarinic inhibitory receptors in pulmonary parasympathetic nerves in the guinea-pig. *Br. J. Pharmacol.* **83**:973-978.

Fryer, A. D., and Maclagan, J. (1987). Ipratropium bromide potentiated bronchoconstriction induced by vagal nerve stimulation in the guinea-pig. *Eur. J. Pharmacol.* **139**:187-191.

Fuller, R. W., Dixon, C. M. S., and Barnes, P. J. (1985). Bronchoconstriction response to inhaled capsaicin in humans. *J. Appl. Physiol.* **58**:1080-1084.

Fuller, R. W., Dixon, C. M. S., Dollery, C. T., and Barnes, P. J. (1986). Prostaglandin D$_2$ potentiated airway responses to histamine and methacholine. *Am. Rev. Respir. Dis.* **133**:252-254.

Fuller, R. W., Dixon, C. M. S., Cuss, F. M. C., and Barnes, P. J. (1987). Bradykinin-induced bronchoconstriction in humans. *Am. Rev. Respir. Dis.* **135**:176-180.

Gold, W. M., Kessler, G.-F., and Yu, D. Y. C. (1972). Role of vagus nerves in experimental asthma in allergic dogs. *J. Appl. Physiol.* **33**:719-725.

Grandordy, B. M., and Barnes, P. J. (1987). Phosphoinositide turnover in airway smooth muscle. *Am. Rev. Respir. Dis.* **136**:17-20.

Grandordy, B. M., Cuss, F. M., Sampson, A. S., Palmer, J. B., and Barnes, P. J. (1986). Phosphatidylinositol response to cholinergic agonists in airway smooth muscle: relationship to contraction and muscarinic receptor occupancy. *J. Pharmacol. Exp. Ther.* **238**:273-279.

Gross, N. J. (1988a). Cholinergic control. In *Asthma: Basic Mechanisms and Clinical Management*. Edited by P. J. Barnes, I. W. Rodger, and N. C. Thomson. London, Academic Press, pp. 381-393.

Gross, N. J. (1988b). Ipratropium bromide. *N. Engl. J. Med.* **319**:486-494.

Gross, N. J., and Skorodin, M. S. (1984). Anticholinergic antimuscarinic bronchodilators. *Am. Rev. Respir. Dis.* **129**:856-870.

Grundstrom, N., and Andersson, R. G. G. (1985). Inhibition of the cholinergic neurotransmission in human airways via prejunctional α_2-adrenoceptors. *Acta Physiol. Scand.* **125**:513-517.

Grundstrom, N., Andersson, R. G. G., and Wikberg, J. E. S. (1981). Prejunctional α_2-adrenoceptors inhibit contraction of tracheal smooth muscle by inhibiting cholinergic neurotransmission. *Life Sci.* **28**:2981-2986.

Hall, A. K., Barnes, P. J., Meldrum, L. A., and Maclagan, J. (1989). Facilitation by tachykinins of neurotransmission in guinea-pig pulmonary parasympathetic nerves. *Br. J. Pharmacol.* **97**:274-270.

Hall, I., and Chilvers, E. R. (1989). Inositol phosphates and airway smooth muscle. *Pulm. Pharmacol.* **2**:113-120.

Higenbottam, T. (1980). Narrowing of glottis opening in humans associated with experimentally-induced bronchoconstriction. *J. Appl. Physiol.* **49**:403-407.

Ichinose, M., Inoue, H., Miura, M., Yafuso, N., Nogami, H., and Takishima, T. (1987). Possible sensory receptor of nonadrenergic inhibitory nervous system. *J. Appl. Physiol.* **63**:923-929.

Ichinose, M., Stretton, C. D., Schwartz, J.-C., and Barnes, P. J. (1989). Histamine H_3-receptors inhibit cholinergic neurotransmission in guinea-pig airways. *Br. J. Pharmacol.* **97**:13-15.

Ind, P. W., Dixon, C. M. S., Fuller, R. W., and Barnes, P. J. (1989). Anticholinergic blockade of beta-blocker-induced bronchoconstriction. *Am. Rev. Respir. Dis.* **139**:1390-1394.

Ito, Y., and Takeda, K. (1982). Non-adrenergic inhibitory nerves and putative transmitters in the smooth muscle of cat trachea. *J. Physiol. Lond.* **330**:497-511.

Ito, Y., and Yoshitomi, T. (1988). Autoregulation of acetylcholine release from vagus nerve terminals through activation of muscarinic receptors in dog trachea. *Br. J. Pharmacol.* **93**:636-646.

Jones, C. A., Madison, J. M., Tom-Moy, M., and Brown, J. K. (1987). Muscarinic cholinergic inhibition of adenylate cyclase in airway smooth muscle. *Am. J. Physiol.* **253**:90-104.

Jonzon, A., Pisarri, T. E., Coleridge, J. C. G., and Coleridge, H. M. (1986). Rapidly adapting receptor activity in dogs is inversely related to lung compliance. *J. Appl. Physiol.* **61**:1980-1987.

Kaliner, M., Orange, R. P., and Austen, K. F. (1972). Immunologic release of histamine and slow reacting substance of anaphylaxis from human lung. IV. Enhancement by cholinergic and alpha-adrenergic stimulation. *J. Exp. Med.* **136**:556-567.

Kaliner, M., Shelthamer, J., Davis, P. B., Smith, L. J., and Venter, J. C. (1982). Autonomic nervous system abnormalities and allergy. *Ann. Intern. Med.* **96**:349-357.

Kallenbach, J. M., Webster, T., Dowdeswell, R., Reinach, S. G., Scott Millar, R. N., and Zwi, S. (1985). Reflex heart rate control in asthma. *Chest* **87**:644-648.

Karczewski, W., and Widdicombe, J. G. (1969). The effect of vagotomy, vagal cooling and efferent vagal stimulation on breathing and lung mechanics of rabbits. *J. Physiol. Lond.* **201**:259-270.

Karlsson, J.-A., and Persson, C. G. A. (1983). Evidence against vasoactive intestinal polypeptide (VIP) as a dilator and in favour of substance P as a constrictor in airway neurogenic responses. *Br. J. Pharmacol.* **79**: 634-636.

Karlsson, J.-A., Sant'Ambrogio, G., and Widdicombe, J. G. (1988). Afferent neural pathways in cough and reflex bronchoconstriction. *J. Appl. Physiol.* **65**:1007-1023.

Konno, A., and Togawa, K. (1979). Role of the vidian neurectomy in nasal allergy. *Am. Otol. Rhinol. Laryngol.* **88**:258-266.

Kroll, F., Karlsson, J.-A., Lundberg, J. M., and Persson, C. G. A. (1990). Capsaicin-induced bronchoconstriction and neuropeptide release in a perfused bronchopulmonary in vitro preparation. (in manuscript).

Laitinen, L. A., and Laitinen, A. (1988). Neural pathways in human airways. In *Asthma: Basic Mechanisms and Clinical Management*. Edited by P. J. Barnes, I. W. Rodger, and N. C. Thomson. London, Academic Press, pp. 341-355.

Laitinen, L. A., Laitinen, A., and Widdicombe, J. G. (1987a). Parasympathetic nervous control of tracheal vascular resistance in dogs. *J. Physiol. Lond.* **385**:135-146.

Laitinen, L. A., Laitinen, M. A., and Widdicombe, J. G. (1987b). Dose-related effects of pharmacological mediators on tracheal vascular resistance in dogs. *Br. J. Pharmacol.* **92**:703-709.

Lammers, J.-W., Minette, P., McCusker, M., and Barnes, P. J. (1989). The role of pirenzepine-sensitive (M1) muscarinic receptors in vagally-mediated bronchoconstriction in humans. *Am. Rev. Respir. Dis.* **139**:446-449.

Leff, A. R. (1988). Endogenous regulation of bronchomotor tone. *Am. Rev. Respir. Dis.* **137**:1198-1216.

Leff, A. R., Stimler, N. P., Munoz, N. M., Shioya, T., Tallet, J., and Dame, C. (1986). Augmentation of respiratory mast cell secretion of histamine caused by vagus nerve stimulation during antigen challenge. *J. Immunol.* **136**:1066-1073.

Lundberg, J. M., and Saria, A. (1982). Bronchial smooth muscle contraction induced by stimulation of capsaicin-sensitive sensory neurons. *Acta Physiol. Scand.* **116**:473-76.

Lundberg, J. M., Lundblad, L., Martling, C.-R., Saria, A., Stjarne, P., and Anggard, A. (1987). Coexistence of multiple peptides and classical transmitters in airway neurons: functional and pathophysiological aspects. *Am. Rev. Respir. Dis.* **136**(Suppl):S16-S22.

Lung, M. A., and Widdicombe, J. G. (1987). Lung reflexes and nasal vascular resistance with anesthetized dog. *J. Physiol. Lond.* **386**:465-474.

Mak, J. C. W., and Barnes, P. J. (1989a). Muscarinic receptor subtypes in guinea-pig and human lung. *Eur. J. Pharmacol.* **164**:223-230.

Mak, J. C. W., and Barnes, P. J. (1989b). Autoradiographic visualization of muscarinic receptor subtypes in human and guinea-pig lung. *Am. Rev. Respir. Dis.* **139**:A74.

Mann, J. S., and George, C. F. (1985). Anticholinergic drugs in the treatment of airways disease. *Br. J. Dis. Chest* **79**:209-228.

Martling, C.-R., Anggard, A., and Lundberg, J. M. (1985). Noncholinergic vasodilatation in the tracheobronchial tree of the cat induced by vagal nerve stimulation. *Acta Physiol. Scand.* **125**:343-346.

Matran, R., Alving, K., Martling, C.-R., Lacroix, J. S., and Lundberg, J. M. (1989). Vagally mediated vasodilatation by motor and sensory nerves in the tracheal and bronchial circulation of the pig. *Acta Physiol. Scand.* **135**:29-37.

McCallister, L. W., McCoy, K. W., Connelly, J. C., and Kaufman, M. P. (1986). Stimulation of groups III and IV phrenic afferents decreases total lung resistance in dogs. *J. Appl. Physiol.* **61**:1346-1351.

McDonald, D. M. (1987). Neurogenic inflammation in the respiratory tract: actions of sensory nerve mediators on blood vessels and epithelium of the airway mucosa. *Am. Rev. Respir. Dis.* **136**(Suppl):S65-S72.

McFadden, E. R., Luparello, T., Lyons, H. A., and Bleaker, E. (1969). The mechanism of action of suggestion in the induction of acute ashtma attacks. *Psychosom. Med.* **31**:134-143.

Michoud, M.-C., Amyot, R., Jeanneret-Grosjean, A., and Couture, J. (1987). Reflex decrease of histamine-induced bronchoconstriction after laryngeal stimulation in humans. *Am. Rev. Respir. Dis.* **136**:618-622.

Michoud, M.-C., Jeanneret-Grosjean, A., Cohen, A., and Amyot, R. (1988). Reflex decrease of histamine-induced bronchoconstriction after laryngeal stimulation in asthmatic patients. *Am. Rev. Respir. Dis.* **138**:1548-1552.

Mills, J. E., Sellick, H., and Widdicombe, J. G. (1969). Activity of lung irritant receptors in pulmonary microembolism, anaphylaxis and drug-induced bronchoconstriction. *J. Physiol. Lond.* **203**:337-357.

Minette, P. A., and Barnes, P. J. (1990). Muscarinic receptor subtypes in airways: function and clinical significance. *Am. Rev. Respir. Dis.* (in press).

Minette, P. A., Lammers, J.-W., and Barnes, P. J. (1988). Is there a defect in inhibitory muscarinic receptors in asthma? *Am. Rev. Respir. Dis.* **137**:239.

Mitchelson, F. (1988). Muscarinic receptor differentiation. *Pharmacol. Ther.* **37**:357-423.

Nadel, J. A. (1980). Autonomic regulation of airway smooth muscle. In *Physiology and Pharmacology of the Airways*. Edited by J. A. Nadel. New York, Marcel Dekker, pp. 217-257.

Nadel, J. A., and Widdicombe, J. G. (1962a). Reflex effects of upper airway irritation on total lung resistance and blood pressure. *J. Appl. Physiol.* **17**:861-865.

Nadel, J. A., and Widdicombe, J. G. (1962b). Effect of changes in blood gas tensions and carotid sinus pressure on tracheal volume and total lung resistance to airflow. *J. Physiol. Lond.* **163**:13-33.

Nadel, J. A., Widdicombe, J. H., and Peatfield, A. C. (1985). Regulation of airway secretions, ion transport and water movement. In *Handbook of Physiology, 3. The Respiratory System, vol. 1.* Edited by A. P. Fishman and A. B. Fisher. Bethesda, MD, American Physiological Society, pp. 419-446.

Neild, J. E., and Cameron, I. R. (1985). Bronchoconstriction in response to suggestion: its prevention by an inhaled anticholinergic agent. *Br. Med. J.* **290**:674.

Nolte, D., and Berger, D. (1983). On vagal bronchoconstriction in asthmatic patients induced by nasal irritation. *Eur. J. Respir. Dis.* **128**(Suppl): S110-S114.

Peatfield, A. C., and Richardson, P. S. (1982). The control of mucin secretion into the lumen of the cat trachea by α- and β-adrenoceptors, and their relative involvement during sympathetic nerve stimulation. *Eur. J. Pharmacol.* **81**:617-626.

Peatfield, A. C., and Richardson, P. S. (1983). Evidence for non-adrenergic non-cholinergic nervous control of mucus secretion in the cat trachea. *J. Physiol. Lond.* **342**:335-345.

Phipps, R. J., Nadel, J. A., and Davis, B. (1980). Effect of α-adrenergic stimulation of mucus secretion and on ion transport in cat trachea in vitro. *Am. Rev. Respir. Dis.* **121**:359-365.

Postma, D. S., Keyzer, J. J., Koeter, G. H., Sluiter, H. J., and De Vries, K. (1985). Influence of the parasympathetic and sympathetic nervous systems on nocturnal bronchial obstruction. *Clin. Sci.* **69**:251-258.

Rebuck, A. S., and Marcus, H. I. (1979). Sch 1000 in psychogenic asthma. *J. Respir. Dis.* **103**(Suppl):186-190.

Rebuck, A. S., Chapman, K. R., Abboud, R., Pare, P. D., Kreisman, H., Wolkove, N., and Vickerson, P. (1987). Nebulized anticholinergic and sympathomimetic treatment of asthma and chronic obstructive airways disease in the emergency room. *Am. J. Med.* **82**:59-64.

Rhoden, K. J., Meldrum, L. A., and Barnes, P. J. (1988). Inhibition of cholinergic neurotransmission in human airways by β-adrenoceptors. *J. Appl. Physiol.* **65**:700-705.

Richardson, P. S., and Somerville, M. (1988). Mucus and mucus-secreting cells. In *Asthma: Basic Mechanisms and Clinical Management.* Edited by P. J. Barnes, I. W. Rodger, and N. C. Thomson. London, Academic Press, pp. 163-186.

Robertson, D. N., Rhoden, K. J., Grandordy, B., Page, C. P., and Barnes, P. J. (1988). The effect of platelet activating factor on histamine and muscarinic receptor function in guinea-pig airways. *Am. Rev. Respir. Dis.* **137**:1317-1322.

Russell, J. A., and Lai-Fook, S. J. (1979). Reflex bronchoconstriction induced by capsaicin in the dog. *J. Appl. Physiol.* **47**:961-967.

Rybicki, K. J., Longhurst, J. C., and Kaufman, M. P. (1983). Stimulation of splanchnic afferents reflexly relaxes tracheal smooth muscle in dogs. *J. Appl. Physiol.* **55**:427-432.

Sahin, G., Webber, S. E., and Widdicombe, J. G. (1987). Lung and cardiac reflex actions on the tracheal vasculature in anaesthetized dogs. *J. Physiol. Lond.* **387**:47-57.

Sant'Ambrogio, G. (1987). Nervous receptors of the tracheobronchial tree. *Ann. Rev. Physiol.* **49**:611-627.

Schultz, H. D., Roberts, A. M., Hahn, H. L., Nadel, J. A., Coleridge, H. M., and Coleridge, J. C. G. (1982). Mechanism of airway constriction and secretion evoked by laryngeal administration of SO_2 in dogs. *Physiologist* **25**:226 (abstract).

Sellick, H., and Widdicombe, J. G. (1970). Vagal deflation and inflation reflexes mediated by lung irritant receptors. *Q. J. Exp. Physiol.* **55**:153-163.

Sellick, H., and Widdicombe, J. G. (1971). Stimulation of lung irritant receptors by cigarette smoke, carbon dust, and histamine aerosol. *J. Appl. Physiol.* **31**:15-19.

Sheller, J. R., Holtzman, M. J., Skoogh, B.-E., and Nadel, J. A. (1982). Interaction of serotonin with vagal and acetylcholine-induced bronchoconstriction in canine lungs. *J. Appl. Physiol.* **52**:964-966.

Simonsson, B. G., Skoogh, B.-E., Berg, N. P., and Andersson, R. (1973). In vivo and in vitro effect of bradykinin on bronchial motor tone in normal subjects and patients with airway obstruction. *Respiration* **30**:378-388.

Skoogh, B.-E., and Svedmyr, N. (1989). $Beta_2$-adrenoceptor stimulation inhibits ganglionic transmission in ferret trachea. *Pulm. Pharmacol.* **1**:167-172.

Stanisz, A., Scicchitano, R., Stead, R., Matsuda, H., Tomiola, M., Denberg, J., and Bienenstock, J. (1987). Neuropeptides and immunity. *Am. Rev. Respir. Dis.* **136**(Suppl):S48-S51.

Stransky, A., Szereda-Przestaszewska, M., and Widdicombe, J. G. (1973). The effect of lung reflexes on laryngeal resistance motoneuron discharge. *J. Physiol. Lond.* **231**:417-438.

Stretton, D., and Barnes, P. J. (1988). Modulation of cholinergic neurotransmission in guinea-pig trachea by neuropeptide Y. *Br. J. Pharmacol.* **93**:672-678.

Szarek, J. L., Gillespie, M. N., Altiere, R. J., and Diamond, L. (1986). Reflex activation of the nonadrenergic noncholinergic inhibitory nervous system in feline airways. *Am. Rev. Respir. Dis.* **133**:1159-1162.

Szereda-Przestaszewska, M., and Widdicombe, J. G. (1973). Reflex effects of chemical irritation of the upper airways on the laryngeal lumen in cats. *Respir. Physiol.* **18**:107-115.

Szolcsanyi, J. (1983). Tetrodotoxin-resistant non-cholinergic neurogenic contraction evoked by capsaicinoids and piperine on the guinea-pig trachea. *Neurosci. Lett.* **42**:83-88.

Tanaka, D. T,m and Grunstein, M. M. (1984). Mechanisms of substance P-induced contraction of rabbit airway smooth muscle. *J. Appl. Physiol.* **57**:1551-1557.

Thomson, N. C. (1987). In vivo versus in vitro human airway responsiveness to different pharmacological stimuli. *Am. Rev. Respir. Dis.* **136**(Suppl): S58-S62.

Todisco, T. (1982). The oto-respiratory reflex. *Respiration* **43**:354-358.

Tomori, Z., and Widdicombe, J. G. (1969). Muscular, bronchomotor and cardiovascular reflexes elicited by mechanical stimulation of the respiratory tract. *J. Physiol. Lond.* **200**:25-49.

Tomori, Z., Korpas, J., and Ivanco, I. (1957). Uber die Bedeutung der afferenten Innervation bei dem aus verschiedenen Gebieten der Luftwege ausgelosten Husten. *Physiol. Bohemoslov.* **6**:175-178.

van Koppen, C. J., Blankensteijn, W. M., Klaasen, A. B. M., Rodrigues de Miranda, F., Beld, A. J., and van Ginneken, C. A. M. (1987). Autoradiographic visualization of muscarinic receptors in human bronchi. *J. Pharmacol. Exp. Ther.* **244**:760-764.

Vidruk, E. H. (1983). Extravagal innervation of canine tracheal stretch receptors. *J. Physiol. Lond.* **338**:11-17.

Vidruk, E. H., Hahn, H. L., Nadel, J. A., and Sampson, S. R. (1977). Mechanisms by which histamine stimulates rapidly adapting receptors in dog lungs. *J. Appl. Physiol.* **43**:397-402.

Ward, M. J., Fentem, P. H., Roderick Smith, W. H., and Davies, D. (1981). Ipratropium bromide in acute asthma. *Br. Med. J.* **282**:590-600.

Webber, S. E. (1989). Receptors mediating the effects of substance P and neurokinin A on mucus secretion and smooth muscle tone of the ferret trachea. *Br. J. Pharmacol.* **98**:1197-1206.

Webber, S. E., and Widdicombe, J. G. (1987). The effect of vasoactive intestinal peptide on smooth muscle tone and mucus secretion from the ferret trachea. *Br. J. Pharmacol.* **91**:139-148.

Widdicombe, J. G. (1986). Reflexes from the upper respiratory tract. In *Handbook of Physiology, 3. The Respiratory System. vol. II.* Edited by N. S. Cherniack and J. G. Widdicombe. Bethesda, MD, American Physiological Society, pp. 363-394.

Widdicombe, J. G., and Nadel, J. A. (1963). Reflex effects of lung inflation on tracheal volume. *J. Appl. Physiol.* **18**:681-686.

Widdicombe, J. G., and Webber, S. E. (1990). Airway mucus secretion. *News Physiol. Sci.* **5**:2-5.

Yan, K., and Salome, C. (1983). The response of the airways to nasal stimulation in asthmatics with rhinitis. *Eur. J. Respir. Dis.* **128**(Suppl):105-108.

13

Role of the Adrenergic Nervous System in Asthma

ALAN R. LEFF

University of Chicago
Chicago, Illinois

Because sympathomimetic drugs are the mainstay of asthma therapy, the physiological role of the autonomic nervous system in regulating bronchomotor tone has been a source of intense interest and investigation in health and in asthmatic disease. Major areas of investigation have focused on (1) the role of beta-adrenoceptor deficiency and alpha-adrenoceptor activation in augmented contractility of asthmatic smooth muscle; (2) the role of sympathetic secretion in downregulation of mast cell degranulating responses; (3) interactions between the sympathetic nervous system (SNS) and other neural influences; and (4) the homeostatic role of sympathetic secretion in the regulation of bronchomotor tone in healthy subjects and patients with asthma. Recent investigations have challenged traditional views in all of these areas and have resulted in a substantial reformulation of the role of the sympathetic component of the autonomic nervous system in the regulation of bronchomotor tone.

I. Anatomical Organization

Sympathetic activation originates in the central nervous system as the result of efferent (visceral sensory) input. The traditional view of the sympathetic

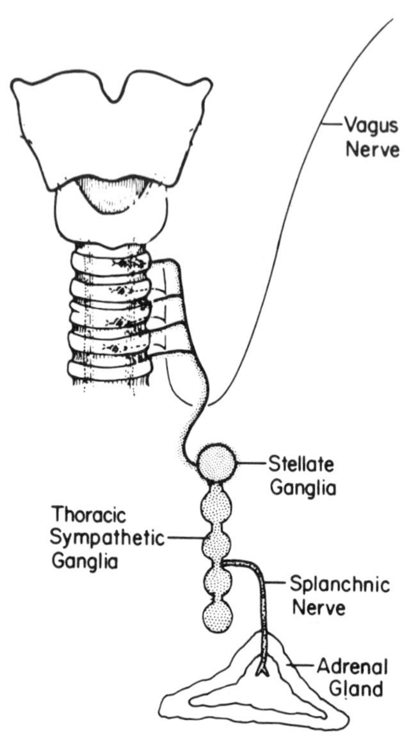

Vagus
Nerve
Stellate
Ganglia
Thoracic
Sympathetic
Ganglia
Splanchnic
Nerve
Adrenal
Gland

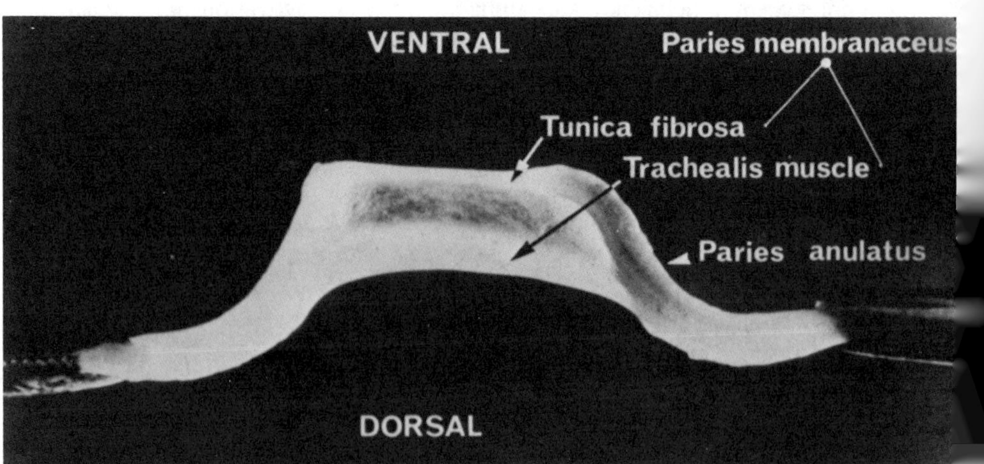

VENTRAL
Paries membranaceus
Tunica fibrosa
Trachealis muscle
Paries anulatus
DORSAL

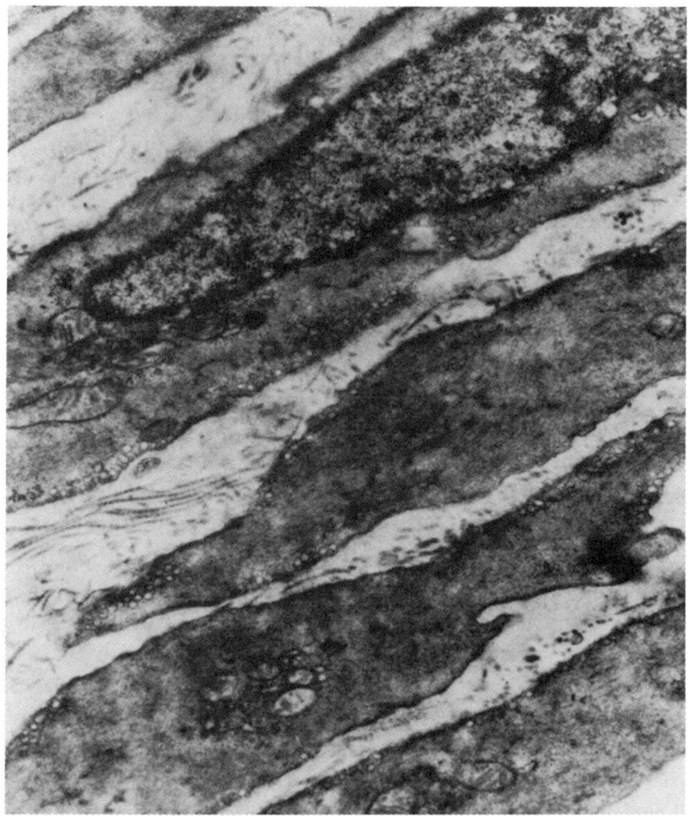

Figure 1 *Above*: Efferent sympathetic secretion. Short preganglionic fibers arising from the spinal cord (not shown) synapse with ganglia in the thoracic sympathetic chains. Multiple synapses arise from each ganglion, providing an amplification factor facilitating the *flight and fright* response. Innervation to organs arise from long postganglionic fibers that traverse the distance between the ganglion and the innervated organ. In contrast, parasympathetic innervation arises from a long preganglionic vagus nerve that synapses directly 1 : 1 in a ganglion contained within the organ that is innervated. A second component of sympathetic activation is adrenal secretion of epinephrine from the adrenal medula, itself a ganglion. Direct sympathetic innervation to airways does not exist in humans and is weak in other species (see Fig. 6). *Below*: Tracheal smooth muscle. In canine trachea and most other species, muscle is localized to the posterior membrane (left). The center portion is relative pure airway smooth muscle with cells running in a transverse plane, the optimal orientation (photomicrograph, right). The ability to obtain pure, relatively homogeneously oriented tissues establishes the trachea as the most widely studied airway smooth muscle for determining the autonomic pharmacology of airways. However, pharmacological response of tracheal muscle differs substantially from that of other airways, even in the same species (see text). (Illustrations from Stephens et al., 1977, with permission from the publisher).

nervous system (SNS) defines a system of global activation, that is, all components are activated at once. The anatomical organization of the SNS (Weiner and Taylor, 1985a) is well suited to *flight and fright* responsiveness (Fig. 1). Preganglionic neurons traverse a short distance from the spinal cord to thoracic and cervical chains of sympathetic ganglia. Each ganglion may give rise to 20 or more postganglionic fibers, which themselves may innervate several different organs. The response may be further amplified by rostrocaudal transmission to other ganglia. This includes transmission through the greater splanic nerve, a preganglionic neuron, to the adrenal medulla, which is itself a ganglion. Stimulation of the adrenal medulla elicits immediate secretion of catecholamine into the circulation, which then perfuses all organs.

Sympathetic activation is mediated by two different mediators (Weiner and Taylor, 1985). These correspond to the anatomical organization of the SNS. The sympathetic neurotransmitter is norepinephrine. Norepinephrine secreted by sympathetic nerve endings into the myoneural junction of vascular smooth muscle is the source of vasomotor tone during SNS activation. Sympathetic neural secretion also may serve to modulate effects of tissues indirectly, for example, by modulation of neural parasympathetic output through downregulation of ganglionic transmission or other effector cells (see below). Norepinephrine is hydroxylated in the 3,4 position and thus is degraded rapidly by the enzyme catecholmethyltransferase (Fig. 2). This rapid degradation is essential to the neurotransmitter function of this mediator, so that stimuli, once initiated, can be attenuated rapidly or amplified by incremental secretion of norepinephrine. Similar rapid degradation at the motor end plate occurs with parasympathetic neurotransmission as acetylcholine is degraded rapidly by cholinesterase enzyme. Norepinephrine has substantial alpha-adrenoceptor activity (alpha$_1$- and alpha$_2$-), substantial beta$_1$-adrenoceptor activity, but little beta$_2$-adrenoceptor activity (Weiner and Taylor, 1985; Leff and Munoz, 1981a). These pharmacological effects correspond closely to the role of this neurotransmitter as a physiological pressor agent (alpha-adrenergic function), inotropic agent (beta$_1$-adrenergic effect), but weak bronchodilator (beta$_2$-effect). In humans, there is no direct innervation of airway smooth muscle by noradrenergic nerves (Richardson and Beland, 1976), although the concept of direct neural regulation airway smooth muscle persists (Weiner and Taylor, 1985).

Epinephrine reaches target tissues directly through the circulation after secretion from the adrenal medulla. It possesses alpha-adrenoceptor activity, as does norepinephrine. However, the addition of a methyl group to the amino-terminal end of the molecule confers this mediator with substantial beta$_2$ as well as beta$_1$-activity (Fig. 2). Epinephrine circulates systemically and possesses beta$_2$-adrenergic activity; it is a potent bronchodilator. Furthermore, because epinephrine is carried by the circulation to tissues associated with airway smooth muscle (mast cells, circulating blood elements, epithelium),

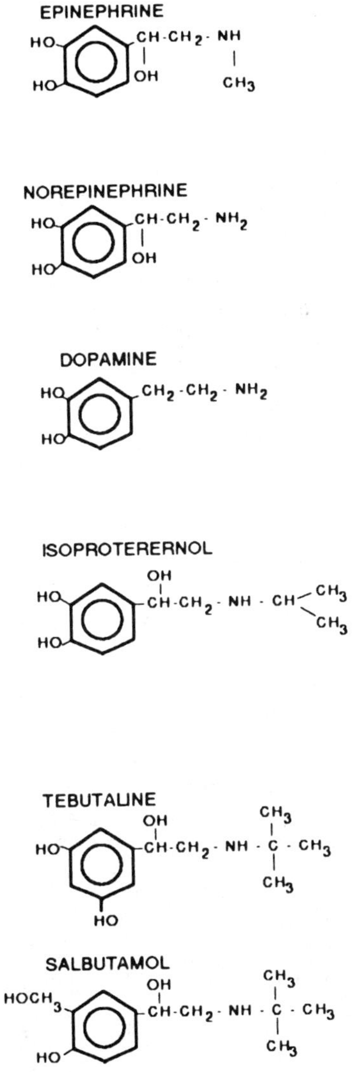

Figure 2 Endogenous catecholamines (epinephrine, norepinephrine, dopamine) and synthetic derivatives. Addition of a single methyl group to the N-terminal end of the norepinephrine molecule confers substantial beta$_1$- and beta$_2$-adrenergic activity on epinephrine. However, metabolism of epinephrine and norepinephrine is rapid because of hydroxylation by ubiquitous methyltransferase enzyme. Addition of methyl groups to the N-terminal end of the molecule further increases beta-adrenergic specificity (isoproterenol) and especially the beta$_2$-specificity (terbutaline) of synthetic derivatives. Terbutaline, which is hydroxylated in the 3,5 rather than 3,4 position, and salbutamol (albuterol), which has a hydroxymethyl group in the 4-position, have substantially longer half-lives in biological fluids than epinephrine, norepinephrine, or isoproterenol.

its secretion also may influence bronchomotor responses. These potential physiological interactions defined by the anatomical organization of the autonomic nervous system and the pharmacological properties of epinephrine and norepinephrine do not specify a physiological role of the adrenergic nervous system in either normal or asthmatic airways. There remains a distinct lack of information about the efferent activation of SNS secretion in airway constrictor responses as well as the role of autonomic secretion in regulation of nonmuscular target tissues.

II. Sympathomimetic Responsiveness of Airway Smooth Muscle and Mast Cells

A. Airway Smooth Muscle

Most studies of receptor pharmacology in airway smooth muscle have examined tracheal smooth muscle (Souhrada and Dickey, 1976; Stephens, 1975, 1976; Stephens et al., 1969; Brown et al., 1980; Kannan and Daniel, 1980; Gunst and Lai-Fook, 1983; Gunst and Russell, 1982). This tissue is ideal for study in some respects: it is easily harvested as a relatively pure tissue (Fig. 3). However, the distribution of airway smooth muscle receptors is heterogeneous throughout the bronchopulmonary tree (Drazen and Schneider, 1977; Hendrix et al., 1983; Souhrada et al., 1983; Shioya et al., 1987). Therefore, estimates of relative receptor or receptor-subtype density or affinity based on a single "prototypic" airway may be misleading (Leff et al., 1982a; Shioya et al., 1987). As such, data regarding adrenergic receptor pharmacology based on studies of tracheal smooth muscle define qualitatively the existence of various receptor types, but may not be extrapolated to define their regional density or affinity of adrenergic receptors in other airways.

Airway smooth muscle contains all four subtypes of postsynaptic adrenergic receptors (alpha$_1$-, alpha$_2$-, beta$_1$-, and beta$_2$) (Weiner and Taylor, 1985; Leff and Munoz, 1981a,b,d; Skoogh et al., 1985). Beta-adrenoceptors, which stimulate relaxation, substantially outnumber alpha-adrenoceptors, which cause airway contraction (Leff and Munoz, 1981b,d; Himori and Taira, 1976; Castro de la Mata et al., 1962; Flavahan and McGrath, 1981; Leff et al., 1985b). The relationship between beta- and alpha-adrenoceptor density is species dependent (Fleisch et al., 1970). In dogs, a substantial alpha-adrenergic response is elicited in tracheal smooth muscle after blockade of the beta-adrenoceptor (Leff and Munoz, 1981b,d; Himori and Taira, 1976; Castro de la Mata et al., 1962). In swine, administration of sympathomimetic agonists after beta-adrenoceptor blockade does not elicit contraction of the tracheal muscle, although a phentolamine-sensitive increase in airway resistance is obtained (Leff et al., 1985a). Alpha-adrenergic contraction has not been demonstrated in normal human airways in vitro; however, in "diseased" human airways, substantial contraction is elicited from excised human airways by norepinephrine, even in the absence of beta-adrenoceptor blockade (Kneussl and Richardson, 1978).

The pharmacological and physiological relevance of alpha-adrenoceptor responses remains controversial. Expression of alpha-adrenergic responsiveness is dependent upon the extent of beta-adrenoceptor blockade (Leff et al., 1986). Prior investigations have indicated possible impairment of beta-adrenoceptor relaxation resulting from airway disease or altered responsiveness resulting from the asthmatic state (Szentivanyi, 1968). Such factors would favor expression of alpha-adrenoceptor responses in human asthma (Boushey et al., 1980; Simonsson et al., 1972; Walden et al., 1984; Patel and Kerr, 1973; Marcelle and Laurent, 1973; Bianco et al., 1974). Phentolamine attenuates the response to exercise-induced asthma (Walden et al., 1984), and there is increased responsiveness to alpha-adrenoceptor agonists in human asthma (Patel and Kerr, 1973; Marcelle and Laurent, 1973; Gross et al., 1974; Bianco et al., 1974). Other experimental models have suggested that alpha-adreno-ceptor expression is affected by endogenous synthesis of prostaglandin in airway smooth muscle (Tallet et al., 1986).

Beta-adrenoceptor stimulation elicits relaxation of airway smooth muscle. The distribution of beta-adrenergic receptors among airway generations is also heterogeneous. There is a diminished gradient of beta-adrenergic receptors from central to peripheral airways (Barnes et al., 1983). The mechanism of transduction of beta-adrenergic stimulation to relaxation is still not fully defined. Beta-adrenergic activation stimulates synthesis of smooth muscle membrane adenylyl cyclase, which in turn augments conversion of adenosine triphosphate (ATP) to 3' 5'- cyclic adenosine monophosphate (cAMP) (Fig. 2). Cyclic AMP is degraded to 5' adenosine monophosphate intracellularly by phosphodiesterase and is inactive in this form. Cyclic AMP causes phosphorylation of cytosolic proteins, which leads to sequestration of intracellular calcium, probably within the sarcoplasmic reticulum. Although smooth muscle is not organized into discrete sarcomeric units, decreased calcium availability to actinomyosin complexes in smooth muscle leads to diminished contractile capacity and, hence, relaxation (Abdel-Latif, 1986; Gunst and Pisoni, 1986; Marthan et al., 1987; Solway and Fanta, 1985; Fish and Norman, 1986; Stephens et al., 1986; Anderson and Nillson, 1975; Anderson, 1972; Triner et al., 1977; Jensen et al., 1986). The temporal correlation between intracellular concentrations of cAMP and physiological decrease in airway smooth muscle tone in vitro is not exact; because physiological relaxation precedes the increase in intracellular cAMP, it has been suggested that cAMP is a modulator rather than a mediator of smooth muscle relaxation and that initial transduction results from alternative mechanisms that sequester intracellular calcium ion (Leff, 1982; Gold, 1977; Villiemoz et al., 1975). Furthermore, some agonists (e.g., histamine) promote intracellular cAMP concentrations in canine lung while eliciting airway contraction (Barnett et al., 1978).

It has been suggested previously that asthma may be the result of deficient beta-adrenoceptor function (Szentivanyi, 1968). Supporting data largely have been indirect and have been based on assay of leukocyte (Conolly and Greenacre, 1976; Morris et al., 1977) or pupillary responses (Henderson et al., 1979). There is no convincing evidence that airway hyperreactivity is the direct result of defective beta-adrenoceptor dysfunction. More recently, re-

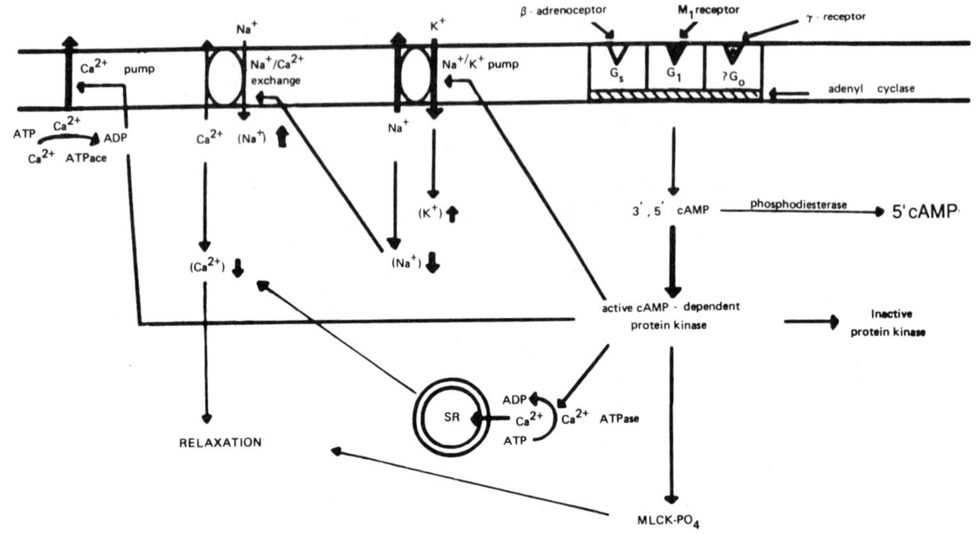

Ca^{2+} pump
Na$^+$
Na$^+$/Ca^{2+} exchange
K$^+$
Na$^+$/K$^+$ pump
β - adrenoceptor
M$_1$ receptor
γ - receptor
G$_s$
G$_1$
?G$_o$
adenyl cyclase
ATP
Ca^{2+}
ADP
Ca^{2+} ATPace
Ca^{2+}
(Na$^+$)
Na$^+$
(K$^+$)
3',5' cAMP
phosphodiesterase
5'cAMP
(Ca^{2+})
(Na$^+$)
active cAMP - dependent protein kinase
Inactive protein kinase
RELAXATION
SR
ADP
Ca^{2+}
ATP
Ca^{2+} ATPase
MLCK-PO$_4$

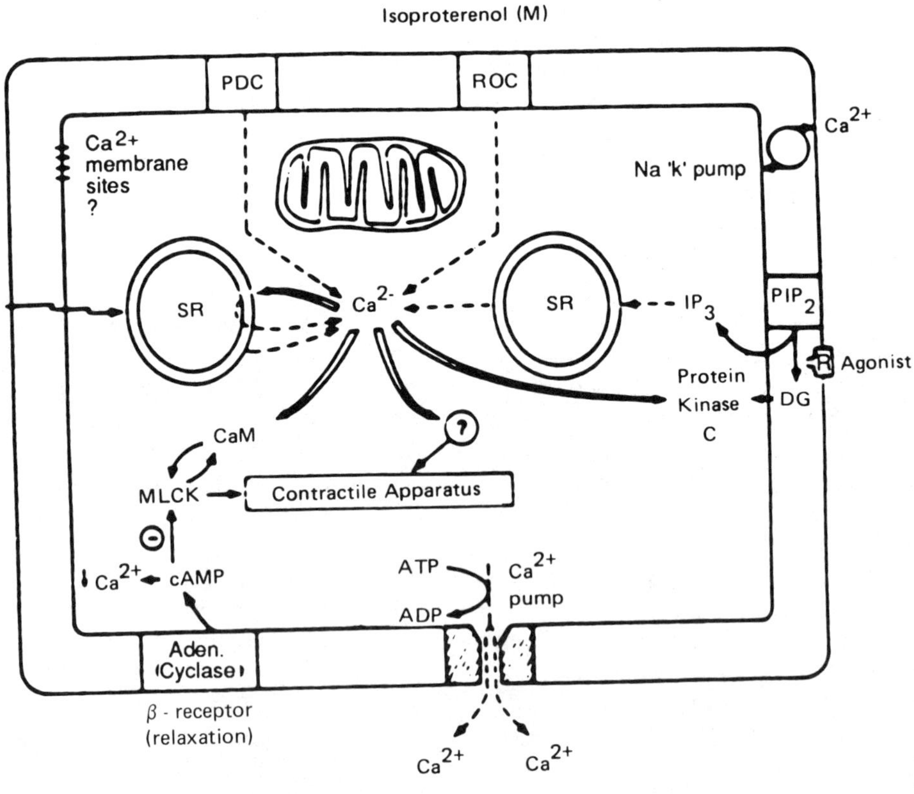

Isoproterenol (M)
PDC
ROC
Ca^{2+}
Ca^{2+} membrane sites ?
Na 'k' pump
SR
Ca^{2-}
SR
IP$_3$
PIP$_2$
Agonist
Protein Kinase C
DG
CaM
?
MLCK
Contractile Apparatus
Ca^{2+}
cAMP
ATP
ADP
Ca^{2+} pump
Aden. (Cyclase)
β - receptor (relaxation)
Ca^{2+}
Ca^{2+}

sistance to beta-adrenergic stimulation has been suggested to be mediator specific (Russell, 1984). Resistance in the asthmatic state to beta-adrenergic relaxation may be caused by the cumulative postsynaptic effects of multiple mediators acting at the same site (Fig. 4) (White et al., 1988a).

Beta-adrenoceptor blockade is a source of prodigious bronchoconstriction in human asthma. Theoretically, this could be the result of removal of functional antagonism of bronchoconstricting influences (Leff and Munoz, 1981d; Castro de le Mata et al., 1962). However, this is not clearly attributable to the degree of beta-adrenoceptor blockade. Nonasthmatic humans receiving massive doses of propranolol do not have substantially augmented airway contractile responses during bronchial challenge despite virtual complete blockade of beta-adrenoceptor influences, while asthmatic individuals may suffer life-threatening beta-adrenoceptor blockade after minimal doses of beta-adrenergic blocking agents. This non-dose-related sensitivity to beta-adrenergic blockade in asthmatic but not nonasthmatic humans has been termed the "propranolol paradox"; its mechanism remains to be defined.

B. Postjunctional Agonist Interactions

Sympathomimetic stimulation elicits complex postjunctional interactions. As for other agonists, the pharmacological activity of sympathomimetic agonists is defined in terms of the tissues being stimulated. The receptor population varies not only topographically with airway generation (Souhrada et al., 1983; Drazen and Schneider, 1977) but also substantially with species. Although $beta_2$-adrenoceptors predominate over $beta_1$-adrenoceptors in most species, ferrets possess only $beta_1$-adrenoceptors, and these elicit air-

---

Figure 3 *Above*: Transduction of airway smooth muscle relaxation elicited by beta-adrenoceptor stimulation in airway smooth muscle membrane: postulated mechanisms. A receptor-specific G_s protein activates membrane adenylyl cyclase and promotes intracellular concentrations of cyclic adenosine monophosphate (3′,5′ cAMP). The cAMP in turn is degraded to inactive adenosine monophosphate (5′AMP) by endogenous phosphodiesterase. Activated protein kinase (1) augments sodium/potassium exchange, (2) augments extracellular extrusion of calcium (Ca^{2+}) ion, and (3) sequesters Ca^{2+} within the sarcoplasmic reticulum (SR). This reduced the amount of Ca^{2+} available for actinomyosin cross-bridges and leads to net relaxation (illustration courtesy of Dr. Steven Koenig, University of Chicago). *Below*: Schema of response in the whole smooth muscle. MCLK, myosin light-chain kinase; PDC, potential-dependent channel; ROC, receptor-operated channel; CaM, calmodulin, a carrier of intracellular Ca^{2+}. Other abbreviations as above. (Illustration from Somerville and Hawthorne, 1986; by permission of the publisher).

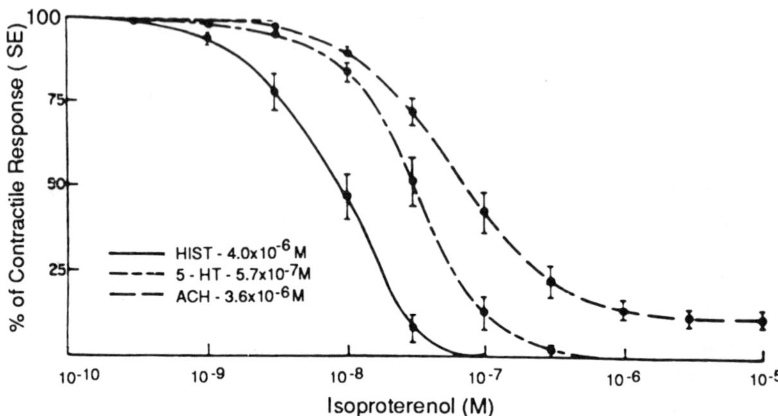

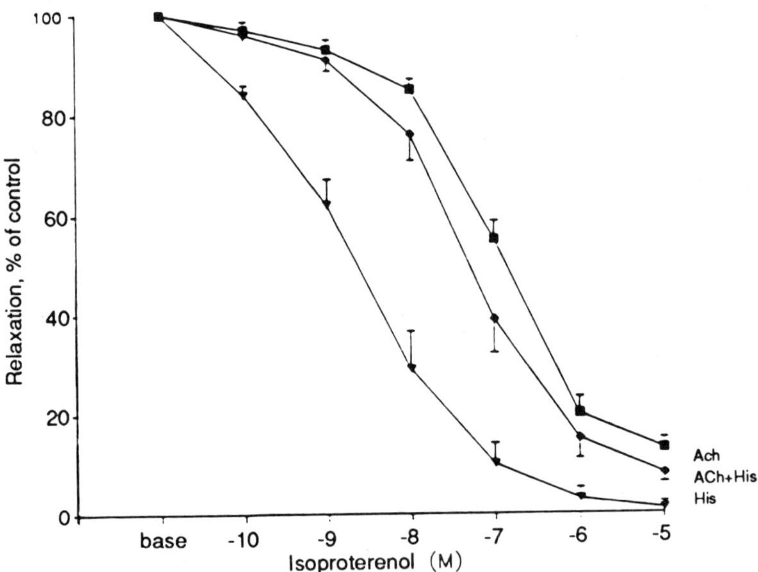

Figure 4   *Above*: Relaxation of canine tracheal muscle by isoproterenol after equivalent contraction by histamine (HIST), serotonin (5-HT), and acetylcholine (ACh). The relaxation response depends substantially upon the agonist contracting the muscle (from Russell, 1984). *Below*: Effect of contraction with multiple agonists. Acetylcholine (ACh) + histamine (His) relaxation response to isoproterenol resembles that of the stronger agonist, ACh, although concentrations of ACh and His were substantially less than for either given alone (reprinted from Leff, 1988 with permission from the publisher).

way relaxation with sympathomimetic stimulation (Skoogh et al., 1985). In humans, beta$_2$-adrenoceptors predominate (Weiner, 1985).

The pharmacological actions of the three endogenously secreted sympathomimetic agonists—epinephrine, norepinephrine, and dopamine—differ substantially. Both epinephrine and norepinephrine possess substantial alpha-adrenergic activity (Weiner and Taylor, 1985; Leff and Munoz, 1981a,b,d; Himori and Taira, 1976). Stimulation with any sympathomimetic agonist elicits simultaneous alpha-adrenergic contraction and beta-adrenoceptor relaxation if airways contain both major receptor types (Leff et al., 1986). However, because of the paucity of alpha-adrenoceptors in airways both epinephrine and norepinephrine elicit net relaxation in the basal state (Leff and Munoz, 1981b; Leff et al., 1986). Because of the predominance of beta$_2$-adrenoceptors in airway smooth muscle, epinephrine is substantially more potent in eliciting airway smooth muscle relaxation than norepinephrine (Leff and Munoz, 1981b). Norepinephrine possesses no significant beta$_2$-adrenergic activity in any tissue. However, because all airways possess beta$_1$-receptors and because the alpha-adrenergic response of airways is weak, norepinephrine elicits relaxation in airways in the absence of beta-adrenergic blockade. Thus, sympathetic neural stimulation in species having sympathetic innervation to airways elicits smooth muscle relaxation.

Dopamine is the third endogenously secreted catecholamine. Dopaminergic receptors have not been found in airway smooth muscle (Koga et al., 1980). Dopamine elicits tyramine-like activity in mammalian airways and causes secretion of norepinephrine from nerve endings in species having direct sympathetic innervation to airway smooth muscle (Koga et al., 1980; Michoud et al., 1984).

The interactions between sympathomimetic stimulation and other mediators are complex. Precontraction with histamine causing minimal changes in active tone substantially diminishes relaxation elicited by sympathomimetic stimulation (Leff and Munoz, 1981b). Histamine also acts synergistically with alpha-adrenergic stimulation in canine airways in eliciting tracheal contraction and bronchoconstriction; similar augmented responsiveness is not observed between postganglionic alpha-adrenergic and cholinomimetic stimulation (Leff and Munoz, 1981c). Beta-adrenoceptor activation is a major source of smooth muscle relaxation. However, the stimulatory effects of beta-adrenoceptor stimulation are augmented by simultaneous activation of adenylyl cyclase by other mediators, such as prostaglandin E$_2$ (Schultz, 1977) or by simultaneous inhibition of the phosphodiesterase enzyme by methylxanthine (Sutherland and Rall, 1958; Butcher and Sutherland, 1962). Some studies have shown augmented bronchodilation by simultaneous muscarinic blockade and sympathomimetic stimulation in asthma (Bryant, 1985), although this has been questioned in a recent clinical trial (Easton et al., 1986).

Recent investigations have elucidated a potential epithelial-derived relaxing factor (EpDRF) that promotes tonic inhibition of airway tone (Flavahan and Vanhoutte, 1985; Flavahan et al., 1985) and thus presumably acts in concert with beta-adrenergic relaxing influences. Inflammatory infiltration eliciting cytotoxic reactions to the epithelium interrupts synthesis of EpDRF, and beta-adrenergic inhibition of canine bronchial smooth muscle contraction is antagonized (Frossard and Muller, 1986). This basal inhibitory role of epithelium augmenting beta-adrenergic relaxation has not been confirmed in in situ investigations in canine trachea (Brofman et al., 1988).

C. Adrenergic Regulation of Mast Cell Secretion

By remarkable coincidence, mast cell secretion is controlled at least in part by a similar adenylyl cyclase system that regulates airway smooth muscle contraction (Lichtenstein and deBarnardo, 1971; Sullivan et al., 1975; Orange et al., 1971; Kaliner et al., 1972; Garrity et al., 1985). It is important to note that immune stimulation of mast cell secretion is an active metabolic process of secretion of preformed mediator (e.g., histamine) and synthesis and secretion of nonpreformed mediators (e.g., lipoxygenase or cycloxygenase products). Secretion is a calcium-dependent process, as is smooth muscle contraction. Promotion of intracellular concentrations of cAMP augments mast cell secretion of mediator, while inhibition of intracellular cAMP augments the effects of IgE-mediated immune activation (Fig. 5) (Kaliner et al., 1972). Both beta-adrenoceptor stimulation and phosphodiesterase inhibition promote intracellular cAMP concentrations and inhibit mast cell degranulation in human lung fragments (Garrity et al., 1985). In mast cells, there is also an antagonistic system that augments IgE-mediated activation of the secretory process (Kaliner et al., 1972; Austen and Orange, 1975). This results from the formation of cyclic guanosine 3'5' monophosphate (cGMP) from guanosine triphosphate in a manner identical to cAMP formation. Alpha-adrenergic and muscarinic receptor stimulation of mast cells promote cGMP formation (Kaliner et al., 1972; Leff et al., 1985b) and augment immune secretion of mediators during IgE-mediated activation in sensitized human lung fragments. (The analogous role of cGMP in airway smooth muscle remains less well defined.) The receptor pharmacology of mast cells, however, varies substantially with both site and species (Garrity et al., 1985). Substantial differences in pharmacological responsiveness of mast cells have been demonstrated among species and between mast cells from the different sites in the same species (Garrity et al., 1985; Munoz et al., 1988; Garrity et al., 1983). While beta-adrenoceptors are uniformly present on mast cells, an alpha-adrenergic response in respiratory mast cells and basophils has not been demonstrated in some studies (White et al., 1988b). A canine mastocy-

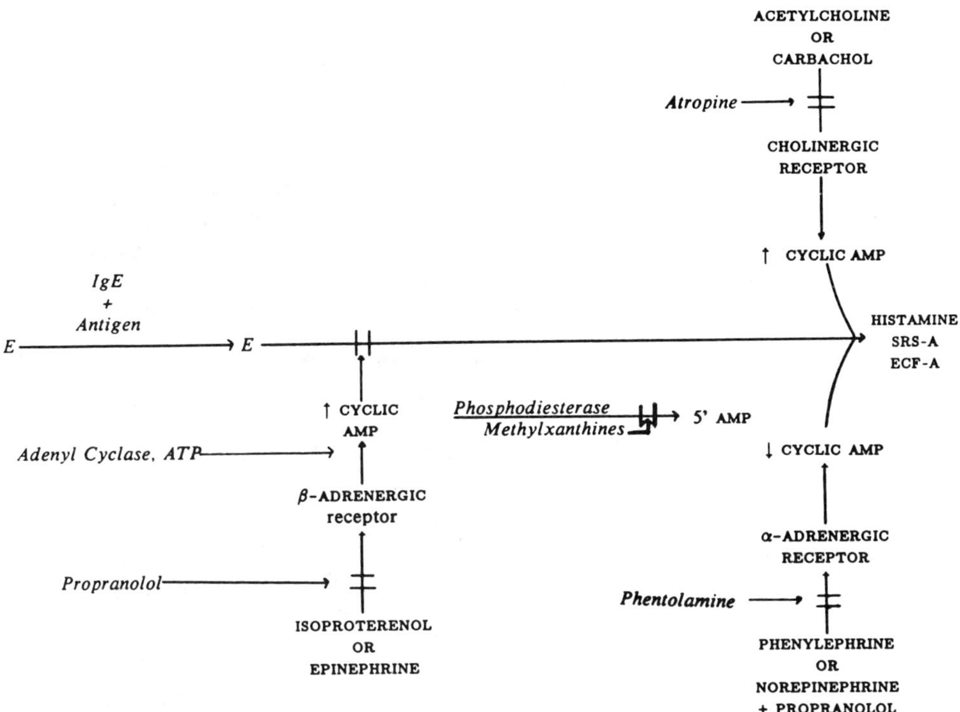

Figure 5 Endogenous modulation of mast cell secretion during immune degranulation. Promotion of intracellular cAMP concentrations downregulates mast cell secretion of formed (histamine) and preformed (SRS-A; leukotrienes) mediators. Cyclic GMP, cyclic guanosine monophosphate; other abbreviations as for previous figures.

toma model (Phillips et al., 1985) has demonstrated neither alpha-adrenergic nor muscarinic receptors; however, dermal reactivity does not predict asthmatic responsiveness in humans, and malignant cell lines while producing pure tissue preparations may have substantially disordered regulatory systems. It is clear that experimental mast cell responsiveness must pertain both to the tissue and the site it models.

It should be noted that the fortuitous similarity between the regulatory systems of respiratory mast cells and the contiguous airway smooth muscle does not imply similar physiological or pharmacological function. It has been estimated that the level of beta-adrenoceptor stimulation to inhibit mast cell secretion is at least 10 times greater than the level needed to elicit airway smooth muscle relaxation (Garrity et al., 1985; Lazarus et al., 1979; Barnett et al., 1978; Chiesa et al., 1975; Nisam et al., 1978; Brown et al., 1982). It is doubtful that usual blood concentrations achieved with therapeutic doses of sympathomimetic agonists are sufficient to alter mast cell secretion, and the therapeutic effects of these agents probably are the sole result of physiological antagonism of bronchomotor tone during asthmatic bronchoconstriction. It is likewise doubtful that nontoxic therapeutic serum concentrations of theophylline are sufficient to induce inhibition of phosphodiesterase in either mast cells or airway muscle, and the mechanism of action of methylxanthine derivatives as therapeutic agents does not appear to be related directly to their in vitro activity (Bergstrand, 1980).

III. Physiological Effects of Sympathetic Nervous System Stimulation

Most investigations of the physiological function of the sympathetic nervous system have examined the effects of efferent stimulation. As such, these studies define potential physiological action and the potential physiological reserve of the SNS in regulating bronchomotor tone and/or airway secretion function. However, results of such studies do not define physiological homeostatic relationships.

A. Sympathetic Neural Stimulation

Airway Smooth Muscle

Global activation of the SNS causes secretion of norepinephrine from sympathetic nerve endings and secretion of epinephrine into the systemic circulation. The extent of SNS innervation to airway smooth muscle varies substantially among species, but always is substantially less than the effects of circulating epinephrine (Fig. 6). Even where SNS innervation is substantial, its modulating influences are weak (norepinephrine is a weak bronchodilator) (Castro de la Mata et al., 1962). Simultaneous stimulation of efferent sympathetic (stellate ganglion) and parasympathetic (vagus) nerves leads to net bronchoconstriction (Cabezas et al., 1971). After adrenalectomy, there is little effective modulation of bronchoconstriction elicited by histamine (Fig. 6). A second inhibitory system exists in some species including humans (Irvin et al., 1982; Richardson and Beland, 1976; Chesrown et al., 1980); airway relaxation is elicited at higher frequencies than for SNS nerves and is obtained in the presence of concentrations of propranolol that block the beta-adrenoceptor. The mediator(s) (probably one or more polypeptides) of airway relaxation elicited by this system has not been identified, and the system thus has been labeled the nonadrenergic-noncholinergic (NANC) inhibitory system. Studies have not quantitated fully the importance of this system as a potential physiological relaxing influence; NANC stimulation has been shown to cause

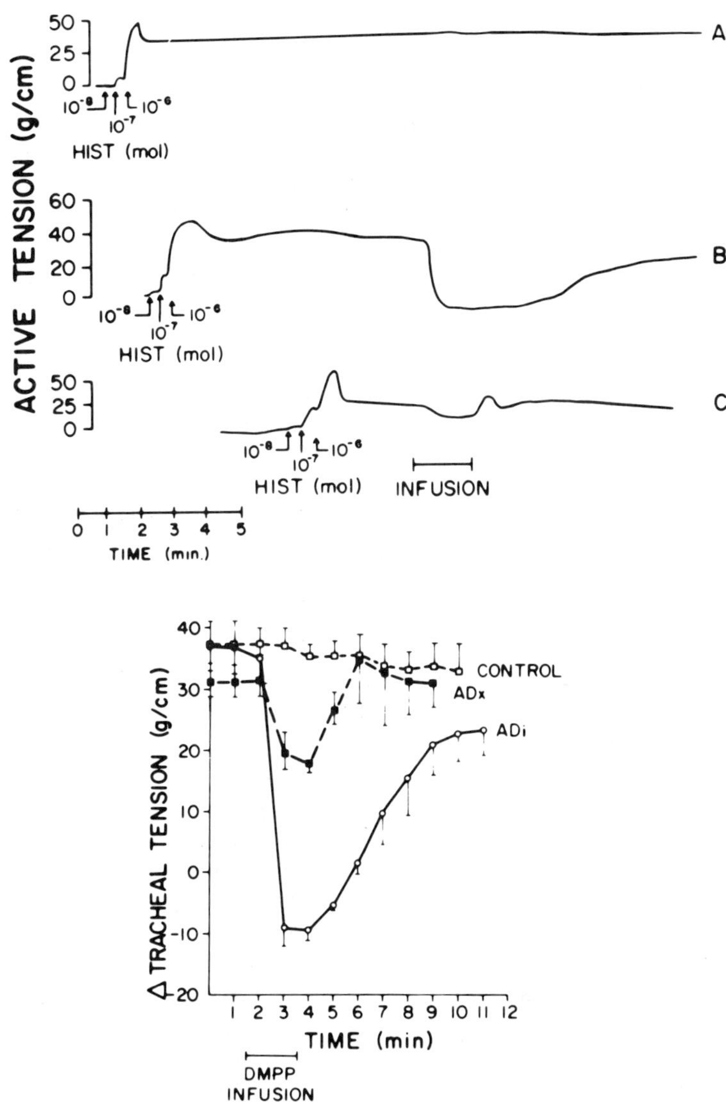

Figure 6 Potential role of sympathetic innervation and adrenal secretion in eliciting airway relaxation. Canine trachea contracted with histamine (A; control) relaxes fully during global sympathetic stimulation elicited by dimethylphenylpiperazinium (DMPP), a ganglionic stimulant (B). Adrenalectomy (ADx) abolishes secretion of epinephrine and leaves only effects of direct noradrenergic innervation. This virtually abolishes the relaxation response caused by the same maximal stimulus (C). *Above*: Illustrative tracings from three different animals. *Below*: Cumulative data for five animals in each group (from Leff et al., 1982b; reprinted with permission of the American Physiological Society).

relaxation equivalent to sympathetic neural relaxation in cats (Irvin et al., 1982); accordingly, it appears that the relaxing influences of this system are rather weak. In humans there is no direct SNS innervation to airway smooth muscle; therefore, all SNS modulating influences are mediated through secretion of epinephrine. Although sympathetic nerves do not innervate airway smooth muscle directly in humans, sympathetic nerves do innervate adjacent parasympathetic ganglia. This regulation is inhibitory (Baker et al., 1983). The potential physiological stimuli initiating this SNS-mediated downregulation of parasympathetic efferent activity and the extent of this inhibition in vivo are unknown.

Mast Cell Secretion

It has been known for some time that sympathomimetic stimulation either augments or inhibits mast cell secretion prior to immune activation in human lung fragments in vitro (Kaliner et al., 1972; Austen and Orange, 1975) (Fig. 5). The potential physiological significance of these observations has been elucidated from several in vivo studies in canine models. Sympathetic stimulation causes complete inhibition of mast cell secretion (Fig. 7), but does not prevent entirely systemic mast cell secretion to anaphylactic doses of antigen (Garrity et al., 1985). These data point to the physiological heterogeneity of mast cell responses from different sites within the same species. Once immune degranulation is initiated, systemic concentrations of histamine remain constant, although SNS stimulation reverses substantially increases in bronchomotor tone and hypotension of anaphylactic shock (Garrity et al., 1985). Thus, the adrenal glands have the physiological potential to synthesize and secrete sufficient quantities of epinephrine to prevent immune activation, but are unable to reverse bronchoconstriction during canine anaphylaxis once immune degranulation has occurred. The level of SNS activity to reverse bronchomotor tone occurring from mediator release during antigen challenge is substantially less than the level required to elicit mast cell inhibition (Garrity et al., 1983, 1985; Lazarus et al., 1979).

The ability of the SNS to inhibit mast cell degranulation and bronchomotor tone is blocked by beta-adrenoceptor blockade (White et al., 1988b). Prior investigations have suggested that pharmacological alpha-adrenergic stimulation augments mast cell secretion in peripheral human lung fragments (Kaliner et al., 1972). However, alpha-adrenoceptor activation does not appear to augment substantially mast cell secretion in the central airways of dogs (White et al., 1988b). Other investigations have not established a uniform presence of alpha-adrenoceptors on respiratory mast cells (Phillips et al., 1985), and the role of the alpha-adrenergic component of SNS stimulation on human respiratory mast cells in the central airways (those most frequently involved in initial asthmatic bronchoconstriction) is unknown.

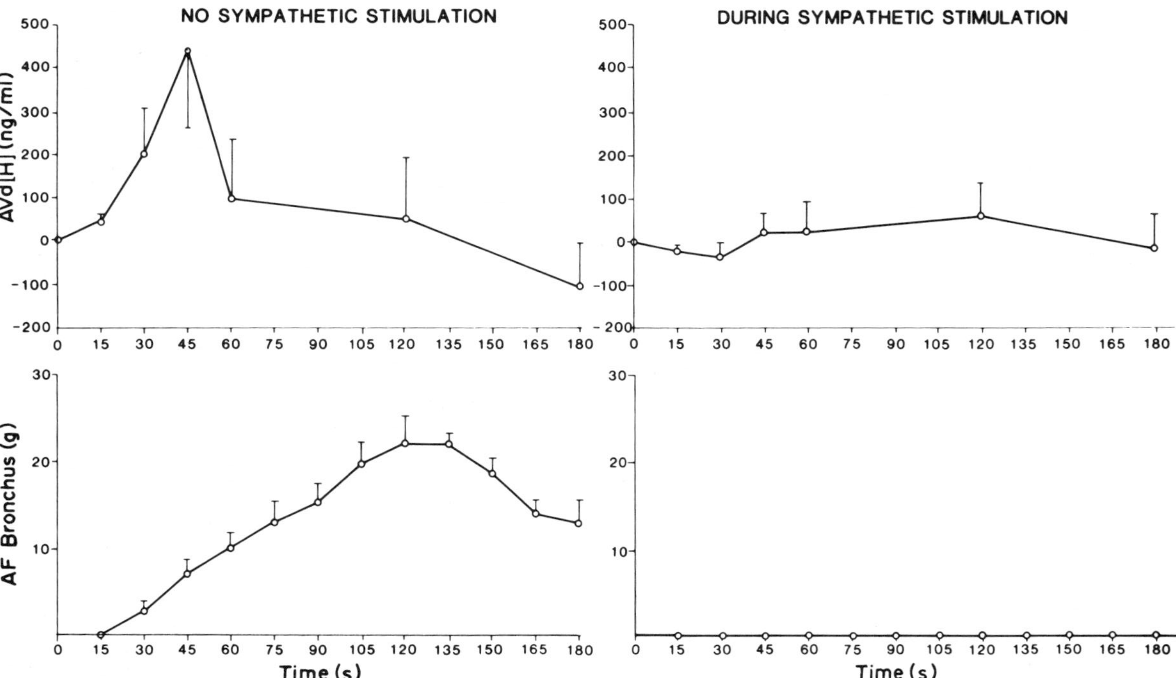

Figure 7 Effect of sympathetic stimulation on bronchial smooth muscle contraction and mast cell degranulation in the dog. Zero time marks administration of a maximal dose of *Ascaris suum* antigen to sensitized animals. Physiological stimulation for 1 min prior to antigen inhibits completely mast cell secretion as measured by the arteriovenous difference (AVd) in histamine concentration [H] across the bronchus and bronchial active force (left). Data from control animals (sympathetic blockade + sham stimulation is shown on the left; from Garrity et al., 1985; with permission from the publisher).

B. Homeostatic Influences

It has been presumed previously that a mutual inhibitory relationship existed between the sympathetic (relaxing) and constricting (parasympathetic, exogenous) components of the bronchomotor response (Weiner and Taylor, 1985). However, exogenous bronchoconstriction does *not* appear to elicit SNS activation. Barnes et al. (1982) found normal plasma catecholamine concentrations in patients with stable asthmatic bronchoconstriction. Sands and co-workers (1985) demonstrated that exogenous bronchoconstriction does not elicit SNS secretion of either norepinephrine (from SNS nerve endings) or adrenal secretion of epinephrine; in contrast, mild orthostatic hypotension elicited by tilt and volume depletion caused substantial increase in the plasma concentration of both catecholamines. White et al. (1987) have demonstrated that even severe bronchoconstriction in swine does not elicit SNS secretion unless accompanied by severe hypoxemia ($PO_2 < 40$ mmHg) or hypotension (decrease of $> 10\%$ in mean arterial blood pressure). The specific nature of the hypotensive stimulus also is a major factor in SNS secretion.

During anaphylactic shock induced by administration of Compound 48/80, a substance causing release of preformed mediators from mast cells, circulating concentrations of epinephrine are substantially greater than for comparable degrees of hypotension induced by direct vasodilation with nitroprusside. In contrast to nitroprusside-induced hypotension, hypotension elicited by mast cell degranulation causes SNS activation even after efferent ganglionic blockade with hexamethonium (White et al., 1988c). These data indicate that circulating mediators of anaphylaxis act directly on the ganglion and bypass normal reflex routes in eliciting secretion of bronchodilating catecholamines. This may account for the relatively minor degree of bronchoconstriction observed during analphylactic shock despite prodigious hypotension. In a porcine model of anaphylaxis, near-lethal shock elicited by Compound 48/80 caused minimal change in airway resistance; after beta-adrenoceptor blockade, however, the bronchoconstrictor response was three to four times greater (White et al., 1988c).

The notion that bronchoconstriction per se does not elicit SNS activity is inconsistent with the clinical state of many asthmatic patients seen with acute severe bronchoconstriction. These patients manifest signs of SNS activation including tachycardia, diaphoresis, and mild hypertension. Furthermore, asthmatic persons generally are mildly hypertensive rather than hypotensive, and severe hypoxemia is rare. In view of current data, it must be concluded that these clinical signs of SNS activation are not the direct result of bronchoconstriction. It is more likely that sympathetic discharge is the concomitant of severe muscular exercise required for ventilation and the associated anxiety of breathing against a high airways resistance. As an alternative, very low concentrations of circulating mediators could account for non-reflex-mediated activation of SNS reaction.

The homeostatic nature of NANC regulation also is not established. Szarek and co-workers (1986) have demonstrated that upper airway stimulation elicits NANC activation. However, no study has demonstrated a NANC response to exogenous bronchoconstriction, and the physiological regulatory role of this system during bronchoconstriction remains undefined.

IV. Summary

The sympathetic nervous system possesses substantial potential for inhibitory modulation of bronchomotor and mast cell responses. However, its precise role in the regulation of bronchomotor responses requires further definition. There is no convincing evidence for beta-adrenoceptor deficiency in asthmatic humans, and the mechanism of the "propranolol paradox" remains undefined. It is not understood why asthmatic humans are so sensitive to small doses of propranolol, while nonasthmatic subjects do not bronchoconstrict even with full beta-adrenoceptor blockade.

The use of congeners of naturally synthesized catecholamines as the mainstay of therapy in asthma is, at least in part, the result of a fortuitous misunderstanding of homeostatic regulation. Asthmatic patients have normal SNS secretion and beta-adrenoceptor populations in airways. Bronchoconstriction per se does not elicit SNS secretion even in nonasthmatic individuals. The homeostatic role of SNS activation in modulating bronchomotor and mast cell secretory responses remains to be defined.

Discussion

Barnes: Beta-blockers can cause severe bronchoconstriction in asthmatic patients, suggesting that a degree of "adrenergic drive" is important in defending against constrictor mechanisms. This is likely to be provided by circulating epinephrine, since there is no convincing evidence for bronchodilator adrenergic nerves in human airways. It is possible that epinephrine acts on cholinergic nerves via beta-2 receptors to inhibit vagal cholinergic tone. Beta-blockers may thus increase cholinergic tone (and anticholinergics can prevent beta-blocker-induced bronchoconstriction, at least in patients with mild asthma). The increase in acetylcholine (Ach) release should be switched off by muscarinic autoreceptors, but we have evidence that they may be dysfunctional in asthma, so that increased release of ACh occurs, giving a bronchoconstriction that could not occur in normal people in whom autoreceptors are intact.

Persson: How effective are anticholinergic drugs in beta-blocker-induced asthma?

Barnes: Pretreatment with an anticholinergic drug will completely prevent propranolol-induced bronchoconstriction in patients with mild asthma, and will also *reverse* beta-blocker bronchoconstriction, although not completely (Ind P, et al. (1989). *Am. Rev. Respir. Dis.* In press). Other mechanisms may be more important in patients with more severe asthma.

Woolcock: In propranolol-induced bronchoconstriction in which the forced expiratory volume in 1s (FEV_1) fell by 30-40%, ipratropium bromide caused partial inhibition of the response in some subjects only.

Tattersfield: We find that once beta-blocker asthma has occurred, ipratropium bromide causes only partial reversal. There are differences according to whether the drug is given before or after the beta-blocker.

Daniel: It may be difficult to conclude that adrenergic innervation is absent in airway smooth muscle. In canine bronchi (third generation or higher) there is extensive evidence of adrenergic innervation to both muscle and nerve endings. Beta-receptors are a mixture of beta-1 and beta-2 subtypes on cholinergic nerves.

Leff: In dogs, there is certainly evidence for direct innervation but not in humans, in whom there is no *functional* evidence for a direct sympathetic innervation.

L. Laitinen: However, at least three groups (Richardson, Jeffery, and ourselves) have demonstrated histochemically that there are catecholamine-positive nerve fibers in human airway smooth muscle.

Leff: But they have not been shown to be *functional*.

O'Byrne: Ind et al. (1985) have shown that circulating epinephrine levels are not increased even in patients with acute severe asthma. Do asthmatic patients give a catecholamine response to stressful stimuli?

Barnes: Old evidence shows that asthmatic persons apparently have a reduced catecholamine response to stress, such as mental arithmetic.

Fuller: We have studied tyramine infusions in normal subjects to see if local endogenous norepinephrine release will affect airway function, and demonstrated no effect. Similarly, Ind and Barnes showed no bronchodilator response in asthmatic subjects. This again suggests that there are no physiologically significant adrenergic nerves in human airways.

Barnes: We also found in vitro that tyramine had no direct bronchodilator effect nor any inhibitory effect on cholinergic neutrotransmission in human bronchi, in contrast to the positive findings in canine bronchi found by Danser et al. (1987). Thus, adrenergic nerves neither directly affect airway smooth muscle nor modulate cholinergic neurotransmission in humans.

Dahl: Are exercise-induced bronchodilatation and nasal dilatation dependent on adrenergic mechanisms?

Leff: Yes, this may be due to catecholamine secretion during exercise.

References

Abdel-Latif, A. (1986). Calcium-mobilizing receptors, polyinositides, and the generation of second messengers. *Pharmacol. Rev.* **38**:227-272.

Anderson, R. (1972). Role of cyclic AMP and Ca^{++} in metabolic and relaxing effects of catecholamines in intestinal smooth muscle. *Acta. Physiol. Scand.* **85**:312-822.

Anderson, R. C. G., and Nillson, K. B. (1975). Role of cyclic nucleotides metabolism and mechanical activity in smooth muscle. In *Advances in Cyclic Nucleotides Research*, vol. 5. Edited by G. Drummond, P. Greengard, and G. S. Robinson. New York, Raven Press, pp. 263-291.

Austen, K. F., and Orange, R. (1975). Bronchial asthma: the possible role of chemical mediators of immediate hypersensitivity in the pathogenesis of subacute chronic disease. *Am. Rev. Respir. Dis.* **112**:423.

Baker, D. G., Basbaum, C. B., Herbert, D. A., and Mitchell, R. A. (1983). Transmission in airway ganglia of ferrets; inhibition by norepinephrine. *Neurosci. Lett.* **41**:139-43.

Barnes, P. J., Ind, P. W., and Brown, M. J. (1982). Plasma histamine and catecholamines in stable asthmatic subjects. *Clin. Sci.* **62**:661-665.

Barnes, P. J., Basbaum, C. B., and Nadel, J. A. (1983). Autoradiographic localization of autonomic receptors in airway smooth muscle. *Am. Rev. Respir. Dis.* **127**:758-762.

Barnett, D. B., Chesrown, S. E., Zbinden, A. F., Nisam, M., Reed, B. R., Bourne, H. R., Melmon, K. L., and Gold, W. M. (1978). Cyclic AMP and cyclic GMP in peripheral lung: regulation in vivo. *Am. Rev. Respir. Dis.* **118**:723-733.

Bergstrand, H. (1980). Phosphodiesterase inhibition and theophylline. *Eur. J. Respir. Dis.* **61**(Suppl. 109):37-44.

Bianco, S., Griffin, J. P., Kamburoff, K. L., and Prime, F. J. (1974). Prevention of exercise-induced asthma by indoramin. *Br. Med. J.* **4**:18-20.

Boushey, H. A., Holtzman, M. J., Sheller, J. R., and Nadel, J. A. (1980). Bronchial hyper-reactivity. *Am. Rev. Respir. Dis.* **121**:389.

Brofman, J. D., Koenig, S. M., Kelly, E., and Leff, A. R. (1989). Epithelial augmentation of trachealis contraction by MBP of eosinophils. *J. Appl. Physiol.* **66**:1867-1873.

Brown, J. K., Leff, A. R., Frey, M. J., Reed, B. R., and Gold, W. M. (1980). Physiological and pharmacological properties of canine trachealis in vivo. *J. Appl. Physiol.* **49**:84-94.

Brown, J. K., Leff, A. R., Frey, M. J., et al. (1982). Characterization of tracheal mast cell reactions in vivo: inhibition by a beta-adrenergic agonist. *Am. Rev. Respir. Dis.* **126**:842-848.

Bryant, D. H. (1985). Nebulized ipratropium in the treatment of acute asthma. *Chest* **88**:24-29.

Butcher, R. W., and Sutherland, E. W. (1962). Adenosine $3'5'$-phosphate in biological materials. *J. Biol. Chem.* **237**:1244-1250.

Cabezas, G. S., Graf, P. D., and Nadel, J. A. (1971). Sympathetic vs parasympathetic nervous regulation of airway in dogs. *J. Appl. Physiol.* **31**:651-665.

Castro de la Mata, R., Penna, M., and Aviado, D. M. (1962). Reversal of sympathomimetic bronchodilation after dicholorisoproterenol. *J. Pharmacol. Exp. Ther.* **135**:197-203.

Chiesa, A., Dain, D., Meyers, G. L., Kessler, G.-F., and Gold, W. M. (1975). Histamine release during antigen inhalation in experimental asthma in dogs. *Am. Rev. Respir. Dis.* **111**:148-156.

Chesrown, S. E., Venugopalan, C. S., Gold, W. M., and Drazen, J. M. (1980). In vivo demonstration of nonadrenergic inhibitory innervation of the guinea pig trachea. *J. Clin. Invest.* **65**:314-320.

Conolly, M. E., and Greenacre, J. K. (1976). The lymphocyte β-adrenoceptor in normal subjects and subjects with bronchial asthma: the effect of different forms of treatment on receptor function. *J. Clin. Invest.* **58**:1307-1316.

Drazen, J. M., and Schneider, M. W. (1977). Comparative response of tracheal spiral and parenchymal strips to histamine and carbachol. *J. Clin. Invest.* **61**:1441-1447.

Easton, P. A., Jadue, C., Dhingra, S., and Anthonisen, N. R. (1986). A comparison of bronchodilating effects of beta-2-adrenergic agent (albuterol) and an anticholinergic agent (ipratroprium bromid) given by aerosol alone. *N. Engl. J. Med.* **315**:735-739.

Fish, J. E., and Norman, P. S. (1986). Effects of the calcium channel blockers, verapamil, on asthmatic airway responses to muscarinic, histaminergic, and allergenic stimuli. *Am. Rev. Respir. Dis.* **133**:730-734.

Flavahan, N. A., and Vanhoutte, P. M. (1985). The respiratory epithelium releases a smooth muscle relaxing factor. *Chest* **87**(Suppl):189-190.

Flavahan, N. A., and McGrath, J. C. (1981). Demonstration of simultaneous α_1-, α_2-, β_1-, β_2-adrenoceptor mediator effects of phenylephrine in the cardiovascular system. *Br. J. Pharmacol.* **72**:585.

Flavahan, N. A., Aarhus, L. L., Rimele, T. J., and Vanhoutte, P. M. (1985). Respiratory epithelium inhibits bronchial smooth muscle tone. *J. Appl. Physiol.* **58**:834-838.

Fleisch, J. A., Maling, H. M., and Brodie, B. (1970). Evidence for the existence of alpha-adrenergic receptors in mammalian trachea. *Am. J. Physiol.* **218**:596-599.

Frossard, N., and Muller, F. (1986). Epithelial modulation of tracheal smooth muscle responses to antigenic stimulation. *J. Appl. Physiol.* **61**:1449-1456.

Garrity, E. R., Stimler, N., Munoz, N. M., Fried, R., Leff, A. R. (1983). Response of bronchial smooth muscle to mast cell degranulation in situ. *J. Appl. Physiol.* **55**:1803-1810.

Garrity, E. R., Stimler, N. P., Munoz, N. M., Tallet, J., David, A. C., and Leff, A. R. (1985). Sympathetic modulation of biochemical and physiological response to immune degranulation in canine bronchial airways in vitrol. *J. Clin. Invest.* **75**:2038-2046.

Gold, W. M. (1977). Neurohumoral interactions in airways. *Am. Rev. Respir. Dis.* **115**:127-137.

Gunst, S. J., and Lai-Fook, S. J. (1983). Effect of inflation on trachealis muscle tone in canine tracheal segments in vitro. *J. Appl. Physiol.* **54**: 906-913.

Gunst, S. J., and Pisoni, J. M. (1986). Effects of extracellular calcium on canine tracheal smooth muscle. *J. Appl. Physiol.* **61**:706-711.

Gunst, S. J., and Russell, J. A. (1982). Contractile force of canine tracheal smooth muscle during continuous stretch. *J. Appl. Physiol.* **52**:655-663.

Henderson, W. R., Shelhamer, J. H., Reingold, D. B., Smith, L. J., Evans, R., III, and Kaliner, M. (1979). Alpha-adrenergic hyper-responsiveness in asthma. *N. Engl. J. Med.* **300**:642-647.

Hendrix, N., Munoz, N. M., and Leff, A. R. (1983). Physiological and pharmacological response of canine bronchial smooth muscle in situ. *J. Appl. Physiol.* **54**:215-224.

Himori, N., and Taira, N. (1976). A method for recording smooth muscle and vascular responses of the blood perfused dog tracheal in situ. *Br. J. Pharmacol.* **56**:293-299.

Irvin, C. G., Martin, R. R., and Macklem, P. T. (1982). Non-purinergic nature and efficacy of nonadrenergic bronchodilation. *J. Appl. Physiol.* **52**:562-569.

Jensen, A. D., Puckett, A. M., Richard, G. A., Torphy, T. J., and Mayer, S. E. (1986). Methacholine sensitivity and cAMP protein kinase in tracheal smooth muscle. *J. Appl. Physiol.* **60**:1043-1053, 1986.

Kaliner, M. A., Orange, R. P., and Austen, K. F. (1972). Immunological release of histamine and slow reacting substances of anaphylaxis from human lung. IV. Enhancement by cholinergic and alpha-adrenergic stimulation. *J. Exp. Med.* **136**:556-557, 1972.

Kannan, M. S., and Daniel, E. E. (1980). Structural and functional study of control of canine tracheal smooth muscle. *Am. J. Physiol.* **238**:C27-33.

Kneussl, M. P., and Richardson, J. B. (1978). Alpha-adrenergic receptors in human and canine tracheal and bronchial smooth muscle. *J. Appl. Physiol.* **45**:307, 1978.

Koga, Y., Downes, H., and Taylor, S. M. (1980). Direct and indirect actions of dopamine on tracheal smooth muscle. *Naunym-Schmiedebergs Arch. Pharmacol.* **315**:15-20.

Lazarus, S. C., Chesrown, S. E., Frey, M. J., Reed, B. R., Mjorndahl, T. O., and Gold, W. M. (1979). Experimental canine anaphylaxis: cyclic nucleotides, histamine, and lung function. *J. Appl. Physiol.* **46**:919-926.

Leff, A. R. (1982). Pathophysiology of asthmatic bronchoconstriction. *Chest* **82**(Suppl):13-21.

Leff, A. R., and Munoz, N. M. (1981a). Evidence for two subtypes of alpha-adrenergic receptors in canine airway smooth muscle. *J. Pharmacol. Exp. Ther.* **218**:530-535

Leff, A. R., and Munoz, N. M. (1981b). Interrelationship between alpha- and beta-adrenergic agonists and histamine in canine airways. *J. Allergy Clin. Immunol.* **68**:300-309.

Leff, A. R., and Munoz, N. M. (1981c). Cholinergic and alpha adrenergic augmentation of histamine-induced contraction of canine airway smooth muscle. *J. Pharmacol. Exp. Ther.* **218**:582-587.

Leff, A. R., and Munoz, N. M. (1981d). Selective autonomic stimulation of canine trachealis with dimethylphenylpiperazinium. *J. Appl. Physiol.* **51**:428-437.

Leff, A. R., Munoz, N. M., and Alderman, B. (1982a). Measurement of airway response by isometric and nonisometric techniques in situ. *J. Appl. Physiol.* **52**:1363-1367.

Leff, A. R., Munoz, N. M., and Hendrix, S. G. (1982b). Sympathetic inhibition of histamine-induced contraction of canine trachealis in vivo. *J. Appl. Physiol.* **53**:21-29.

Leff, A. R., Munoz, N. M., Tallet, J., and David, A. C. (1985a). Autonomic response characteristic of porcine smooth muscle in vivo. *J. Appl. Physiol.* **58**:1176-1188.

Leff, A. R., Stimler, N. P., Munoz, N. M., Shioya, T., Tallet, J., and Dame, C. (1985b). Augmentation of respiratory mast cell secretion of histamine caused by vagus nerve stimulation during antigen challenge. *J. Immunol.* **136**:1066-1073.

Leff, A. R., Tallet, J., Munoz, N. M., and Shoulberg, N. (1986). Physiological antagonism caused by adrenergic stimulation of canine tracheal muscle. *J. Appl. Physiol.* **60**:216-224.

Lichtenstein, L. M., and DeBernardo, R. (1971). The immediate allergic response: in vivo action of cyclic AMP-active and other drugs on the two stages of histamine release. *J. Immunol.* **107**:1131-1136.

Marcelle, R., and Laurent, B. (1973). Reactivité des bronches humaines in vitro. *Arch. Int. Physiol. Biochem.* **81**:901-920.

Marthan, R., Armour, C. L., Johnson, R. A., and Black, J. L. (1987). The calcium channel agonist BAY K8644 enhances the responsiveness of human airway muscle to KC1 and histamine but not to carbachol. *Am. Rev. Respir. Dis.* **135**:185-189.

Michoud, M. C., Anyot, R., and Jeanneret-Grosjean, A. (1984). Dopamine effect on bronchomotor tone in vivo. *Am. Rev. Respir. Dis.* **130**:755-758.

Morris, H. G., Rusnak, S. A., Selner, J. C., et al. (1977). Adrenergic desensitization in leukocytes of normal and asthmatic subjects. *J. Cyclic Nucleotide Res.* **3**:438-446.

Munoz, N. M., Chang, S.-W., Murphy, T. M., Stimler-Gerard, N. P., Blake, J., Mack, M., Irvin, C., Volke, N., and Leff, A. R. (1989). Distribution of bronchoconstrictor responses in isolated-perfused central and peripheral airways of the rat. *J. Appl. Physiol.* **66**:202-209.

Nisam, M. R., Zbinden, A., Chesrown, S., Barnett, D., and Gold, W. M. (1978). Distribution and pharmacological release of histamine in canine lung in vivo. *J. Appl. Physiol.* **44**:455-463, 1978.

Orange, R. P., Austen, W. G., and Austen, K. F. (1971). Immunological release of histamine and slow-reacting substance of anaphylaxis from human lung. I. Modulation by agents influencing cellular levels of cyclic 3',5'-adenosine monophosphate. *J. Exp. Med.* **134**(Suppl):136-148.

Patel, K. R., and Kerr, J. W. (1973). Airways response to phenylephrine after blockade of alpha and beta receptors in extrinsic bronchial asthma. *Clin. Allergy* **3**:939-448.

Phillips, M. J., Barnes, P. J., Gold, W. M. (1985). Characterization of purified dog mastocytoma cells: autonomic membrane receptors in pharmacologic modulation of histamine release. *Am. Rev. Respir. Dis.* **132**: 1019-1026.

Richardson, J. B., and Beland, J. (1976). Nonadrenergic inhibitory nervous system in human airways. *J. Appl. Physiol.* **41**:764-471.

Russell, J. A. (1984). Differential inhibitory effect of isoproterenol on contractions of canine airways. *J. Appl. Physiol.* **57**:801-807, 1984.

Sands, M. F., Douglas, F. L., Green, J., Banner, A., Robertson, G. L., and Leff, A. R. (1985). Homeostatic regulation of bronchomotor tone by sympathetic activation during bronchoconstriction in normal and asthmatic humans. *Am. Rev. Respir. Dis.* **131**:995-998.

Schultz, G. (1977). Calcium and cyclic nucleotide inter-relations. In *Asthma: Physiology, Immunopharmacology, and treatment.* Edited by L. M. Lichtenstein and K. F. Austine. New York, Academic Press, pp. 77-91.

Shioya, T., Solway, J., Munoz, N. M., Mack, M., and Leff, A. R. (1987). Distribution of airway contractile responses within the major diameter bronchi during exogenous bronchoconstriction. *Am. Rev. Respir. Dis.* **135**:1105-1111.

Simonsson, B. G., Svedmyr, N., Skoogh, B.-E., Anderson, R., and Bergh, N. P. (1972). In vivo and in vitro studies on alpha-receptors in human airways. Potentiation with bacterial endotoxin. *Scand. J. Respir. Dis.* **53**:227-236.

Skoogh, B.-E., Löfdahl, C.-G., and Svedmyr, N. (1985). Beta-adrenoceptors in ferret tracheal smooth muscle subtyped as beta-1. *Am. Rev. Respir. Dis.* **131**:A284 (abstr).

Solway, J., and Fanta, C. H. (1985). Differential inhibition of bronchoconstriction by the calcium channel blockers verapamil and nifedipine. *Am. Rev. Respir. Dis.* **132**:666-670.

Souhrada, J. F., and Dickey, D. W. (1976). Mechanical activities on trachea as measured in vitro and in vivo. *Respir. Physiol.* **26**:27.

Souhrada, M., Klein, J., Berend, N., and Souhrada, J. F. (1983). Topographical differences in the physiological response of canine airway smooth muscle. *Respir. Physiol.* **52**:245-258.

Stephens, M. L., Kroeger, E., and Mehta, J. A. (1969). Force-velocity characteristics of respiratory airway smooth muscle. *J. Appl. Physiol.* **26**:685.

Stephens, N. L. (1975). Physical properties of contractile system. In *Method in Pharmacology.* Edited by E. E. Daniel and D. M. Patton. New York, Plenum Press, pp. 265-296.

Stephens, N. L. (1976). Airway smooth muscle. In *Lung Cells in Disease.* Edited by A. Bouhouys. New York, Elsevier North-Holland, p. 113.

Stephens, N. L., Morgan, G., Kepron, W., and Seow, C. Y. (1986). Changes in cross-bridge properties of sensitized airway smooth muscle. *J. Appl. Physiol.* **61**:492-498.

Sullivan, T. J., Parker, K. L., Eisen, S. A., and Parker, C. W. (1975). Modulation of cyclic AMP in purified rat mast cells. II. Studies on the relationship between intra-cellular cyclic AMP concentrations and histamine release. *J. Immunol.* **114**:1480-1485.

Sutherland, E. W., and Rall, T. W. (1958). Fractionation and characterization of a cyclic adenine ribonucleotide formed by tissue particles. *J. Biol. Chem.* **232**:1077-1091.

Szarek, J. L., Gillespie, M. N., Altiere, R. J., and Diamond, L. (1986). Reflex activation of the nonadrenergic non-cholinergic inhibitory nervous system in feline airways. *Am. Rev. Respir. Dis.* **133**:1159-1162.

Szentivanyi, A. (1968). Beta-adrenergic theory of the atopic abnormality in bronchial asthma. *J. Allergy* **42**:203-232.

Tallet, J., Munoz, N. M., Fried, R., and Leff, A. R. (1986). Endogenous modulation of α-adrenergic contraction in canine tracheal muscle. *J. Appl. Physiol.* **61**:464-471.

Triner, L., Vulliemoz, Y., and Verosky, M. (1977). Cyclic 3',5'-adenosine monophosphate and bronchial tone. *Eur. J. Pharmacol.* **41**:37-46.

Villiemoz, Y., Verosky, M., and Triner, L. (1975). The cyclic adenosine 3',5'-monophosphate system in bronchial tissue. In *Advances in Cyclic Nucleotide Research,* vol. 5. Edited by G. Drummond, P. Greengard, and G. A. Robinson. New York, Raven Press, pp. 293-327.

Walden, S. M., Bleecker, E. R., Chahal, K., Britt, E. J., Mason, P., and Permutt, S. (1984). Effect of alpha-adrenergic blockade on exercise-induced asthma and conditioned cold air. *Am. Rev. Respir. Dis.* **130**: 357-362.

Weiner, N. (1985). Norepinephrine, epinephrine and the sympathomimetic amines. In *The Pharmacological Basis of Therapeutics*, 7th ed. Edited by Gilman, A. G., L. S. Goodman, T. W. Rall, and F. Murad. New York, Macmillan, pp. 145-180.

Weiner, N., and Taylor, P. (1985). Neurohumoral transmission: the autonomic and somatic motor nervous system. In *The Pharmacological Basis of Therapeutics,* 7th ed. Edited by A. G. Gilman, L. S. Goodman, T. W. Rall, and F. Murad. New York, Macmillan, pp. 66-99.

White, S. R., and Leff, A. R.)1988). The relationship of chronic obstructive pulmonary disease to asthma. In *Chronic Obstructive Lung Disease.* Edited by N. S. Cherniak.

White, S. R., Popovich, K. J., Mack, M., Munoz, N. M., and Leff, A. R. (1988a). Antagonism of relaxation to isoproterenol caused by postjunctional agonist interactions. *J. Appl. Physiol.* **64**:2501-2507.

White, S., Stimler-Gerard, N. P., Munoz, N. M., Popovich, K. J., Murphy, T. M., Blake, J. A., Mack, M., and Leff, A. R. (1988b). Effect of beta-adrenergic blockade and sympathetic stimulation on the canine mast cell response to immune degranulation in vivo (abstr). *Am. Rev. Respir. Dis.* **133**:A173.

White, S., Blake, J. S., Murphy, T. M., Mack, M. M., Munoz, N. M., and Leff, A. R. (1989). Effect of vasomotor and mediator-induced hypotension on bronchomotor tone in swine. *J. Appl. Physiol.* **66**:1852-1859.

White, S. R., Sands, M. F., Murphy, T. M., et al. (1987). Homeostatic regulation of airway smooth muscle tone by catecholamine secretion in swine. *J. Appl. Physiol.* **62**:972-977.

14

Airway Neuropeptides and Asthma

PETER J. BARNES

National Heart and Lung Institute
London, England

JAN M. LUNDBERG

Karolinska Institute
Stockholm, Sweden

I. Introduction

The abundant presence and potent effects of neuropeptides on various aspects of airway function suggest that they may be involved in controlling airway smooth muscle, blood flow, vascular permeability, and exocrine secretion (Polak and Bloom, 1986; Uddman and Sundler, 1987; Barnes, 1987b). Asthma, which is characterized by bronchial hyperreactivity, or excessive "twitchiness" of the airways, was attributed to abnormal nervous mechanisms until the middle of the present century, when immunological and mediator theories of pathogenesis gained favor (Barnes, 1986a). The demonstration of an extensive network of nerve fibers containing potent peptides, in addition to classic neurotransmitters, in the airways has revived interest in possible neural abnormalities in asthma. Recent experimental and clinical studies suggest that asthma and bronchial hyperreactivity may be associated with an inflammatory response in the airway wall. Neural and neuropeptide control mechanisms might be involved in, as well as influenced by, this airway inflammation.

II. Nonadrenergic-Noncholinergic Nerves in Airways

Neural control of airways is far more complex than previously recognized (Barnes, 1986a, 1988; Lundberg and Saria, 1987). In addition to the classic cholinergic and adrenergic mechanisms, neural pathways that are nonadrenergic-noncholinergic (NANC) have been described. Both excitatory (bronchoconstrictor) and inhibitory (bronchodilator) NANC mechanisms have been described in airways of animals and humans (Richardson, 1981; Anderson and Grundstrom, 1983; Barnes, 1986b; Martling, 1987). NANC nerves also regulate tracheobronchial vascular resistance and blood flow (Martling et al., 1987a; Alving et al., 1988; Salonen et al., 1988), microvascular leakage (Lundberg et al., 1983), and mucus secretion (Peatfield & Richardson, 1983). The physiological role of these nervous pathways is likely to remain obscure until specific blockers become available, however.

It was once believed that neuropeptides were localized to their own "peptidergic" nerves in airways, but it is increasingly apparent that neuropeptides occur as cotransmitters within classic adrenergic, cholinergic, and sensory nerves and may interact with these nerves in a complex way (Lundberg et al., 1988).

III. Vasoactive Intestinal Peptide

A. Effects on Tracheobronchial Smooth Muscle

Vasoactive intestinal peptide (VIP), a 28 amino acid peptide, is the neuropeptide found in highest concentrations in human lung and is localized to efferent nerves (Polak and Bloom, 1986; Uddman and Sandler, 1987; Lundberg et al., 1984a). VIP-immunoreactive nerve fibers are associated with airway smooth muscle (particularly in large airways), mucus glands, airway blood vessels, and parasympathetic ganglia (which contain VIP-immunoreactive nerve cell bodies). VIP relaxes human bronchi in vitro and is almost 100 times more potent than isoproterenol, making it the most potent endogenous bronchodilator discovered so far (Palmer et al., 1986a). In asthmatic patients nebulized VIP is rather disappointing, since it has no bronchodilator effect and provides only weak protection against histamine-induced bronchospasm, probably because little of the nebulized peptide can reach receptors in airway smooth muscle (Barnes and Dixon, 1984). VIP similarly has no bronchodilator effect when infused in normal subjects (who bronchodilate with isoproterenol), probably because the profound hypotensive and vasodilator effects of the peptide limit the dosage that can be given to human subjects (Palmer et al., 1986b). In asthmatic patients, a small bronchodilator response to intravenous VIP has been reported (Morice et al., 1983), although this could be due to a reflex reduction in vagal tone resulting from the cardiovascular response.

VIP is the most favored candidate for the neurotransmitter of NANC inhibitory nerves, since in animal airways it mimics the electrophysiological changes produced by NANC nerve stimulation (Cameron et al., 1983), it is released when these nerves are stimulated electrically (Matsuzaki et al., 1980), and when tolerance is induced by exposure to high concentrations of VIP, the NANC inhibitory nerve effects (but not sympathetic inhibitory effects) are reduced (Ito and Takeda, 1982).

Histochemical studies show that VIP-immunoreactive nerves diminish in the smaller airways and are virtually absent from bronchioles (Lundberg et al., 1984a; Polak and Bloom, 1986). Autoradiographic mapping of VIP receptors has demonstrated that while smooth muscle of large airways has VIP receptors, they are absent in smooth muscle of peripheral airways (Carstairs and Barnes, 1986a). An interesting finding is that nonadrenergic relaxation, evoked by electrical field stimulation, is almost absent in small airways, which fail to relax with VIP, although isoprotenerol is effective (Palmer et al., 1986a). Taken together, the evidence points to VIP as a neurotransmitter of NANC inhibitory nerves, but certain proof must await the development of specific receptor antagonists.

B. Other Airway Effects

In animals, VIP is also a potent stimulant of airway mucus secretion (Peatfield et al., 1983), and of fluid transport across airway epithelium (Nathanson et al., 1983), which suggests that VIP-ergic nerves may also regulate airway secretions. VIP is a very potent vasodilator and, in the tracheal circulation, might play an important role in regulating perfusion of the airways (Laitinen et al., 1987). In the trachea, noncholinergic vasodilator mechanisms of parasympathetic origin predominate (Martling et al., 1987a; Matran et al., 1989a). By contrast, the vagal neural control of the bronchial circulation seems to involve mainly afferent nerves. VIP is more potent as a vasodilator in the tracheal than the bronchial circulation (Matran et al., 1989a,b).

Autoradiographic mapping of VIP receptors in human and guinea pig lung has confirmed the presence of receptors on airway glands, epithelium, and vascular smooth muscle (Carstairs and Barnes, 1986a). Vascular smooth muscle appears to have the highest density of VIP receptors, which is in agreement with the demonstration that VIP is a potent vasodilator.

C. Cotransmission with Acetylcholine

Electron microscopic studies have indicated that VIP may be present in cholinergic nerves in the airways, and may therefore function as a cotransmitter with acetylcholine (Laitinen et al., 1985b). VIP reduces the contractile effect of acetylcholine on airway smooth muscle in vitro and may therefore act as a "braking" mechanism to cholinergic bronchoconstriction (Barnes,

1987a). It is possible that VIP is coreleased only under certain patterns of neural activation, such as high-frequency firing (Lundberg et al., 1988), thus acting as a protective mechanism. Another possible physiological role for VIP could involve regulation of local blood flow. If cholinergic nerve activity causes bronchoconstriction, release of VIP from activated cholinergic nerves may have an effect on nearby vessels, so that blood flow increases as smooth muscle contracts, thus supplying more nutrients to active smooth muscle cells under metabolic demand (Barnes, 1988).

D. Peptide Histidine Methionine

Peptide histidine isoleucine (PHI) is a 27 amino acid protein with marked structural similarities to VIP and coded by the same gene (Tatemoto, 1984). In humans there is a terminal methionine, giving the name peptide histidine methionine (PHM). PHI/PHM is present in the same nerves as VIP (Lundberg et al., 1984a) and has similar effects. PHM is equipotent to VIP as a relaxant of airway smooth muscle (Palmer et al., 1986a), although is less potent as a vasodilator than VIP, suggesting that it might act on different receptors or have a different rate of degradation. Peptide histidine valine (PHV-42) is a precursor of VIP and is also a potent bronchodilator in vitro (Yiangou et al., 1987), but whether it is released from airway nerves is still unknown. Like VIP, it has no effect on airway function in human subjects (Chilvers et al., 1988).

E. NANC Inhibitory Nerves and Asthma

Whether any abnormality in NANC inhibitory nerves or VIP might contribute to bronchial hyperresponsiveness is uncertain. NANC inhibitory nerves have been demonstrated ion human airways in vitro by electrical field stimulation (Richardson and Beland, 1976; Taylor et al., 1984; Palmer et al., 1986a) and, in the absence of demonstrable sympathetic bronchodilator nerves, this is the only neural bronchodilator mechanism. NANC bronchodilator nerves have also been demonstrated in normal human subjects in vivo by a variety of means (Michoud et al., 1987; Lammers et al., 1988a; Ichinose et al., 1988). However, patients with mild asthma have no apparent defect in this neural bronchodilator pathway (Lammers et al., 1988b). However, it is possible that abnormal function of NANC bronchodilator nerves only becomes apparent in more severe asthma, when there is presumably a greater degree of inflammation. A defect in the inhibitory control of airway smooth muscle tone would certainly account for some of the features of bronchial hyperreactivity. A primary defect in NANC innervation seems unlikely, since there is no obvious abnormality in gastrointestinal sphincter function or motility in asthmatic patients, which would be expected in a generalized defect of this system. However, it is possible that a functional defect might develop as a result of airway inflammation. Inflammatory cells identified in the asthmatic airway, such as neutrophils, eosinophils, and mast cells, may release a variety of peptidases (e.g., mast cells releases tryptase) that would rapidly break down VIP and PHM. Indeed, VIP is a good substitute for mast cell tryptase (Caughey et al., 1988). This may be like taking the brake off cholingeric nerves, resulting in exaggerated reflex cholinergic bronchoconstriction, at least in the larger airways (Fig. 1). Although this is unlikely to be the primary cause of asthma, it could contribute to the bronchial hyperresponsiveness associated with airway inflammation.

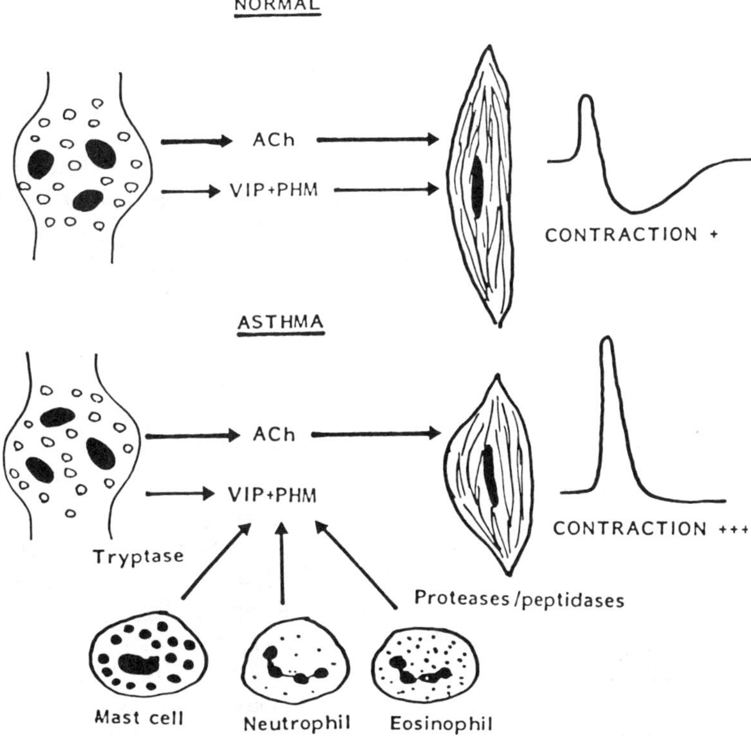

Figure 1 Release of VIP and PHM normally counteracts the bronchoconstrictor effect of acetylcholine (ACh), but in asthma peptidases released from inflammatory cells (such as tryptase from mast cells) may increase degradation of these peptides, leading to unopposed cholinergic bronchoconstriction (from Barnes, 1987a).

III. Peptides in Sensory Nerves

A. Substance P

Substance P (SP) is localized to unmyelinated sensory nerves (C-fibers) in airways (Polak and Bloom, 1986; Uddman and Sundler, 1987; Lundberg et al., 1984b), and has several effects reminiscent of the inflammatory response of asthma (Lundberg et al., 1987; Martling, 1987). SP exerts its effects on target cells via specific receptors, which have been localized by autoradiography to smooth muscle of all airways, from trachea to small bronchioles; therefore, it may regulate the caliber of peripheral airways (Carstairs and Barnes, 1986b). In addition to contraction of airway smooth muscle, SP also potently stimulates airway mucus secretion (Coles et al., 1984; Rogers et al., 1988b), increases airway microvascular permeability and exudation of plasma into the airway lumen (Lundberg et al., 1983b; Rogers et al., 1988a), and causes vasodilatation in the tracheobronchial circulation (Matran et al., 1989b). SP also degranulates mast cells of the skin (Foreman et al., 1983), although this has not been demonstrated conclusively in lung and may have chemotactic effects on inflammatory cells. SP also degranulates eosinophils, although this is not mediated by classic tachykinin receptors (Kroegel et al., 1989).

Noncholinergic bronchoconstrictor nerves have been demonstrated in vitro and in vivo in guinea pigs (Andersson and Grundstrom, 1983). These nerves are antagonized by SP analogs with tachykinin antagonist activity (Lundberg et al., 1983b), which suggest that SP or a related tachykinin may be the excitatory neurotransmitter. These studies raise the possibility that SP might be released from sensory nerve endings by an axon reflex mechanism. Such axon reflex mechanisms are well established in the skin (Szolcsanyi, 1988).

Capsaicin, the hot extract of pepper, releases SP from unmyelinated sensory nerve endings (Buck and Burks, 1986) and, in rats and guinea pigs, this pungent agent causes acute bronchoconstriction and airway microvascular leakiness (Lundberg et al., 1987). Chronic treatment with capsaicin leads to depletion of SP immunoreactivity and other tachykinins as well as calcitonin gene-related peptide (see below) and can, therefore, be used as a tool to investigate the contribution of peptides in C-fiber afferent nerves to airway responses. Depletion of peptides from sensory nerves is associated with a reduced bronchoconstrictor and vasodilator response to allergen in sensitized animals (Lundberg and Saria, 1987; Alving et al., 1988), and prevents irritants, such as cigarette smoke or mechanical stimulation of the airway, from causing airway microvascular leakage (Lundberg and Saria, 1983).

Although these local effects of SP innervation are clearly demonstrable in rodents, the relevance of these findings to human airways is less certain. Reports of SP innervation of human airways are conflicting (Laitinen et al.,

1983; Lundberg et al., 1984), but human lungs obtained at surgery are usually from older smokers in whom SP content may be reduced (Lundberg et al., 1988). Nevertheless, SP causes contraction of human airways in vitro, and capsaicin causes similar contraction, which suggests the release of SP from nerves within airway smooth muscle (Lundberg et al., 1983a). It has been established that capsaicin causes the release of SP (and other peptides) from guinea pig lung (Saria et al., 1988). Inhalation of capsaicin in human volunteers also causes bronchoconstriction, although this is only transient and may be due to a laryngeal reflex (Fuller et al., 1985). Inhalation of SP has no effect (Fuller et al., 1987b), even in asthmatic patients, presumably because the peptide is metabolized by airway epithelial cells and is not able to reach receptors on bronchial smooth muscle.

B. Other Tachykinins

Using a series of related naturally occurring peptides derived from nonmammalian species (called tachykinins because they all have rapid contractile effects on smooth muscle), it has been possible to characterize at least three types of response that appear to be mediated by different tachykinin receptors (Buck & Burcher, 1986; Regoli, 1987). In some tissues SP is most potent (SP-P or NK-1 receptor), whereas in others eledoisin (derived from octopus skin) is most potent (SP-E or NK-2 receptor). A tachykinin selective for this NK-2 receptor, neurokinin A (NKA), has recently been isolated from the mammalian nervous system and is found in the same airway nerves that contain SP (Martling et al., 1987b); it is coded by the same gene (Nawa et al., 1983). NKA is far more potent than SP in contracting airway smooth muscle (Martling et al., 1987b; Advenier et al., 1987; Palmer and Barnes, 1987), which suggests that the receptors on airway smooth muscle are of the NK-2 type. By contrast, SP is more potent than NKA as a vasodilator and in causing airway microvascular leakage (Hua et al., 1984; Rogers et al., 1988a; McCormack et al., 1988), which indicates that NK-1 receptors are present on the vasculature. SP is also more potent than NKA in stimulating mucus secretion from human bronchi, which indicates that NK-1 receptors regulate airway secretions (Rogers et al., 1988b). When SP and NKA are infused into volunteers, SP causes marked cardiovascular effects, whereas NKA has less marked vascular effects but causes bronchoconstriction (Fuller et al., 1987b; Evans et al., 1988). Nebulized NKA, but not SP, also causes bronchoconstriction in asthmatic patients (Joos et al., 1987). NKA also facilitates cholinergic neurotransmission in guinea pig airways and would thus tend to exaggerate cholinergic reflex bronchoconstriction (Hall et al., 1989).

Both NKA and SP are released from guinea pig by histamine and bradykinin (Saria et al., 1988). Another mammalian tachykinin, neurokinin B, appears to activate a third receptor subtype (NK-3 receptor) (Buck and Burcher, 1986; Regoli, 1987), but NKB has not yet been identified in airway nerves (Hua et al., 1985). A fourth tachykinin receptor has also been proposed in guinea pig trachea (McKnight et al., 1989), but does not appear to be present on human bronchi (Rhoden K, Barnes PJ, unpublished data).

C. Role of Epithelium

Recent research suggests that airway epithelium modulates the bronchoconstrictor effect of many spasmogens, possibly by releasing a relaxant substance similar to (but not the same as) endothelium-derived relaxant factor (Cuss and Barnes, 1987; Vanhoutte, 1988). This is particularly relevant in asthma, since airway epithelium is shed or damaged even in patients with mild asthma (Laitinen et al., 1985). Epithelium removal markedly potentiates the bronchoconstrictor effect of tachykinins (Tschirhart and Landry, 1986; Grandordy et al., 1988). For NKA this can be explained by the fact that the major metabolizing enzyme for tachykinins, neutral endopeptidase (enkephalinase) (Sekizawa et al., 1987), is localized to airway epithelium (Johnson et al., 1985). Inhibition of this enzyme by specific inhibitors, such as phosphoramidon or thiorphan, potentiates bronchoconstriction to the same extent as epithelial removal (Frossard et al., 1989). For SP it is more complex, since SP also appears to release relaxant factors from airway epithelium via NK-1 receptors on epithelial cells (Frossard et al., 1989) (Fig. 2). Thus, if epithelium is shed in asthma the tachykinins released from sensory nerves in the airways are likely to have much more pronounced effects, not only on bronchoconstriction but also on microvascular leakage and mucus secretion.

D. Calcitonin Gene-Related Peptide

Another peptide that has recently been localized to sensory nerves is calcitonin gene-related peptide (CGRP), which may also be costored and coreleased with SP (Lundberg et al., 1985). CGRP has no consistent effects on guinea pig airways (Martling et al., 1988) but contracts human airways in vitro (Palmer et al., 1987), although perhaps a more important effect is the regulation of airway blood flow, since it produces intense and long-lasting vasodilation in skin (Brain et al., 1985). It is also a potent vasodilator of bronchial vessels both in vivo and in vitro (Salonen et al., 1988; McCormack et al., 1988). Receptor mapping studies have shown that CGRP receptors are localized predominantly to bronchial vessels in animal and human airways (Mak and Barnes, 1988), which further suggests that CGRP may be an important regulator of bronchial blood flow, perhaps contributing to the hyperemic appearance of asthmatic airways. CGRP does not cause microvascular leakage in airways (Martling et al., 1987; Rogers et al., 1988a), but

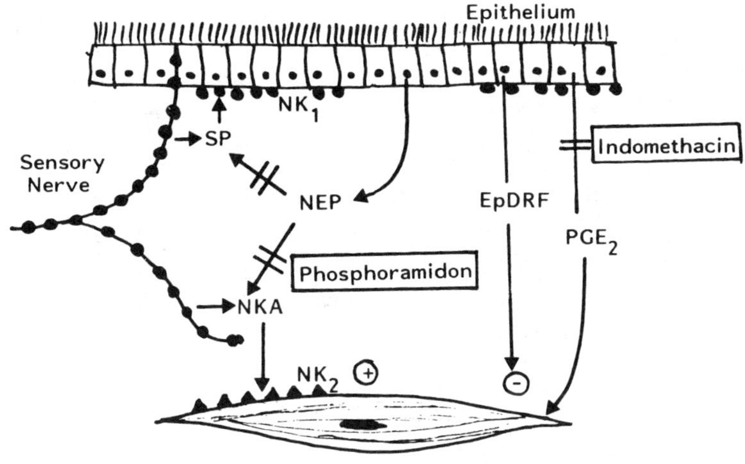

Figure 2 Interaction between tachykinins and airway epithelium. Neurokinin A (NKA) released from sensory nerves acts on NK2-receptors on airway smooth muscle, but is degraded by neutral endopeptidase/enkephalinase (NEP) from airway epithelium. Substance P (SP) may act on NK1 receptors on airway epithelium to release a relaxant factor (EpDRF) as well as prostaglandin E2 (PGE2) to counteract its constrictor action on airway smooth muscle (from Barnes, 1989).

could increase the leakage produced by other agents. CGRP potentiates the leakage produced by SP in skin (Gamse and Saria, 1985), but this does not occur in airways, possibly because blood flow is higher than in skin (Rogers et al., 1988a).

E. Axon Reflex Mechanisms in Asthma

Because neuropeptides such as SP, NKA, and CGRP produce many of the features of asthma, it is tempting to speculate that they may be involved in its pathogenesis, and the idea of neurogenic inflammatory mechanisms in asthma is attractive (Barnes, 1986; Lundberg et al., 1987). Damage to airway epithelium may occur even in patients with relatively mild asthma, thereby exposing afferent nerve endings (Laitinen et al., 1985a). These nerve endings may then be stimulated by inflammatory mediators in the airway lumen. Bradykinin, an inflammatory peptide formed by enzymatic cleavage from a plasma precursor, is likely to be found in the asthmatic airway by the action of enzymes released from inflammatory cells on exuded plasma. Bradykinin selectively stimulates C-fiber nerve endings (Kaufman et al., 1980) and may release sensory neuropeptides (Saria et al., 1988). Bradykinin is a potent bronchoconstrictor in asthmatic patients (Fuller et al., 1987a) and may result in the release of sensory neuropeptides such as SP, NKA, and CGRP from collateral branches of sensory nerves via an axon reflex. This could result in bronchoconstriction, mucus hypersecretion, and microvascular leakage leading to edema of the airway wall and extravasation of plasma in the lumen (Fig. 3). Furthermore, epithelial shedding would lead to loss of neutral endopeptidase so that any tachykinins released would have a greater effect (Frossard et al., 1989). Axon reflexes may then amplify the inflammatory response and spread inflammatory changes in the airway mucosa from patchy areas of epithelial damage. It follows that treatments that reduce axon reflex mechanisms might be beneficial in patients with asthma.

F. Modulation of Neurogenic Inflammation: Future Asthma Therapy?

Several drugs appear to modulate the release of sensory neuropeptides from sensory nerves (Fig. 4). The alpha-2 agonist, clonidine, inhibits NANC bronchoconstriction in guinea pigs (Grundstrom and Anderson, 1985). Opioids, which inhibit the release of SP in the CNS, are also very effective in inhibiting

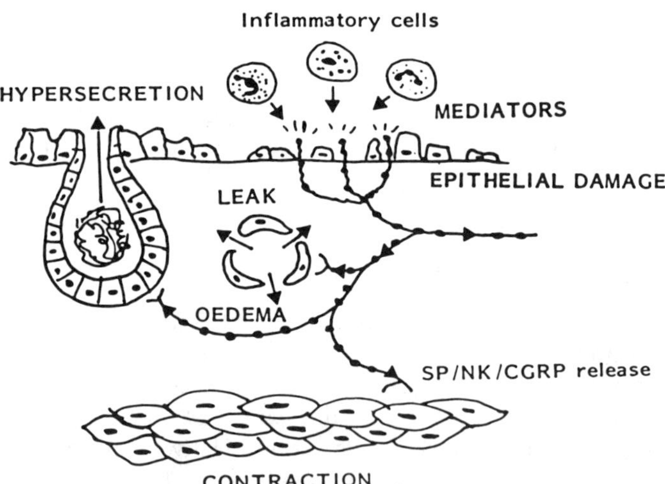

Figure 3 Axon reflex mechanisms in asthma. Damage to airway epithelium exposes sensory nerve endings, which, when activated by inflammatory mediators (e.g., bradykinin), leads to release of sensory peptides from sensory nerves such as substance P (SP), neurokinin A (NK), and calcitonin gene-related peptide (CGRP). This leads to spread and amplification of mucosal inflammation (from Barnes, 1986c).

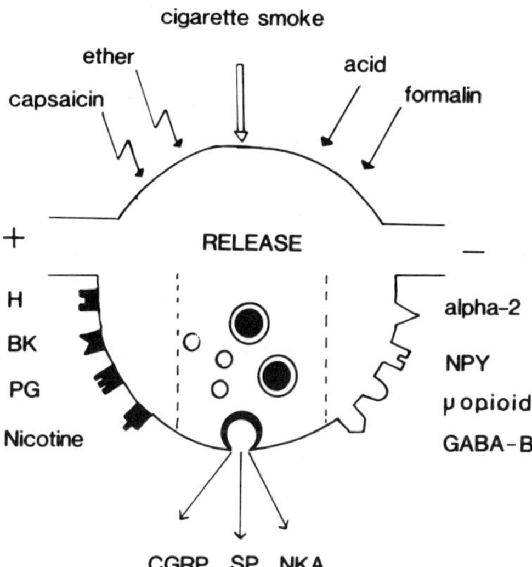

Figure 4 Schematic illustration of the regulation of release of multiple peptides (SP, NKA, and CGRP) from peripheral branches of capsaicin-sensitive afferents in the airways. Inhalation of irritant agents, such as capsaicin, HCl, ether, formalin, or the vapor phase of cigarette smoke will activate sensory nerves and elicit both local axon reflexes with peptide release and centrally mediated parasympathetic reflexes. Certain substances, such as histamine (H), bradykinin (BK), nicotine, and prostaglandins (PG), facilitate release from these sensory nerves. Conversely, activation of α2-adrenergic, μ-opioid, GABA-B, or NPY receptors will inhibit peptide release from capsaicin-sensitive sensory nerves elicited by nerve stimulation.

NANC bronchoconstriction, both in vitro and in vivo (Frossard and Barnes, 1987; Belvisi et al., 1988) and airway neurogenic microvascular leakage (Belvisi et al., 1989b), acting via μ-opioid receptors on sensory nerve endings. Recent evidence suggests that the inhibitory neurotransmitter gamma-aminobutyric acid (GABA) acting via $GABA_B$-receptors may also inhibit tachykinin release from airway sensory nerves (Belvisi et al., 1989a). Furthermore, neuropeptide Y is also effective (Matran et al., 1989c). Cromoglycate (cromolyn sodium) is an antiasthma drug whose mode of action is unknown. It is remarkably effective in reducing the dyspnea and bronchoconstriction due to inhaled bradykinin in asthmatic patients (Fuller et al., 1987a; Dixon and Barnes, 1989), which suggests a possible effect on sensory nerves. This is in agreement with early experimental studies that demonstrated that cromoglycate reduced the firing of airway C-fibers (Dixon et al., 1979).

IV. Other Neuropeptides

Several other neuropeptides have been identified in human airway nerves (Table 1), although their physiological role is far from certain (Barnes, 1990).

A. Neuropeptide Y

Neuropeptide Y (NPY) is colocalized with norepinephrine in adrenergic nerves of the lung (Sheppard et al., 1984; Lundberg et al., 1988). It may play a role in regulating bronchial blood flow and modulating airway ganglia, rather than airway smooth muscle directly, since sympathetic nerves are relatively sparse in airway smooth muscle in humans. Recent studies suggest that NPY may modulate cholinergic and NANC neurotransmission in airways (Stretton and Barnes, 1988; Matran et al., 1989c), as well as in reducing tracheal blood flow (Salonen et al., 1988).

B. Cholecystokinin Octapeptide

Cholecystokinin octapeptide (CCK8) has been found in lung in low concentrations (Ghatei et al., 1982). CCK8 is a potent constrictor of proximal human and guinea pig airways in vitro, acting directly on receptors in airway smooth

Table 1 Neuropeptides in Airways

Peptide	Nerve type	Cotransmitter
Vasoactive intestinal peptide	Motor	Acetylcholine
Peptide histidine isoleucine/methionine/valine		
Substance P	Sensory	Occur together
Neurokinin A		
Neuropeptide K		
Calcitonin gene-related peptide		
Neuropeptide Y	Motor	Norepinephrine
Galanin	Motor	?VIP, ?ACh
Gastrin releasing peptide (bombesin)	?	?
Cholecystokinin octapeptide	?	?
Somatostatin	?	?
Enkephalins	?	?

muscle. These receptors are potently antagonized by the peripheral CCK antagonist L 363,851, thus indicating that they may belong to the CCK-A receptor type (Stretton and Barnes, 1989).

CCK8 does not appear to influence either ganglionic transmission or postganglionic cholinergic nerves in guinea pig. The constrictor effect of CCK-8 is enhanced by epithelium removal and by phosphoramidon, suggesting that, like the tachykinins, it is metabolized by neutral endopeptidase in airway epithelium (Stretton and Barnes, 1989). It is interesting that the responses to CCK are similarly enhanced in sensitized animals after exposure to allergen, which is presumably explained by epithelial dysfunction.

V. Future Directions

There has been an explosion of knowledge about the effects of neuropeptides in animal and human airways, yet we still know very little about the physiological role of these peptides in the regulation of airway function, and even less about their role in airway diseases such as asthma. This information will only come with the development of specific antagonists for neuropeptides. Although there has been some progress, the development of peptide antagonists is beset by problems in clinical practice because of instability or difficulty in delivering them to target cell receptors. Nonpeptide antagonists would be preferable but progress in their development has been slow. A highly potent and specific CCK-8 antagonists has now been synthesized (Evans et al., 1986) and it is hoped that similar antagonists will eventually be derived from neuropeptides of interest in the airways, particularly tachykinins.

Another area that requires further development is an understanding of the synthesis and metabolism of airway neuropeptides. Little is known of the factors that influence neuropeptide synthesis, particularly in the local nerves in lung. In situ hybridization studies using cDNA probes for neuropeptides should give further insight into the expression of neuropeptide genes, and such approaches should give insights into the plasticity of the peripheral nervous system. Thus, neural activation causes increased formation of messenger RNA for peptides (Schalling et al., 1988). Nerve growth factor, which might be released from inflammatory cells, such as mast cells in the airways, results in increased synthesis of mRNA for preprotachykinin B, which is the precursor of SP and NKA, in sensory neurons (Lindsay and Harmar, 1989). It thus seems likely that in a chronic inflammatory disease such as asthma there will be factors that influence both the expression of neuropeptides and the growth of nerves, and that this could contribute to the altered responsiveness of the airways in this condition.

Further understanding of the enzymatic degradation of neuropeptides is also needed. Identification of the critical enzymes and study of their expression and control are important directions for future research.

The ultimate goal of research into airway neuropeptides is to provide new approaches to therapy. Perhaps the most fruitful area may be in investigating drugs that inhibit the release of multiple neuropeptides via prejunctional receptors on sensory nerve endings. Such drugs could be expected to have a beneficial action in asthma by reducing neurogenic inflammation.

Discussion

Sybrecht: Why is the major adverse effect of ACE inhibitors cough rather than symptoms of asthma?

Barnes: ACE is important in degrading *circulating* bradykinin and tachykinins, since it is predominantly localized to vascular endothelial cell surface membranes. Thus, ACE inhibitors do not affect the bronchoconstrictor response to bradykinin. NEP is more important in breaking down these peptides in tissues.

Fuller: ACE inhibitor-induced cough appears to be due to prostaglandins not bradykinin, since it can be blocked by a cycloxygenase inhibitor.

Persson: If epithelial enzymes catabolizing tachykinins are leaking in asthma, these mediators would be more active compared to other mediators in asthma, but they are not.

Barnes: Epithelium shedding in asthma is patchy, so enough may remain to metabolize any inhaled tachykinin and this would explain why even high dosages of inhaled substance P are inactive in patients with asthma. However, patchy loss of epithelium may still mean that endogenously released tachykinins may not be broken down in the area of damage.

Irvine: Is NEP effective in degrading dilator peptides, such as VIP?

Barnes: We have found that NEP does degrade VIP in guinea pig airways, but the effect is not as striking as for tachykinins. Caughey and Nadel have shown that mast cell tryptase is more active in degrading VIP.

Kaliner: We find that capsaicin-induced sensory denervation in rats failed to inhibit allergen-induced microvascular leak in airways.

Lundberg: The vasodilator component of the acute allergic reaction seems to be dependent on local mediator release from sensory nerves, both in human skin and pig bronchi. The protein extravasation response may not involve sensory nerves.

Widdicombe: Is it possible that sensory nerves may affect airway parasympathetic ganglia via a local reflex, as has been described in the gut?

Barnes: We have demonstrated that tachykinins (especially NKA) facilitate postganglionic cholinergic nerves in guinea pig, but we could not clearly demonstrate effects at a ganglionic level.

Lundberg: We find that capsaicin pretreatment, which inhibits NANC bronchoconstriction, also reduces vagal cholinergic bronchoconstriction, indicating that endogenous tachykinins could facilitate cholinergic neurotransmission.

Sertl: We have shown by autoradiography that there are SP-receptors on cholinergic nerves in bronchi.

Leff: What is the origin of sensory nerves in airways?

Lundberg: The peptide-containing capsaicin-sensitive nerves to the trachea are mainly of vagal origin, while in lung both vagal and spinal afferents contribute.

Woolcock: Since sodium cromoglycate and nedocromil inhibit SO_2 and metabisulfite (MBS)-induced challenge, what does this imply about their mode of action?

Barnes: Both may block the *activation* of sensory nerves in the airways. They will block the bronchoconstriction and dyspnea induced by SO_2, MBS, and bradykinin. Their molecular mode of action is not known, but we have shown that they do not block tachykinin release from sensory nerves as opiates do.

Woolcock: Our preliminary studies suggest that asthmatic airways have increased numbers of SP-immunoreactive nerves in the basement membrane and in the lamina propria compared to nonasthmatic airways.

Karlsson: Inhaled capsaicin, which stimulates sensory nerves, stimulates transient bronchoconstriction, which can be blocked by an anticholinergic and its effects are not increased in patients with asthma. Why?

Barnes: Capsaicin induces intense coughing and may stimulate a laryngeal reflex bronchoconstriction. Perhaps a high enough concentration cannot be delivered to lower airways. Certainly, asthmatic patients do not show any increased response. Different populations of unmyelinated sensory nerves are now being recognized: some will respond to bradykinin, and perhaps they also respond to SO_2 rather than to low-doseage capsaicin.

Acknowledgment

We thank Madeleine Wray for her careful preparation of the manuscript.

References

Advenier, C., Naline, E., Drapean, G., and Regoli, D. (1987). Relative potencies of neurokinins in guinea-pig and human bronchus. *Eur. J. Pharmacol.* **139**:133-137.

Alving, K., Matran, R., Lacroix, J. S., and Lundberg, J. M. (1988). Allergen challenge induces vasodilatation in pig bronchial circulation via a capsaicin sensitive mechanism. *Acta Physiol. Scand.* **134**:571-572.

Andersson, R. G. G., and Grundstrom, N. (1983). The excitatory non-cholinergic, non-adrenergic nervous system of the guinea-pig airways. *Eur. J. Respir. Dis.* **64**:141-157.

Barnes, P. J. (1986a). State of art. Neural control of human airways in health and disease. *Am. Rev. Respir. Dis.* **134**:1289-1314.

Barnes, P. J. (1986b). Non-adrenergic non-cholinergic neural control of human airways. *Arch. Int. Pharmacodyn.* **280**(Suppl):208-228.

Barnes, P. J. (1986c). Asthma as an axon reflex. *Lancet* **1**:242-245.

Barnes, P. J. (1987a). Airway neuropeptides and asthma. *Trends Pharmacol. Sci.* **8**:24-27.

Barnes, P. J. (1987b). Neuropeptides in the lung: localization, function and pathophysiologic implications. *J. Allergy Clin. Immunol.* **79**:285-295.

Barnes, P. J. (1988). Neuropeptides and airway smooth muscle. *Pharmacol. Ther.* **36**:119-129.

Barnes, P. J. (1990). Neuropeptides and asthma. *Am. Rev. Respir. Dis.* In press.

Barnes, P. J., and Dixon, C. M. S. (1984). The effect of inhaled vasoactive intestinal peptide on bronchial hyperreactivity in man. *Am. Rev. Respir. Dis.* **130**:162-166.

Belvisi, M. G., Chung, K. F., Jackson, D. M., and Barnes, P. J. (1988). Opinoid modulation of non-cholinergic neural bronchoconstriction in guinea-pig *in vivo. Br. J. Pharmacol.* **95**:413-418.

Belvisi, M. G., Ichinose, M., and Barnes, P. J. (1989a). Modulation of non-adrenergic non-cholinergic neural bronchoconstriction in guinea pig airways via GABA B receptors. *Br. J. Pharmacol.* **97**:1225-1231.

Belvisi, M. G., Rogers, D. F., and Barnes, P. J. (1989b). Neurogenic plasma extravasation: inhibition by morphine in guine pig airways in vivo. *J. Appl. Physiol.* **66**:268-272.

Brain, S. D., Williams, T. J., Tippins, J. R., Morris, H. R., and MacIntyre, I. (1985). Calcitonin gene-related peptide is a potent vasodilator. *Nature* **313**:54-56.

Buck, S. H., and Burcher, E. (1986). The tachykinins: a family of peptides with a brood of "receptors." *Trends Pharmacol. Sci.* **7**:65-68.

Buck, S. H., and Burks, T. F. (1986). The neuropharmacology of capsaicin: a review of some recent observations. *Pharmacol. Rev.* **38**:179-226.

Cameron, A. R., Johnston, C. D., Kirkpatrick, C. T., and Kirkpatrick, M. C. A. (1983). The quest for the inhibitory neurotransmitter in bovine tracheal smooth muscle. *Q. J. Exp. Psychol.* **68**:413-426.

Carstairs, J. R., and Barnes, P. J. (1986a). Visualization of vasoactive intestinal peptide receptors in human and guinea pig lung. *J. Pharmacol. Exp. Ther.* **239**:249-255.

Carstairs, J. R., and Barnes, P. J. (1986b). Autoradiographic mapping of substance P receptors in lung. *Eur. J. Pharmacol.* **127**:295-296.

Caughey, G. H., Leidig, F., Viro, N. F., and Nadel, J. A. (1988). Substance P and vasoactive intestinal peptide degradation by mast cell tryptase and chymase. *J. Pharmacol. Exp. Ther.* **244**:133-137.

Chilvers, E. R., Dixon, C. M. S., Yiangou, Y., Bloom, S. R., and Ind, P. W. (1988). Effect of peptide histidine valine on cardiovascular and respiratory function in normal subjects. *Thorax* **43**:750-755.

Coles, S. J., Neill, K. H., and Reid, L. M. (1984). Potent stimulation of glycoprotein secretion in canine trachea by substance P. *J. Appl. Physiol.* **57**:1323-1327.

Cuss, F. M., and Barnes, P. J. (1987). Epithelial mediators. *Am. Rev. Respir. Dis.* **136**:S32-35.

Dixon, C. M. S., and Barnes, P. J. (1989). Bradykinin induced bronchoconstriction: inhibition by nedocromil sodium and sodium cromoglycate. *Br. J. Clin. Pharmacol.* **27**:831-836.

Dixon, M., Jackson, D. M., and Richards, I. M. (1979). The effect of sodium cromoglycate on lung irritant receptors and left ventricular receptors in anaesthetised dog. *Br. J. Pharmacol.* **67**:569-574.

Evans, B. E., Bock, M. G., Rittle, K. E., Di Pard, R. M., Whitter, W. L., Veber, D. F., Anderson, P. S., and Friedinger, R. M. (1986). Design of potent orally effective nonpeptidal antagonist of the peptide hormone cholecystokinin. *Proc. Nat. Acad. Sci.* **83**:4918-4922.

Evans, T. W., Dixon, C. M. S., Clarke, B., Conradson, T.-B., and Barnes, P. J. (1988). Comparison of neurokinin A and substance P on cardiovascular and airway function in man. *Br. J. Clin. Pharmacol.* **25**:273-275.

Foreman, J. C., Jordan, C. C., Oehme, P., and Renner, H. (1983). Structure-activity relationships for some substance P-related peptides that cause wheal and flare reactions in human skin. *J. Physiol.* **335**:449-465.

Frossard, N., and Barnes, P. J. (1987). μ-Opioid receptors modulate noncholinergic constrictor nerves in guinea-pig airways. *Eur. J. Pharmacol.* **141**:519-522.

Frossard, N., Rhoden, K. J., and Barnes, P. J. (1989). Influence of epithelium on guinea pig airway responses to tachykinins: role of endopeptidase and cyclooxygenase. *J. Pharmacol. Exp. Ther.* **248**:292-298.

Fuller, R. W., Dixon, C. M. S., and Barnes, P. J. (1985). The bronchoconstrictor response to inhaled capsaicin in humans. *J. Appl. Physiol.* **85**: 1080-1084.

Fuller, R. W., Dixon, C. M. S., Cuss, F. M. C., and Barnes, P. J. (1987a). Bradykinin-induced bronchoconstriction in man: mode of action. *Am. Rev. Respir. Dis.* **135**:176-180.

Fuller, R. W., Maxwell, D. L., Dixon, C. M. S., McGregor, G. P., Barnes, V. F., Bloom, S. R., and Barnes, P. J. (1987b). The effects of substance P on cardiovascular and respiratory function in human subjects. *J. Appl. Physiol.* **62**:1473-1479.

Gamse, R., and Saria, A. (1985). Potentiation of tachykinin-induced plasma protein extravasation by calcitonin gene-related peptide. *Eur. J. Pharmacol.* **114**:61-66.

Ghatei, M. A., Sheppard, M., O'Shaunessy, D. J., Adrian, T. E., MacGregor, J. M., Polak, J. M., and Bloom, S. R. (1982). Regulatory peptides in the mammalian respiratory tract. *Endocrinology* **111**:1248-1254.

Grandordy, B. M., Frossard, N., Rhoden, K. J., and Barnes, P. J. (1988). Tachykinin-induced phosphoinositide breakdown in airway smooth muscle and epithelium: relationship to contraction. *Mol. Pharmacol.* **33**:515-519.

Grundstrom, N., and Andersson, R. G. G. (1985). In vivo demonstration of alpha$_2$-adrenoceptor mediated inhibition of the excitatory non-cholinergic neurotransmission in guinea-pig airways. *Naunyn-Schmiedebergs Arch. Pharmacol.* **328**:236-240.

Hall, A. K., Barnes, P. J., Meldrum, L. A., and Maclagan, J. (1989). Facilitation by tachykinins of neurotransmission in guinea-pig pulmonary parasympathetic nerves. *Br. J. Pharmacol.* **97**:274-280.

Hua, X., Lundberg, J. M., Thodorsson-Norheim, E., and Brodin, E. (1984). Comparison of cardiovascular and bronchoconstrictor effects of substance P, substance K and other tachykinins. *Naunyn-Schmiedebergs Arch. Pharmacol.* **328**:196-201.

Hua, X.-Y., Theodorsson-Norheim, E., Brodin, E., Lundberg, J. M., and Hokfelt, T. (1985). Multiple tachykinins (neurokinin A, neuropeptide K and substance P) in capsaicin-sensitive sensory neurons in the guinea-pig. *Regul. Peptides* **13**:1-19.

Ichinose, M., Inoue, H., Miura, M., and Takishima, T. (1988). Nonadrenergic bronchodilation in normal subjects. *Am. Rev. Respir. Dis.* **138**:31-34.

Ito, Y., and Takeda, K. (1982). Non-adrenergic inhibitory nerves and putative transmitters in the smooth muscle of cat trachea. *J. Physiol.* **330**:497-511.

Johnson, A. R., Ashton, J., Schulz, W. W., and Erdos, E. G. (1985). Neutral metalloendopeptidases in human lung tissue and cultured cells. *Am. Rev. Respir. Dis.* **132**:564-568.

Joos, G., Pauwels, R., and van der Straeten, M. (1987). Effect of inhaled substance P and neurokinin A on the airways of normal and asthmatic subjects. *Thorax* **42**:779-783.

Kaufman, M. P., Coleridge, H. M., Coleridge, J. C. G., and Baker, D. G. (1980). Bradykinin stimulates afferent vagal C-fibers in intrapulmonary airways of dogs. *J. Appl. Physiol.* **48**:511-517.

Kroegel, C., Yukawa, T., and Barnes, P. J. (1989). Substance P induces degranulation of eosinophils. *Am. Rev. Respir. Dis.* **139**:A238.

Laitinen, L. A., Laitinen, A., Panula, P. A., Partanen, M., Tervo, K., and Tervo, T. (1983). Immunohistochemical demonstration of substance P in the lower respiratory tract of the rabbit and not of man. *Thorax* **38**: 531-536.

Laitinen, L. A., Heino, M., Laitinen, A., Kava, T., and Haahtela, T. (1985a). Damage of the airway epithelium and bronchial reactivity in patients with asthma. *Am. Rev. Respir. Dis.* **131**:599-606.

Laitinen, A., Partanen, M., Hervonen, A., Peto-Huikko, M., and Laitinen, L. A. (1985b). VIP-like immunoreactive nerves in human respiratory tract. Light and electron microscopic study. *Histochemistry* **82**:313-319.

Laitinen, L. A., Laitinen, A., Salonen, R. O., and Widdicombe, J. G. (1987). Vascular actions of airway neuropeptides. *Am. Rev. Respir. Dis.* **136**: S59-64.

Lammers, J.-W., Minette, P., McCusker, M. T., Chung, K. F., and Barnes, P. J. (1988a). Nonadrenergic bronchodilator mechanisms in normal human subjects *in vivo*. *J. Appl. Physiol.* **64**:1817-1822.

Lammers, J.-W., Minette, P., McCusker, M., Chung, K. F., and Barnes, P. J. (1988b). Non-adrenergic non-cholinergic bronchodilatation stimulated by capsaicin inhalation in normal and asthmatic subjects. *Am. Rev. Respir. Dis.* **134**(Suppl):240.

Lindsay, R. M., and Harmar, A. J. (1989). Nerve growth factor regulates expression of neuropeptide genes in adult sensory neurons. *Nature* **337**: 362-364.

Lundberg, J. M., and Saria, A. (1983). Capsaicin-induced desensitization of the airway mucosa to cigarette smoke, mechanical and chemical irritants. *Nature* **302**:251-253.

Lundberg, J. M., and Saria, A. (1987). Polypeptide-containing neurons in airway smooth muscle. *Annu. Rev. Physiol.* **49**:557-572.

Lundberg, J. M., Martling, C.-R., and Saria, A. (1983a). Substance P and capsaicin-induced contraction of human bronchi. *Acta Physiol. Scand.* **119**:49-53.

Lundberg, J. M., Saria, A., Brodin, E., Rusells, S., and Folkers, R. (1983b). A substance P antagonist inhibits vagally induced increase in vascular permeability and bronchial smooth muscle contraction in the guinea-pig. *Proc. Na. Acad. Sci.* **80**:1120-1124.

Lundberg, J. M., Fahrenkrug, J., Hokfelt, T., Martling, C.-R., Larsson, O., Tatemoto, K., and Anggard, A. (1984a). Coexistence of peptide H1 (PH1) and VIP in nerves regulating blood flow and bronchial smooth muscle tone in various mammals including man. *Peptides* **5**:593-606.

Lundberg, J. M., Hokfelt, T., Martling, C.-R., Saria, A., and Cuello, C. (1984b). Substance P-immunoreactive sensory nerves in the lower respiratory tract of various mammals including man. *Cell Tissue Res.* **235**: 251-261.

Lundberg, J. M., Anders, F.-C., Hua, X., Hokfelt, T., and Fisher, J. A. (1985). Coexistence of substance P and calcitonin gene-related peptide-like immunoreactivities in sensory nerves in relation to cardiovascular and bronchoconstrictor effects of capsaicin. *Eur. J. Pharmacol.* **108**: 315-319.

Lundberg, J. M., Saria, A., Lundblad, L., Angaard, A., Martling, C.-R., Theodorsson-Norheim, E., Stjarne, P., and Hokfelt, T. (1987). Bioactive peptides in capsaicin-sensitive C-fiber afferents of the airways: functional and pathophysiological implications. In *The Airways: Neural Control in Health and Disease*. Edited by M. A. Kaliner and P. J. Barnes. New York, Marcel Dekker, pp. 417-445.

Lundberg, J. M., Martling, C.-R., and Hokfelt, T. (1988). Airways, oral cavity and salivary glands: classical transmitters and peptides in sensory and autonomic motor neurons. In *Handbook of Chemical Neuroanatomy vol. 6. Peripheral Nervous System*. Edited by A. Bjorklund, T. Hokfelt and C. Owman. Amsterdam, Elsevier, pp. 391-444.

Mak, J. C. M., and Barnes, P. J. (1988). Autoradiographic localization of calcitonin gene-related peptide binding sites in human and guinea pig lung. *Peptides* **9**:957-964.

Martling, C.-R. (1987). Sensory nerves containing tachykinins and CGRP in the lower airways. Functional implications for bronchoconstriction, vasodilatation and protein extravasation. *Acta Physiol. Scand.* **63**:1-57.

Martling, C.-R., Gazelius, B., and Lundberg, J. M. (1987a). Nervous control of tracheal blood flow in the rat measured by the laser Doppler technique. *Acta Physiol. Scand.* **130**:409-417.

Martling, C.-R., Theordorsson-Norheim, E., and Lundberg, J. M. (1987b). Occurrence and effects of multiple tachykinins: substance P, neurokinin A, neuropeptide K in human lower airways. *Life Sci.* **40**:1633-1643.

Martling, C.-R., Saria, A., Fischer, J. A., Hokfelt, T., and Lundberg, J. M. (1988). Calcitonin gene-related peptide and the lung: neuronal coexistence with substance P, release by capsaicin and vasodilatory effect. *Regul. Peptides* **20**:125-139.

Matran, R., Alving, K., Martling, C.-R., Lacroix, J. S., and Lundberg, J. M. (1989a). Vagally mediated vasodilation by motor and sensory nerves in the tracheal and bronchial circulation of the pig. *Acta Physiol Scand.* **135**:29-37.

Matran, R., Alving, K., Martling, C.-R., Lacroix, J. S., and Lundberg, J. M. (1989b). Effects of neuropeptides and capsaicin on tracheo bronchial blood flow in the pig. *Acta Physiol. Scand.* In press.

Matran, R., Martling, C.-R., and Lundberg, J. M. (1989c). Neuropeptide Y and alpha2-receptor inhibition of cholinergic and non-adrenergic, non-cholinergic bronchoconstriction. *Eur. J. Pharmacol.* **163**:15-23.

Matsuzaki, Y., Hamasaki, Y., and Said, S. I. (1980). Vasoactive intestinal peptide: a possible transmitter of nonadrenergic relaxation of guinea pig airways. *Science* **210**:1252-1253.

McCormack, D. G., Salonen, R. O., Widdicombe, J. G., and Barnes, P. J. (1988). Sensory neuropeptides are potent vasodilators of canine bronchial arteries *in vitro*. *Am. Rev. Respir. Dis.* **137**:369.

McKnight, A. T., Maguire, J. J., Varney, M. A., and Williams, B. J. (1989). Characterization of receptors for tachykinins using selectivity of agonists and antagonists: evidence for an NK-4 receptor in guinea-pig isolated trachea. *J. Physiol.* **409**:30.

Michoud, M.-C., Amyot, R., Jeanneret-Grosjean, A., and Couture, J. (1987). Reflex decrease of histamine-induced bronchoconstriction after laryngeal stimulation in humans. *Am. Rev. Respir. Dis.* **136**:618-622.

Morice, A., Unwin, R. J., and Sever, P. S. (1983). Vasoactive intestinal peptide causes bronchodilatation and protects against histamine-induced bronchoconstriction in asthmatic subjects. *Lancet* **2**:1225-1226.

Nathanson, I., Widdicombe, J. H., and Barnes, P. J. (1983). Effect of vasoactive intestinal peptide on ion transport across dog tracheal epithelium. *J. Appl. Physiol.* **55**:1844-1848.

Nawa, H., Hirose, T., Takashima, H., Inayama, S., and Nakanishi, S. (1983). Nucleotide sequences of cloned cDNAs for two types of bovine brain substance P precursor. *Nature* **306**:32-36.

Palmer, J. B. D., and Barnes, P. J. (1987). Neuropeptides and airway smooth muscle function. *Am. Rev. Respir. Dis.* **136**:50-54.

Palmer, J. B., Cuss, F. M. C., and Barnes, P. J. (1986a). VIP and PHM and their role in non-adrenergic inhibitory responses in isolated human airways. *J. Appl. Physiol.* **61**:1322-1328.

Palmer, J. B. D., Cuss, F. M. C., Warren, J. B., and Barnes, P. J. (1986b). The effect of infused vasoactive intestinal peptide on airway function in normal subjects. *Thorax* **41**:663-666.

Palmer, J. B. D., Cuss, F. M. C., Mulderry, P. K., Ghatei, M. A., Springall, D. R., Cadieux, A., Bloom, S. R., Polak, J. M., and Barnes, P. J. (1987). Calcitonin gene-related peptide is localised to human airway nerves and potently constricts human airway smooth muscle. *Br. J. Pharmacol.* **91**:95-101.

Peatfield, A. C., and Richardson, P. S. (1983). Evidence for non-cholinergic, non-adrenergic nervous control of mucus secretion into the cat trachea. *J. Physiol.* **342**:335-345.

Peatfield, A. C., Barnes, P. J., Bratcher, C., Nadel, J. A., and Davis, B. (1983). Vasoactive intestinal peptide stimulates tracheal submucosal gland secretion in ferret. *Am. Rev. Respir. Dis.* **128**:89-93.

Polak, J. M., and Bloom, S. R. (1986). Regulatory peptides of the gastro-intestinal and respiratory tracts. *Arch. Int. Pharmacodyn.* **280**:16-49.

Regoli, D. (1987). Pharmacological receptors for substance P and neuro-kinins. *Life Sci.* **403**:66-76.

Richardson, J., and Beland, J. (1976). Nonadrenergic inhibitory nervous system in human airways. *J. Appl. Physiol.* **41**:764-771.

Richardson, J. B. (1981). Nonadrenergic inhibitory innervation of the lung. *Lung* **159**:315-322.

Rogers, D. F., Belvisi, M. G., Aursudkij, B., Evans, T. W., and Barnes, P. J. (1988a). Effects and interactions of sensory neuropeptides on airway microvascular leakage in guinea pigs. *Br. J. Pharmacol.* **95**:1109-1116.

Rogers, D. F., Carstairs, J. R., Alton, E. W. F. W., Dewar, A., and Barnes, P. J. (1988b). Tachykinins and mucus secretion in human bronchi *in vitro*. *Am. Rev. Respir. Dis.* **137**(Suppl):12.

Salonen, R. O., Webber, S. E., and Widdicombe, J. G. (1988). Effects of neuropeptides and capsaicin on the canine tracheal vasculature *in vivo*. *Br. J. Pharmacol.* **95**:1262-1270.

Saria, A., Martling, C.-R., Yan, Z., Theordorson-Norheim, E., Gamse, R., and Lundberg, J. M. (1988). Release of multiple tachykinins from capsaicin-sensitive sensory nerves in the lung by bradykinin, histamine, dimethylphenyl piperazinium and vagal nerve stimulation. *Am. Rev. Respir. Dis.* **137**:1330-1335.

Schalling, M., Franco-Cereceda, A., Hokfelt, T., Persson, H., and Lundberg, J. M. (1988). Increased neuropeptide Y messenger RNA and peptide in sympathetic ganglia after reserpine pretreatment. *Eur. J. Pharmacol.* **156**:419-420.

Sekizawa, K., Tamaoki, J., Graf, P. D., Basbaum, C. B., Borson, D. B., and Nadel, J. A. (1987). Enkephalinase inhibitor potentiates mammalian tachykinin-induced contraction in ferret trachea. *J. Pharmacol. Exp. Ther.* **243**:1211-1217.

Sheppard, M. N., Polak, J. M., Allen, J. M., and Bloom, S. R. (1984). Neuropeptide tyrosine (NYP): a newly discovered peptide is present in the mammalian respiratory tract. *Thorax* **39**:326-330.

Stretton, D., and Barnes, P. J. (1988). Modulation of cholinergic neurotransmission in guinea-pig trachea by neuropeptide Y. *Br. J. Pharmacol.* **93**:672-678.

Stretton, C. D., and Barnes, P. J. (1989). Cholecystokinin octapeptide constricts guinea-pig and human airways. *Br. J. Pharmacol.* **97**:675-682.

Szolcsanyi, J. (1988). Antidromic vasocilatation and neurogenic inflammation. *Agents Actions* **23**:5-11.

Tatemoto, K. (1984). PHI—a new brain-gut peptide. *Peptides* **5**:151-154.

Taylor, S. M., Pare, P. D., and Schellenberg, R. (1984). Cholinergic and nonadrenergic mechanisms in human and guinea pig airways. *J. Appl. Physiol.* **56**:958-965.

Tschirhart, E., and Landry, Y. (1986). Epithelium releases a relaxant factor: demonstration with substance P. *Eur. J. Pharmacol.* **132**:103-104.

Uddman, R., and Sundler, F. (1987). Neuropeptides in the airways: a review. *Am. Rev. Respir. Dis.* **136**:S3-8.

Vanhoutte, P. M. (1988). Epithelium-derived relaxing factor: myth or reality. *Thorax* **43**:665-668.

Yiangou, Y., Di Marzo, V., Spokes, R. A., Panico, M., Morris, H. R., and Bloom, S. R. (1987). Isolation, characterization, and pharmacological actions of peptide histidine valine 42, a novel prepro-vasoactive intestinal peptide-derived peptide. *J. Biol. Chem.* **262**:14010-14013.

15

Mast Cells and Asthma

MARTHA V. WHITE and MICHAEL A. KALINER

National Institute of Allergy and Infectious Disease
National Institutes of Health
Bethesda, Maryland

Allergy is a component of asthma in about 90% of children, 70% of adults under age 30 years, and 50% of adults above this age. Although not every episode of wheezing can be directly attributed to a recognized exposure to an allergen, mast cell activation is probably a factor in those patients with concomitant allergy and asthma.

I. Mast Cell Distribution

In humans, the mast cell is found in the loose connective tissue of all organs, especially around blood vessels, nerves, and lymphatics. Mast cells are most abundant in the skin, upper and lower respiratory tract, and in the gastrointestinal and reproductive mucosa (Metcalfe et al., 1981). In the lung, they occur in concentrations of $1\text{-}7 \times 10^6$ cells/g lung tissue (Wasserman, 1980), and constitute as much as 2% of alveolar tissue (Fox et al., 1981). About half the mast cells in the human lung are found on the lining of the bronchioles and bronchi, beneath the basement membrane; the other half are in the intralveolar septa (Friedman and Kaliner, 1987). Both types are adjacent to capillaries. The mast cells in the alveoli are about 10-20 μm long and are only about 2 μm away from the airway. These mast cells probably play little or no role in asthma. Depending on the size of the airway, mast cells in the lining of the airway are about 200 μm from the airway in the bronchi and 15-50 μm from the airway in the bronchioles. Because their exposure to antigen would be limited, these mast cells may be triggered in part by antigen and in part by other factors, such as neuropeptides.

II. Resting Mast Cell Morphology

Lung mast cells in situ may appear oval, triangular, or trapezoidal in electron micrographic sections and average 10-12 μm in maximum diameter, or they may be flattened and highly elongate, reaching more than 20 μm in length (Fig. 1). The former shapes are commonly observed in loose connective tissue and the alveolar septa, whereas the latter are common in the lamina propria of bronchioles, sandwiched between layers of fibroblasts and extracellular fibers beneath the airway's basal lamina. Isolated mast cells in suspension are rounded. The nucleus roughly mimics the cell in shape, and may possess clefts or indentations on electron micrographs. Rough endoplasmic reticulum, ribosomes, and mitochondria are present. Other cytoplasmic organelles include the Golgi apparatus, vesicles, lipid droplets, and rare microtubules. Microfilaments are numerous, approximately 83-100 Å in diameter, and are most apparent in areas devoid of granules (Kawanami et al., 1979; Ts'ao et al., 1977; Caulfield et al., 1980). Modest numbers of narrow cytoplasmic projections, or filopodia, extend from the cell surface. In electron micrographs of resting, connective tissue mast cells, the ubiquitous, densely stained, secretory granules are roughly spherical, and most are 0.2-0.5 μm in diameter. Most granules are comprised of a dense, amorphous matrix material with embedded or interspersed crystalline constituents in the form of scrolls, gratings, or lattices (Friedman and Kaliner, 1987). Scrolls are found most commonly, and appear as concentric rings or whorls when viewed in cross section, and as tubular groups of parallel tracks when viewed in longitudinal section. Gratings are found less often, and appear as parallel electron dense lines separated by lucent areas. Lattices, which may make up approximately 2% of the resting granules (Caulfield et al., 1980), appear as two sets of parallel electron-dense lines running in different directions and overlying each another. These patterns are thought to represent storage forms of granule substances and to typify resting mast cells (Nisam et al., 1978; Caulfield et al., 1980).

It should be noted that even in experimentally unstimulated nasal and lung tissues, variable numbers of degranulating mast cells are present. In unstimulated nasal epithelium, one-third of mast cells may be degranulated

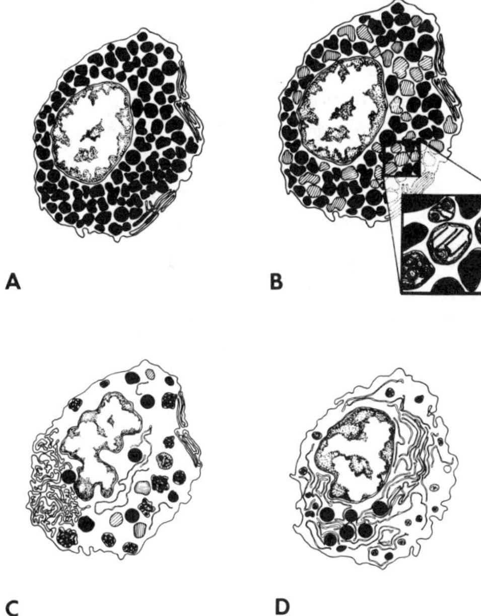

Figure 1 Schematic depiction of human lung mast cell degranulation. A resting mast cell (A) contains about 1000 granules, which are noted to be homogeneous in appearance in resting cells. As the cell becomes activated after antigen challenge, the granules take on a scroll-like structure (B, inset). After about 15 min, the granules have largely dissolved intracytoplasmically, leaving residual vacuoles, representing empty granules and prominent lipid bodies, which appear as dark granule-like structures (C). After about 30 min, the mast cell is largely devoid of recognizable granules except for the lipid bodies (D) (from Friedman and Kaliner, 1987).

(Kawabori and Unno, 1983) and the percentage progressively increases from the lamina propria to the mucosal surface (Dvorak et al., 1983). In resting lung, the percentage of degranulated mast cells progressively increases from parenchyma to bronchial mucosa to bronchial lumen (Ts'ao et al., 1977). It is unlikely that degranulation observed in unstimulated tissue is entirely an artifactual finding (Lamb and Lumsden, 1982). It more likely suggests that there is some degree of constant mast cell degranulation (Fox et al., 1981; Kawanami et al., 1979).

III. Morphology of Degranulating Mast Cells

Early events following IgE-mediated stimulation of human lung mast cells include granule swelling with loss of stainable matrix, an increase in the proportion of granules demonstrating a scroll pattern, and the appearance of electron-dense clumps in the granules. Perigranular membranes fuse with each other or with the plasma membrane to form deep degranulation channels throughout the cytoplasm (Trotter and Orr, 1973; Caulfield et al., 1980; Dvorak et al., 1983), which open to the external environment at points of fusion with the plasma membrane. By 3 min after stimulation, granule material may already be extruded from the cell surface (Caulfield et al., 1980; Dvorak et al., 1985). Unlike the skin mast cell, extruded granules are never observed intact in the external environment of the degranulated lung mast cell. Two patterns of degranulation occur in human lung mast cells: (1) gradual degranulation has been observed in situ in lung and other human tissues; (2) rapid degranulation has been seen in suspensions of enzymatically digested mast cells containing human tissues. The former may or may not be associated with the formation of cytoplasmic degranulation channels, while the latter is always associated with the formation of these channels.

The fate of degranulated mast cells has not been determined. It has been speculated that degranulated mucosal mast cells may migrate into the epithelium to become intraepithelial mast cells, which ultimately may be shed into the lumen where they might be observed in bronchial lavage fluid (Patterson et al., 1980). Degranulated mast cells in situ may possess residual secretory granules and have an intact biosynthetic apparatus, which suggests the capacity for granule repletion (Friedman and Kaliner, 1987).

IV. Mast Cell Secretagogues

Degranulation of human mast cells and basophils can be induced by a variety of immunological and nonimmunological secretagogues (Fig. 2). The best-studied secretagogue, IgE, binds high-affinity FC_E receptors on mast cells and basophils. When cross-linked by anti-IgE or by specific antigen, IgE induces degranulation through aggregation of FC_E receptors (Segal et al., 1977; Ishizaki et al., 1972). Thus, IgE provides a mechanism for specific antigen-mediated mast cell degranulation.

Numerous other agents of potential importance in human disease also cause mast cell degranulation. Opioids, such as morphine, cause cutaneous mast cell degranulation through a naloxone-sensitive receptor (Casale et al., 1984). Hypoxia can also induce mast cell degranulation (Haas and Bergofsky, 1972), potentially recruiting mast cell participation in hypoxic conditions such as adult respiratory distress syndrome. Various complement byproducts such as C5a, C4a, and C3a cause receptor-mediated mast cell degranulation (Gorski et al., 1979; Cochran and Muller-Eberhard, 1968) and thus might be capable of recruiting mast cell participation in immune complex diseases. Certain drugs, such as the antibiotics polymyxin B, and amphotericin B, the neuromuscular agents D-tubocurare and succinylcholine, and iodinated contrast media (Metcalfe et al., 1981), are also capable of inducing mast cell degranulation.

Secretagogues of research interest include compound 48/80 (Morrison and Henson, 1978); concanavalin A, which cross-links IgE (Margo, 1974);

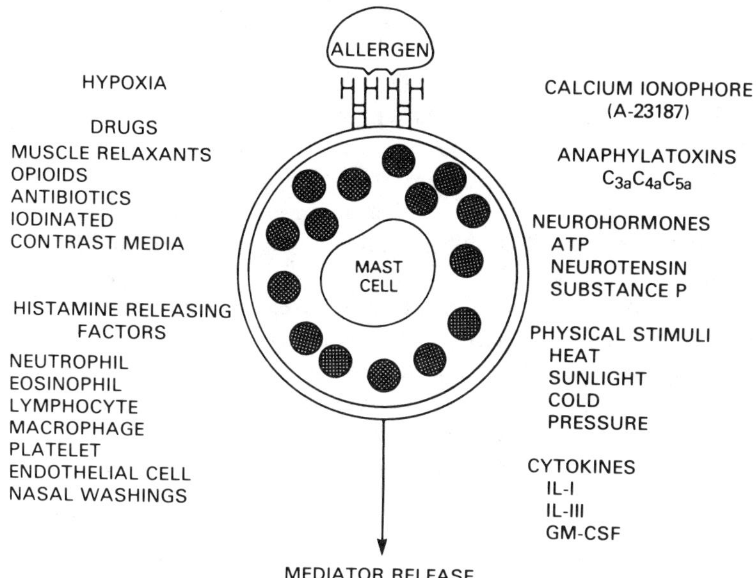

Figure 2 Mast cell secretagogues.

and the calcium ionophore A23187, which induces mast cell secretion by enhancing calcium transport into the cell (Foreman et al., 1973). Certain physical stimuli, such as heat, sunlight, cold, vibration, and pressure, also cause mast cell degranulation (Soter et al., 1979; Kaplan, 1983; Keahey et al., 1987; Huston et al., 1986; Casale et al., 1986); however, the mechanism is obscure.

Nonimmunological mast cell secretagogues of potential importance in asthma include histamine-releasing factors derived from human nasal washings (MacDonald et al., 1987), mononuclear cells (Theuson et al., 1979; Baeza et al., 1989; Schulman et al., 1988), human lung macrophages (Schulman et al., 1985), eosinophils (O'Donnell et al., 1983), neutrophils (White and Kaliner, 1987; White et al., 1989a), and platelets (Orchard et al., 1986). In addition, cytokines such as IL-I, IL-III, and GM-CSF have been reported to cause basophil histamine release (Haak-Frendscho, 1988; Submaranian, 1987). These factors may be instrumental in recruiting mast cell (or basophil) participation in pulmonary late phase allergic reactions as well as chronic nonallergic asthma.

Several of the neuropeptides may also play a role in asthma. The best studied, substance P, induces human cutaneous mast cell degranulation when present at nanomolar concentrations (Haegermark et al., 1978), and at higher concentrations causes human lung mast cell degranulation (Church, personal communication). The effect on human lung mast cells of other neuropeptides, neurokinin A, somatostatin, neurotensin, and calcitonin gene-related peptide, carried in sensory neurons with substance P, is unknown; however, all but neurotensin are capable of inducing mast cell degranulation in the rat (White et al., 1989b). Thus it is possible that some neuropeptides may activate mast cells during asthma triggered by infection, irritants, and possibly exercise. Another neuropeptide, vasoactive intestinal peptide (VIP), may actually inhibit bronchoconstriction, but it is not known whether VIP inhibits human lung mast cell activation.

Thus, a number of physiological agents are capable of activating mast cells. IgE-induced mast cell activation is essential during the early phase of allergic asthma and plays at least a permissive role during the late phase of allergic asthma. The agents most likely to recruit mast cell participation in nonallergic and late-phase allergic asthma include the inflammatory cell derived histamine-releasing factors, neuropeptides, and, in severe cases, hypoxia.

V. Mast Cell Mediators and Asthma

After death from status asthmaticus, the lungs remain inflated and may even spill out of the chest when the thorax is opened. Muscles, like all contractile tissues, relax at the time of death. The lung has considerable elastic recoil and should relax back to its resting state. Thus airflow obstruction in fatal asthma is not caused by muscle spasm alone. In status asthmaticus, the airflow obstruction is fixed as a result of mucus inspissation and blockage of the airways, as well as edema and inflammation.

Four factors have been identified as causes of airway obstruction in asthma: muscle spasm, mucosal edema, mucosal inflammation or cellular infiltration, and mucus secretion. Let us examine these four factors more closely in terms of the mast-cell-derived mediators that may be involved (Table 1). Release of mast cell mediators in conjunction with the infiltration of inflammatory cells into the airway wall (e.g., neutrophils and eosinophils) provides a potent stimulus for the pathological changes characteristic of asthma.

A. Bronchospasm

It is difficult to conceive of any mechanisms of airway obstruction other than spasm of the muscle layers encircling the airways that would be capable of rapid onset as well as a rapid reversal. Of the mast cell-derived mediators, histamine, bradykinin, leukotrienes C, D, and E (LTC4, LTD4, and LTE4), prostaglandins PGG_2, PGF_{2a}, and PDG_2, platelet-activating factor (PAF), and thromboxane A_2 (TXA_2) are capable of causing bronchial obstruction.

Table 1 Pathological Changes in Asthma and the Mediators That May Be Responsible

Bronchial smooth muscle contraction	Histamine (H-1 response) Leukotrienes C4, D4, E4 Prostaglandins and thromboxane A2 Bradykinin PAF
Mucosal edema	Histamine (H-1 response) Leukotrienes C4, D4, E4 Prostaglandin E2 Bradykinin PAF
Cellular infiltration (airway hyper-reactivity)	Inflammatory factors of anaphylaxis Eosinophil chemotactic factors Neutrophil chemotactic factors Leukotriene B4 PAF
Mucus secretion	Histamine (H-2 response) Prostaglandins Monohydroxyeicosatetraenoic acids Leukotrienes C4, D4, E4 PAF Chymase

Two cellular receptors for histamine have been identified, designated H_1 and H_2. Histamine induces airway obstruction through stimulation of H_1 receptors on muscle fibers. Analysis of histamine-induced constriction in vivo reveals that histamine acts directly on muscles (Rosenthal et al., 1977) and, in addition, may have a vagally mediated reflex parasympathetic action (Yu et al., 1972). Histamine also dilates small radicles of the pulmonary vascular tree through an H_1 receptor and increases the distance between endothelial cells of the venules, thereby increasing the potential for transduction of plasma and for extravasation of leukocytes (Wasserman, 1980).

The prostaglandins are generated during human lung anaphylaxis and appear in parallel with histamine (Dawson et al., 1976; Kaliner, 1980). Histamine, through stimulation of H_1 receptors is responsible for about 50% of the prostaglandins generated (Platshon and Kaliner, 1978). The rest are stimulated by airway muscle contraction (Steel et al., 1979), prostaglandin-generating factor of anaphylaxis (PGF-A), leukotrienes, and bradykinin (Steel and Kaliner, 1981).

In the human, products of arachidonic acid metabolism via a cycloxygenase-dependent pathway constitute the vast majority of prostaglandins (PG). At present, the exact role for PG generation in asthma is unclear; $PGF2_a$, PGD_2, and TXA_2 cause bronchospasm while PGE_2 and PGI_2 are bronchodilators. It is conceivable that a balance between these opposing influences may affect bronchial tone and play a role in allergic bronchospasm.

The leukotrienes C, D, and E are a series of closely related conjugated trienes derived from arachidonic acid through the 5-lipoxygenase pathway. In vivo experiments comparing their effects on airway resistance and lung compliance, and in vitro studies of lung and parenchymal strips indicate that these agents are more active in contracting small airways and peripheral lung tissue than larger airways (Spannhake et al., 1981). Studies on human bronchial muscle (Dahlen et al., 1980) indicate that LTC4 and LTD4 are 1,000 times more potent than histamine and 500 times more potent than PGF_{2a} on a molar basis. Experiments by other investigators (Paterson et al., 1981; Burka and Paterson, 1980; Hitchcock and Kokolis, 1981) support the hypothesis that in the sensitized lung, cycloxygenase inhibitors may enhance allergic tracheal contraction by diverting arachidonic acid through the lipoxygenase pathway toward the production of leukotrienes. Experiments in normal humans revealed inhalation of LTC4 and LTD4 to be 3,800-6,000 times more potent than histamine in causing specific, dose-related decrements in flow rates at 30% of vital capacity (Griffin et al., 1983). Moreover, asthmatic subjects are 25-100 times more sensitive to the bronchoconstrictive effects of LTD4 than are normal subjects (Smith et al., 1985). These studies suggest that in humans LTC4 and LTD4 are the most potent bronchoconstrictor substances yet described and that their prolonged duration of action (15-20 min) is consistent with a possible role in the mediation of IgE-mediated bronchoconstriction.

All normal bronchial tone is mediated by vagal constrictive influences. In experimental animals, mediators such as histamine are capable of stimulating vagal afferent nerves found interlaced among the epithelial cell lining of the airways (Karczewski and Widdicombe, 1969). In asthmatic patients, the inhalation of muscarinic blocking agents causes bronchodilation (Storms et al., 1975), which suggests that parasympathetic discharge of neurotransmitters might be contributing to the bronchoconstriction. The potential mechanisms by which cholinergic efferent discharges may be induced in asthma include both mediator-stimulated reflex discharges and increased cholinergic hyperreactivity as a reflection of disturbed autonomic balance in asthma (Kaliner et al., 1982).

Kinins are released in parallel with histamine during both immediate and late-phase responses to allergen challenge in the nose (Proud et al., 1986).

Anti-IgE challenge of partially purified human lung mast cells leads to a dose-dependent release of a kininogenase (Proud et al., 1985). This factor may participate in IgE-mediated asthma by the production of bradykinin.

B. Mucosal Edema

Edema of airway mucosa is due to increased capillary permeability, with leakage of serum proteins into interstitial areas. In addition, it has recently been appreciated that plasma protein-rich edema fluid moves rapidly through the epithelium and enters the airwáy lumen. Thus, vascular permeability causes part of the increased tracheobronchial secretions seen in asthma. Histamine, PAF, PGE, LTC, LTD, LTE, and bradykinin are all capable of causing increased capillary permeability. The neuropeptide, substance P, which can be released from sensory nerves in response to mast cell mediators, is a potent stimulator of increased vascular permeability, with resultant mucosal edema (Kowalski and Kaliner, 1988). Thus, complete pharmacological prevention of vascular permeability would require inhibition of the generation and/or activity of all of these peptides.

C. Cellular Infiltrates

The mucosa of patients who have died in status asthmaticus contain mixed cellular infiltrates consisting of eosinophils, neutrophils, macrophages, monocytes, and plasma cells (Kaliner et al., 1976). In the airway lumen, admixed in the abundant secretions, are eosinophils, neutrophils, and desquamated epithelial cells. Mast cell degranulation leads to the rapid appearance of histamine, eosinophil chemotactic factor of anaphylaxis (ECF-A), neutrophil chemotactic factor of anaphylaxis (NCF), and arachidonic acid metabolites (such as LTC, LTD, and LTE), which may initiate the characteristic eosinophil and neutrophil infiltration prominent in the histopathological findings characteristic of status asthmaticus. Also, the mast cell granule matrix may be a source of mediators such as inflammatory factor of anaphylaxis (IF-A), which could elicit cellular infiltrates appearing up to 24 h after the initial antigen-induced mast cell degranulation event (Tannenbaum et al., 1980). All of the inflammatory cells identified in asthma release factors capable of causing recrudescent mast cell degranulation. Thus, a cycle may be activated in asthma involving mast cell degranulation followed by infiltration of inflammatory cells, release of histamine-releasing factors, and further mast cell degranulation, and so on (Fig. 3). Interruption of this cycle would require either mast cell stabilizing agents, such as cromolyn sodium, or anti-inflammatory agents, such as corticosteroids, both of which are known to be effective in treating chronic asthma.

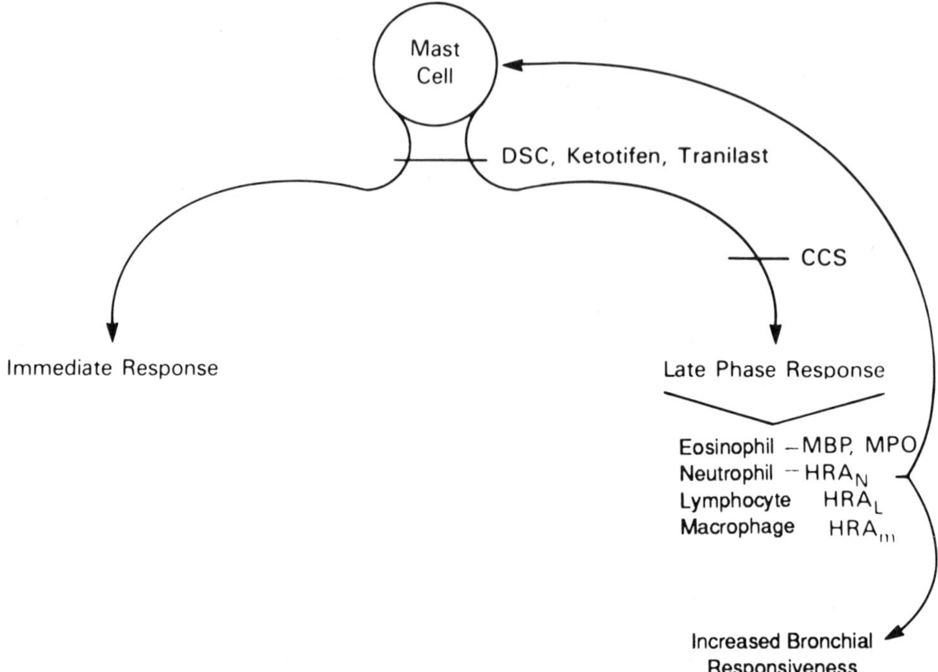

Figure 3   Interrelationship between inflammatory cell infiltration and mast cell activation. Mast cells attract inflammatory cells to the site of mediator release as a consequence of chemotactic factors being released. The infiltrating cells have the capacity to generate their own histamine-releasing factors, which might reactivate mast cells (or possibly basophils, which might infiltrate the area together with the other inflammatory cells). Eosinophils are known to release both eosinophil peroxidase and major basic protein, which can stimulate histamine release, whereas neutrophils, lymphocytes, macrophages, and other cell types release distinct histamine-releasing factors. The cycle could continue until arrested by mast-cell-stabilizing drugs such as cromoglycate (DSC), ketotifen, and tranilast, or the inflammatory process is broken with corticosteroids (CCS).

D. Mucus Secretion

Pathological examinations of fatal cases of status asthmaticus almost always reveal diffuse secretions of mucus, which appear to contribute significantly to the airways obstruction (Table 2) (Messer et al., 1960). The primary sources of the mucus component of these secretions are submucosal glands and goblet cells. Parasympathetic fibers innervate submucosal glands, stimulating smooth muscle contraction and glandular secretion. Asthma is characteristically asso-

Table 2 Drugs Capable of Affecting Late-Phase Asthmatic Responses

Antihistamines	
H1	+
H2	?
H1 & H2	?
Cromolyn sodium	+ +
Corticosteroids	+ +
Sympathomimetics	NE

+, Significant effect; + +, marked effect; NE, no effect; ?, data not available.

ciated with hyperplasia of goblet cells, which, in contrast to mucous glands, appear devoid of innervation (Kaliner, 1985).

Allergic pulmonary reactions in vivo lead to airway constriction and mucous secretion, while in vitro lung anaphylaxis leads to mediator release and increased mucous glycoprotein secretion from cultured human airways. The precise mechanisms responsible for increased mucus production are not clear, although the association between allergic pulmonary reactions and mucorrhea suggest that immediate hypersensitivity reactions may lead to the release or generation of secretagogues. To identify factors capable of influencing mucus secretion, a model was developed (Shelhamer et al., 1980; Marom et al., 1981) that used human airways cultured in the presence of radiolabeled aminosugars. The labeled glycoproteins synthesized in vitro may be quantitated and potential modulating influences examined using this model, we determined that the order of potency of mediators of anaphylaxis on mucus secretion is (Shelhamer et al., 1981): LTD4 (pg/ml) $\geqslant$ LTC4 (pg/ml) > hydroxyeicosatetranoic acids (nM) > PGF_{2a} = PGD2 = PGI2 = PGE1 = PGA2 (μM) > histamine stimulation (μM).

Mucus secretion in response to histamine involves H_2 receptors in the lung. The airway produces 5- and 15-HETEs spontaneously; during inflammation, this production increases dramatically. Because leukotrienes do not appear to be produced spontaneously by the airways, we must assume that the HETEs are more important in the normal regulation of mucus secretion than are leukotrienes, whereas the latter would be more important when allergic mechanisms are involved. The PGF-A molecule released from mast cells during their activation contributes to the production of HETEs and prostaglandins (Kaliner, 1989).

The autonomic nervous system is also capable of inducing mucus secretion in two ways: through parasympathetic stimulation involving the muscarinic receptors, which results in both serous and mucus secretion; and through alpha-adrenergic stimulation, which tends to be responsible only for serous secretion (Shelhamer et al., 1980). Of the neuropeptides, substance P and gastrin-releasing peptide are potent stimuli for mucus secretion (Lundgren et al., 1988; Baraniuk, in press). Eosinophil-derived proteins are also potent secretagogues. Finally, the macrophage/monocyte can synthesize a molecule known as macrophage-dervied mucus secretagogue (MMS). This molecule has been identified in bronchoalveolar lavage fluid in chronic bronchitis, and may play a role in mucus secretion among smokers with bronchitis (Marom et al., 1985).

D. Desquamation of Surface Epithelium, Thickening of the Basement Membrane, and Goblet Cell Hyperplasia

Denudation of airway epithelial surfaces with the appearance of epithelial clumps (Creola bodies) in expectorated secretions accompanies severe asthma. The denuded epithelial surfaces may be replaced by goblet cells, resulting in goblet cell hyperplasia. The mechanism for this desquamation has not been systematically examined, although several mast cell mediators might contribute to this process. Mast cell degranulation is accompanied by the production of the superoxide anion, O_2^- (Henderson and Kaliner, 1978), which may lead to the production of H_2O_2, OH^-, singlet oxygen, and other highly destructive oxygen radicals. These molecules are able to damage cell membranes and thereby contribute to denudation of the epithelium. Granule matrix-derived proteolytic enzymes may also help release epithelial cells from the basal layer by weakening intercellular bonds. In addition, edema formation in the interstitium leads to fluid movement through the basement membrane and resultant weakening of epithelial attachment. The continued movement of edema fluid towards the airway lumen appears to contribute to lifting the epithelium off the basement membrane and results in desquamation.

IV. Evidence for Mast Cell Participation in Asthma: Early and Late Phase Allergic Reactions

Following antigen challenge, isolated immediate, isolated late, and dual asthmatic reactions may occur (Lemanske and Kaliner, 1988). The immediate reaction generally occurs within minutes after antigen exposure or challenge and is characterized by airway obstruction that generally resolves 30-60 min later. Late-phase reactions (LPR) begin 3-4 h following exposure or challenge, airway obstruction peaks by 4-8 h, and the response resolves in 12-24 h.

Biopsy specimens of human cutaneous LPR reveal early infiltration of neutrophils and eosinophils followed later by mononuclear cells (Keahey et al., 1988). Ethical and technical considerations limit investigation of human pulmonary LPR to bronchoalveolar lavage fluid, which may not always reflect the mediators and cell present in the tissues, nonetheless, the cellular findings in BAL are similar to those of the skin (Fick et al., 1987).

Dual asthmatic reactions are characterized clinically by a biphasic period of asthmatic symptoms consisting of wheezing, coughing, and shortness of breath. Despite a single antigen exposure or challenge, the intensity of the airway obstruction developed during the late response is more prolonged and usually more severe than that observed during the immediate reaction. A variety of antigens, as well as exercise and administration of distilled water, have been noted to cause pulmonary LPR (Lemanske and Kaliner, 1988).

The presence of inflammatory cells during pulmonary LPR suggests that immune complexes may play a pathogenic role. However complement levels, which fall during type II hypersensitivity pneumonitis (Baur et al., 1980), are unaltered during the development of pulmonary LPR (Baur et al., 1980; Stalenheim and Machado, 1985). Moreover, depletion of complement in a rat model of LPR failed to affect the generation of LPR (Lemanske and Kaliner, 1988). Thus, the late pulmonary response does not appear to be secondary to IgG or IgM immune complexes.

In contrast, a large body of evidence exists to suggest that pulmonary early and late asthmatic reactions developing after antigen challenge are primarily due to IgE-dependent mast-cell-mediated mechanisms. Several investigators have reported that patients who experience pulmonary LPR following antigen challenge have positive immediate skin test responses, but not precipitating antibody to the challenge antigen (Robertson et al., 1974; Franz et al., 1971). Moreover, the patients with dual asthmatic responses tend to have the highest levels of IgE-dependent sensitivity (Boulet et al., 1984; Robertson et al., 1974), and immunotherapy, which is thought to raise IgG blocking antibody, protects against pulmonary LPR (Warner, 1976; Warner et al., 1978). Moreover, animal experiments in a rabbit model of LPR demonstrate that passive administration of antigen-specific IgG antibody attenuates the development of the late asthmatic reaction in IgE-primed animals (Behrens et al., 1984). These data provide indirect evidence that allergic LPR are dependent upon allergic sensitivity to the inciting antigens and thus are mediated, at least in part, by mast cell activation.

More direct evidence of mast cell involvement in LPR can be obtained by studying mediators released during LPR. Inhalation challenge with antigen leads to both early and late asthmatic responses. Elevations in plasma (Durham et al., 1984; Casale et al., 1987), but not urinary (Keyzer et al., 1984), levels of the mast cell mediator, histamine, can be measured during the late response. Other investigators have detected a second mast cell mediator, neutrophil chemotactic activity, during both early and late asthmatic responses following exercise (Lee et al., 1983) and antigen inhalation challenge (Nagy et al., 1982). These data suggest that mast cells (or basophils) are activated to secrete during allergic as well as nonallergic early and late asthmatic responses, and are responsible, at least in part, for mediating these reactions.

VII. Pharmacological Modulation of Asthma

Analysis of the effects of various medications on the development of experimentally induced immediate and late-phase asthmatic responses can provide a better understanding of the possible pathogenesis of asthma (Table 2). If the mast cell is an important mediator of both early- and late-phase asthmatic responses, mast cell stabilizing drugs should inhibit both phases of asthma. The effects of antagonists of specific mast cell mediators should be variable, and would depend on the importance of the mediator in question in the pathogenesis of asthma. It follows that at least some of the medications useful for asthma management should inhibit either mast cell degranulation or should antagonize the effects of mast cell mediators. Let us examine the data for antihistamines, corticosteroids, disodium cromoglycate, and beta agonists individually.

A. Antihistamines

Chlorpheniramine, an H1 antagonist, has been studied extensively. Nathan and co-workers (1981) and Schachter and associates (1982) found that a single 8 mg dose of chlorpheniramine inhibits histamine-induced bronchial obstruction in asthmatic as well as in normal subjects. Multiple doses given orally over a 2 day period also caused improvement in baseline forced expiratory volume in 1s (FEV_1) and forced expiratory flow (FEF_{25-75}) in asthmatic subjects. Eiser et al. (1981) found that a single 20 mg dose of chlorpheniramine delivered intravenously inhibited the bronchial obstructive response to inhaled histamine in both asthmatic and nonasthmatic subjects, improved specific airway conductance, and prevented bronchial obstruction after inhaled antigen challenge in asthmatics. In similar fashion, the H1 antagonist mepyramine inhibited the development of antigen-induced late asthmatic reactions (Booij-Noord et al., 1972). Inhaled chlorpheniramine and clemastine both caused bronchodilation in a group of pediatric asthmatic patients (Hodges et al., 1983) as well as adult asthmatic patients (O'Byrne et al., 1983).

While the evidence suggests that histamine is involved in mediating asthma, large clinical trials with antihistamines have been disappointing (Gobel, 1978; Henry et al., 1983). This is not surprising, since histamine is only one of several mast cell mediators capable of participating in the pathogenesis of asthma. Furthermore, antihistamine trials have been limited in dosage by these agents' sedative effects. Two new nonsedating antihistamines, terfenadine and astemizole, have been studied. Orally administered terfenadine has been shown to inhibit exercise-induced asthma (Patel, 1984), while oral astemizole inhibits antigen-, histamine-, and exercise-induced asthma (Holgate et al., 1985; Clee et al., 1984). These nonsedating antihistamines can be used at higher dosages than classic antihistamines and thus their effect on asthma deserves further study.

B. Corticosteroids

Corticosteroids are one of the most potent classes of drugs available for the treatment of asthma, although their precise mechanism of action in asthma is not completely clear. Cockcroft and Murdock (1987) studied the effect of single-dose inhaled beclomethasone on the asthmatic response to inhaled antigen. The topical steroid had no effect on the immediate asthmatic response, but inhibited both the late asthmatic response and the resultant increased airways hyperreactivity.

Human basophils incubated overnight with dexamethasone, or other corticosteroids, release less histamine in response to anti-IgE than control cells (Schleimer et al., 1981). However, basophils obtained from asthmatic subjects receiving oral steroids chronically released similar amounts of histamine compared to patients with non-steroid-dependent asthma and controls. Basophils obtained from asthmatic subjects who required oral corticosteroids were less responsive to the inhibitory effects of in vitro dexamethasone exposure (Lampl et al., 1985). These data were interpreted as suggesting that the steroid-sensitive basophils had been sequestered from the bloodstream. However, an alternative explanation might be that the steroid-dependent asthmatic patients originally had more reactive basophils, which were partly inhibited by steroid administration. Although dexamethasone had no effect on histamine release induced by agents other than IgE, the effect was thought to be mediated through a steroid receptor rather than the IgE receptor (Schleimer et al., 1982). In contrast, when isolated human lung mast cells were incubated overnight with dexamethasone, no inhibition of IgE-mediated histamine or arachidonic acid metabolism occurred (Schleimer et al., 1983). These data have been interpreted collectively as suggesting that steroids work by inhibiting inflammation and possibly basophil activation associated with LPR, but not mast cell reactivity.

There is a growing body of evidence to suggest, however, that chronic steroid administration may inhibit mast cell activation. Van der Star and colleagues (1976) studied the effect of 1 and 6 days of pretreatment with inhaled beclomethasone diproprionate (BDP) on the early and late asthmatic response following antigen challenge. After 1 day of BDP only the late asthmatic response was inhibited, but after 6 days of pretreatment both the early and the late response were inhibited. The inhibitory effect of chronic steroid administration on the early asthmatic response was confirmed by Martin et al. (1980) after oral prednisolone and by Burge et al. (1982) after inhaled BDP.

Similar experiments have been performed in the nasal mucosa. Although single-dose administration of corticosteroid had no effect on the immediate response to nasal antigen challenge, 1 week of topical flunisolide protected against both immediate and late nasal symptoms. In these experiments, flunisolide also inhibited mast cell histamine release during both the early- and late-phase response following antigen challenge (Pipkorn et al., 1987). Bascom et al. (1988), using a similar protocol, biopsied human nasal mucosae 1 and 11 h after antigen challenge and found that 1 week of topical fluonisolide pretreatment inhibited the antigen-induced influx of basophils into the nasal mucosa. Topical steroids administered for only 2 days lowered the nasal responsiveness to antigen and inhibited the priming effect normally seen on rechallenge (Andersson et al., 1988). Thus, while acute steroid administration inhibits only the late asthmatic response, and has no apparent effect on mast cells or the immediate asthmatic response, chronic administration inhibits nasal, and probably pulmonary, mast cell activation as well as both the early and the late asthmatic response. These data may help to explain the clinical observation that topical corticosteroids generally require weeks of administration before their full beneficial effects are appreciated.

Whether the effect of chronic corticosteroid therapy on the reduction of mediator release and symptoms during the immediate allergic response is due to mast cell stabilization or to a toxic effect on mast cells is uncertain. Pipkorn and Everback (1987) found that topical budesonide had no effect on the increase in nasal mast cell numbers normally observed after birch season in birch-sensitive patients with allergic rhinitis; however, tissue histamine levels were decreased. These data suggest that corticosteroids downregulate mast cell metabolism. However, following 6 weeks of topical steroids, cutaneous mast cells are undetectable by electron microscopic examination, and tissue histamine levels are also reduced, suggesting a toxic effect on mast cells. More data are needed to resolve this question.

C. Cromolyn

Disodium cromoglycate inhibits IgE-dependent in vitro degranulation of human lung mast cells obtained from lung fragments (Church et al., 1983), dispersed lung cell preparations (Church and Ko, 1983), bronchoalveolar lavage fluid (Flint, 1985) and from antigen-stimulated human jejunal mucosal mast cells (Selbekk, 1979). One would expect, therefore, that if mast cells are important mediators of early- and late-phase asthma, cromolyn should block both components of the asthmatic reaction. This is indeed the case. Cromolyn administered prior to allergen challenge inhibits not only the immediate asthmatic response (Frith, 1981) but also the delayed response (Pepys et al., 1968, 1974; Booij-Noord, 1971; Booij-Noord et al., 1972; Feldman et al., 1982; Hegardt et al., 1981). Similar results have been found by investigators studying the effect of cromolyn on nasal allergen challenge. Pelikan (1982) found that cromolyn administered immediately prior to nasal antigen challenge inhibited both the early and the late allergic response. Acute administration of cromolyn prior to challenge has been shown to inhibit the human asthmatic response to nonimmunological stimuli as well, including exercise (Davies, 1968), airway cooling (Fanta, 1981; Breslin, 1980), sulfur dioxide (Sheppard et al., 1981), and ultrasonically nebulized distilled water or fog (Godden et al., 1983; Fuller and Collier, 1984). The mechanism by which airway cooling induces asthma may involve mast cell activation, since cold, dry air challenge to the nose results in the release of histamine and PGD2 (Togias et al., 1985).

Chronic administration of cromolyn also reduces bronchial reactivity. Not all clinical trials have demonstrated this. The negative studies tend to be of short duration: 1 (Cockroft et al., 1977) or 2 (Ryo et al., 1970) weeks, while the positive studies are of at least 6 weeks duration. Altounyan (1970) and Dixon (1979) treated subjects for 6 weeks and 1 year, respectively, and were able to demonstrate a significant reduction in bronchial reactivity to histamine. Using a model of natural allergen exposure, Lowhagen and Rak (1985) studied the effect of cromolyn on the increased bronchial reactivity normally occurring in birch-sensitive asthmatic patients after the pollen season. A 6 week trial of cromolyn during the birch season completely inhibited the normal postseasonal increase in bronchial reactivity to histamine. Thus cromolyn, like corticosteroids, inhibits both early- and late-phase asthmatic responses to allergen- as well as antigen-induced increases in bronchial reactivity.

The major mechanism by which cromolyn inhibits asthma is thought to be mast cell stabilization. Atkins and colleagues (1978) showed that a single dose of cromolyn blocked not only the bronchospastic response to antigen but also the release of the mast cell mediator NCA. Furthermore, when bronchoalveolar lavage fluid was examined, an asthmatic patient who had a clinical response to a 1 month trial with cromolyn had fewer eosinophils, and less allergen-specific IgE, which suggested a lower level of mast cell activation. Whether cromolyn works by mechanisms other than mast cell stabilization is unclear. It has some anti-inflammatory properties, since it also inhibits the activation of leukocytes (Moqbel et al., 1986; Kay and Barnes, 1985). Cromolyn also has been shown to inhibit histamine-induced excitatory responses of sensory nerve C fibers, which initiate reflex bronchoconstriction in the dog lung (Dixon et al., 1980; Harries, 1981). In addition, cromolyn inhibits vagally mediated bronchoconstriction initiated by leukotriene D4 (Advenier et al., 1983).

D. Sympathomimetics

Beta agonists are smooth muscle relaxants and are classically used to prevent and reverse the symptoms of asthma. Administered before antigen inhalation challenge, they effectively block the early asthmatic response, but have no effect on the late asthmatic response (Booij-Noord et al., 1972; Hegardt et al., 1981; Feldman et al., 1982). In fact, late asthmatic responses are relatively resistant to treatment with bronchodilators. Only one in vivo study suggests that beta agonists inhibit histamine release after antigen inhalation challenge (Howarth et al., 1987), and that study suffers from the serious flaw that the evidence is based on histamine measurements below the limits of sensitivity of the assay used. Thus, the evidence suggests that beta agonists work in asthma by causing bronchodilation, not by inhibiting mast cell activation.

VIII. Conclusion

Asthma induced by allergen or cold dry air inhalation is associated with release of the mast cell mediator, histamine. These data support a role for mast cells in the pathogenesis of allergic and nonallergic asthma. Allergen-induced asthma occurs in two phases, both of which are associated with histamine release. If mast cells are important mediators of both phases of asthma, mast-cell-stabilizing drugs should inhibit both reactions. As expected, the mast-cell-stabilizing medications, corticosteroids (chronic administration only) and cromolyn, inhibit both early- and late-phase allergic asthma. Short-term corticosteroids and beta agonists, which have no mast-cell-stabilizing effects, inhibit only the late and early phases, respectively, while antihistamines have a mild effect on the early phase asthmatic response. Thus, the evidence based upon direct measurement of mast cell activation, as well as pharmacological modulation of mast cell activation, indicate that mast cells play a critical role in acute and chronic asthma. The recent findings that IgE levels are closely correlated with asthma, even in nonallergic individuals (Burrows et al., 1989), and that cromolyn is effective in patients with carefully evaluated intrinsic (nonallergic) asthma (Petty et al., 1989), suggest that mast cells are likely to contribute to all forms of asthma.

Discussion

Kay: We found a decrease in mast cells in BAL after LPR. We attribute this to the possible presence of cytokines with histamine-releasing activity. Are the mast cells playing a central or secondary role?

Kaliner: Allow me to remind you that LPR was described as a late sequela to allergen challenge in the skin, nose, or lungs. LPR may be passively transferred with IgE antibody, which transfers sensitivity to the recipient for a prolonged period. Mast cell degranulating agents such as 48/80 also induce LPR, and have no recognized effect on other cell types. Moreover, several mast-cell-derived mediators, including the inflammatory factors of anaphylaxis, have the capacity to elicit LPR upon injection into recipients. Thus, the weight of evidence overwhelmingly indicates that the mast cell is central to LPR.

Dahl: Only a portion of allergen challenges elicit a LPR. Mast cells may be involved in the early reaction, but if mast cells were involved in LPR why do all allergic reactions not lead to LPR?

Kaliner: LPR are a dose-dependent response. Thus, one can elicit sufficient mediator release to cause an early reaction in individuals with increased airway hyperactivity, but insufficient to cause a clinically apparent LPR. Even in these subclinical cases, histological analysis will show microscopic inflammation. In other subjects, with less airway hyperreactivity, more mediator release is required to cause an early reaction, and because more inflammatory factors are released, there is now clinically apparent LPR.

Fuller: Why do beta adrenergic agonists not inhibit mast cells in vivo?

Kaliner: Systemic beta agonists fail to achieve a sufficient concentration to affect mast cells in vivo. Thus, we can skin test in the presence of beta agonists without any inhibitory effect. Other than Howarth et al.'s (1987) article, there is no evidence that inhaled beta agonists reduce mast cell reactions in the lung. Since that evidence is based on measurements of histamine below the level of sensitivity of the assay used, we have questions about the accuracy of the levels published.

Fish: We have recently completed studies showing that both the EAR and LAR can be inhibited by oral colchicine. Intravenous colchicine given after the EAR but before the LPR had no effect on the subsequent LPR. However, when we studied the effect of colchicine on human lung mast cell histamine release, we found no effect. Have you any explanation?

Kaliner: Colchicine inhibits mast cell and basophil histamine release, but only after disaggregation of microtubules. Thus, if you were to chill the mast cells to 4 °C prior to exposure to the colchicine, it will inhibit the reaction.

Schleimer: Have you tested HRA-N on human mast cells?

Kaliner: HRA-N activates isolated human cutaneous mast cells in vitro and causes positive immediate skin test reactions in humans in vivo. It also elicits LPR in humans in vivo.

Schleimer: Did Warren Gold not show inhibition of mast cell reaction in vivo in dogs?

Leff: Yes. While I was with Dr. Gold, we showed that intravenous isoproterenol could inhibit allergen-induced histamine release in vivo. In my lab in Chicago, we also showed that sympathetic stimulation was capable of inhibiting mast cell degranulation in vivo in dogs.

Platts-Mills: The correlation between the development of asthma and allergen exposure is strictly with those subjects who have IgE antibody. IgE has a far greater affinity for mast cells than for any other cell, and thus it is far more likely that mast cells would be activated after allergen exposure than any other cell.

A. Capron: It should be kept in mind that the affinity of IgE for FCE RII, which is 2×10^7 M-1 for monomeric IgE, is increased to 5×10^8 M-1 for dimeric IgE and IgE complexes. Extensive in vivo studies performed on atopic or parasitized patients have shown by flow cytometry that 10-50% of the cells bind IgE in vivo. The binding of IgE has also been shown by elution of membrane-bound IgE. Taken together, these studies demonstrate that cells with low-affinity IgE receptors do bind IgE in vivo.

Kaliner: Several American studies have failed to find that alveolar macrophages obtained from atopic humans release mediators upon exposure to allergen. Current work from Gleich's group, just published in the *Journal of Immunology* (Abu-Ghazaleh, 1989), fails to show activation of eosinophil degranulation through IgE mechanisms, although IgA is very efficient. These data, all performed in humans, fail to demonstrate that cells with low-affinity IgE receptors respond to antigen ex vivo.

Church: Let me add two pieces of data to this discussion. Nadel's group in San Francisco showed that mast cell tryptase sensitized smooth muscle to hyperresponsiveness to histamine. Second, canine mast cell tryptase was shown to be able to metabolize VIP but not substance P. This differential capability might influence response to neuropeptides released as a consequence of allergic reactions.

Church: You showed that HRA-N released histamine but not PGD2 or LTC4. We have published findings that a variety of secretagogues including VIP, SP, somatostatin, poly-L-lysine, morphine, and compound 48/80 all have the same property. However, all of these agents work only on skin, and not lung, mast cells.

Kaliner: We have not studied HRA-N on human lung mast cells yet.

Barnes: Single doses of inhaled corticosteroids have no effects on the EAR but may completely block the LAR. This supports the view that steroids have no direct effect on mast cells and that mast cells may not be crucial to LPR. Can you reconcile this observation with your concept of the central role of the mast cell?

Kaliner: The mast cell orchestrates the inflammation, which causes the LPR. Thus, short-term corticosteroid exposure might not affect the immediate response of mast cell degranulation, but might still reduce the inflammation. Thus, corticosteroids may act by reducing the influx of neutrophils and eosinophils, reducing edema formation, reducing secretions, and eventually by reducing both mast cell numbers and reactivity.

Kay: How do you account for the fact that several drugs developed in the 1970s, which were powerful inhibitors of mast cell degranulation, were without effect in clinical trials of asthma?

Kaliner: Many candidate drugs have actions in animals, and even in vitro in human tissues, but fail in clinical trials.

References

Abu-Ghazaleh, R. I., Fujisawa, T., Mestecky, J., Kyle, R. A., and Gleich, G. J. (1989). IgA induced eosinophil degranulation. *J. Immunol.* **142:** 2393-2400.

Advenier, C., Cerrina, J., Dukroux, P., Floch, A., Pradel, J., and Renier, A. (1983). Sodium cromoglycate, verapamil and nicardipine antagonism to leukotriene D4 bronchoconstriction. *Br. J. Pharmacol.* **78:**301-306.

Altounyan, R. E. C. (1970). Changes in histamine and atropine responsiveness as a guide to diagnosis and evaluation of therapy in obstructive airways disease. In *Disodium Cromoglycate in Allergic Airways Disease.* Edited by J. Pepys, and A. W. Frankland. London, Butterworth, pp. 105-120.

Andersson, M., Andersson, P., and Pipkorn, U. (1988). Topical glucocorticosteroids and allergen-induced increase in nasal reactivity: relationship between treatment time and inhibitory effect. *J. Allergy Clin. Immunol.* **82:**1019-1026.

Atkins, P. C., Norman, M. E., and Zweiman, B. (1978). Antigen-induced neutrophil chemotactic activity in man. Correlation with bronchospasm and inhibition by disodium cromoglycate. *J. Allergy Clin. Immunol.* **62:**149-155.

Baeza, M. L., Reddigari, S., Haak-Frendscho, M., and Kaplan, A. P. (1989). Purification and further characterization of human mononuclear cell histamine releasing factor. *J. Clin. Invest.* **83**:1204-1210.

Baraniuk, J. N., Lundgren, J. D., Goft, J., Peden, D., Merida, M., Shelhamer, J., and Kaliner, M. (1989). Gastrin releasing peptide (GRP) in human nasal mucosa. *J. Clin. Invest.* **85**:998-1005.

Bascom, R., Wachs, M., Naclerio, R. M., Pipkorn, U., Galli, S. J., and Lichtenstein, L. M. (1988). Basophil influx occurs after nasal antigen challenge: effects of topical corticosteroid pretreatment. *J. Allergy Clin. Immunol.* **81**:580-589.

Baur, X., Dorsch, W., and Becker, T. (1980). Levels of complement factors in human serum during immediate and late asthmatic reactions and during actue hypersensitivity pneumonitis. *Allergy* **35**:383-390.

Behrens, B. L., Clark, A. F., Marsh, W., and Larsen, G. (1984). Modulation of the late asthmatic response by antigen-specific immunoglobulin G in an animal model. *Am. Rev. Respir. Dis.* **130**:1134-1139.

Booij-Noord, H., Orie, N. G. M., and Devries, K. (1971). Immediate and late bronchial obstructive reactions to inhalation of house dust and protective effects of disodium cromoglycate and prednisolone. *J. Allergy Clin. Immunol.* **48**:344-354.

Booij-Noord, H., de Vries, K., Sluiter, H. J., and Orie, N. G. (1972). Late bronchial obstructive reaction to experimental inhalation of house dust extract. *Clin. Allergy* **2**:43-61.

Boulet, L. P., Roberts, R. S., Dolovich, J., and Hargreave, F. E. (1984). Prediction of late asthmatic responses to inhaled allergen. *Clin. Allergy* **14**:379-385.

Breslin, F. J., McFadden, E.R., and Ingram, R. H. Jr. (1980). The effect of cromolyn sodium on the airway response to hypernea and cold air in asthma. *Am. Rev. Respir. Dis.* **122**:11-16.

Burge, P. S., Efthimiou, J., Turner-Warwick, M., and Nelmes, P. T. J. (1982). Double blind trial of inhaled beclomethasone diproprionate and fluocortin butyl ester in allergen induced immediate and late asthmatic reactions. *Clin. Allergy* **12**:523-531.

Burka, J. F., and Paterson, N. A. M. (1980). Evidence for lipoxygenase pathway involvement in allergic tracheal contraction. *Prostaglandins* **19**:499-515.

Burrows, B., Martinez, F. D., Halonen, M., Barbee, R. A., and Cline, M. G. (1989). Association of asthma with serum IgE levels and skin-test reactivity to allergens. *N. Engl. J. Med.* **320**:271-277.

Casale, T. B., Bowman, S., and Kaliner, M. (1984). Induction of human cutaneous mast cell degranulation by opiates and endogenous opioid peptides: evidence for opiate and nonopiate receptor participation. *J. Allergy Clin. Immunol.* **73**:775-780.

Casale, T. B., Keahey, T. M., and Kaliner, M. (1986). Exercise-induced anaphylactic syndromes. *JAMA* **255**:2049-2053.

Casale, T. B., Wood, D., Richerson, H. B., Zehr, B., Zavala, D., and Hunninghake, G. W. (1987). Direct evidence of a role for mast cells in the pathogenesis of antigen-induced bronchoconstriction. *J. Clin. Invest.* **80**:1507-1511.

Caulfield, J. P., Lewis, R. A., Hein, A., and Austen, K. F. (1980). Secretion in dissociated human pulmonary mast cells. *J. Cell. Biol.* **85**:299-311.

Church, M. K., Holgate, S. T., and Pao, G. J. (1983). Histamine release from mechanically and enzymatically dispersed human lung mast cells: Inhibition by salbutamol and cromoglycate (abstract). *Br. J. Pharmacol.* **79**:374.

Church, M. K., and Young, K. O. (1983). The characteristics of inhibition of histamine release from human lung fragments by sodium cromoglycate, salbutamol and chlorpromazine. *Br. J. Pharmacol.* **78**:671-679.

Clee, M. D., Ingram, C. G., Reid, P. C., and Robertson, A. S. (1984). The effect of astemizole on exercise-induced asthma. *Br. J. Dis. Chest* **78**: 180-183.

Cochran, C. G., and Muller-Eberhard, H. J. (1968). The derivation of the two distinct anaphylatoxin activities from the third and fifth components of human complement. *J. Exp. Med.* **127**:371-377.

Cockroft, D. W., Killian, D. N., Mellan, J. J. A., and Hargreave, F. E. (1977). Protective effect of drugs on histamine-induced asthma. *Thorax* **32**:429-437.

Cockroft, W. D., and Murdock, K. Y. (1987). Comparative effects of inhaled salbutamol, sodium cromoglycate, and beclomethasone dipropionate on allergen-induced early asthmatic responses, late asthmatic responses, and increased bronchial responsiveness to histamine. *J. Allergy Clin. Immunol.* **79**:734-740.

Dahlen, S. E., Hedqvist, P., Hammarstrom, S., and Samuelsson, B. (1980). Leukotrienes are potent constrictors of human bronchi. *Nature* **288**: 484-486.

Davies, S. E. (1968). Effect of disodium cromoglycate on exercise-induced asthma. *Br. Med. J.* **3**:593-599.

Dawson, W., Boot, J. R., Cockerell, A. F., Mallen, D. N. B., and Osbourne, D. J. (1976). The release of novel prostaglandins and thromboxanes after immunologic challenge of guinea pig lung. *Nature* **262**:699-703.

Dixon, W. A. (1979). One-year's trial of Intal compound in 24 children with severe asthma. In *Disodium Cromoglycate in Allergic Airways Disease.*

Edited by J. Pepys and A. W. Frankland. London, Butterworth, pp. 105-120.

Dixon, M., Jackson, D. M., and Richards, I. M. (1980). The action of sodium cromoglycate on "C" fiber endings in the dog lung. *Br. J. Pharmacol.* **70**:11-13.

Durham, S. R., Lee, T. H., Cromwell, O., Shaw, R. J., Merrett, J., Cooper, P., and Kay, A. B. (1984). Immunologic studies in allergen-induced asthmatic reactions. *J. Allergy Clin. Immunol.* **74**:49-60.

Dvorak, A. M., Galli, S. J., Schulman, E. S., Lichtenstein, L. M., and Dvorak, H. F. (1983). Basophil and mast cell degranulation: ultrastructural analysis of mechanisms of mediator release. *Fed. Proc.* **2**:2510-2515.

Dvorak, A. M., Schulman, E. S., Peters, S. P., MacGlashan, D. W., Jr., Newball, H. H., Schleimer, R. P., and Lichtenstein, L. M. (1985). Immunoglobulin E-mediated degranulation of isolated human lung mast cells. *Lab. Invest.* **53**:45-56.

Eiser, N. M., Mills, J., Snashall, P. D., and Guz, A. (1981). The role of histamine receptor antagonists in normal and asthmatic subjects. *Thorax* **35**:428-34.

Fanta, C. H., McFadden, E. R., and Ingram, R. H. Jr. (1981). Effects of cromolyn sodium on the response to respiratory heat loss in normal subjects. *Am. Rev. Respir. Dis.* **123**:161-164.

Feldman, C. H., Fox, J., Kraut, E., Feldman, B. R., Davies, W. J. (1982). Exercise induced asthma (EIA): treatment for early and late responses (abstract). *Am. Rev. Respir. Dis.* **125**(pt 2):191.

Fick, R. B., Jr., Richerson, H. B., Zavala, D. C., and Hunninghake, G. W. (1987). Bronchoalveolar lavage in allergic asthmatics. *Am. Rev. Respir. Dis.* **135**:1204-1209.

Flint, K. C., Leung, K. B. P., Pearce, F. L., Hudspith, B. N., Brostoff, J., and Johnson, N. M. (1985). *Clin. Sci.* **68**:427-432.

Foreman, J. C., Mongar, J. L., and Gomperts, B. D. (1973). Calcium ionophores and movement of calcium ions following physiologic stimulus to a secretory process. *Nature (London)* **245**:249-251.

Fox, B., Bull, T. B., and Guz, A. (1981). Mast cells in the human alveolar wall: an electron microscopic study. *J. Clin. Pathol.* **34**:1333-1342.

Franz, T., McMurrain, K. D., Brooks, S., and Bernstein, I. L. (1971). Clinical, immunologic and physiologic observations in factory workers exposed to *B. subtilis* enzyme dust. *J. Allergy* **47**:170-180.

Friedman, M. M., and Kaliner, M. A. (1987). Mast cells and asthma. *Am. Rev. Respir. Dis.* **135**:157-164.

Frith, P. A., Ruffin, R. E., Juniper, E. F., Dolovich, J., and Hargreave, F. E. (1981). Inhibition of allergen-induced asthma by three forms of sodium cromoglycate.

Fuller, R. W., and Collier, J. C. (1984). Sodium cromoglycate and atropine block the fall in FEV$_1$ but not the cough induced by hypotonic mist. *Thorax* **39**:766-770.

Gobel, P. P. (1978). The protective effect of ketotifen in bronchial asthma. *J. Int. Med. Res.* **6**:79-85.

Godden, D., Jamieson, S., and Higenbottan, T. (1983). "Fog"-induced bronchoconstriction is inhibited by sodium cromoglycate but not lignocain or ipratropium. *Thorax* **38**:226-227.

Gorski, J. P., Hugli, T. E., and Muller-Eberhard, H. J. (1979). The third anaphylatoxin of the human complement system. *Proc. Natl. Acad. Sci. (USA)* **76**:5299-5304.

Griffin, M., Weiss, J. W., Leitch, A. G., McFadden, E. R. Jr. Corey, E. J., Austen, K. F., and Drazen, J. M. (1983). Effects of leukotriene D on the airways in asthma. *N. Engl. J. Med.* **308**:436-439.

Haas, F., and Bergofsky, E. H. (1972). Role of the mast cell in the pulmonary pressor response to hypoxia. *J. Clin. Invest.* **51**:3143-3162.

Haegermark, O. E., Hoekfelt, T., and Pernow, B. (1978). Flare and itch induced by substance P in human skin. *J. Invest. Dermatol.* **71**:233-235.

Harries, M. G. (1981). Bronchial irritant receptors and a possible new action for cromolyn sodium. *Ann. Allergy* **46**:156-158.

Hegardt, B., Pauwels, R., and Van der Straaten, M. (1981). Inhibitory effect of KWO 2131, terbutaline and DSCG on the immediate and late allergen-induced bronchoconstriction. *Allergy* **36**:115-122.

Henderson, W. R., and Kaliner, M. (1978). Immunologic and nonimmunologic generation of superoxide from mast cells and basophils. *J. Clin. Invest.* **61**:187-196.

Henry, R. L., Hodges, I. G., Milner, A. D., and Stokes, G. M. (1983). Bronchodilator effects of the H$_1$ receptor antagonist-clemastine. *Arch. Dis. Child.* **58**:304-305.

Hitchcock, M., and Kokolis, N. A. (1981). Arachidonic acid metabolism and modulation of *in vitro* anaphylaxis by 5, 8, 11, 14-eicosatetranoic acid and 9a, 12a-octadecadiynoic acid. *Br. J. Pharmacol.* **72**:689-695.

Hodges, I. G., Milner, A. D., and Stokes, G. M. (1983). Bronchodilator effects of two inhaled H1-receptor antagonists, clemastine and chlorpheniramine, in wheezy school children. *Br. J. Dis. Chest* **77**:270-275.

Holgate, S. T., Emanuel, M. B., and Howarth, P. H. (1985). Astemizole and other H$_1$-antihistaminic drug treatment of asthma. *J. Allergy Clin. Immunol.* **76**:375-380.

Howarth, P. H., Durham, S. R., Kay, A. B., and Holgate, S. T. (1987). The relationship between mast cell-mediator release and bronchial reactivity in allergic asthma. *J. Allergy Clin. Immunol.* **80**:703-711.

Huston, D. P., Bressler, R. B., Kaliner, M., Sowell, L. K., and Baylor, M. W. (1986). Prevention of mast-cell degranulation by ketotifen in patients with physical urticarias. *Ann. Intern. Med.* **104**:507-510.

Ishizaka, T., Chang, T. H., Taggart, M., and Ishizaka, K. (1972). Histamine release from rat mast cells by antibodies against rat basophilic leukemic cell membrane. *J. Immunol.* **108**:339-345.

Kaliner, M. A. (1980). Mast cell-derived mediators and bronchial asthma. In *Airway Reactivity*. Edited by F. E. Hargreave. Mississauga, Ontario, Canada, Astra Pharmaceuticals Canada LTD, pp. 175-187.

Kaliner, M. (1985). Mast cell mediators and asthma. *Chest* **87S**:2-5.

Kaliner, M. (1989). Asthma and mast cell activation. *J. Allergy Clin. Immunol.* **83**:510-520.

Kaliner, M., Blennerhassett, J., and Austen, K. F. (1976). Bronchial asthma. In *Textbook of Immunopathy*. Edited by P. A. Meischer and H. J. Muller-Eberhard. New York, Grune & Stratton, pp. 387-402.

Kaliner, M., Shelhamer, J. H., Davis, P. B., Smith, L. J., and Venter, J. C. (1982). Autonomic nervous system abnormalities and allergy. *Ann. Intern. Med.* **96**:349-357.

Kaplan, A. P. (1983). Urticaria and angioedema. In *Allergy Principles and Practice*, 2nd ed. Edited by E. Middleton, C. S. Reed, and E. S. Ellis. St. Louis, C. V. Mosby, pp. 1341-1360.

Karcezewski, W., and Widdicombe, J. G. (1969). The role of the vagus nerves in the respiratory and circulatory reactions of anaphylaxis in rabbits. *J. Physiol. (Lond.)* **201**:293-304.

Kawabori, S., and Unno, T. (1983). Degranulation of nasal epithelial mast cells after challenge of allergen. *J. Submicrosc. Cytol.* **15**:823-832.

Kawanami, O., Ferrans, V. J., Fulmer, J. D., and Crystal, R. G. (1979). Ultrastructure of pulmonary mast cells in patients with fibrotic lung disorders. *Lab. Invest.* **40**:717-735.

Kay, A. B., and Barnes, P. J. (1985). Pharmacologic modulation of the asthmatic response. In *Current Perspectives in the Immunology of Respiratory Diseases*. Edited by A. B. Kay and E. J. Goetzl. New York, Churchill Livingstone, pp. 30-38.

Keahey, T. M., Indrisano, J. M., Lavaker, R. M., and Kaliner, M. A. (1987). Delayed vibratory angioedema: insights into pathophysiologic mechanisms. *J. Allergy Clin. Immunol.* **80**:831-838.

Keyzer, J. J., Kauffman, H. F., de Monchy, J. G., Keyzer-Udding, J. J., and de Vries, K. (1984). Urinary N-tau methylhistamine during early and late allergen-induced bronchial-obstructive reactions. *J. Allergy Clin. Immunol.* **74**:240-245.

Kowalski, M. L., and Kaliner, M. A. (1988). Neurogenic inflammation, vascular permeability, and mast cells. *J. Immunol.* **140**:3905-3911.

Lamb, D., and Lumsden, A. (1982). Intra-epithelial mast cells in human airway epithelium: evidence for smoking-induced changes in their frequency. *Thorax* **37**:334-342.

Lampl, K. L., Lichtenstein, L. M., and Schleimer, R. P. (1985). *In vitro* resistance to dexamethasone of basophils from patients receiving long-term steroid therapy. *Am. Rev. Respir. Dis.* **132**:1015-1018.

Lee, T. H., Nagakura, T., Papageorgiou, N., Iikuray, I., and Kay, A. B. (1983). Exercise-induced late asthmatic reactions with neutrophil chemotactic activity. *N. Engl. J. Med.* **308**:1502-1505.

Lemanske, R. F., and Kaliner, M. A. (1988). Late-phase allergic reactions. In *Allergy Principles and Practice*, 3rd ed. Edited by E. Middleton, C. E. Reed, E. F. Ellis, N. F. Adkinson, and J. W. Yunginger. Washington, D. C., C. V. Mosby.

Lowhagen, O., and Rak, I. (1985). Modification of bronchial hyperreactivity after treatment with sodium cromoglycate in atopic asthmatic patients not exposed to relevant allergens. *J. Allergy Clin. Immunol.* **75**:343-347.

Lundgren, J. D., Wiedermann, C. J., Logun, C., Plutchok, J., Kaliner, M., and Shelhamer, J. (1988). Substance P mediated secretion of respiratory glycoconjugate from feline airways *in vitro*. *Exp. Lung. Res.* **15**:17-29.

MacDonald, S. M., Lichtenstein, L. M., Proud, D., Plaut, M., Naclerio, R. M., MacGlashan, D. W., and Kagey-Sobotka, A. (1987). Studies of IgE-dependent histamine releasing factors: heterogeneity of IgE. *J. Immunol.* **139**:506-512.

Margo, A. M. (1974). Involvement of IgE in Con-A induced histamine release from human basophils *in vitro*. *Nature (London)* **249**:572-574.

Marom, Z., Shelhamer, J. H., and Kaliner, M. (1981). The effects of arachidonic acid, monohydroxyeicosatetrenoic acid, and prostaglandins on the release of mucous glycoproteins from human airways *in vitro*. *J. Clin. Invest.* **67**:1695-1702.

Marom, Z., Shelhamer, J. N., and Kaliner, M. (1985). Human monocyte-derived mucus secretagogue. *J. Clin. Invest.* **75**:191-198.

Martin, G. L., Atkins, P. S., Dunsky, E. H., and Zweiman, B. (1980). Effects of theophylline, terbutaline and prednisolone on antigen-induced bronchospasm and mediator release. *J. Allergy Clin. Immunol.* **66**:204-212.

Messer, J. W., Peters, G. A., and Bennett, W. A. (1960). Causes of death and pathologic findings in 304 cases of bronchial asthma. *Chest* **38**:616-624.

Metcalfe, D. D., Kaliner, M. A., and Donlon, M. A. (1981). The mast cell. *CRC Crit. Rev. Immunol.* **3**:23-74.

Moqbel, R., Durham, S. R., Shaw, R. J., Walsh, G. M., MacDonald, A. J., MacKay, J. A., Carroll, M., and Kay, A. B. (1986). Enhancement of leukocyte cytotoxicity after exercise-induced asthma. *Am. Rev. Respir. Dis.* **133**:609-613.

Morrison, D. C., and Henson, P. M. (1978). Release of mediators from mast cells and basophils induced by different stimuli. In *Immediate Hypersensitivity—Modern Concepts and Development.* Edited by M. K. Bach. New York, Marcel Dekker, pp. 431-502.

Nagy, L., Lee, T. H., and Kay, A. B. (1982). Neutrophil chemotactic activity in antigen-induced late asthmatic reactions. *N. Engl. J. Med.* **306**:497-501.

Nathan, R. A., Segali, N., and Schocket, A. L. (1981). A comparison of the actions of H1 and H2 antihistamines on histamine-induced bronchoconstriction and cutaneous wheal response in asthmatic patients. *J. Allergy Clin. Immunol.* **67**:171-177.

Nissam, M. R., Zbinden, A., Chestown, S., Barnett, N., and Gold, W. M. (1978). Distribution and pharmacologic release of histamine in canine lung *in vivo. J. Appl. Physiol.* **44**:455-463.

O'Byrne, P. M., Thomson, N. C., Morris, M., Roberts, R. S., Daniel, E. E., and Hargreave (1983). The protective effect of inhaled chlorpheniramine and atropine on bronchoconstriction stimulated by airway cooling. *Am. Rev. Respir. Dis.* **126**:611-617.

O'Donnell, M. C., Ackerman, S. J., Gleich, G. L. J., and Thomas, L. L. (1983). Activation of basophil and mast cell histamine release by eosinophil granule major basic protein. *J. Exp. Med.* **157**:1981-1991.

Orchard, M. A., Kagey-Sobotka, A., Proud, D., and Lichtenstein, L. M. (1986). Basophil histamine release induced by a substance from stimulated human platelets. *J. Immunol.* **136**:2240-2244.

Patel, K. R. (1984). Terfenadine in exercise-induced asthma. *Br. Med. J.* **288**:1496-1497.

Patterson, R., Ts'ao, C.-H., and Susko, I. M. (1980). Heterogeneity of bronchial lumen mast cells which are homogeneous by electron microscopy. *J. Allergy Clin. Immunol.* **65**:278-284.

Paterson, N. A. M., Burka, J. F., and Craig, I. D. (1981). Release of slow reacting substance of anaphylaxis from dispersed pig lung cells: effect of cyclo-oxygenase and lipoxygenase inhibitors. *J. Allergy Clin. Immunol.* **67**:426-434.

Pelikan, Z. (1982). The effects of disodium cromoglycate and beclomethasone dipropionate on the late nasal mucosa reponse to allergen challenge. *Ann. Allergy* **49**:200-212.

Pepys, J., Chan, M., Hargreave, F. E., and McCarthy, D. S. (1968). Inhibitory effects of disodium cromoglycate on allergen-inhalation tests. *Lancet* **2**:134-137.

Pepys, J., Davies, R. J., Breslin, A. B., Hendrick, D. J., and Hutchcrost, B. J. (1974). The effects of inhaled beclomethasone dipropionate (Becotide) and sodium cromoglycate on asthmatic reactions to provocation tests. *Clin. Allergy* **4**:13-24.

Petty, T. L., Rollins, D. R., Christopher, K., Good, J. T., and Oakley, R. (1989). Cromolyn sodium is effective in adult chronic asthmatics. *Am. Rev. Respir. Dis.* **139**:694-701.

Pipkorn, U., and Enerback, L. (1987). Nasal mucosal mast cells and histamine in hay fever: effect of topical glucocorticoid treatment. *Int. Arch. Allergy Appl. Immunol.* **84**:123-128.

Pipkorn, U., Proud, D., Lichtenstein, L. M., Kagey-Sobotka, A., Norman, P. S., and Naclerio, R. M. (1987). Inhibition of mediator release in allergic rhinitis by pretreatment with topical glucocorticosteroids. *N. Engl. J. Med.* **316**:1506-1510.

Platshon, L., and Kaliner, M. (1978). The effect of the immunologic release of histamine upon human lung cyclic nucleotide levels and prostaglandin generation. *J. Clin. Invest.* **62**:1113-1121.

Proud, D., Baumgarten, C. R., Naclerio, R. M., and Lichtenstein, L. M. (1986). The role of kinins in human allergic disease. *NER Allergy Proc.* **7**:213-218.

Robertson, D. G., Kerigan, A. T., Hargreave, F. E., Chalmers, R., and Dolovich, J. (1974). Late asthmatic responses induced by ragweed pollen allergen. *J. Allergy Clin. Immunol.* **54**:244-254.

Rosenthal, R. R., Norman, P. S., Summer, W. R., and Permutt, S. (1977). Role of the parasympathetic system in antigen-induced bronchospasm. *J. Appl. Physiol.* **42**:600-606.

Ryo, U. Y., Kang, B., and Townley, R. C. (1970). Cromolyn therapy in patient with bronchial asthma: effect of inhalation challenge with allergen, histamine and methacholine. *JAMA* **236**:927-931.

Schacter, E. N., Brown, S., Lach, E., and Gerstenhaber, B. (1982). Histamine blocking agents in healthy and asthmatic subjects. *Chest* **82**:143-147.

Schleimer, R. P., Lichtenstein, L. M., and Gillespie, E. (1981). Inhibition of basophil histamine release by anti-inflammatory steroids. *Nature* **292**:454-455.

Schleimer, R. P., MacGlashan, D. W., Gillespie, E., and Lichtenstein, L. M. (1982). Inhibition of basophil histamine release by anti-inflammatory steroids II. Studied on the mechanism of action. *J. Immunol.* **129**:1632-1636.

Schleimer, R. P., Schulman, E. S., MacGlashan, D. W. M., Jr., Peters, S. P., Hayes, E. C., Adams, G. K., III., Lichtenstein, L. M., and Adkinson, N. F. (1983). Effects of dexamethasone on mediator release from human lung fragments and purified human lung mast cells. *J. Clin. Invest.* **71**: 1830-1835.

Schulman, E. S., Liu, M. C., Proud, D., MacGlashan, D. W., Lichtenstein, L. M., and Plaut, M. (1985). Human lung macrophages induce histamine release from basophils and mast cells. *Am. Rev. Respir. Dis.* **131**:230-235.

Schulman, E. S., McGettigan, M. C., Post, T. J. M., Vigderman, R. J., and Shapiro, S. S. (1988). Human monocytes generate basophil histamine releasing activities. *J. Immunol.* **140**:2369-2375.

Segal, D. M., Taurog, J. D., and Metzger, H. (1977). Dimeric immunoglobulin E serves as a unit signal for mast cell degranulation. *Proc. Natl. Acad. Sci. USA* **74**:2993-2998.

Selbekk, B. H. (1979). The effect of disodium cromoglycate on *in vitro* mast cell degranulation in human jejunal mucosa. *Allergy* **34**:283-288.

Shelhamer, J. H., Marom, Z., and Kaliner, M. (1980). Immunologic and neuropharmacologic stimulation of mucous glucoprotein release from human airways *in vitro*. *J. Clin. Invest.* **66**:1400-1408.

Shelhamer, J. H., Marom, Z., Sun, F., Black, M. K., and Kaliner, M. (1981). The effects of arachinoids and leukotrienes on the release of mucus from human airways. *Chest* **81**S:36-37.

Sheppard, D., Nadel, J. A., and Boushey, H. A. (1981). Inhibition of sulfur dioxide-induced bronchoconstriction by disodium cromoglycate in asthmatic subjects. *Am. Rev. Respir. Dis.* **124**:257-259.

Smith, L. J., Greenberger, P. A., Patterson, R., Krell, R. D., and Bernstein, P. R. (1985). The effect of inhaled leukotriene D4 in humans. *Am. Rev. Respir. Dis.* **131**:368-372.

Soter, N. A., Wasserman, S., Pathak, M. A., Parish, J. A., and Austen, K. F. (1979). Solar urticaria: release of mediators into the circulation after experimental challenge. *J. Invest. Dermatol.* **72**:282 (abstr).

Spannhake, E. W., Hyman, A. L., and Kadowitz, P. J. (1981). Bronchoactive metabolites of arachidonic acid and their role in airway function. *Prostaglandins* **22**:1013-1026.

Stalenheim, G., and Machado, L. (1985). Late allergic bronchial reactions and the effect of allergen provocation on the complement system. *J. Allergy Clin. Immunol.* **75**:508-512.

Steel, L., and Kaliner, M. A. (1981). Prostaglandin-generating factor of anaphylaxis-identification and isolation. *J. Biol. Chem.* **256**:12592-12598.

Steel, L., Platshon, L., and Kaliner, M. A. (1979). Prostaglandin generation by human and guinea pig lung tissue: comparison of parenchymal and airway responses. *J. Allergy Clin. Immunol.* **64**:287-293.

Storms, W. W., DoPico, G. A., and Reed, C. E. (1975). Aerosol SCH 1000-an anticholinergic bronchodilator. *Am. Rev. Respir. Dis.* **11**:419-422.

Tannenbaum, S., Oertel, H., Henderson, W., and Kaliner, M. (1980). The biologic activity of mast cell granules. I. Elicitation of inflammatory responses in rat skin. *J. Immunol.* **125**:325-335.

Theuson, D. O., Speck, L. S., Lett-Brown, A., and Grant, J. A. (1979). Histamine-releasing activity (HRA). I. Production by mitogen or antigen stimulated human mononuclear cells. *J. Immunol.* **123**:626-632.

Togias, A. G., Naclerio, R. M., Proud, D., Fish, J. E., Adkinson, N. F., Kagey-Sobotka, A., Norman, P. S., and Lichtenstein, L. M. (1985). Nasal challenge with cold, dry air results in release of inflammatory mediators. Possible mast cell involvement. *J. Clin. Invest.* **76**:1375-1381.

Trotter, C. M., and Orr, R. S. C. (1973). A fine structure study of some cellular components in allergic reactions. *Clin. Allergy* **3**:411-425.

Ts'ao, C., Patterson, R., McKenna, J. M., and Suzko, I. M. (1977). Ultrastructural identification of mast cells obtained from human bronchial lumens. *J. Allergy Clin. Immunol.* **59**:320-326.

Van der Star, J. G., Berg, W. C., Steenhuis, E., and de Vries, K. (1976). The effect of beclomethasone diproprionate aerosol on bronchial obstruction after the inhalation of house dust. *Ned. Tijdschr. Geneekd.* **120**:1928-1932.

Warner, J. O. (1976). Significance of late reactions after bronchial challenge with house dust mite. *Arch. Dis. Child.* **51**:905-911.

Warner, J. O., Soothill, J. F., Price, J. F., and Hey, E. N. (1978). Controlled trial of hyposensitization to *Dermatophagoides pteronyssius* in children with asthma. *Lancet* **2**:912-915.

Wasserman, S. I. (1980). The lung mast cell: its physiology and potential relevance to defense of the lung. *Environ. Health Perspect.* **35**:153-164.

White, M. V., and Kaliner, M. A. (1987). Neutrophils and mast cells I. Human neutrophil-derived histamine-releasing activity. *J. Immunol.* **139**:1624-1630.

White, M. V., Kaplan, A. P., Haak-Frendscho, M., and Kaliner M. (1988). Neutrophils and mast cells. Comparison of cells responsive to neutrophil derived histamine releasing activity (HRA-N) with other histamine releasing factors. *J. Immunol.* **141**:3575-3583.

White, M. V., Kowalski, M., and Kaliner, M. A. (1989). Mast cell secretagogues. In *Biochemistry of the Acute Allergic Reaction*, Fifth International Symposium. Edited by B. Wintroub, F. Tauber, and A. S. Simon. New York, Alan R. Liss.

Yu, D. Y. C., Galant, S. P., and Gold, W. M. (1972). Inhibition of antigen-
    induced bronchoconstriction by atropine in asthmatic patients. *J. Appl.
    Physiol.* **32**:832-843.

16

Role of Neutrophils in the Pathogenesis of Airway Hyperresponsiveness and Asthma

PAUL M. O'BYRNE and EDWIN E. DANIEL

McMaster University,
Hamilton, Ontario, Canada

I. Introduction

Over the past 40-50 years, airway hyperresponsiveness—the ability of the airways of asthmatic subjects to constrict when exposed to small concentrations of inhaled bronchoconstrictor mediators (Weiss et al., 1932; Curry, 1947) or naturally occurring bronchoconstrictor stimuli (Anderson, 1985; O'Byrne et al., 1982)—has been described and extensively investigated. Airway hyperresponsiveness is now considered a characteristic feature of current, symptomatic asthma (Hargreave et al., 1981).

In the past, studies examining the pathogenesis of airway hyperresponsiveness and symptomatic asthma have focused on inhaled stimuli that cause airway hyperresponsiveness, such as allergen or occupational sensitizing agents, and mediators released from cells in asthmatic airways, such as mast cells. Studies attempting to implicate specific mediators have been difficult to perform, because of difficulties in measuring the mediators at their site of action in the airways, and have not been definitive, mostly because of a lack of potent and specific mediator antagonists.

More recently, studies examining the pathogenesis of asthma have focused on the role of airway inflammation (O'Byrne et al., 1987). The knowledge that severe airway inflammation was present in the airways of patients with severe, fatal asthma is not new. Indeed, William Osler described in the first edition of his book, *The Principles and Practice of Medicine*, "bronchial asthma... in many cases is a special form of inflammation of the smaller bronchioles" (Osler, 1982). A more complete description of airway inflammation and asthma was provided by Dunnill and colleagues (1969) in the 1960s, again in patients dying of acute asthma.

Airway inflammation is now believed to be important in causing both stable asthma and acute exacerbations of asthma. Studies have focused on the inflammatory cells present in asthmatic airways, as well as the mediators that attract the cells into the airways and the state of activation of the cells.

II. Airway Hyperresponsiveness in Asthma

Asthma is now defined as a disease characterized by both reversible airway narrowing and airway hyperresponsiveness (American Thoracic Society, 1962). The release of constrictor mediators in airways and hyperresponsiveness to these mediators are both important in the clinical manifestations of asthma.

Airway hyperresponsiveness can be stable over several years in many asthmatic subjects (Juniper et al., 1982). However, inhalation of a number of stimuli such as allergens (Cartier et al., 1982; Cockcroft et al., 1977; Boulet et al., 1983), ozone (Golden et al., 1978), and low-molecular-weight chemical sensitizers, such as toluene diisocyanate (TDI) (Yeung et al., 1985; Fabbri et al., 1985), or plicatic acid from western red cedar (Chan-Yeung 1982) can cause airway hyperresponsiveness in human subjects. This is associated with an increase in symptoms of asthma and in the amount of treatment required to control symptoms (Juniper et al., 1981). Therefore, in many asthmatic subjects inhaled allergens or other stimuli are an important cause of asthma morbidity. Furthermore, Cockcroft (1983) has suggested that in many patients with asthma who are also allergic to commonly encountered environmental allergens, such as house dust mite, their persisting symptoms are caused by regular allergen exposure. This hypothesis has been supported by several studies showing that allergen avoidance in patients with persisting asthma can improve both airway hyperresponsiveness and symptoms of asthma (Platts-Mills et al., 1982; Murray and Ferguson, 1983; Doward et al., 1988).

III. Airway Hyperresponsiveness in Animal Models

There is no animal model of human asthma. However, the stimuli known to cause airway hyperresponsivness in humans also cause airway hyperresponsiveness in a number of animal species. This has allowed experimental studies to be carried out in animal models, to investigate the pathogenesis of airway hyperresponsiveness, and has allowed hypothesis to be generated, some of which could be subsequently tested in human subjects.

The initial studies that suggested that some component(s) of acute airway inflammation is responsible for the development of transient airway hyperresponsiveness were performed in dogs after administration of inhaled ozone (Holtzman et al., 1983b) and allergen (Chung et al., 1985). Several other animal preparations of airway hyperresponsiveness have been described. These have included rabbits after allergen (Marsh et al., 1985); in guinea pigs after ozone (Murlas and Roum, 1985b), allergen (Hutson et al., 1988), and toluene diisocyanate (TDI) (Gordon et al., 1985); and sheep after allergen (Lanes et al., 1985). Each of these stimuli can cause acute airway inflammation, presumably through initiating the release of mediators chemotactic for inflammatory cells. The cells drawn into the airways subsequently release mediators that change airway responsiveness to bronchoconstrictor mediators. The precise role of individual inflammatory cells and mediators in initiating airway hyperresponsiveness is controversial and appears to vary between species and with the inciting stimulus.

IV. Neutrophils and Airway Hyperresponsiveness in Animal Models

The studies that have implicated neutrophils in the pathogenesis of airway hyperresponsiveness were initially performed in dogs after inhaled ozone. These studies demonstrated a temporal association between the development of airway hyperresponsiveness and the presence of neutrophils in the airways (Holtzman et al., 1983a). Inhaled ozone causes transient airway hyperresponsiveness in dogs, which is maximal several hours after exposure and has completely recovered by 1 week (Holtzman et al., 1983b). Biopsies of the central airways of dogs before and after inhaled ozone demonstrated a large influx of neutrophils after inhaled ozone, when the dogs had airway hyperresponsiveness, and that both the influx of neutrophils and the airway hyperresponsiveness had resolved at 1 week (Holtzman et al., 1983a). The influx of neutrophils was also demonstrated in bronchoalveolar lavage fluid from dogs after inhaled ozone (Fabbri et al., 1984). Other investigators have confirmed that neutrophils are present in the airways when airway hyperresponsiveness has developed in dogs (Chung et al., 1985) and rabbits after inhaling allergen (Marsh et al., 1985).

More recently, we have examined the ultrastructure of airways from dogs with airway hyperresponsiveness after inhaled ozone and compared this to findings in control dogs. These studies were performed on airways from the trachea to fifth-order bronchi. The prominent findings were a marked increase in the numbers of neutrophils, cells resembling mast cells, and platelets in the interstitial space between the epithelium and the smooth muscle. Also, some of the neutrophils and those resembling mast cells had migrated into the epithelium at 1-2 h after ozone administration. At this time, the epithelium had evidence of focal damage to ciliated epithelial cells. However, extensive desquamation of the mucosal layer was not seen. There were no qualitative structural changes in the innervation or the smooth muscle after administration of ozone.

The temporal associations between the presence of neutrophils and the presence of airway hyperresponsiveness do not prove causality. To test further the hypothesis that neutrophils are important in the pathogenesis of airway hyperresponsiveness, dogs were depleted of circulating neutrophils using intravenous hydroxyurea and exposed to ozone (O'Byrne et al., 1984b). During the period of neutropenia, ozone inhalation did not lead to airway hyperresponsiveness. When the neutrophil counts had recovered, all dogs developed airway hyperresponsiveness after ozone administration.

Similar studies have been performed in rabbits sensitized to *Alternaria tenuis*. The development of late responses and airway hyperresponsiveness after inhaled allergen is associated with the presence of polymorphonuclear leukocytes and mononuclear cells in the airways (Marsh et al., 1985). In addition, leukocyte depletion abolished both of these responses. Lastly, repletion of cells by infusion of neutrophil-rich cell suspensions restored the ability to develop late responses and airway hyperresponsiveness (Murphy et al., 1986).

The chemotactic mediator(s) that attracts neutrophils into the airways after inhaled ozone or allergen in dogs has not been identified. Neutrophils, which were present in airway biopsies 3 h after inhaled ozone, were predominantly seen in the airway epithelium, with fewer cells in the submucosa (Holtzman et al., 1983a). This suggested that the chemotactic mediator(s) was originating in the airway lumen or the epithelium. Holtzman et al. (1983c) have identified that canine epithelial cells can release the neutrophil chemoattractant, leukotriene (LT)B$_4$. In addition, inhaled LTB$_4$ can cause both neutrophil chemotaxis and airway hyperresponsiveness in dogs (O'Byrne et al., 1985). Therefore, LTB$_4$ may be an important proinflammatory mediator, released from alveolar macrophages (Lewis and Austen, 1984) or epithelial cells (Holtzman et al., 1983c) after inhaled stimuli such as ozone or allergen in dogs.

These studies, taken together, have provided a working hypothesis of the development of airway hyperresponsiveness after stimuli such as ozone or allergen, which is demonstrated in Figure 1. This hypothesis suggests that influx and activation of neutrophils into the airways causes the release not only of a variety of potentially damaging substances but also of enzymes that can metabolize the chemotactic mediators, such as LTB$_4$, and thereby modulate the inflammatory reaction.

HYPOTHESIS

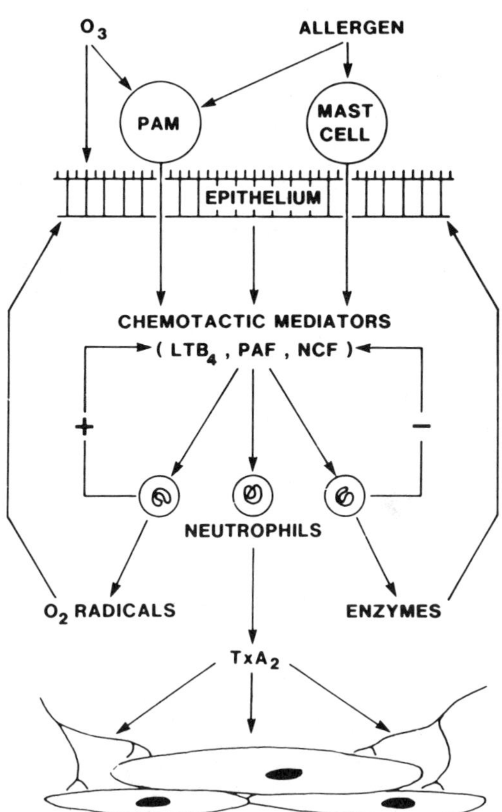

Figure 1 A hypothesis to explain the pathogenesis of airway hyperresponsiveness after inhaled ozone or allergen in dogs. Chemotactic mediators, released from cells in the airway lumen or epithelium, cause influx and activation of neutrophils. Release of mediators (such as thromboxane), oxygen radicals, and enzymes causes tissue damage. Neutrophils also have the capacity to up- or downregulate the inflammatory response by releasing chemotactic mediators (such as LTB_4) or enzymes that deactivate these mediators.

The importance of neutrophils in the development of airway hyperresponsiveness appears to be species specific. For example, neutrophil depletion using cyclophosphamide does not inhibit airway hyperresponsiveness in guinea pigs after inhalation of ozone (Murlas and Roum, 1985a) or TDI (Thompson et al., 1986). In sensitized guinea pigs, inhaled allergen causes influx of both neutrophils and eosinophils into airways (Hutson et al., 1988). However, only the presence of eosinophils appears to be necessary for the development of late responses.

A major problem, however, with all studies in which neutrophil depletion has been performed is the lack of specificity of the drug used to deplete neutrophils. Therefore, while the studies in dogs (O'Byrne et al., 1984b) suggested that neutrophils were involved in the development of airway hyperresponsiveness after ozone, and in rabbits (Murphy et al., 1986) that poly-morphonuclear leukocytes were involved in the development of airway hyperresponsiveness after allergen, they did not provide proof. To clarify further the ability of neutrophils to induce airway hyperresponsiveness, human neutrophils were isolated (>95% pure preparations) and stimulated with arachidonic acid and the calcium ionophore A23187. Inhalation of the supernatant fluid from the stimulated neutrophils caused airway hyperresponsiveness in dogs, while inhalation of arachidonic acid and A23187 alone did not. Also, inhaled supernatants from stimulated human neutrophils (Irvin et al., 1986), but not eosinophils (Uchida et al., 1987), cause airway hyperresponsiveness in allergic rabbits. These studies indicate that human neutrophils have the capacity to release mediators that cause airway hyperresponsiveness in dogs and rabbits.

To summarize the animal studies, all studies agree that some component(s) of an acute airway inflammatory response are important in the pathogenesis of airway hyperresponsiveness after inhaled stimuli such as allergen, ozone, and TDI. These studies have suggested, however, that the important effector cell and possibly mediators for the development of airway hyperresponsiveness may vary between species, or according to the stimulus used to cause airway hyperresponsiveness.

V. Inflammatory Mediators Released from Neutrophils

Mediators released from inflammatory cells are responsible for the events that cause airway narrowing in asthma. These mediators can be considered in three groups:

1. Mediators that cause transient bronchoconstriction, such as histamine or acetylcholine

2. Mediators that cause influx of inflammatory cells and possibly activation of cells in the airways, such as platelet-activating factor (PAF) or LTB_4

3. Mediators that are released from inflammatory cells and cause airway hyperresponsiveness

The importance of thromboxane in causing airway hyperresponsiveness in dogs has come from studies in which airway hyperresponsiveness occurred following inhalation of ozone (Aizawa et al., 1985), allergen (Chung et al., 1986a), LTB_4 (O'Byrne et al., 1985), and PAF (Chung et al., 1986b). These studies have been done by both inhibition of the production of mediators, using specific synthetase inhibitors, and measurement of levels of mediators in lavage fluid at a time when airway hyperresponsiveness was present. Indomethacin, an inhibitor of the cycloxygenase pathway of arachidonate metabolism, was initially demonstrated to prevent airway hyperresponsivness after administration of ozone in dogs (O'Byrne et al., 1984a). This suggested that a prostaglandin or thromoboxane was involved in the pathogenesis of airway hyperresponsiveness after this stimulus. Indomethacin has also been demonstrated to prevent airway hyperresponsiveness after administration of C5a in rabbits (Berend et al., 1985) and after inhaled allergen in sheep (Lanes et al., 1986).

Measurement of cycloxygenase products in lavage fluid when airway hyperresponsiveness was present after inhaled LTB_4 in dogs demonstrated an increase in thromboxane B_2 levels compared to controls (O'Byrne et al., 1985). Inhibition of thromboxane synthesis using OKY-046 prevented the rise in thromboxane in lavage and airway hyperresponsiveness after LTB_4 (O'Byrne et al., 1985) as well as the increases in airway responsiveness after ozone (Aizawa et al., 1985), allergen (Chung et al., 1986a), and PAF (Chung et al., 1986b) administration in dogs. Lastly, pretreatment with the thromboxane mimetic U46619 can increase airway responsiveness (Aizawa et al., 1985). Therefore, thromboxane appears to be an important mediator for the development of airway hyperresponsiveness in dogs.

Neutrophils have been demonstrated to release thromboxane, when stimulated ex vivo (Goldstein et al., 1978). However, it is extremely difficult to obtain preparations of neutrophils that are not contaminated by platelets, which also release thromboxane. One elegant study has suggested that neutrophils do release thromboxane at inflammatory sites. Higgs et al. (1983) demonstrated that platelets were the source of thromboxane in blood, but that neutrophils were the source of thromboxane at inflammatory sites caused by carrageenan-impregnated sponges in rats. Therefore, it is at least conceivable that neutrophils are the cells of origin of thromboxane in dog airways after inhaled inflammatory stimuli, such as ozone.

Activated neutrophils also have the capacity to release a number of other products that can damage the airway. These include the oxygen radicals O_2, H_2O_2, and hydroxyl radical, which are known to be highly toxic to a variety of tissues in the lungs (Tate and Repine, 1983). Also, neutrophil granules contain a variety of substances, including myeloperoxidase, elastase, collagenase, cationic proteins, and lysozyme, which are known to damage lung tissues (Tate and Repine, 1983). There is no information yet available that implicates any of these products in the pathogenesis of airway hyperresponsiveness.

VI. Neutrophils and Airway Hyperresponsiveness in Humans

The association between the presence of inflammatory cells in the airways and airway hyperresponsiveness has also been investigated in human subjects.

In these studies, numbers of cells and the cellular differential have been measured in bronchoalveolar lavage fluid before and after subjects have inhaled stimuli known to cause airway hyperresponsiveness, such as ozone (Stelzer et al., 1986), the occupational sensitizing agents TDI (Fabbri et al., 1987) and western red cedar (Lam et al., 1985), and allergen (De Monchy et al., 1985). All of these studies have demonstrated an acute inflammatory response in the airways associated with the development of airway hyperresponsiveness. In addition, these studies have suggested that the stimulus that initiates airway hyperresponsiveness may determine the cellular response.

Stelzer et al. (1986) demonstrated that inhaled ozone causes both airway hyperresponsiveness and an increase in neutrophils in bronchoalveolar lavage fluid in human subjects. There was no significant increase in any other inflammatory cells. In addition, a large increase in neutrophils and a smaller increase in eosinophils has been demonstrated in bronchoalveolar lavage fluid in subjects with airway hyperresponsiveness after exposure to TDI (Fabbri et al., 1987).

In contrast to the studies with ozone or TDI, an increase in eosinophils but not neutrophils was demonstrated in lavage fluid after allergen inhalation in some studies (De Monchy et al., 1985) and in western-red-cedar-induced asthma (Lam et al., 1985). In another study, however, levels of both eosinophils and neutrophils were elevated after inhaled allergen (Metzger et al., 1987), although measurements were made at different times. Therefore, although these studies have suggested that components of the airway inflammatory response cause airway hyperresponsiveness, the cellular responses may differ between stimuli or at different times during the response. However, as with the animal studies, all of these investigations have, at best, demonstrated a temporal association between the presence of the cells and airway hyperresponsiveness.

VII. Airway Inflammation and Stable Asthma

Several studies have provided information on cell populations in lavage fluid of patients with stable asthma who have persisting airway hyperresponsiveness (Flint et al., 1985; Tomioka et al., 1984; Kirby et al., 1987; Wardlaw et al., 1988). These studies have all demonstrated the presence of inflammatory cells and have suggested that an increase in mast cells (Flint et al., 1985; Tomioka et al., 1984; Kirby et al., 1987) and/or eosinophils (Kirby et al., 1987; Wardlaw et al., 1988) exists in asthmatic airways. In addition, close correlations exist between numbers of mast cells and eosinophils and the degree of airway hyperresponsiveness in these patients with mild, stable asthma (Kirby, 1987).

In a more recent study, Kelly et al. (1988) also showed correlations between the numbers of neutrophils and airway hyperresponsiveness. They also demonstrated that the activity of both the neutrophils and alveolar macrophages, as indicated by luminol-enhanced chemiluminescence, was increased in asthmatic subjects compared to control subjects. Therefore, this study not only demonstrated the presence of inflammatory cells in asthmatic airways but also that the cells are metabolically active, which suggests that they play a role in asthma.

All of these studies have been consistent with the hypothesis that even in patients with mild stable asthma, airway hyperresponsiveness is maintained as a consequence of some component of the inflammatory response and that this response may involve mast cells, eosinophils, or neutrophils. Mediators released from the inflammatory cells can cause not only bronchoconstriction and airway hyperresponsiveness but also mucosal edema and release of secretions, all of which play a role in causing airway narrowing (Fig. 2).

The close associations between the presence of inflammatory cells and the level of airway hyperresponsiveness in asthmatic subjects also suggest that measurements of airway hyperresponsiveness may be used as an indication,

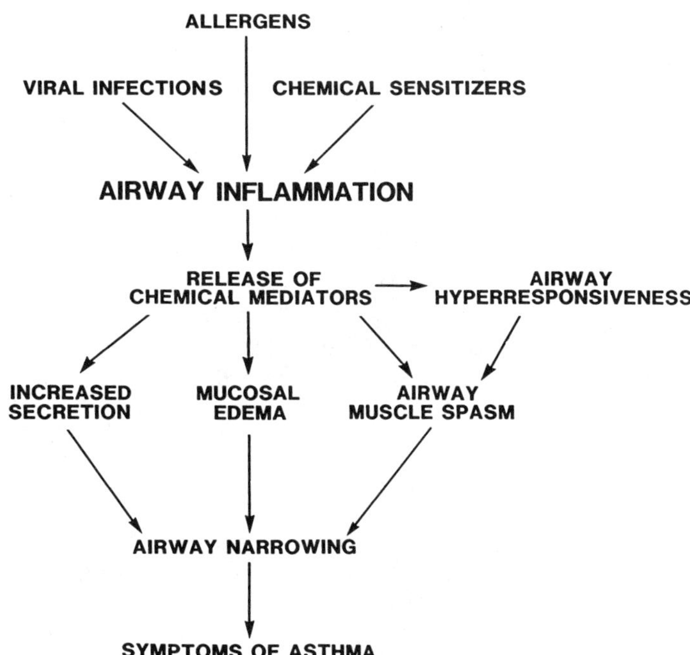

Figure 2   The central role of airway inflammation in causing symptomatic asthma.

albeit indirect, of the presence and severity of airway inflammation in these subjects. This concept is useful in that no other noninvasive method exists to indicate the presence of airway inflammation in asthmatic subjects, and improvements in airway hyperresponsiveness after appropriate treatment may reflect improvements in the degree of airway inflammation, although this remains to be proven.

VIII. Conclusions

It is now widely accepted that some component(s) of an acute airway inflammatory response is responsible for the development of airway hyperresponsiveness after stimuli such as allergens and occupational sensitizing agents, leading to the development of symptomatic asthma. The sequence of events leading to airway hyperresponsiveness is partially understood in some animal species; however the importance of different inflammatory cells and mediators between species is still being debated.

In dogs and rabbits, but not guinea pigs, neutrophils appear to be the important inflammatory cell leading to airway hyperresponsiveness. Studies using human neutrophils have demonstrated that they have the capacity to release mediators that can cause airway hyperresponsiveness in animals. Also, neutrophils are present in human airways after inhaled stimuli that cause airway hyperresponsiveness. However, no more direct evidence exists that would implicate neutrophils in causing airway hyperresponsiveness. In addition, while several studies have supported the hypothesis that airway inflammation also results in airway hyperresponsiveness in patients with stable asthma, the predominant cells demonstrated in the airways of these subjects are mast cells and eosinophils.

It is clear that a great deal more research is necessary to elucidate fully the interactions between the important cells and mediators involved. However, this improved understanding of the role of airway inflammation in patients with asthma has already provided improved rationale for the earlier use of anti-inflammatory drugs, such as inhaled glucocorticoids, in the management of asthma.

Discussion

Irwin: We have performed similar experiments, administering neutrophils supernatants to intact rabbits. The rabbits did not develop acute airflow obstruction, but did develop hyperresponsiveness. The responsible factors were analyzed and found to be a neutral lipid and/or a phospholipid, which was not PAF.

I would also like to comment on the potential dangers of counting inflammatory cells as a means of quantifying inflammation. Cell numbers do not necessarily reflect cell activation or granule release, and do not account for the traffic of cells into and out of an area. Neutrophils are efficient at rapidly infiltrating an area and may leave quickly as well. Therefore, static counts may be very misleading.

Chung: One must also consider the possibility that neutrophils may be beneficial in asthma. In a recent study, the presence of neutrophils in BAL correlated inversely with the capacity of inhaled PAF to cause increases in airway hyperactivity. Thus, neutrophils may actually metabolize mediators.

Schleimer: I am surprised that you did not mention the recent description by Gleich that some lungs obtained from patients dying in status asthmaticus demonstrate neutrophil elastase staining.

We have also examined the capacity of supernatants obtained from human neutrophils activated by exposure to zymosan to affect guinea pig airway reactivity. Exposure of guinea pig trachea overnight to these supernatants increased the reactivity of some specimens, but not others. We decided not to pursue this area.

Woolcock: What relationship exists between the dose-response curve to allergen-induced increases in airway hyperactivity in your model and those found in humans?

O'Byrne: The dog model has very similar dose-response relations to those found after allergen challenge of humans. Animal models are essential to test hypotheses before attempting them in humans.

Church: In the guinea pig we have conclusively demonstrated that neutrophils are not involved in the pathogenesis of LAR, although they are increased in the BAL after challenge.

Kay: In our experience, neutrophils are found in the same number in BAL from normal and asthmatic subjects, if studied in a resting state. Neutrophils do appear in the BAL after LPR but do not appear to be related to the magnitude of the response.

Kerribijn: In cyctic fibrosis, chronic neutrophil-rich airway inflammation is prominent, but these patients may have normal or only slightly increased hyperresponsiveness. Can you comment?

O'Byrne: It had been documented that airway hyperresponsiveness is increased in patients with cystic fibrosis.

Acknowledgment

Dr. O'Byrne is the recipient of a Medical Research Council of Canada Scholarship.

References

Aizawa, H., Chung, K. F., Leikauf, G. D., et al. (1985). Significance of thromboxane generation in ozone-induced airway hyperresponsiveness in dogs. *J. Appl. Physiol.* **59**:1918-1923.

American Thoracic Society. (1962). Definition of asthma. *Am. Rev. Respir. Dis.* **134**:704-707.

Anderson, S. D. (1985). Exercise-induced asthma. The state of the art. *Chest* **87S**:191-195.

Berend, N., Armour, C. L., and Black, J. L. (1985). Indomethacin inhibits C5a des arg-induced airway hyperresponsiveness in the rabbit. *Am. Rev. Respir. dis.* **131**:24A.

Boulet, L. P., Cartier, A., and Thomson, N. C. (1983). Asthma and increases in nonallergic bronchial responsiveness from seasonal pollen exposure. *J. Allergy Clin. Immunol.* **71**:399-406.

Cartier, A., Thomson, N. C., and Frith, P. A. (1982). Allergen-induced increase in bronchial responsiveness to histamine: relationship to the late asthmatic response and change in airway caliber. *J. Allergy Clin. Immunol.* **70**:170-177.

Chan-Yeung, M., Lam, S., and Koener, S. (1982). Clinical features and natural history of occupational asthma due to western red cedar (*Thuja plicata*). *Am. J. Med.* **72**:411-15.

Chung, K. F., Becker, A. B., and Lazarus, S. C. (1985). Antigen-induced airway hyperresponsiveness and pulmonary inflammation in allergic dogs. *J. Appl. Physiol.* **58**:1347-1353.

Chung, K. F., Aizawa, H., and Becker, A. B. (1986a). Inhibition of antigen-induced airway hyperresponsiveness by a thromboxane synthetase inhibitor (OKY 046) in allergic dogs. *Am. Rev. Respir. Dis.* **134**:258-261.

Chung, K. F., Aizawa, H., and Leikauf, G. D. (1986b). Airway hyperresponsiveness induced by platelet-activating factor: role of thromboxane generation. *J. Pharmacol. Exp. Ther.* **236**:580-584.

Cockcroft, D. W. (1983). Mechanism of perennial allergic asthma. *Lancet* **2**:253-256.

Cockcroft, D. W., Ruffin, R. E., Dolovich, J., and Hargreave, F. E. (1977). Allergen-induced increase in non-allergic bronchial reactivity. *Clin. Allergy* **7**:503-513.

Curry, J. J. (1947). Comparative action of acetyl-beta-methyl choline and histamine on the respiratory tract in normals, patients with hay fever and subjects with bronchial asthma. *J. Clin. Invest.* **26**:430-438.

De Monchy, J. G. R., Kauffman, H. F., Venge, P., et al. (1985). Bronchoalveolar eosinophilia during allergen-induced late asthmatic reaction. *Am. Rev. Respir. Dis.* **131**:373-376.

Dorward, A. J., Colloff, M. J., MacKay, N. S., et al. (1988). Effect of house dust mite avoidance measures on adult atopic asthma. *Thorax* **43**:98-102.

Dunnill, M. S., Massarell, G. R., and Anderson, J. A. (1969). A comparison of the quantitive anatomy of the bronchi in normal subjects, in status asthmaticus, in chronic bronchitis and in emphysema. *Thorax* **24**:176-179.

Fabbri, L. M., Aizawa, H., Alpert, S. E., et al. (1984). Airway hyperresponsiveness and changes in cell counts in bronchoalveolar lavage after ozone exposure in dogs. *Am. Rev. Respir. Dis.* **129**:288-291.

Fabbri, L. M., Chiesura-Corona, P., Dal Vecchio, L., et al. (1985). Prednisone inhibits late asthmatic reactions and the associated increase in airway responsiveness induced by toluene diisocyanate in sensitized subjects. *Am. Rev. Respir. Dis.* **132**:1010-1014.

Fabbri, L. M., Boschetto, P., Zocca, E., et al. (1987). Bronchoalveolar neutrophilia during late asthmatic reactions induced by toluene diisocyanate. *Am. Rev. Respir. Dis.* **136**:36-42.

Flint, K. C., Leung, K. B. P., Hudspith, B. N., et al. (1985). Bronchoalveolar mast cells in extrinsic asthma: a mechanism for the initiation of antigen specific bronchoconstriction. *Br. Med. J.* **291**:923-926.

Golden, J. A., Nadel, J. A., and Boushey, H. A. (1978). Bronchial hyperirritability in healthy subjects after exposure to ozone. *Am. Rev. Respir. Dis.* **118**:287-294.

Goldstein, I. M., Malmsten, C. L., Kindahl, H., et al. (1978). Thromboxane generation by human peripheral blood polymorphonuclear leukocytes. *J. Exp. Med.* **148**:787-792.

Gordon, T., Sheppard, D., McDonald, D., et al. (1985). Airway hyperresponsiveness and inflammation induced by toluene diisocyanate in guinea pigs. *Am. Rev. Respir. Dis.* **132**:1106-1112.

Hargreave, F. E., Ryan, G., Thomson, N. C., et al. (1981). Bronchial responsiveness to histamine or methacholine in asthma: measurement and clinical significance. *J. Allergy Clin. Immunol.* **68**:347-355.

Higgs, G. A., Moncada, S., Salmon, J. A., and Seager, K. (1983). The source of thromoboxane and prostaglandins in experimental inflammation. *Br. J. Pharmacol.* **79**:863-868.

Holtzman, M. J., Fabbri, L. M., O'Byrne, P. M., et al. (1983a). Importance of airway inflammation for hyperresponsiveness induced by ozone. *Am. Rev. Respir. Dis.* **127**:686-690.

Holtzman, M. J., Fabbri, L. M., Skoogh, B.-E., et al. (1983b). Time course of airway hyperresponsiveness induced by ozone in dogs. *J. Appl. Physiol.* **55**(4):1232-1236.

Holtzman, M. J., Aizawa, H., Nadel, J. A., and Goetzl, E. J. (1983c). Selective generation of leukotriene B_4 by tracheal epithelial cells from dogs. *Biochem. Biophys. Res. Commun.* **114**:1071-1076.

Hutson, P. A., Church, M. K., Clay, T. P., et al. (1988). Early and late-phase bronchoconstriction after allergen challenge of nonanaesthetized guinea pigs. *Am. Rev. Respir. Dis.* **137**:548-557.

Irvin, C., Baltopoulos, G., Honour, J., et al. (1986). Lipid mediators released by activated human neutrophils which increase airway reactivity. *Am. Rev. Respir. Dis.* **133**:A175.

Juniper, E. F., Frith, P. A., and Hargreave, F. E. (1981). Airway responsiveness to histamine and methacholine: relationship to minimum treatment to control symptoms of asthma. *Thorax* **36**:575-579.

Juniper, E. F., Frith, P.A., and Hargreave, F. E. (1982). Long term stability of bronchial responsiveness to histamine. *Thorax* **37**:288-291.

Kelly, C., Ward, C., Stenton, C. S., et al. (1988). Number and activity of inflammatory cells in bronchoalveolar lavage fluid in asthma and their relation to airway responsiveness. *Thorax* **43**:684-692.

Kirby, J., Hargreave, F. E., Gleich, G. J., and O'Byrne, P. M. (1987). Bronchoalveolar cell profiles of asthmatic and nonasthmatic subjects. *Am. Rev. Respir. Dis.* **136**:379-383.

Lam, S., Chan-Yeung, M., Le Riche, J., et al. (1985). Cellular changes in bronchial lavage fluid following late asthmatic reactions in patients with red cedar asthma. *Am. Rev. Respir. Dis.* **131**:42A.

Lanes, S., Stevenson, J. S., Codias, E., et al. (1985). Effects of busesonide on late bronchial response and the associated airway hyperresponsiveness in allergic sheep. In *Glucocorticoids, Inflammation and Bronchial Hyperreactivity*. Edited by J. C. Hogg, R. Ellul-Micallef, and R. Brattsand. New York, Excerpta Medica, pp. 38-50.

Lanes, S., Stevenson, J. S., Codias, E., et al. (1986). Indomethacin and FPL 55321 inhibit antigen-induced airway hyperresponsiveness in sheep. *J. Appl. Physiol.* **61**:864-872.

Lewis, R. A., and Austen, K. F. (1984). The biologically active leukotrienes. Biosynthesis, metabolism, receptors, functions and pharmacology. *J. Clin. Invest.* **73**:889-897.

Marsh, W. R., Irvin, C. G., and Murphy, K. R. (1985). Increases in airway reactivity to histamine and inflammatory cells in bronchoalveolar lavage after the late asthmatic response in an animal model. *Am. Rev. Respir. Dis.* **131**:875-879.

Metzger, W. J., Zavala, D., and Richerson, H. B. (1987). Local allergen challenge and bronchoalveolar lavage of allergic asthmatic lungs. *Am. Rev. Respir. Dis.* **135**:433-440.

Murlas, C., and Roum, J. H. (1985a). Bronchial hyperreactivity occurs in steroid-treated guinea pigs depleted of leukocytes by cyclophosphamide. *J. Appl. Physiol.* **58**:1630-1637.

Murlas, C. G., and Roum, J. H. (1985b). Sequence of pathological changes in the airway mucosa of guinea pigs during ozone-induced bronchial hyperreactivity. *Am. Rev. Respir. Dis.* **131**:875-879.

Murphy, K. R., Wilson, M. C., Irvin, C. G., et al. (1986). The requirement for polymorphonuclear leukocytes in the asthmatic response and heightened airways reactivity in an asthmatic model. *Am. Rev. Respir. Dis.* **134**:62-68.

Murray, A. B., and Ferguson, A. C. (1983). Dust-free bedrooms in the treatment of asthmatic children with house dust or house dust mite allergen: a controlled trial. *Pediatrics* **71**:418-422.

O'Byrne, P. M., Ryan, G., Morris, M., et al. (1982). Asthma induced by cold air and its relation to nonspecific bronchial responsiveness to methacholine. *Am. Rev. Respir. Dis.* **125**:281-285.

O'Byrne, P. M., Walters, E. H., Aizawa, H., et al. (1984a). Indomethacin inhibits the airway hyperresponsiveness but not the neutrophil influx induced by ozone in dogs. *Am. Rev. Respir. Dis.* **130**:220-224.

O'Byrne, P. M., Walters, E. H., Gold, B. D., et al. (1984b). Neutrophil depletion inhibits airway hyperresponsiveness induced by ozone exposure. *Am. Rev. Respir. Dis.* **130**(2):14-19.

O'Byrne, P. M., Leikauf, G. D., Aizawa, H., et al. (1985). Leukotriene B4-induced airway hyperresponsiveness in dogs. *J. Appl. Physiol.* **59**:1941-1946.

O'Byrne, P. M., Kirby, J. G., and Hargreave, F. E. (1987). Airway inflammation and hyperresponsiveness. *Am. Rev. Respir. Dis.* **136**:S35-S37.

Osler, W. (1982). *The Principles and Practice of Medicine.* New York, Appleton and Co., p. 497.

Platts-Mills, T. A., Mitchell, E. B., Nock, P., et al. (1982). Reduction of bronchial hyperreactivity during prolonged allergen avoidance. *Lancet* 675-678.

Stelzer, J., Bigby, B. G., Stulbarg, M., et al. (1986). Ozone-induced changes in bronchial reactivity to methacholine and airway inflammation in humans. *J. Appl. Physiol.* **60**:1321-1326.

Tate, R. M., and Repine, J. E. (1983). Neutrophils and the adult respiratory distress syndrome. *Am. Rev. Respir. Dis.* **128**:552-559.

Thompson, J. E., Scypinski, L. A., Gordon, T., and Sheppard, D. (1986). Hydroxyurea inhibits airway hyperresponsiveness in guinea pigs by a granulocyte-independent mechanism. *Am. Rev. Respir. Dis.* **134**:1213-1218.

Tomioka, M., Ida, S., Shindoh, Y., et al. (1984). Mast cells in bronchoalveolar lumen of patients with bronchial asthma. *Am. Rev. Respir. Dis.* **129**:1000-1005.

Uchida, D. A., Kimani, G., Larsen, G. L., and Irvin, C. G. (1987). Effects on airway function of supernatants from phagocytosing eosinophils. *Am. Rev. Respir. Dis.* **135**:A178.

Wardlaw, A. J., Dunnette, S., Gleich, G. J., et al. (1988). Eosinophils and mast cells in bronchoalveolar lavage in subjects with mild asthma. *Am. Rev. Respir. Dis.* **137**:62-69.

Weiss, S., Robb, G. P., and Ellis, L. B. (1932). The systemic effects of histamine in man. *Arch. Intern. Med.* **49**:360-396.

Yeung, M., Lam, S., and Tse, K. S. (1985). Measurement of airway responsiveness in occupational asthma. In *Airway Responsiveness*. Edited by F. E. Hargreave and A. J. Woolcock. Mississauga, Ontario, Canada, Pharmaceuticals, pp. 129-134.

17

Participation of Fc Epsilon RII-Positive Macrophages and Eosinophils in Asthma

MONIQUE CAPRON and ANDRÉ-BERNARD TONNEL

Institut Pasteur,
Lille, France

Many of the characteristics of bronchial asthma may be linked to inflammatory processes induced by mediators released after antigen-IgE interaction. A classic view of the mechanisms responsible for allergic diseases is that the initial high-affinity binding of free (monomeric) IgE antibody to specific cell surface receptors (Fcε receptors) on mast cells and basophils is followed, upon reexposure to the corresponding antigen, by cross-linking of the IgE receptors. The clustering of Fcε receptors is considered to be the triggering signal for cell activation, leading to the discharge of an array of proinflammatory mediators. The rapid release of mast cell-associated mediators is likely to play a major role in the early clinical manifestations of asthma, and immediate reactions are largely the result of bronchoconstriction consecutive to the release of histamine, prostaglandin (PG) D2 or leukotrienes. However, inflammatory reactions are complex and result from the participation of many bioactive mediators and many different cell types, not necessarily acting all together at a given time. Although most mediators responsible for bronchoconstriction, bronchial hyperreactivity, and infiltration of airways with inflammatory cells have initially been considered as derived from mast cells, considerable doubt now exists about their cellular sources. For some time, it was believed that other cells also found at the site of anaphylactic reactions were merely recruited by mast cell and basophil-derived factors and could only participate as a source of so-called secondary mediators to enhance the inflammatory reaction. However, by studying the properties and cell sources of the mediators of anaphylaxis, it was shown that most of these mediators are also produced by neutrophils, macrophages, eosinophils, and platelets.

The characterization of a second class of IgE Fc receptors (FcεRII) on proinflammatory cells has broadened our current understanding of the role of cells such as mononuclear phagocytes, eosinophils, and platelets, all of which are found to infiltrate the airways in allergic asthma (A. Capron et al., 1986). One must therefore consider the participation of proinflammatory cells in the development of the local inflammatory response that occurs after repeated exposure to allergens or during the late-phase reaction, leading progressively to bronchial hyperresponsiveness. After a survey of the general characteristics of FcεRII, the present review will focus on the involvement of FcεRII-positive macrophages and eosinophils in patients with asthma.

I. Second Receptor for IgE [FcεRII] on Macrophages and Eosinophils

The study of IgE receptors on inflammatory cells came from convergent observations made in our laboratory during the investigation of immunity in human schistosomiasis. These parasitic models are characterized, as are many other helminthic infections, by a massive production of antiparasite IgE, part of which is complexed with circulating schistosome antigens. One of the major issues concerning the participation of IgE in immune reactions, whether protective against parasites or contributing to allergy, is the mechanism of its interaction with macrophages, eosinophils, and platelets. Observations made in ADCC systems pointed to a cytophilic binding of IgE, which prompted studies on the binding of this molecule to these cell populations (Capron and Dessaint, 1985).

A. Fcε Receptor on Mononuclear Phagocytes

The specific binding of IgE to the surface of macrophages can be demonstrated. When fixed erythrocytes are coated with myeloma IgE protein and used as the basis of a rosette assay, it can be shown that mononuclear phagocytes and macrophage/monocytic cell lines form IgE rosettes in rats, mice, and humans. The percentages of Fcε receptor positive cells vary in different species and in cells from different anatomical locations: monocytes show lower percentages than peritoneal or alveolar macrophages (reviewed in Spiegelberg, 1984).

An interesting finding is that monocytes or alveolar macrophages from healthy donors form a lower percentage of IgE rosettes than cells from patients with severe allergic disorders. Likewise in the rat, infection by helminthic parasites is associated with elevated percentages of Fcε-receptor-positive macrophages and the role of IgE in inducing this increase is demonstrated *in vivo* as well as *in vitro* (reviewed in Spiegelberg, 1984). Besides IgE itself, the expression of Fcε receptors on a human monocytic cell line (U937) and on macrophages can be increased by lymphokines such as γ-interferon or IL4- (Naray-Fejes Toth and Cuyre, 1984; Boltz-Nitulescu et al., 1988a,b; Vercelli et al., 1988). With respect to allergy, glucocorticoids can decrease Fcε receptor expression by U937 cells (Naray-Fejes Toth et al., 1985).

Saturation binding of radiolabeled monomeric IgE to human rat or mouse mononuclear phagocytes can be demonstrated, which is specifically inhibited by native IgE or its Fcε fragment but not by IgG. The average association constant for unaggregated IgE is 0.8 to 6 $\times$ 10^7/M, but monomeric IgE dissociates rapidly from the cells ($t_{1/2}$ = 2-3 min) (Spiegelberg, 1984; Finbloom and Metzger, 1982; Dessaint et al., 1983). Therefore, complexed IgE or IgE-opsonized particles would not be hindered by monomeric IgE fixed to macrophages. Indeed, dimeric IgE binds to rat macrophages with a higher association constant (2.3 $\times$ 10^8/M) than monomers, and IgE dimers dissociate with a much slower rate ($t_{1/2}$ = 94 min) (Finbloom and Metzger, 1982). Accordingly, when the Fcε-receptor-positive human monocytic cell line U937 is incubated with radiolabeled IgE monomers or dimers, the binding of each label is competitively inhibited by a moderate ($\times$ 50) excess of unlabeled dimers, but IgE monomers do not inhibit significantly in these conditions (Dessaint et al., 1983).

B. Fcε Receptors on Eosinophils

By using homologous IgE-coated erythrocytes, the rosetting of a significant proportion of rat or human eosinophils is obtained, and the specificity of the binding is shown by inhibition experiments using aggregated IgE or IgG. The binding of IgE to the eosinophil surface is also confirmed by ultrastructural studies (M. Capron et al., 1981). In order to determine the quantitative aspects of eosinophil IgE receptor, experiments involving binding of radiolabeled IgE were performed. Myeloma human IgE previously aggregated with dimethylsuberimidate (DMSI) and labeled with ^{125}I is able to bind to purified human eosinophils (M. Capron et al., 1981). Heating at 56°C for 3 h predictably destroys the ability of labeled IgE to bind to eosinophils. Moreover, the binding of [^{125}I]IgE is inhibited by unlabeled aggregated IgE in a dose-dependent manner (M. Capron et al., 1981). Further experiments using radiolabeled monomeric IgE were performed to estimate the total number of FcE RII per eosinophil. When hypodense eosinophils are incubated with varying concentrations of ^{125}I-labeled human myeloma IgE (ND) for 90 min at $+4\,^\circ$C, saturation of the binding can be detected which allows to estimate the mean number of receptors per cell in the range of 10^5. The binding constant, determined by equilibrium measurement and plotting the data in the form of Scatchard plots, is in the range of 10^7/M (reviewed in M. Capron et al., 1989b).

In both hypereosinophilic patients and *S. mansoni*-infected rats, an increase in the percentage of Fcε-receptor-positive eosinophils is observed, which is an indication of a possible *in vivo* modulation of the expression of the receptor for IgE. Incubation of normal rat eosinophils with either purified myeloma IgE protein or the heat-labile antibodies of infected rat serum indeed leads to a dose-dependent increase in the proportion of Fcε-receptor-positive eosinophils (Capron et al., 1983). Besides IgE itself, other factors seem to control the expression of eosinophil receptors for IgE. Through the release of their mediators, mast cells can enhance the expression of the Fcε receptors by eosinophils. ECF-A tetrapeptides can, in particular, induce a significant increase in the proportion of eosinophils forming IgE rosettes (M. Capron et al., 1981, 1983).

Another factor accounting for variations in the expression of Fcε receptors by eosinophils is related to the heterogeneity of these cells, notably in hypereosinophilic patients. In such patients, and particularly in those with parasitic infections or with the hypereosinophilic syndrome, blood eosinophils are mainly formed of light-density cells with a reduced size of specific granules. Yet these "hypodense" eosinophils express Fcε receptors at a higher number per cell and with increased affinity for IgE than the normodense cells (M. Capron et al., 1984). Moreover, it was shown that the IgE-dependent cytotoxic capacity was apparently restricted to these hypodense blood eosinophils from highly hypereosinophilic patients (blood counts greater than 3000/mm^3) and to the hypodense eosinophils found in tissues (M. Capron et al., 1984).

C. Characteristics of Fcε Receptors on Macrophages and Eosinophils

Investigations performed in several laboratories since 1975 demonstrate that subpopulations of cells classically associated with inflammatory reactions (mononuclear phagocytes, eosinophils, and platelets) carry IgE-specific cell membrane receptors that differ in many ways from the Fcε receptor on mast cells and basophils. In parallel, studies on the control of the IgE response also indicate that B- and T-cell subsets bear IgE receptors and participate in the isotypic regulation of IgE production.

The most striking property of these new receptors is that they bind monomeric IgE with a relatively low affinity compared to the "classic" Fcε receptor on basophils and mastocytes, from which monomeric IgE dissociates slowly. The lower affinity of that second receptor does not, however, lessen its biological significance. In fact, the affinity for monomeric IgE ($Ka10^7$/M) is comparable with or even higher than the affinity generally reported for the IgG receptors. Moreover, the increased affinity for IgE dimers or complexes ($Ka10^8$/M) gives to this class of receptors a particular significance in all situations where IgE complexes are produced. This is the case not only in parasitic infections (A. Capron and Dessaint, 1985) but also in various allergic diseases including asthma (Stevens and Bridts, 1984). In addition, the number of FcεRII-bearing cells increases in all pathological or experimental situations associated with elevated IgE levels (A. Capron et al., 1986; Spiegelberg, 1984).

Compared to the properties of the classic IgE receptor on mast cells and basophils, both the binding parameters and the circumstances in which the Fcε receptors are modulated on mononuclear phagocytes, eosinophils, and platelets appear sufficiently different to justify the separate recognition of a second class of Fcε receptors (FcεRII) expressed by subpopulations of proinflammatory cells and lymphoid cells (A. Capron et al., 1986).

An antiserum prepared against lymphocyte Fcε receptors has been shown to inhibit the binding of IgE to human monocytes and to U937 monocytic cells. This antiserum precipitates two surface components from U937 cells of approximately 47 and 23 kDa. The comparison made between human mononuclear phagocytes and lymphocytes indicates that both cells bear trypsin-sensitive Fcε receptors of similar structure and antigenicity, which differ from the high-affinity monovalent receptor for IgE on basophils or mast cells (Spiegelberg, 1984). The same antiserum specifically inhibits both the formation of IgE rosettes and the IgE-dependent cytotoxicity by eosinophils from hypereosinophilic patients (M. Capron et al., 1984). Thus, the second class of IgE receptor shares common features with the various FcεRII positive cell subpopulations, clearly distinct from those of the FcεRII on mast cells and basophils.

More recently, a monoclonal antibody (BB10) specific for FcεRII has been obtained by immunization with FcεRII-positive hypodense blood and lung eosinophils. The use of this antibody has confirmed the sharing of antigenic specificity of the IgE receptor on mononuclear phagocytes, eosinophils, and platelets (M. Capron et al., 1986). By using affinity chromatography with the anti-FcεRII monoclonal antibody or with IgE, it is possible to identify two major specific bands of approximately 45-50 and 23 kDa for U937 monocytic cells, 43-45 and 31kDa for platelets (M. Capron et al., 1986) and three polypeptide fragments at 45-50, 23, and 15 kDa for eosinophils (Jouault et al., 1988). Similar results were recently obtained by immunoprecipitation, and, moreover, eosinophil FcεRII was compared to CD23. Whereas BB10 precipitates three polypeptides of 45-50, 20-25, and 15 kDa on eosinophils and on a B-cell line (WIL-2WT), an mAb anti-CD23 (mAb135 kindly provided by Dr. G. Delespesse, University of Montreal, Canada) binds to a major 45-50 kDa component of both eosinophils and WIL-2WT cells. This study together with previous results, confirms the existence of a common structure between FcεRII present on eosinophils, platelets, macrophages, and B lymphocytes (Grangette et al., 1989).

A direct indication of the cytophilic binding of IgE to proinflammatory cells has been obtained by *ex vivo* studies. When one compares macrophages collected by bronchoalveolar lavage from normal controls and from patients with allergic asthma, a higher percentage of rosettes was obtained in the allergic donors using indicator erythrocytes coated with anti-IgE antibody (Joseph et al., 1983). Flow microfluorometry was also used to investigate the presence of cytophilic IgE on eosinophils from hypereosinophilic patients. In most cases, it was possible to detect IgE bound to the purified eosinophils, and a significant association was found between cytophilic IgE and elevated serum IgE levels (M. Capron et al., 1985).

These observations therefore support the hypothesis that when IgE levels are elevated, Fcε receptors on proinflammatory cells can be occupied despite the relatively low affinity of their surface receptors. A striking result of these studies directly demonstrating *in vivo* binding of IgE to inflammatory cells is the inconstant and low detection of cytophilically bound IgG on these cells. One may assume therefore that preferential occupation of FcεRII rather than Fcγ receptors may confer an operational superiority on surface-bound IgE in triggering the cell.

II. Alveolar Macrophages and Asthma

Mast cells probably initiate type I hypersensitivity reactions, but bronchial asthma cannot be fully explained by this cell type only. Less than 0.25% of the cells recovered from the airway lumen by bronchoalveolar lavage (BAL) are mast cells and, paradoxically, the highest levels of mast cells and histamine are recovered from patients with interstitial pulmonary diseases (Rankin et al., 1987). In fact, the most abundant cell type present in the lumen of the respiratory tract is the alveolar macrophage (AM). Indeed, AM are present not only at the level of alveoli but also throughout the bronchial tree at the surface of bronchiolar and bronchial mucosa. With the use of a new technique to isolate a human large airway *in vivo*, cellular components largely different from BAL were detected in bronchial wash, with two prominent cell types, macrophages and neutrophils, that together represent almost 60% of the total cell count (Rankin et al., 1988).

A. Involvement of Alveolar Macrophages in Allergic Asthma

Several studies have identified the presence of receptors for IgE on the mononuclear phagocyte surface and their increased numbers in patients with atopic disorders. Concerning alveolar macrophages, the percentage of human AM expressing the Fcε receptor was found to be 18-20% in patients with allergic asthma, compared with 6-8% in controls (Joseph et al., 1983). Additional evidence for the presence of surface IgE on AM was provided by electron microscopic examination with colloidal gold conjugated anti-IgE (Fuller et al., 1986).

Following the binding of IgE of the appropriate molecular form (i.e., at least dimers), signs of cell activation can be detected in the various populations concerned. Besides products such as oxygen metabolites that are commonly generated, more specialized mediators are released depending on the particular cell subset. In the case of macrophages, together with the discharge of oxygen metabolites and of lysosomal enzymes, IgE triggers the secretion of sulfidopeptide leukotrienes, leukotriene B4, prostaglandins, and platelet-activating factor (PAF) (A. Capron et al., 1986; Joseph et al., 1983; Ferreri et al., 1986; Rankin et al., 1984; Rouzer et al., 1982). An interesting finding was that human alveolar macrophages successively incubated with the serum from allergic patients and with anti-human IgE specifically released β-glucuronidase, excreted neutral proteases, and produced the superoxide anion O_2 (Joseph et al., 1983). The release is dependent on IgE antibody in patients' sera, as shown by the disappearance of the anti-IgE-induced changes after heating at 56 °C or after the depletion of IgE of the sensitizing serum. Alveolar macrophages collected from allergic patients or cultured with the serum from patients allergic to house mites or to grass pollen selectively release lysosomal enzymes after the addition of the specific allergen (+ 830% increase), and the depletion of IgE but not of IgG prevents enzyme release by the corresponding allergen (Joseph et al., 1983). In humans after AM stimulation with anti-IgE, the secretion of TxB_2, PGF_2, and LTB_4 appears within the first 15 min (Fuller et al., 1986). The data suggest that the *in vivo* release might effectively occur within the time span necessary to initiate bronchospasm after challenge in sensitive patients. AM retrieved from asthmatic patients were also shown to be potent producers of PAF (Arnoux et al., 1980), a lipid-derived mediator known to act as a chemotactic factor for human eosinophils and as an inducer of severe and prolonged bronchial hyperreactivity when given by inhalation in humans. After incubation with anti-IgE or specific allergens, AM are also able to secrete a low-molecular-weight chemotactic factor for neutrophils and eosinophils, probably related to LTB_4 (Gosset et al., 1984). In addition, human lung macrophages have been shown to secrete a factor susceptible to induce calcium-dependent histamine release from human basophils and lung mast cells (Schulman et al., 1985). Therefore all these findings point to the human alveolar macrophage as a potential source of mediators implicated in the local inflammatory response, especially since some of them can be released after local bronchial challenge test (Tonnel et al., 1983).

B. Alveolar Macrophages and Monokine Production After IgE-Dependent Stimulation

The role of AM in allergic asthma is not restricted to the secretion of lipid-derived mediators: AM can also act as regulatory cells. In order to study the possible role of AM in the development of the local immune response, our interest was recently focused on monokine production, interleukin 1 (IL_1) and tumor necrosis factor α (TNFα) after IgE-dependent stimulation. Mononuclear phagocytes are known to produce IL1, a molecule considered to play a crucial role in inflammatory processes and in lymphocyte proliferation. To appreciate the possible role of AM in the local response to inhaled allergens, we compared IL_1 production by peripheral blood monocytes and AM from patients with allergic asthma and controls (Gosset et al., 1988). When stimulated by polysaccharides, AM and blood monocytes released IL_1 in similar amounts (148 $\pm$ 47 and 160 $\pm$ 78 IL_1 units/ml), but in response to anti-IgE or allergens at variance with monocytes that generated significant amounts of IL_1, AM supernatants contained no detectable IL_1 activity. In contrast in the same experimental conditions, AM secreted preferentially an IL_1 inhibitory factor, independent from prostaglandin E_2, with a molecular weight of 40-50 kDa. These results demonstrate that unlike some stimuli such as endotoxins that are able to induce IL_1 production, AM after IgE-dependent stimulation deliver a negative signal for lymphocyte proliferation, suggesting an potential *in situ* limitation of the immune response to common inhaled allergens. In parallel with IL1, another monokine (TNFα) has been recently investigated. AM directly retrieved from the lung of asthmatic patients released significantly more TNFα (0.96 $\pm$ 0.50 ng/ml) than AM from controls. After IgE-dependent stimulation, performed *in vitro* by addition of allergen or anti-IgE, the levels of TNFα present in supernatants was increased up to 2.8 $\pm$ 0.9 ng/ml). It is also interesting to note a significant amplification ($\times$3) of monokine production in the case of costimulation with interferon γ. These results on the measurements of TNFα production were clearly corroborated by the elevation of TNFα mRNA expression. These high levels of TNFα secretion seen in patients with asthma as well as its potentiation by IFNγ suggest a possible interaction with lymphocytes present in airways. The recruitment of T lymphocytes after inhalation challenge (Gonzales et al., 1987) and the presence of a high proportion of activated T lymphocytes, with a predominant CD4 "helper-inducer" subset, shown in blood of patients with acute severe attack of asthma (Corrigan et al., 1988), raise the possibility of interactions between AM and T lymphocytes present in airways. These interactions may contribute to a subsequent activation of other cells recruited in the respiratory tract.

III. Eosinophils and Asthma

Although peripheral blood eosinophilia is currently associated with allergic disorders, the contribution of eosinophils has yet to be fully appreciated. Early studies centered on its ability to downregulate immediate hypersensitivity reactions, but convincing data have more recently focused interest on the role of eosinophils as effector cells for killing parasites and also for causing bronchial and/or lung damage.

A. Eosinophil Fcε Receptor and IgE-Dependent Mediator Release

Eosinophils are known to express surface receptors for IgE, the demonstration of which was obtained after binding of labeled myeloma IgE, by rosette formation and by flow-microfluorometry, with a significant correlation between all methods (M. Capron et al., 1989b). The proportion of eosinophils bearing Fcε receptors could be evaluated: in humans 20-55% of blood eosinophils express the IgE receptor. A rise in Fcε-RII-bearing eosinophils seems linked to the activation by chemotactic factors such as ECF-A or PAF-acether, which may enhance the receptor expression on normal eosinophils (reviewed in M. Capron et al., 1989b). Cytophilically bound IgE is detected by flow microfluorometry with anti-IgE on about 75% of eosinophils from patients with hypereosinophilia. A significant increase in the percentage of IgE-bearing cells is found in patients with elevated serum IgE levels (> 240 KU/L). In patients with the pulmonary infiltration with eosinophils (PIE) syndrome, eosinophils collected by bronchoalveolar lavage shows higher percentages of surface-bound IgE than circulating eosinophils (M. Capron et la., 1985; Prin et al., 1986). The presence of a large proportion of hypodense eosinophils with surface bound IgE suggests that an increased expression of Fcε receptor might represent one of the markers of eosinophil activation, and indicates, moreover, the functionality of eosinophil IgE receptor.

The demonstration of surface IgE, cytophilically bound to hypodense eosinophils present in the blood, but also on tissue eosinophils (in the lungs) (M. Capron et al., 1985; Prin et al., 1986), led us to investigate the role of cytophilic IgE in mediator release. Surface IgE-bearing eosinophils purified from hypereosinophilic patients are able to release granule proteins such as eosinophil peroxydase (EPO) or major basic protein (MBP) (Khalife et al., 1986; Capron and Capron, 1987), in contrast to eosinophilic cationic protein (ECP), which is hardly liberated by IgE-dependent reactions (Khalife et al., 1986; M. Capron et al., 1989c). PAF is also generated by human eosinophils in response to activation by IgE but not by IgG (M. Capron et al., 1988a). In fact, this apparent selectivity in mediator release may be related to eosinophil heterogeneity: the particular subset of human eosinophils, sometimes found in blood, but prominent in lung, characterized by low density on metrizamide gradients (hypodense cells), high expression of IgE receptors, and binding of the BB10 monoclonal antibody, also has the selective capacity to release EPO and MBP by anaphylactic antibody challenge. In contrast, eosinophils with normal density ("normodense" cells) are activated by IgG antibodies to release mainly cationic proteins (MBP, ECP) together with low amounts of PAF (reviewed in M. Capron et al., 1989b). The selectivity in mediator release might be linked to different kinetics of activation through IgE versus IgG receptors. This was reported for rat macrophages (Pestel et al., 1984) and more recently suggested for human eosinophils (M. Capron et al., 1989c).

The release of potent proinflammatory mediators by eosinophils under IgE-dependent stimulation suggests that FcεRII-bearing eosinophils can contribute to allergic reactions.

B. Participation of Fcε-Positive Hypodense Eosinophils in Asthma

A series of recent clinical studies, focused either on peripheral blood eosinophils or on resident eosinophils recovered by bronchoalveolar lavage, has resulted in interesting data on eosinophil involvement in asthma.

Based on density and metabolic activity, peripheral blood eosinophils appear as a heterogeneous population in allergic disorders (Prin et al., 1986; Shult et al., 1988). A significantly higher proportion of hypodense eosinophils is observed in the blood of patients with allergic asthma (40.8 ± 5.8% hypodense eosinophils) or allergic rhinitis (30 ± 5%) than in controls (9 ± 2%). In addition, an increased percentage of hypodense eosinophils is detected more often in patients with severe symptoms, suggesting a possible connection between hypodense cells and the development of symptoms.

The eosinophil is known to release a large variety of substances able to cause cellular and tissue damage in bronchial asthma. Among cationic proteins, MBP mediates damage that mimics the pathological changes of asthma. MBP concentrations as low as 10 μg/ml produced ciliostasis with disruption of the epithelium and damage to the cells present in the lumen. With higher MBP concentrations (50-100 μg/ml), ciliated cells were progressively exfoliated to the level of the basal membrane. In parallel, measurements of MBP showed that patients with acute asthma had high levels of MBP in sputum, compatible with the cell alterations observed *in vitro* (Gleich and Adolphson, 1986).

Other eosinophil-derived products are potentially active in asthma, such as eosinophil peroxidase (EPO) localized in the granule matrix, which can, in the presence of H_2O_2 and halide, induce mast cell degranulation and also direct lung injury (Davis et al., 1984).

After the demonstration of a specific release of EPO and MBP through the Fcε receptor, in the case of parasite-infected patients (Khalife et al., 1986; Capron and Capron, 1987), similar data have been recently confirmed in patients sensitized to common inhaled allergens (M. Capron et al., 1989a,c). Blood eosinophils purified from patients with asthma are able to release EPO after triggering with the specific related allergen: grass pollen and/or *Dermatophagoides pteronyssinus*. The specificity of EPO release is suggested by a parallel mediator release in the presence of anti-IgE and allergen, while anti-IgG antibodies were uneffective. In a control group of nonatopic patients with high eosinophilia (mean blood eosinophil count, 42%, range 8-85%; compared to 12.5%, range 5-20%, in asthmatic patients) no EPO was detected after allergen stimulation, which renders highly probable mediator release through the Fcε receptor.

Eosinophil heterogeneity in atopy is also reflected in differences in lipid-derived mediator production. Hypodense eosinophils produce more PAF-acether in response to calcium ionophore than cells with normal density (M. Capron et al., 1988a). Lung eosinophils obtained by BAL produce 1000 times more PAF after incubation with anti-IgE than the corresponding blood eosinophils from the same patients (Bruynzeel and Verhagen, 1989).

These results support the concept of a functional heterogeneity among human eosinophils, specifically in respect to IgE-dependent mediator release. Moreover, they indicate that eosinophils, considered for a long time as secondary cells only able to be mobilized at the sites of the allergen conflict, can be also directly triggered through their specific IgE receptors to release various pharmacologically active mediators.

The exact contribution to allergic reactions, of eosinophils, through their activation by anaphylactic antibodies, remains to be evaluated, but it should be remembered that the same eosinophil subset (i.e., hypodense cells) is identified in the tissue lesions of the hypereosinophilic syndrome and demonstrates a greater cytotoxic capability in the presence of IgE. It is in these patients that eosinophils seem to participate in immunopathological lesions in inducing tissue lysis, and tissue eosinophils such as pleural or pulmonary cells are predominantly found as cells with lower density and granule content than blood eosinophils. Moreover, IgE-dependent eosinophilic cytotoxicity was incriminated in chronic eosinophilic pneumonia (Mc Evoy et al., 1988). Indeed, eosinophils from such patients were found to bear IgE but not IgG on their surface (M. Capron et al., 1985b; Prin et al., 1986). The selectivity of the mediators released after IgE or IgG-dependent activation (Capron et al., 1989c) is consistent with *in vivo* findings showing that release of MBP is often linked to hypersensitivity states (asthma, atopic skin diseases), whereas ECP levels are lower in asthmatic patients than in patients with eosinophilia not associated with asthma (reviewed in Gleich and Adolphson, 1986). One can therefore speculate that differences in organ injury seen in various hypereosinophilic disorders could be due to differences in the stimulus responsible for cell activation (Capron and Capron, 1987).

IV. Therapeutic Implications

Some antiallergic drugs including disodium cromoglycate (DSCG) have been demonstrated to exert an inhibitory action on IgE-dependent activation of cell populations expressing Fcε receptors of low affinity (FcεRII). Alveolar macrophages and eosinophils from patients with allergic diseases were tested. In humans, preliminary observations show that DSCG inhibited β-glucuronidase release by human alveolar macrophages in response to IgE-dependent stimulation (Tsicopoulos et al., 1988). This inhibitory effect is dose-dependent (optimal inhibitory concentration: $2.10^7/M$). Kinetic studies of DSCG's effects showed that it appeared at 15 min *in vitro* and was superposable to the duration of its *in vivo* activity in allergic diseases (between 4 and 6 hr). DSCG also inhibits the release of neutrophil chemotactic activity by alveolar macrophages observed after IgE triggering. No effect is observed when preformed chemotactic factors are incubated with the drug, showing that DSCG does not influence neutrophil chemotaxis and that the alveolar macrophage is indeed the DSCG target in these experiments. These *in vitro* observations are consistent with DSCG pharmacokinetics: after inhalation of a 20 ng DSCG capsule by normal subjects, peak plasma levels observed 5-30 min later are 44 ± 24 ng/ml. For asthmatic subjects, these levels are lower and more variable (16 ± 5 ng/ml). However, the *in vitro* concentration used in our experiments was of 100 ng/ml, which is close to the *in vivo* concentrations obtained with usual drug administration.

The participation of eosinophils in the cellular network during allergy and more generally inflammatory reactions has led to new therapeutic approaches to decrease or abolish the deleterious effects of eosinophils and their mediators. Three major steps in eosinophil activation might represent the targets of such drugs: the attraction of eosinophils by chemotactic factors, the stage of activation by various stimuli, and the release of mediators. Very recently, the strong inhibitory effect of a new antihistamine, antiallergic drug (Cetirizine), on eosinophil chemotaxis induced by PAF or by FMLP has been reported (Leprevost et al., 1988). The specific gingkolide-derived PAF antagonist, BN52021, strongly inhibited the PAF-induced chemotaxis (Kurihara et al., 1989). These two drugs have limited effects on neutrophils. Selective inhibition of the activation signal due to IgE triggering is a possible alternative. Indeed, DSCG was shown to inhibit the chemiluminescence reaction induced by addition of anti-IgE but not by anti-IgG or phorbol esters, to eosinophils from asthmatic patients. It is noteworthy to point out that DSCG has similar effects on macrophages and platelets (Tsicopoulos et al., 1988), whereas the inhibition of IgE-dependent release of mediators from human lung mast cells is surprisingly weak (reviewed in Kay et al., 1987). It could therefore be considered that the action of antiallergic drugs such as DSCG is not restricted to their effects on mast cells and basophils, but also interferes with Fcε-RII positive cells, leading to a potential reduction of the inflammatory response in allergic diseases and opening new insights into the mechanisms of action of these drugs in allergic asthma. Finally, the potent inhibition of eosinophil-mediated IgE-dependent cytotoxicity, but at a lesser extent of IgG-mediated cytotoxicity by PAF-antagonists (Capron et al., 1988b), tends to support our working hypothesis of the selectivity of mediator release.

Corticosteroids are the most effective drugs for the treatment of chronic asthma. However, hypereosinophilic patients do not always respond favorably to corticosteroïd therapy, especially patients with malignant hypereosinophilic syndrome (HES). We have recently shown that eosinophils from corticoresistant patients were lacking the receptor for corticosteroïds. We used both radiolabeled hormone binding assay and a specific antireceptor monoclonal antibody (Prin et al., 1989). These data provide evidence that the presence of corticosteroïd receptors is a prerequisite for corticosteroïd activity on eosinophils and may provide valuable information on corticosteroïd sensitivity.

V. Concluding Comments

The demonstration that the expression of the second class of receptors for IgE is increased in allergic patients and that FcεRII can possibly be upregulated by IgE indicates that immediate-type hypersensitivity can no longer be viewed as a mere breakthrough in IgE production. Instead, multiple changes in many reactive cells are in fact involved in allergy, resulting in an upgraded response potential. The production of many proinflammatory mediators by mononuclear phagocytes and eosinophils, in response to IgE immune complexes, indicates that mast cells and basophils cannot be considered as the unique targets in IgE-dependent reactions. It points to the primary effector function of cell populations, until now considered as only involved in nonspecific inflammatory responses. In immediate-type hypersensitivity, where there is an increased production of IgE and the formation of IgE complexes, FcɛRII behaves as an essential signaling structure. Local formation of IgE immune complexes capable of binding with higher affinity to FcɛRII, and of activating proinflammatory cells, may also be assumed, resulting from local exposure to allergens when (free) IgE antibodies circulate. Thus, although monomeric IgE rapidly dissociates from the cell surface, preformed or newly formed IgE immune complexes will persist and give FcɛRII-positive cells a direct role in the pathophysiology of asthma. Besides their potential value in a global view of allergic reactions, these results might have a particular importance in terms of predictive diagnosis and perhaps therapy. Identification of the second class of Fcɛ receptors on proinflammatory cells, as an important functional structure of these cells, has opened an entirely new field of knowledge that is bound to have a rapid and important influence on many areas of human pathology, especially in allergic or putatively allergic diseases.

Discussion

Fuller: It is important to discuss the pharmacology of the macrophage. We have shown that although the macrophage is sensitive to forskolin, it may show no inhibition by β-agonists. However, therapeutic concentrations of dexamethasone inhibit TxB_2 release from macrophages.

Schleimer: I believe that La Cronique et al. have claimed to show IgE-dependent IL-1 secretion from human alveolar macrophages. Why do you think your results differ from theirs? Second, you have demonstrated an inhibitor of IL-1 induced thymocyte proliferation in the supernatants of BAL macrophages. You suggest that BAL macrophages do not release IL-1. Have you directly demonstrated this by separating any IL-1 present from the putative inhibitor?

Capron: We have shown that alveolar macrophages under IgE-dependent stimulation did not produce IL-1, but we have not looked at macrophages from other sources, or after stimulation with other immunological stimuli (such as IgG or complement).

Woolcock: What is the effect of steroids on mediated release from macrophages and on the FcɛRII receptor expression?

Capron: It has been previously shown that corticosteroids were able to inhibit the expression of Fc RII IgE receptor on macrophages and on U937 monocyte cell lines.

Sertl: Can you inhibit monocyte IL-1 production by supernatant of alveolar macrophages of allergic patients?

Capron: The presence of an IL-1 inhibitory factor in the supernatants of IgE-dependent stimulated alveolar macrophages was included in measuring the inhibition of an IL-1 dependent proliferation of thymocytes, whereas the IL2-dependent proliferation of cytotoxic T-cell lines was not affected.

Kaliner: Do you have data indicating that alveolar macrophages will react to antigen unless they are sensitized ex vivo with IgE? Can you tell us of the reactivity of nonatopic alveolar macrophages? Can you suggest how nonatopic macrophages could participate in asthma in the "intrinsic" asthmatic patient?

Capron: Allergen can induce activation of alveolar macrophages either directly when macrophages were obtained from asthmatic patients or indirectly after passive sensitization of normal alveolar macrophages with the serum of asthmatic persons (Joseph et al., 1983).

Barnes: Does IgE bind to alveolar macrophages in vivo?

Capron: IgE does bind to alveolar macrophages in vivo, as shown by flow cytometry studies using IgE antibodies. The binding of IgE is also confirmed by the activation induced by anti-IgE antibodies. One must recall that the affinity of FcεRII increased for polymeric IgE, which is the molecular form of IgE immune complexes in allergic disorders.

Dahl: Can you give other characteristics of the Fcε receptor-bearing alveolar macrophage. Is it a younger cell or more mature cell? Does it have other special functions or metabolic functions? Does the number of FcεRII bearing cells increase in response to allergen, during a pollen season, or after a challenge test? Finally, is there a similar cell function in the nose?

Capron: It is likely that alveolar macrophages represent a heterogeneous population, similar to eosinophils. Concerning the expression of IgE receptors, they appear to be present in more mature cells (since their expression is increased by the variety of interleukins or growth factors).

Pipkorn: In the comparison between the presence of cells, a major difference is that you find very low numbers of macrophages on the nasal mucosal surface compared to the lower airways. Still, you have allergic airway disease.

Capron: We have not performed studies on macrophages in other locations than the peritoneum or alveolae.

References

Arnoux, B., Duval, D., and Benveniste, J. (1980). Release of platelet activating factor (PAF-acether) from alveolar macrophages by the calcium ionophore A 23187 and phagocytosis. *Eur. J. Clin. Invest.* **10**:437-441.

Boltz-Nitulescu, G., Nemet, H., Pernersdorfer, T., Gessl, A., Wiltscke, C., and Förster, O. (1988a). Enhancement of IgE receptor expression on rat macrophages by murine recombinant interleukin 4 and tumor necrosis factor. *FASEB J.* **2**:A12148, abstract 5536.

Boltz-Nitulescu, G., Wiltscke, C., Langer, K., Nemet, H., Holzinger, C., Gessl, A., Förster, O., and Penner, E. (1988b). Augmentation of IgE receptor expression and IgE receptor-mediated phagocytosis of rat bone marrow-derived macrophages and murine interferons. *Immunology* **63**: 529-535.

Bruynzeel, P. L. B., and Verhagen, J. (1989). Lipid metabolism by eosinophils. In *Eosinophils in Asthma*. Edited by J. Morley. London, Academic Press.

Capron, A., and Dessaint, J. P. (1985). Effector and regulatory mechanisms in immunity to schistosomes: a heuristic view. *Annu. Rev. Immunol.* **3**:455-476.

Capron, A., Dessaint, J. P., Capron, M., Joseph, M., Ameisen, J. C., and Tonnel, A. B. (1986). From parasites to allergy: the second receptor for IgE (FcεR2). *Immunol. Today* **7**:15-18.

Capron, M., and Capron, A. (1987). The IgE receptor of human eosinophils. In *Allergy and Inflammation*. Edited by A. B. Kay. London, Academic Press, pp. 151-159.

Capron, M., Capron, A., Dessaint, J. P., Torpier, G., Johansson, S. G. O., and Prin, L. (1981). Fc receptors for IgE on human and rat eosinophils. *J. Immunol.* **126**:2087-2092.

Capron, M., Capron, A., Joseph, M., and Verwaerde, C. (1983). IgE receptors on phagocytic cells and immune response to schistosome infection. *Monogr. Allergy* **18**:33-44.

Capron, M., Spiegelberg, H. L., Prin, L., Bennich, H., Butterworth, A. E., Pierce, R. J., Ouaissi, M. A., and Capron, A. (1984). Role of IgE receptors in effector function of human eosinophils. *J. Immunol.* **232**:462-468.

Capron, M., Kusnierz, J. P., Prin, L., Spiegelberg, H. L., Ovlaque, G., Gosset, P., Tonnel, A. B., and Capron, A. (1985). Cytophilic IgE on human blood and tissue eosinophils: detection by flow microfluorometry. *J. Immunol.* **134**:3013-3018.

Capron, M., Jouault, T., Prin, L., Joseph, M., Ameisen, J. C., Butterworth, A. E., Papin, J. P., Kusnierz, J. P., and Capron, A. (1986). Functional study of a monoclonal antibody to IgE Fc receptor (FcεR2) of eosinophils, platelets and macrophages. *J. Exp. Med.* **164**:72-89.

Capron, M., Benveniste, J., Braquet, P., and Capron, A. (1988a). Role of PAF-acether in IgE-dependent activation of eosinophils. In *New Trends in Lipid Mediators Research*, vol. 2. Edited by P. Braquet. Basel, Karger, pp. 10-17.

Capron, M., Benveniste, J., Grzych, J. M., Butterworth, A. E., and Capron, A. (1988b). PAF-acether and eosinophil-mediated cytotoxicity: inhibition by the PAF-acether antagonist BN 52021 and related ginkgolides. In *Ginkgolides—Chemistry, Biology, Pharmacology and Clinical Perspectives*, Vol. 1. Edited by P. Braquet. Barcelona, Prous Science, pp. 205-215.

Capron, M., Leprevost, C., Prin, L., Tomassini, M., Torpier, G., MacDonald, S., and Capron, A. (1989a). Immunoglobulin-mediated activation of eosinophils. In *Eosinophils in Asthma*. Edited by J. Morley. London, Academic Press.

Capron, M., Leprevost, C., Torpier, G., and Capron, A. (1989b). The second receptor for IgE in eosinophil effector function. In *Chemical Immunology Structures and Fucntions of Low-Affinity Fc Receptors*. Edited by W. H. Fridman. Karger, Basel, vol. 47, pp. 128-178.

Capron, M., Tomassini, M., Torpier, G., Kusnierz, J. P., MacDonald, S., and Capron, A. (1989c). Selectivity of mediators released by eosinophils. *Int. Arch. Allergy Apply. Immunol.* **88**:54-58.

Corrigan, C. J., Hartnell, A., and Kay, A. B. (1988). T lymphocyte activation in acute severe asthma. *Lancet* **1**:1129-1132.

Davis, B. W., Fells, A. G., Xiu-Hong, S., Gadek, E. J., Venet, A., and Crystal, R. G. (1984). Eosinophil-mediated injury to lung parenchymal cells and interstitial matrix. *J. Clin. Invest.* **74**:269-278.

Dessaint, J. P., Capron, A., Joseph, M., Auriault, C., and Pestel, J. (1983). Macrophage-mediated IgE ADCC to helminth parasites and IgE-dependent macrophage activation. In *Macrophage-Mediated Antibody-Dependent Cellular Cytotoxicity*. Edited by H. S. Koren. New York, Marcel Dekker, pp. 315-338.

Finbloom, D. S., and Metzger, H. (1982). Binding of immunoglobulin E to the receptor on rat peritoneal macrophages. *J. Immunol.* **129**:2004-2008.

Fuller, R. W., Morris, P. K., Richmond, R., Sykes, D., Varndell, I. M., Kemeny, D. M., Cole, P. J., Doller, C. T., and MacDermot, J. (1986). Immunoglobulin E-dependent stimulation of human alveolar macrophages: significance in type I hypersensitivity. *Clin. Exp. Immunol.* **65**:416-426.

Gleich, C. J., and Adolphson, C. R. (1986). The eosinophilic leukocyte. *Adv. Immunol.* **39**:177-253.

Gonzales, C., Diaz, P., Galleguillos, F., Ancic, P., Cromwell, O., and Kay, A. B. (1987). Allergen-induced recruitment of bronchoalveolar helper (OKT4) and suppressor (OKT8) cells in asthma. Relative increases in OKT8 cells in single early responders compared with those in late phase responders. *Am. Rev. Respir. Dis.* **136**:600-604.

Gosset, P., Tonnel, A. B., Joseph, M., Prin, L., Mallart, A., Charon, J., and Capron, A. (1984). Secretion of a chemotactic factor for neutrophils and eosinophils by alveolar macrophages patients. *J. Allergy Clin. Immunol.* **74**:827-834.

Gosset, P., Lassalle, P., Tonnel, A. B., Dessaint, J. P., Wallaert, B., Prin, L., Pestel, J., Capron, A. (1988). Production of an interleukin 1 inhibitory factor by human alveolar macrophages from normal and allergic patients. *Am. Rev. Respir. Dis.* **138**:40-46.

Grangette, C., Gruart, V., Ouaissi, M. A., Rizvi, F., Delespesse, G., Capron, A., and Capron, M. (1989). IgE receptor on human eosinophils (FcεRII): comparison with B cell CD23 and association with an adhesion molecule. *J. Immunol.*, submitted.

Joseph, M., Tonnel, A. B., Torpier, G., Capron, A., Arnoux, B., and Benveniste, J. (1983). Involvement of IgE in the secretory processes of alveolar macrophages from asthmatic patients. *J. Clin. Invest.* **71**:221-230.

Jouault, T., Capron, M., Balloul, J. M., Ameisen, J. C., and Capron, A. (1988). Quantitative and qualitative analysis of the Fc receptor for IgE (FcεRII) on human eosinophils. *Eur. J. Immunol.* **18**:237-241.

Kay, A. B., Walsh, G. M., Moqbel, R., MacDonald, A. J., Nagakura, T., Carroll, M. P., and Richerson, H. B. (1987). Disodium cromoglycate inhibits activation of human inflammatory cells *in vitro*. *J. Allergy Clin. Immunol.* **80**:1-8.

Khalife, J., Capron, M., Cesbron, J. Y., Taelman, H., Prin, L., and Capron, A. (1986). Role of specific IgE antibodies in peroxidase (EPO) release from human eosinophils. *J. Immunol.* **137**:1659-1664.

Kurihara, K., Wardlaw, A. J., Moqbel, R., and Kay, A. B. (1989). Inhibition of PAF-induced chemotaxis and PAF-binding to human eosinophils and neutrophils, by the specific gingkolide derived PAF antagonist, BN 52021. *J. Allergy Clin. Immunol.* in press.

Leprevost, C., Capron, M., De Vos, C., Tomassini, M., and Capron, A. (1988). Inhibition of eosinophil chemotaxis by a new antiallergic compound (Cetirizine). *Int. Arch. Allergy Appl. Immunol.* **87**:9-13.

Mc Evoy, J. D. S., Donald, K. J., and Edwards, P. L. (1978). Immunoglobulin level and electron-microscopy in eosinophil pneumonia. *Am. J. Med.* **64**:529-535.

Naray-Fejes-Toth, A., and Cuyre, P. M. (1984). Recombinant human immune interferon induces increased IgE receptor expression on the human monocyte cell line U937. *J. Immunol.* **133**:1914-1918.

Naray-Fejes-Toth, A., Cornwell, G. G., and Guyre, P. M. (1985). Glucocorticoids inhibit IgE receptor expression on the human monocyte cell line U937. *Immunology* **56**:359-363.

Pestel, J., Dessaint, J. P., Joseph, M., Bazin, H., and Capron, A. (1984). Macrophage triggering by aggregated immunoglobulins. II. Comparison of IgE and IgG aggregates or immune complexes. *Clin. Exp. Immunol.* **57**:404-408.

Prin, L., Capron, M., Gosset, P., Wallaert, B., Kusnierz, J. P., Bletry, O., Tonnel, A. B., and Capron, A. (1986). Eosinophilic lung disease: immunological studies of blood and alveolar eosinophils. *Clin. Exp. Immunol.* **63**:249-257.

Prin, L., Lefebvre, P., Gruart, V., Capron, M., Tonnel, A. B., Formstecher, P., Loiseau, S., and Capron, A. (1989). Variability in the expression of eosinophil glucorticoïd receptors: correlation with corticoresistance in hypereosinophilic patients. *Clin. Exp. Immunol.* **78**:383-389.

Rankin, J. A., Hitcock, M., Merrill, W. W., Huand, S. S., Braschler, J. R., Bach, M. K., and Askenase, P. W. (1984). IgE immune complexes induced immediate and prolonged release of leukotriene C4 (LTC4) from rat alveolar macrophages. *J. Immunol.* **132**:1993-1997.

Rankin, J. A., Kaliner, M., and Reynolds, H. Y. (1987). Histamine levels in bronchoalveolar lavage from patients with asthma, sarcoidosis and idiopathic pulmonary fibrosis. *J. Allergy Clin. Immunol.* **79**:371-377.

Rankin, J. A., Marcy, T., Smith, S., Olchowski, J., Sussman, J., and Merrill, W. W. (1988). Human airway lining fluid (ALF): cellular and protein constituents. *Am. Rev. Respir. Dis.* **137**:5 (Abstract).

Rouzer, C. A., Scott, W. A., Hamill, A. L., Liu, F. T., Katz, D. H., and Cohn, Z. A. (1982). Secretion of leukotriene C4 and other arachidonic acid metabolites by macrophages challenged with IgE immune complexes. *J. Exp. Med.* **156**:1077-1082.

Schulman, E. S., Liu, M. C., Proud, D., MacGlashan, D. W., Lichtenstein, L. M., and Plaut, M. (1985). Human lung macrophages induce histamine release from basophils and mast cells. *Am. Rev. Respir. Dis.* **131**:230-235.

Shult, P. A., Lega, M., Jadidi, S., Vrtis, R., Warner, T., Graziano, F. M., and Busse, W. W. (1988). The presence of hypodense eosinophils and diminished chemiluminescence response in asthma. *J. Allergy Clin. Immunol.* **81**:429-437.

Spiegelberg, H. L. (1984). Structure and function of Fc receptors for IgE on lymphocytes, monocytes and macrophages. *Adv. Immunol.* **35**:61-88.

Stevens, W. J., and Bridt, C. H. (1984). IgG containing and IgE-containing circulating immune complexes in patients with asthma and rhinitis. *J. Allergy Clin. Immunol.* **73**:276-280.

Tonnel, A. B., Gosset, P., Joseph, M., Fournier, E., and Capron, A. (1983). Stimulation of alveolar macrophages in asthmatic patients after local provocation test. *Lancet* **1**:1406-1408.

Tsicopoulos, A., Lassalle, P., Joseph, M., Tonnel, A. B., Thorel, T., Dessaint, J. P., and Capron, A. (1988). Effect of disodium cromoglycate on inflammatory cells bearing the FcεRII. *Int. J. Immunopharmacol.* **10**:227-236.

Vercelli, D., Jabara, H. H., Lee, B. W., Woodland, N., Geha, R. S., and
    Leung, D. Y. M. (1988). Human recombinant IL4 induces FcεRII/CD23
    on normal human monocytes. *J. Exp. Med.* **167**:1406-1416.

18

The Eosinophil and Asthma

PER VENGE and LENA HÅKANSSON

University Hospital
Uppsala, Sweden

I. Introduction

The eosinophil granulocyte was discovered in blood by Paul Ehrlich more than 100 years ago. During the following decades, the study of the function of the eosinophil attracted a considerable number of investigators and it was revealed that high counts of eosinophils in blood often were associated with diseases such as asthma and with parasitic infestations (Ellis, 1908; Huber and Koessler, 1922). It was even concluded that the massive tissue eosinophilia found in patients dying from status asthmaticus "...would undoubtedly greatly elucidate the pathogenesis of asthma." In spite of this, however, the interest in the eosinophil faded away and few reports emerged during the following 50 years. One conclusion drawn from that knowledge was that the eosinophil plays an important role in the protection of the organism against parasites and against the many harmful effects of the mast cell in the allergic reaction (Olsson and Venge, 1979; Weller and Goetzl, 1980; Gleich and Adolphson, 1986), a view still widely held in modern textbooks.

During the last decade the view of the eosinophil, however, has gradually changed. Today the eosinophil is regarded as a potent proinflammatory cell with considerable tissue-injuring capacity, possibly casually involved in the development of diseases such as asthma. This change in the view of the eosinophil has been prompted by the isolation of several highly cytotoxic secretory proteins from the eosinophil (Venge, 1985; Gleich and Adolphson, 1986) and the demonstration in several studies of direct correlations between eosinophil numbers and activities on one hand and the severity of diseases such as asthma on the other hand (Horn et al., 1975; Durham and Kay, 1985; Frigas and Gleich, 1986; Dahl et al., 1988).

In this chapter we will briefly review the present knowledge of the biochemistry and function of the human eosinophil and our knowledge of the relation of the eosinophil to human disease, notably asthma: is asthma an eosinophil disease? (Fig. 1). More details about the eosinophil can be found in the excellent monograph by Spry (1988).

II. Proteins of the Human Eosinophil Granulocyte

The human eosinophil is characterized morphologically by its content of eosin-staining granules, some of which contain typical crystalloid formations visible under the electron microscope. The protein content of the granules is dominated by four proteins (Venge, 1985; Gleich and Adolphson, 1986; Spry, 1988)

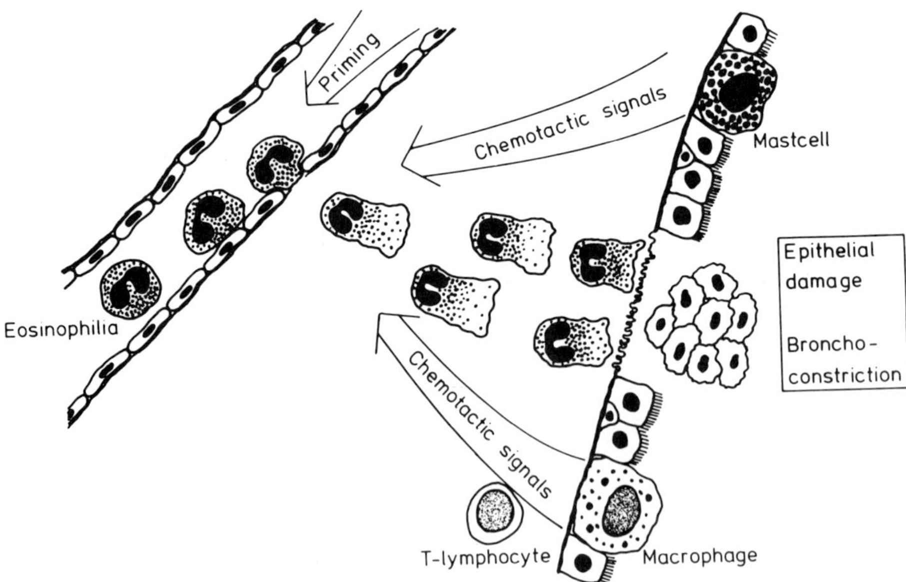

Figure 1 Asthma: an eosinophil disease?

(Fig. 2). These are the eosinophil cationic protein (ECP), eosinophil peroxidase (EPO), eosinophil protein X or eosinophil derived neurotoxin (EPX/EDN), and major basic protein (MBP), of which the latter is part of the crystalloids and the others are contained in the matrix of the granules. In addition to these four proteins, a protein that forms Charcot-Leyden crystals in tissues has been purified from the human eosinophil (Ackerman et al., 1980; Weller et al., 1980). The location of this protein is mainly the plasma membrane. Probably ECP and EXP/EDN are unique to the eosinophil (Slifman et al., 1989). MBP and the Charcot-Leyden crystal protein, however, are both found in basophils as well and enough MBP is found even in placental x-cells and giant cells. EPO has also been found in the uterus. Whether this reflects the fact that EPO is produced by other cells as well or merely that eosinophils are frequent cells in the uterus has not been established. Among blood cells, EPO is found uniquely in eosinophils.

The major characteristics of the four granule proteins are their high isoelectric points, above pH 11 for some of them. The first proteins to be purified were ECP and MBP. All four proteins have subsequently been purified both from normal eosinophils and from eosinophils of patients with the hypereosinophilic syndrome or chronic myeloid leukemia (Olsson and Venge,

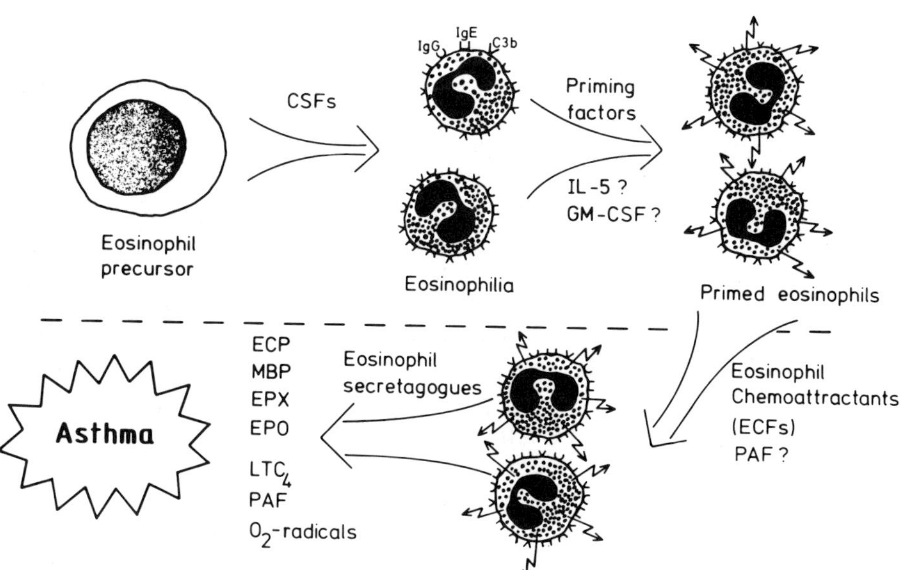

Figure 2 A working hypothesis on the relationship between the eosinophil and asthma.

1974; Gleich et al., 1976; Durack et al., 1981; Olsson et al., 1977; Carlson et al., 1985; Peterson and Venge, 1983; Peterson et al., 1988). The relative content of the four granule proteins varies with the source of eosinophils. In normal eosinophils, however, the content seems to be of a similar magnitude: around 10 μg/10^6 eosinophils.

ECP is a heterogeneous, but single-chained, protein with molecular weights ranging from 18 to 21 kDa. The heterogeneity is probably due to differences in glycosylation since various measures to eliminate the carbohydrates from the protein produces one single band on electrophoresis. Moreover N-terminal amino acid sequencing has suggested the presence of only one peptide sequence. ECP is very rich in basic amino acids such as arginine, which explains the high isoelectric point of the protein. ECP is a zinc-binding protein, binding approximately 2 moles of zinc per mole of protein. This zinc-binding property may explain the demonstration of eosinophil granules as organelles particularly rich in zinc. The N-terminal amino acid sequence revealed two important homologies. One was a 40% homology with EPX/ EDN and the other was a lesser, but significant, homology with the sequence of pancreatic ribonuclease. The latter homology suggested that ECP might have ribonuclease activity, which was also confirmed (Gleich et al., 1986; Gullberg et al., 1986). The homology with EPX/EDN indicates a close relationship and may explain why one of the monoclonal antibodies, EG2, produced against ECP also reacts with EPX/EDN (Tai et al., 1984).

Besides having a weak ribonuclease activity, ECP has been shown to have a number of other interesting biological activities. First, ECP is a cytotoxic molecule, which has the capacity to kill both mammalian and nonmammalian cells (see below and Venge and Peterson, 1989). ECP has also been demonstrated to affect a number of cellular activities in a noncytotoxic way. These include recent observations of the induction of histamine release from mast cells and basophils (Bergstrand et al., 1985) and the fact that ECP stimulates the hyaluronic acid production by human fibroblasts (Särnstrand et al., 1988). These findings relate to the role of eosinophil in allergic inflammation and tissue repair, respectively. Another finding of potentially great interest is the capacity of ECP to inhibit T-lymphocyte proliferation as a response to mitogens, but also in mixed leukocyte reactions (Peterson et al., 1986). The latter experiments were prompted by observations that ECP potently inhibited the response to purified protein derivative (PPD) (i.e., the tuberculin response) when injected into the skin of normal individuals (unpublished findings by Dahl and Venge). Hence, by virtue of its granule proteins, the eosinophil may regulate cellular-mediated immunological reactions.

One of the major clinical manifestations of patients with the hypereosinophilic syndrome is thromboembolism. It was therefore of interest that ECP, under certain conditions, had the capacity to shorten the coagulation time of plasma by mechanisms related to the enhancement of the activity of factor XII (Venge et al., 1979). In another study, the effect on fibrinolysis was investigated since earlier reports had suggested that eosinophils contained plasminogen-activating properties (Riddle and Barnhard, 1965). Thus, ECP was demonstrated to preactivate plasminogen, which means that the subsequent exposure of plasminogen to a plasminogen activator such as urokinase resulted in a considerable enhancement of the fibrinolytic activity (Dahl and Venge, 1979). The relevance of this finding is still uncertain, since no further indications have been obtained that link the eosinophil to the human fibrinolytic system. Finally, it should be mentioned that ECP, under certain conditions, is bound in complex with alpha-2-macroglobulin, probably to the site where the binding of proteolytic enzymes takes place (Peterson and Venge, 1987). In fact, the ECP binding to this site seems to require the prior exposure of alpha-2-macroglobulin to a limited proteolytic attack. Such proteolytic attack may be the consequence of the release of proteases from inflammatory cells (e.g., cathepsin G) from the neutrophils, or the consequence of protease formation during activation (e.g. thrombin) of the coagulation cascade and may represent an important means of neutralizing the actions of ECP.

EPX and EDN were purified independently (Durack et al., 1981; Peterson and Venge, 1983) and have now been shown to be identical proteins (Slifman et al., 1989). EPX/EDN is a single-chained protein. On gel filtration, EPX/EDN is a 23 kDa protein but on sodium dodecyl sulfate (SDS)-polyacrylamide gel electrophoresis the molecular weight is about 18 kDa. The difference in molecular weight is probably due to glycosylation of the protein molecule. As noted above, EPX/EDN has a 40% homology with ECP and shares at least one epitope with ECP as recognized by the monoclonal antibody EG2 (Tai et al., 1984). EPX/EDN is slightly less basic than ECP, which is partly reflected by the lower content of basic amino acids. EPX/EDN is a potent ribonuclease and about 100 times more active than ECP in this respect (Gullberg et al., 1986). Besides this activity, EPX/EDN also harbors some cytotoxic capacity (see below). As with ECP, EPX/EDN also potently inhibits T-lymphocyte proliferation in a noncytotoxic fashion and at concentrations similar to those of ECP (Peterson et al., 1986).

EPO is a two-chained protein with a heavy chain of 52 kDa and a light chain of 15 kDa (Carlson et al., 1985). EPO is distinct from the myeloperoxidase of neutrophils and antibodies prepared against either of the proteins do not show any cross-reactivity between the proteins. The amino acid composition is dominated by basic amino acids and the pH of EPO is above 11. EPO is a potent peroxidase and constitutes a potent cytotoxic mechanism in combination with a halide and H_2O_2 (see below). In addition, EPO may degranulate mast cells in a noncytotoxic manner (Henderson et al., 1980). Recently EPO was shown to be taken up by neutrophils. The uptake was specific and probably receptor related. It was speculated that this uptake might constitute an important regulatory mechanism that actively neutralizes the toxic effects of the peroxidase (Zabucchi et al., 1986).

MBP is a one-chained protein with a unique amino acid sequence. Based on the total amino acid sequence, the molecular weight has been estimated to be 13.8 kDa and the pI 10.9 (Wasmoen et al., 1988). The cDNA coding for MBP has been identified recently and indicated that MBP is translated as a preproprotein with a molecular weight of 25.2 kDa. The pro-portion is an acidic sequence and the properties of the pro-portion of the proMBP suggested that it may mask the cytotoxic activity of MBP and protect the eosinophil from damage during packing and processing of MBP. MBP is not unique to the eosinophil, but is also found in several other cells. The major biological function of the eosinophilic MBP is related to its cytotoxic activities (see below). In addition MBP, as ECP and EPO, degranulates mast cells (Gleich and Adolphson, 1986).

In addition to the four proteins ECP, EPO, EPX/EDN, and MBP, the human eosinophil contains a number of less well characterized substances (Venge, 1985; Gleich and Adolphson, 1986; Spry, 1988). These are an arylsulfatase, a collagenase, a histaminase, and a phosphoplipase D. The putative function of some of these enzymes is the neutralization of mast cell mediators such as the sulfidopeptide leukotrienes, histamine, and platelet-activating factor (PAF). These activities have formed the basis for the hypothesis that the function of the eosinophil would be primarily to regulate the activities of the mast cell in the allergic reaction.

III. Secretion of Preformed and Nonpreformed Components of the Human Eosinophil

A. Granule Proteins

The granules of human eosinophils show a great morphological heterogeneity. Histochemical staining has demonstrated two different populations: one made up of peroxidase-positive large, crystalloid-containing granules and another by small peroxidase-negative granules containing no crystals. ECP and EPO were shown to be present in the large, crystalloid-containing granules (Egesten et al., 1986). In addition, ECP was observed in the small peroxidase-negative granules. In preliminary experiments, eosinophil granules were separated on sucrose density gradients and showed at least four peaks containing eosinophil proteins (Peterson et al., 1989). The densest peak contained all the EPO that was found and approximately 40% of either ECP and EPX. The two intermediate peaks contained together approximately 40% of ECP and 30% of EPX. The least dense peak, which coincided with the membrane fraction, contained approximately 10% of ECP and 20% of EPX. Hence the granules of human eosinophils seems to be made up of two distinct populations: one peroxidase-negative and one peroxidase-positive, of which the former may be present in more than one subpopulation.

Early investigations showed that optimal ECP release from human eosinophils was achieved when the cells were exposed to large particles such as Sephadex G-15 and that the opsonin required, presumably C3b, was derived from the incubation of the particles in serum (Winqvist et al., 1984). Others demonstrated the release of peroxidase and MBP but not ECP after exposure of hypodense cells to IgE complexes, in contrast to the release of ECP that occurred when the eosinophils were exposed to IgG complexes (Khalife et al., 1986). Two conclusions were drawn from these studies. One was that optimal release of granule proteins from eosinophils requires the presence of the opsonin on a surface. The other was that release of eosinophil granule proteins may occur differentially, depending on the stimulus to which the cell is exposed. The question of differential release of eosinophil granule proteins was studied further by simultaneous measurement of ECP, EPX/EDN, and EPO after exposure of normal eosinophils to various stimuli. When serum-opsonized or unopsonized Sephadex particles were used, significant amounts of ECP and EPX/EDN were released. The release of these two proteins was completely parallel, in contrast to the release of EPO, which was negligble (Peterson et al., 1989). However, when the release was initiated by the particular protein kinase C active lipid IpOCOC$_9$, the release of EPX/EDN was on average three to four times that of ECP: 30-40% versus 10% of the total cellular content. With IpOCOC$_9$, 3-5% of the total cellular content of EPO was released. These data support the view that differential release of granule proteins from human eosinophils does take place.

B. Other Components

The eosinophils share many of the properties of neutrophils. Thus, both cell types respond to chemotactic signals and are able to phagocytose opsonized particles, although the capacity of the eosinophil in the latter respect seems to be inferior to that of the neutrophil. Also both cells respond to certain stimuli by an oxidative burst, which is the enhanced uptake of oxygen and the formation of various oxygen-derived toxic metabolites such as O_2^-, H_2O_2, and $OH^.$ (Pincus et al., 1981). Most studies indicate that eosinophils and neutrophils, among inflammatory cells, are the two most potent producers of such toxic metabolites. Another consequence of the receptor-mediated stimulation of eosinophils is the production and secretion of various lipid mediators including prostaglandins, leukotrienes, and platelet-activating factor (PAF) (Lee et al., 1984). PGE$_2$ was first described as the eosinophil-derived inhibitor (EDI) of mast cell secretion of histamine (Hubscher, 1975). Eosinophils seem to produce only directly acting leukotrienes such as LTC_4, in contrast to the neutrophils, which primarily seem to produce the chemotactic leukotriene LTB_4 (Shaw et al., 1984; Verhagen et al., 1984; Bruynzeel et al., 1986). It is notable that the production of LTC_4 and PAF by eosinophils is of the same magnitude as that of other cells, such as the mast cell.

IV. Cytotoxic Activities of the Human Eosinophil

One of the most conspicuous features of the eosinophil is its cytotoxic potential, with the capacity to cause injury to almost any mammalian or non-mammalian cell. The cytotoxic property of the eosinophil is dependent on both oxygen-dependent and oxygen-independent mechanisms. The former is made up of the toxic oxygen metabolites and EPO, and the latter by the three granule proteins ECP, EPX/EDN, and MBP. These two principally different mechanisms most likely to have different targets and probably work together to obtain maximal effects. Thus it has been demonstrated that the helminthotoxic activity of ECP is greatly enhanced by previous or simultaneous exposure of the helminth to nontoxic concentrations of toxic oxygen metabolites and vice versa (Yazdanbakhsh et al., 1987).

ECP, EPO, and MBP kill the schistosomula of *Schistosoma mansoni* in vitro (Butterworth et al., 1979; McLaren et al., 1981, 1984; Jong et al., 1981). EPO needs the presence of H_2O_2 and a halide to kill schistosomula efficiently. Since H_2O_2 is one of the products formed during activation of the eosinophil in contact with an opsonized parasite, it is reasonable to postulate that this mechanism might occur in vivo as well. The killing of schistosomula by ECP occurred at considerably lower concentrations than the concentrations needed for MBP, which suggests that ECP in this particular model is more cytotoxic than MBP (Ackerman et al., 1985). If lung-stage larvae of *Schistosoma mansoni* were used as target organisms instead, ECP was almost without any effect. This was in contrast to EPX, since this protein, which was without any appreciable effects on the schistosomula, quite efficiently killed the lung-stage larvae. The reason for these differences in cytotoxic activities towards the two different forms of *Schistosoma mansoni* is not known but indicates that their modes of action in killing parasites are different. In addition, EPO and MBP were shown to kill other parasites such as *T. cruzi* and *T. spiralis* (Gleich and Adolphson, 1986). Even *P. falciparum* was killed by eosinophils by a mechanism partly dependent on ECP (Kierszenbaum et al., 1986). With the possible exception of EPO and the toxic oxygen metabolites, the granule proteins do not seem to be able to kill bacteria.

Over 50 years ago Gordon described the development of ataxia and other symptoms in rabbits after injection of extracts of lymph node material from patients with Hodgkin's disease into the ventricles of the brain (Gordon, 1932). The most conspicuous histological finding was destruction of the Purkinje cells of the cerebellum. More recent findings suggested that the neurotoxic effect of the lymph node material was related to the number of eosinophils present in the extract (Durack et al., 1979). Attempts were made to define the neurotoxic agent of the eosinophils. The protein thus identified was purified and given the name eosinophil-derived neurotoxin (EDN) (Durack et al., 1981). In other experiments, the purified proteins ECP and EPX were injected into the ventricles of the brains of experimental animals (Fredans et al., 1982). These experiments showed that both proteins were capable of producing the clinical symptoms described by Gordon and the typical histological picture with Purkinje cell destruction. In these experiments, ECP was about 100 times more potent than EPX/EDN and induced the Gordon phenomenon within some weeks after injection of as little as 60 ng protein. Hence, both ECP and EPX/EDN are capable of producing the phenomenon described by Gordon; however, this effect is nonspecific and unselective since, depending on the deposition of the material, the proteins would destroy any cell or structure (Fredans et al., 1985).

Few studies in humans have actually confirmed the neurotoxic activity of the eosinophil in vivo. It is therefore of interest that very high ECP levels were demonstrated in the cerebrospinal fluid of those patients who had a poor outcome after bacterial infections of the brain (Hällgren et al., 1983). It is also noteworthy that many patients with the hypereosinophilic syndrome have both central nervous and peripheral nervous symptoms as indications of the neurotoxic activity of the eosinophil (Spry, 1988). Recently some interesting findings were published from a patient with esophageal achalasia secondary to gastric cancer. In this patient, a massive infiltration of activated eosinophils was seen in the muscalaris of the esophagus with signs of secretion of large amounts of ECP. Simultaneously, a nearly total absence of the neurotransmittors vasoactive intestinal peptide (VIP), substance P, and acetylcholinesterase (AChE) was observed (Fredans et al., 1989).

Most studies of the toxic effects of eosinophil products on cells of the respiratory tract have been performed with MBP. Micromolar concentrations of MBP caused detachment and injury to pneumocytes (Ayars et al., 1985) and the epithelium was extensively damaged, producing a histological picture reminiscent of the pathological changes seen in human bronchial asthma (Frigas et al., 1980). Also, MBP impairs ciliary beating and may, through its epithelial actions, be involved in the development of bronchial hyperreactivity (Gleich et al., 1988). Instillation of small amounts of ECP produced results similar to those with MBP: epithelial cell damage and patchy denudation of the epithelial cell layer in both the trachea and bronchi, and cell plugging (Dahl et al., 1988). Both ECP and MBP were demonstrated by immunohistochemical techniques in the lung tissue of patients who died from asthma (Frigas and Gleich, 1986; Dahl et al., 1988). The staining suggested extracellular deposition of the proteins mainly in association with destroyed epithelium. More recently, paranasal tissues from patients with bronchial asthma and chronic sinusitis were examined (Harlin et al., 1988). This examination showed extensive infiltration of eosinophils and a striking association between the presence of extracellular deposition of MBP and damage to the sinus mucosa. More direct evidence of secretion of ECP was obtained when elevated levels of ECP were measured in bronchoalveolar lung fluid obtained during the late asthmatic reaction after allergen inhalation challenge of asthmatic individuals (DeMonchy et al., 1985) and similarly in nasal washings in patients with allergic rhinitis (Linder et al., 1987).

Further evidence of the cytotoxic activities of the eosinophil granule proteins has come from the study of patients with diseases of the gastrointestinal tract, such as Crohn's disease and adult celiac disease, and also from the direct demonstration of the toxic affect of guinea pig MBP on intestinal cells (Gleich and Adolphson, 1986). Intestinal fluid was obtained from the small intestine of patients with Crohn's disease and adult celiac disease. These fluids showed in some cases highly elevated concentrations of ECP compared to normals (Hällgren et al., 1989). Biopsy specimens were also taken from the jejunal cell wall of patients with adult celiac disease. These showed a remarkable infiltration of eosinophils in areas with ulceration. Staining for ECP suggested a heavy extracellular deposition of ECP in these areas, consistent with active degranulation of the eosinophils. This picture was in contrast with areas of undamaged intestinal wall where eosinophils were also present but extracellular deposition of ECP was not observed. The eosinophil had probably taken part in the processes leading to ulceration of the intestinal wall in adult celiac disease, and ulceration might have been caused by, among other things, the cytotoxic eosinophil granule proteins. Few indications of neutrophil involvement (i.e., cathepsin-G-staining cells) were observed in the areas of damaged tissues, suggesting the selective involvement of eosinophils in the processes.

The examples cited above demonstrate that the eosinophil may have the capacity to destroy almost any cell, mammalian or nonmammalian. To study the mechanism of action of the cytotoxicity of the granule proteins, a lipid vesicle permeability assay was used. This assay demonstrated that the proteins ECP and EPX/EDN caused leakiness of the vesicles to monovalent ions and, to a certain extent, also to divalent ions (Ding-E. Young et al., 1986).

Further studies with phospholipid planar lipid bilayers showed typical changes in the conductance when exposed to ECP, which indicated opening of individual channels in the membrane. These pores were remarkably resistant to closing by high transmembrane voltage, similarly to poly-C9 channels. Further experiments with human eosinophils indicated that ECP was the dominating pore-forming granular protein, with EPX causing leakage by cross-linking membrane structures instead of making pores. Ultrastructural studies of ECP-exposed lipid bilayers have identified ringlike structures in liposomes approximately 40 Å wide (Ding-E. Young, unpublished data). ECP therefore belongs to the growing family of pore-forming proteins produced by a variety of cells such as cytotoxic T lymphocytes (Ding-E. Young, 1985).

V. Eosinophils in Asthma

A role for the eosinophil in asthma has been assumed since the beginning of this century based on the demonstration of blood and lung eosinophilia in patients with asthma. A specific role, good or bad, however, has remained elusive. Horn et al. (1975) demonstrated a relationship between the extent of blood eosinophilia and severity of asthma as measured by several tests of lung function. Our own studies demonstrated that the eosinophils secreted their granule proteins, such as ECP, in both blood (Dahl et al., 1978) and the lung (DeMonchy et al., 1985) when the asthmatic patient was challenged by inhalation of an allergen, which would suggest an active participation of the eosinophil in the processes involved in asthma. Other indications of active participation are the studies showing huge concentrations of the granule protein MBP in sputum from asthmatic patients (Dor et al., 1984).

Recent studies have extended the observations by Horn et al. (1975) and demonstrated close relationships between the reactivity of the airways and the activity and number of eosinophils. Positive correlations between eosinophil counts and serum levels of ECP and the reactivity of the lung after allergen challenge have been found, and it was suggested that measurements of ECP or EPX might be used to predict the occurrence of a late asthmatic reaction (Venge et al., 1988). Serum levels of ECP and EPX were significantly raised before challenge in those patients who developed a definite LAR. Also in patients with an equivocal LAR the protein levels were significantly raised above those obtained in patients who had no tendency to develop LAR. In another study, a highly significant linear correlation was found between the extent of exercise-induced asthma and serum ECP levels before exercise, suggesting a relationship between the activity of the eosinophil and this hyper-reactivity of the asthmatic lung (Venge et al., 1989a). As was also demonstrated after allergen inhalation challenge, the ECP levels increased initially in some patients after exercise. This increment was, however, replaced by a reduction of ECP and the levels 60 min after exercise were even significantly lower than the prechallenge levels. In asthmatic patients without exercise-induced asthma (EIA), the prechallenge levels of ECP were significantly lower than in the EIA group and exercise induced no reduction of serum ECP. A reduction in serum ECP levels that is seen also after allergen challenge (Dahl et al., 1978; Venge et al., 1983, 1988) has been suggested to be due to an enhanced rate of elimination of ECP. This could be due to binding of ECP to some structure produced as a consequence of the processes involved in the asthmatic process.

Binding to alpha-2-macroglobulin has been suggested as one such principle, since ECP forms complexes with alpha-2-macroglobulin under conditions that may be operative during an acute allergic process (Peterson and Venge, 1987) (see above). The glucocorticosteroid budesonide and, to a lesser degree, disodium cromoglycate but not beta-2-agonists seem to prevent the challenge-induced reduction in serum ECP. No reduction was seen after histamine or metacholine challenge, which indicates that the reduction is not a mere consequence of the bronchoconstriction as such.

Other indications of a relationship between lung hyperreactivity in asthma and the activity of eosinophils have come from studies on atopic individuals with seasonal allergic symptoms. In this group of patients, serum ECP levels rose significantly during the pollen season (Rak et al., 1988). Lung reactivity as measured by histamine PC_{20} also increased during the season and correlated significantly with the ECP levels. In that same study, a group treated by immunotherapy exhibited no changes in ECP, a lower level of expressed hyperresponsiveness, and diminished use of mediation during the season. Increased numbers of eosinophils and somewhat higher levels of ECP were also present in the lavage fluids obtained in the untreated patients, whereas among the group receiving immunotherapy no such increments were seen (Rak et al., 1989a). In a number of other lavage studies involving asthmatic patients, signs of eosinophil accumulation and activation in the lung have been obtained and been related to the development of LAR, increased airway reactivity to histamine, and increased number of sloughed bronchial epithelial cells (Diaz et al., 1984; Lam et al., 1987; Wardlaw et al., 1988). It should, however, be pointed out that selective lung eosinophilia is not invariably found in asthma. Thus, in patients challenged with toluene diisocyanate the presence of neutrophils was marked with only slight infiltration of eosinophils (Mapp et al., 1987).

Suggestions have been made that the eosinophil counts might differentiate between allergic and nonallergic asthma. However, as in allergic asthma, the blood eosinophil count is almost invariably raised in nonallergic, intrinsic asthma (Venge et al., 1977; Azevedo et al., 1980; Dahl and Venge, 1982; Azofra et al., 1986; Frigas and Gleich, 1986). Blood eosinophil counts were inversely correlated to both histamine PC_{20} and forced expiratory volume in 1s (FEV_1) but with no difference between the two groups of asthmatic patients (Taylor and Luksza, 1987). The function of the eosinophils with respect to their capacity to produce LTC_4 was identical to that of cells from patients with extrinsic and intrinsic asthma (Taniguchi et al., 1985). We studied serum ECP levels in the two groups and found a huge variation in the group of patients with intrinsic asthma with both very high and, as in the group with extrinsic asthma, often unexpectedly low levels. From this study, it was apparent that the variation in serum ECP was much greater than in the group with allergic asthma, and the results included a higher proportion of patients with these very low ECP levels. One possible explanation for these unexpectedly low ECP levels is discussed above and may by itself be an indication of an active process in the lung. The huge variations in ECP levels may, in fact, suggest that the group of patients with intrinsic asthma is more heterogeneous than the group with allergic asthma. One identified subgroup of patients with intrinsic asthma may actually be acetylsalicylic-acid (ASA)-sensitive patients (Mullarkey et al., 1986). BAL fluids obtained in these patients contain much higher numbers of eosinophils than in BAL from patients with allergic asthma (Godard et al., 1982).

VI. Attraction of Eosinophils to the Asthmatic Lung

The formation of eosinophil chemotactic activity in allergic processes was suggested by a number of findings during the early 1970s. A tetrapeptide, eosinophil chemotactic factor A (ECF-A), showed some eosinophil chemotactic property (reviewed in Weller and Goetzl, 1980), but its relevance has been questioned. Eosinophil chemotactic activity (ECA) has recently been demonstrated in the serum of patients with asthma after allergen challenge (Metzger et al., 1986; Håkansson et al., 1989a). Since the major ECA has salient similarities to heat-labile neutrophil chemotactic activity (HL-NCA) and therefore most likely is identical to HL-NCA, we will describe some of the important findings related to this latter activity.

Heat-stable NCA was first discovered in serum after inhalation challenge of asthmatic patients in 1977 (Atkins et al., 1977). We discovered some years later the formation also of HL-NCA in serum after inhalation challenge (Venge et al., 1982). HL-NCA eluted at a position corresponding to a molecular weight of about 150 kDa (Håkansson et al., 1989b). Our present data suggest that the activity is a complex made up by at least one large molecule (150 kDa) that serves as a cofactor and one small molecule (400 D), which appears to be the actual chemotactic principle (Håkansson and Venge, to be published). In contrast to HS-NCA, which seems to parallel the changes in lung function HL-NCA peaks in serum well after the early airway reaction: 30-120 min after allergen provocation (Venge et al., 1982, 1987). HL-NCA does not appear in serum after exercise-induced asthma or after challenge of asthmatic patients with bronchoconstrictors such as histamine and metacholine (Venge et al., 1989b). The former is clearly in contrast to the findings with HS-NCA. The origin of HL-NCA is unknown. A correlation to serum lysozyme levels after allergen inhalation challenge suggested that it might be released from monocytes/macrophages (Venge et al., 1982). Both HL-NCA and HS-NCA levels are raised in patients with mastocytosis (Granérus et al., 1988) suggesting the possibility of a relation to the mast cell, either direct or indirect. Others have demonstrated the production of eosinophil chemotactic activities by alveolar macrophages from asthmatic patients (Gosset et al., 1984).

The peak activity of HL-NCA after inhalation challenge was closely correlated to the extent of the ensuing late asthmatic reaction, although these two variables were not related in time (Venge et al., 1987). Hence one prerequisite for the subsequent attraction of inflammatory cells to the lung and the development of the late reaction may be the formation of HL-NCA. The pharmacological inhibition of the late reaction after challenge was also associated with a significant reduction in HL-NCA in serum. Finally, HL-NCA was normal in atopic asthmatic patients out of season whereas the activity during a pollen season rose significantly to levels, in many cases, above those seen after allergen inhalation challenge in the laboratory (Håkansson et al., 1989a). It was interesting that immunotherapy completely abrogated this rise during pollen season (Rak et al., 1989a). The prevention of the formation of HL-NCA by immunotherapy was accompanied by a clear reduction in the patients' use of medication, which further suggests the relevance of this particular chemotactic activity.

As indicated above, the ECA found in serum of asthmatic patients after allergen challenge behaved almost identically to the HL-NCA and led to the hypothesis that the two activities might be identical. Further studies demonstrated that ECA was heat-labile and that 80% of the eosinophil chemotactic activity cochromatographed on gel filtration with HL-NCA. Thus the major ECA also had a molecular weight of about 150 kDa (Håkansson et al., 1989). The remaining 20% of the activity eluted in the void volume and at a position corresponding to about 40 kDa. The former activity was also heat-stable, suggesting a resemblance to HS-NCA. The important implications of our conclusion is that the clinical observations with HL-NCA probably are valid for ECA as well.

All the above results on chemotactic activities in serum of asthmatic patients were obtained in studies in which patients had been challenged by their allergen either in the laboratory as a single provocation or during a defined pollen season. The question of whether these activities are present also in day-to-day asthma has only recently been addressed. Thus, in one study on 57 patients with an asthmatic disease of varying severities, significantly raised ECA was found (Håkansson et al., 1989). HL-NCA, on the other hand, appeared to be unaltered, which differentiates these results from those discussed above. The reason for this is not clear but may relate to the sensitivity of the methods. Raised chemokinetic activities for both eosinophils and neutrophils were observed, with a significant negative correlation between the eosinophil chemokinetic activity and lung function as measured by PEF. In this study no differences were found between patients with allergic and non-allergic asthma. These results therefore suggest that eosinophil chemotactic and chemokinetic activities found in the circulation are parts of the processes involved in the creation of inflammation in the asthmatic lung.

The studies on serum chemotactic activities in patients with asthma raise some important questions. Are the chemotactic activities actually produced in the lung and is their production related to the inflammatory cell accumulation in the lung? These questions have been addressed in two clinical studies that used bronchoalveolar lavage. In one study a small group of asthmatic individuals were lavaged twice after inhalation allergen challenge (DeMonchy et al., in preparation): once before taking any medication and once after a period of inhalation of the glucocorticosteroid budesonide. Previous studies had shown that inhalation challenge would produce a selective accumulation of eosinophils in the BAL fluid and an increment in extracellular concentrations of ECP (DeMonchy et al., 1985). After pretreatment with budesonide there was a tendency towards a reduction in eosinophil numbers and a significant reduction in ECP concentrations in BAL fluid. Large amounts of ECA were found in BAL fluids before treatment. After budesonide treatment the ECA was significantly reduced. Thus the effects of budesonide on ECA in BAL fluids were similar to those observed earlier in serum after allergen challenge (Venge et al., 1987). The reduction in ECA in BAL samples was closely related to the inhibition of the late reaction by budesonide. In the second study (Rak et al., 1989b), another group of patients with allergic asthma were subjected to bronchoalveolar lavage before and during the pollen season. Half of the patients were treated by immunotherapy. Before the season, low numbers of inflammatory cells were recovered in BAL fluids. During the season, the number of eosinophils rose more than 400% with no alteration in the number of neutrophils. The concentration of ECP was slightly increased whereas the concentration of myeloperoxidase, as a marker of neutrophils, was unaltered, thus supporting the selective accumulation of eosinophils during season. Eosinophil and neutrophil chemotactic activities, however, were both significantly raised in BAL fluids during season. Again immunotherapy completely abrogated the formation of any chemotactic activity. Also, the number of eosinophils and the ECP concentration remained unaltered during season in the patients receiving immunotherapy.

These results clearly support the hypothesis expressed above of a causal relationship between the formation of chemotactic activities and the accumulation of inflammatory cells to the lung and the development of asthmatic symptoms. It is also of interest that the ECA recovered in the BAL fluid were linearly and positively correlated to the activity measured in serum of the same patients, which suggests that these activities are closely related. One study showed the production of both eosinophil and neutrophil chemotactic activity by alveolar macrophages from asthmatic patients (Gosset et al., 1984). The rough characterization of these activities suggested a relationship to LTB_4. Another chemotactic agent, PAF, is produced by alveolar macrophages and is a more potent chemotactic stimulus to eosinophils than is LTB_4 (Wardlaw et al., 1986; Håkansson et al., 1987).

Thus both eosinophil and neutrophil chemotactic activities were increased in the BAL fluids, but only the eosinophils accumulated. This apparent paradox may be explained by the observations that eosinophils but not neutrophils obtained from asthmatic patients showed an enhanced chemotactic and chemokinetic response to asthmatic serum containing HL-NCA, normal complement-activated serum (i.e., predominantly C5 fragments), and the tripeptide fMLP (Håkansson et al., 1989). These results demonstrate that asthmatic eosinophils may be primed and that one explanation for the selective accumulation of eosinophils in the lung may be related to this. Furthermore, the chemokinetic responsiveness of the eosinophils was positively correlated to the serum ECP levels, which indicate that similar mechanism are operative in the priming of the chemokinetic and the secretory response of the eosinophil. In addition, the increased responsiveness was reduced in those patients who experienced improvement in their asthma after 5 weeks of treatment, suggesting the relevance of the priming phenomenon and that the chemotactic responsiveness of the asthmatic eosinophils was related to blood eosinophil numbers. These facts could suggest that the mechanisms that accelerate eosinophil production are identical or related to those that prime mature cells. Thus, colony-stimulating factors (CSFs) and other hormone-like compounds such as the interleukins (ILs), notably IL5, which are believed to be important components of eosinophilopoiesis, have been shown to prime eosinophils in vitro (Hamblin, 1988). We therefore hypothesize that one important mechanism in vivo for achieving selective accumulation of inflammatory cells is the selective priming of inflammatory cells rather than the production of selective chemotactic signals.

VII. Conclusion

A variety of circumstantial evidence suggests that the eosinophil is intimately involved in the inflammatory process in the lung of asthmatic individuals. The precise role of the eosinophil, however, is still not well understood. Our own working hypothesis is depicted in Figure 2 and assumes that the eosinophil is causally involved in the creation of the major symptoms of asthma, such as reversible bronchoconstriction and airway hyperresponsiveness to both immunological and nonimmunological stimuli. However, eosinophil involvement may not be more than one of many components of the inflammatory process of the asthmatic lung, which can develop such symptoms. The virtual absence of eosinophil infiltration in some patients dying of asthma and the fact that the neutrophil in some situations seem to be the predominant cell tell us that the process is much more complex than depicted in Figure 2.

Blood eosinophilia is almost invariably found in patients with asthma and is probably a consequence of the production of various factors by T lymphocytes and macrophages such as CSFs and ILs. These same components also have the capacity to prime mature eosinophils to an enhanced responsiveness that is manifest in several ways. One is the enhanced response to chemotactic and chemokinetic stimuli and another is the enhanced propensity to secrete toxic oxygen metabolites and granule proteins. The selective accumulation in the lung of eosinophils requires the production of some kind of signals tentatively termed chemotactic factors. The molecular identity of these is uncertain, but they probably include both high-molecular-weight protein molecules and molecular-weight peptides and lipids, such as PAF. The chemotactic signals may originate from several sources such as macrophages, mast cells, T lymphocytes, and epithelial cells.

Discussion

Kay: In our experience, T-cell products (including cytokines) are not chemotactic for eosinophils, at least not compared to PAF. They do, however, prime eosinophils for PAF-induced migration.

Venge: The inhibition of T-lymphocyte proliferation by ECP is not restricted to the case when you stimulate with PHA, but also takes place in a mixed leukocyte reaction. The effect is not due to the binding of ECP to PPD and PHA.

Fuller: Could you tell me what the effects are of commonly used antiasthma treatments on eosinophil function?

Barnes: We have demonstrated that β-agonists have no inhibitory effect on eosinophil degranulation. Furthermore, theophylline has no inhibitory effect at therapeutic concentrations. These findings are consistent with the view that eosinophils may be important in bronchial hyperreactivity, since neither β-agonists nor theophylline are effective in reducing hyperreactivity.

Venge: We have shown that budesonide potently inhibits ECP release. However, we have been unable to demonstrate any appreciable effect of budesonide on eosinophil migration. β-Agonists and cromoglycates seem to have limited effects. We have also heard that the antihistamine Cetirizin inhibits eosinophil chemotaxis.

Schleimer: We have performed studies that support the hypothesis that selective recruitment of eosinophils may be related to priming of the leukocyte rather than the release of specific chemoattractants. Thus all chemoattractants and endothelial activators tested induce a nonselective adherence of leukocytes in an in vitro adherence model, which suggests that selectivity may not be expressed at the level of either the factor or the endothelial cell.

Is it possible that other types of heterogeneity (e.g., density or state of maturity), rather than the state of priming, may explain the differences in chemotaxis and chemokinesis of blood eosinophils between allergic and normal patients?

Venge: We do not know whether the priming of the eosinophils is related to the density. It might be so that the hypodense are the more responsive.

Kay: The real question is "How do eosinophils accumulate at the site of allergic tissue reaction?" Present evidence suggests that there may be at least three important mechanisms:

1. Hyperadhesiveness of eosinophils to vascular endothelium through the elaboration of agents such as PAF and IL5
2. Priming of eosinophils by IL5 for selective locomotion (to PAF for instance)
3. Increased tissue survival of eosinophils (GM-CSF, IL3, IL5).

Acknowledgment

Parts of the studies cited in this chapter were supported by grants from the Swedish Medical Research Council, The Swedish National Environment Protection Board, and AB Draco, Lund.

References

Ackerman, S. J., Loegering, D. A., and Gleich, G. J. (1980). The human eosinophil Charcot-Leyden crystal protein: biochemical characteristics and measurements by radioimmunoassay. *J. Immunol.* **125**:2118-2117.

Ackerman, S. J., Gleich, G. J., Loegering, D. A., Richardson, B. A., and Butterworth, A. E. (1985). Comparative toxicity of purified human eosinophil granule cationic proteins for schistosomula of *Schistosoma mansoni*. *Am. J. Trop. Med. Hyg.* **34**:735-745.

Atkins, P. C., Norman, M., Weiner, H., and Zweiman, B. (1977). Release of neutrophil chemotactic activity during immediate hypersensitivity reactions in humans. *Am. Intern. Med.* **86**:415-418.

Ayars, G. H., Altman, L. C., Gleich, G. J., Loegering, D. A., and Baker, C. B. (1985). Eosinophil- and eosinophil granule-mediated pneumocyte injury. *J. Allergy Clin. Immunol.* **76**:595-604.

Azevedo, M., Castel-Branco, M. G., Mendes, A., Oliveira, J. F., Carvalho, A. S., Almeida, J., and Grenha, F. I. (1980). T and B lymphocytes, total serum IgE and peripheral eosinophils in bronchial asthma. *Allergol. Immunopathol.* **8**:189-196.

Azofra, J., Sastre, J., Gomez, B., Rivas, F., and Sastre, A. (1986). Some cytological aspects of bronchial asthma. *Allergol. Immunopathol.* **14**: 295-301.

Bergstrand, H., Lundquist, B., Peterson, B.-Å., Peterson, C. G. B., and Venge, P. (1985). Eosinophil derived cationic proteins and human leukocyte histamine release. In *Inflammation. Basic Mechanisms, Tissue Injuring Principles and Clinical Models*. Edited by P. Venge and A. Lindbom. Stockholm, Almqvist & Wiksell International, pp. 361-366.

Bruynzeel, P. L. B., Kok, P. T. M., Vitor, R. J., and Verhagen, J. (1986). On the optimal conditions of LTC4 formation by human eosinophils in vitro. *Prostaglandin Leuktrienes Med.* **20**:11-16.

Butterworth, A. E., Wassom, D. L., Gleich, G. J., Loegering, D. A., and David, J. R. (1979). Damage to schistosomula of *Schistosoma mansoni* induced directly by eosinophil major basic protein. *J. Immunol.* **122**: 221-229.

Carlson, M. G. Ch., Peterson, C. G. B., and Venge, P. (1985). Human eosinophil peroxidase: purification and characterization. *J. Immunol.* **134**:1875-1879.

Dahl, R., and Venge, P. (1979). Enhancement of urokinase-induced plasminogen activation by the cationic protein of human granulocytes. *Thromb. Res.* **14**:599-608.

Dahl, R., and Venge, P. (1982). Role of the eosinophil in bronchial asthma. *Eur. J. Respir. Dis.* **63**(suppl. 122):23-28.

Dahl, R., Venge, P., and Olsson, I. (1978). Variations of blood eosinophils and eosinophil cationic protein in serum in patients with bronchial asthma. Studies during inhalation challenge tests. *Allergy* **33**:211-215.

Dahl, R., Fredens, K., Marcussen, C., and Venge, P. (1985). Eosinophils and bronchial injury. Annual Meeting, European Academy of Allergology and Clinical Immunology, abstract no. 63976.

Dahl, R., Venge, P., and Fredens, K. (1988). The eosinophil. In *Asthma: Basic Mechanisms and Clinical Management*. Edited by P. J. Barnes, I. Rodger, and N. Thomson. London, Academic Press, pp. 115-130.

DeMonchy, J. G. R., Kauffman, H. F., Venge, P., Koter, G. H., Jansen, H. M., Sluiter, H. J., and DeVries, K. (1985). Bronchoalveolar eosinoophilia during allergen-induced late asthmatic reactions. *Am. Rev. Respir. Dis.* **131**:373-376.

Diaz, P., Galleguillos, F. R., Gonzalez, M. C., Pantin, C., and Kay, A. B. (1984). Bronchoalveolar lavage in asthma: the effect of disodium cromoglycate (cromolyn) on leukocyte counts, immunoglobulins, and complement. *J. Allergy Clin. Immunol.* **74**:41-48.

Ding-E Young, J. (1985). Cytolytic proteins. In *Inflammation*. Edited by P. Venge and A. Lindbom. Stockholm, Almqvist & Wiksell International, pp. 329-340.

Ding-E Young, J., Peterson, C. G. B., Venge, P., and Cohn, Z. A. (1986). Mechanism of membrane damage mediated by human eosinophil cationic protein. *Nature* **321**:613-616.

Dor, P. J., Ackerman, S. J., and Gleich, G. J. (1984). Charot-Leyden crystal protein and eosinophil granule major basic protein in sputum of patients with respiratory disease. *Am. Rev. Respir. Dis.* **130**:1072-1077.

Durack, D. T., Sumi, S. M., and Klebanoff, S. J. (1979). Neurotoxicity of human eosinophils. *Proc. Natl. Acad. Sci. U.S.A.* **76**:1443-1447.

Durack, D. T., Ackerman, S. J., Loegering, D. A., and Gleich, G. J. (1981). Purification of human eosinophil-derived neurotoxin. *Proc. Natl. Acad. Sci. U.S.A.* **78**:5165-5169.

Durham, S. R., and Kay, A. B. (1985). Eosinophils, bronchial hyperreactivity and late-phase asthmatic reactions. *Clin. Allergy* **15**:411-418.

Egesten, A., Alumets, J., von Mecklenburg, C., Palmegren, M., and Olsson. I. (1986). Localization of eosinophil cationic protein, major basic protein, and eosinophil peroxidase in human eosinophils by immunoelectron microscopic technique. *J. Histochem. Cytochem.* **34**:1399-1403.

Ellis, A. G. (1908). The pathologic anatomy of bronchial asthma. *Am. J. Med. Sci.* **136**:407.

Filley, W. V., Holley, K. E., Kephart, G. M., and Gleich, G. J. (1982a). Identification by immunofluorescence of eosinophil granule major basic protein in lung tissues of patients with bronchial asthma. *Lancet* **2**:11-16.

Fredens, K., Dahl, R., and Venge, P. (1982). The Gordon phenomenon induced by the eosinophil cationic protein and eosinophil protein x. *J. Allergy Clin. Immunol.* **70**:361-366.

Fredens, K., Dahl, R., and Venge, P. (1985). Eosinophils and cellular injury. *NER Allergy Proc.* **6**:346-351.

Fredens, K., Tottrup, A., Kristensen Bayer, I., Dahl, R., Jacobsen, N. O., Funch-Jensen, P., and Thommesen, P. (1989). Severe destruction of esophageal nerves in a patient with achalasia secondary to gastric cancer. A possible role of eosinophil neurotoxic proteins. *Dig. Dis. Sci.* **34**:297-303.

Frigas, E., and Gleich, G. J. (1986). The eosinophil and the pathophysiology of asthma. *J. Allergy Clin. Immunol.* **77**:527-537.

Frigas, E., Loegering, D. A., Solley, G. O., Farrow, G. M., and Gleich, G. J. (1981). Elevated levels of the eosinophil granule major basic protein in the sputum of patients with bronchial asthma. *Mayo Clin. Proc.* **56**: 345-353.

Frigas, E., Loegering, D. A., and Gleich, G. J. (1980). Cytotoxic effects of the guinea pig eosinophil major basic protein in tracheal epithelium. *Lab. Invest.* **42**:35-43.

Gleich, G. J., and Adolphson, C. R. (1986). The eosinophil leukocyte: structure and function. *Adv. Immunol.* **39**:177-253.

Gleich, G. J., Loegering, D. A., Mann, K. G., and Maldonado, J. E. (1976). Comparative properties of the Charcot-Leyden crystal protein and the major basic protein from human eosinophils. *J. Clin. Invest.* **57**:633-640.

Gleich, G. J., Loegering, D. A., Bell, M. P., Chekel, J. L., Ackerman, S. J., and McKean, D. J. (1986). Biochemical and functional similarities between human eosinophil-derived neurotoxin and eosinophil cationic protein: homology with ribonuclease. *Proc. Natl. Acad. Sci. U.S.A.* **83**: 3146-3150.

Gleich, G. J., Motojima, S., Frigas, E., Kephart, G. M., Fujisawa, T., and Kravi, L. (1987). The eosinophilic leukocyte and the pathology of fatal bronchial asthma: evidence for pathologic heterogeneity. *J. Allergy Clin. Immunol.* **80**:412-415.

Gleich, G. J., Flavahan, N. A., Fujisawa, T., and Vanhoutte, P. M. (1988). The eosinophil as a mediator of damage to respiratory epithelium: a model for bronchial hyperreactivity. *J. Allergy Clin. Immunol.* **81**:776-781.

Godard, P., Chaintreuil, J., Damon, M., Coupe, M., Flandre, O., Crastes de Paulet, A., and Michel, F. B. (1982). Functional assessment of alveolar macrophages: comparison of cells from asthmatics and normal subjects. *J. Allergy Clin. Immunol.* **70**:88-93.

Gordon, M. H. (1932). *Studies of the Aetiology of Lymphadenoma*. Bristol, England, John Wright and Sons Ltd., pp. 7-76.

Gosset, P., Tonnel, A. B., Joseph, M., Prin, L., Mallart, A., Charon, J., and Capron, A. (1984). Secretion of a chemotactic factor for neutrophils and eosinophils by alveolar macrophages from asthmatic patients. *J. Allergy Clin. Immunol.* **74**:827-834.

Granérus, G., Håkansson, L., Roupe, G., and Venge, P. (1988). Serum levels of NCF and ECF in mastocytosis. The European Histamine Research Society 17th Meeting, abstract.

Gullberg, U., Widegren, B., Arnason, U., Egesten, A., and Olsson, I. (1986). The cytotoxic eosinophil cationic protein (ECP) has ribonuclease activity. *Biochem. Biophys. Res. Commun.* **139**:1239-1242.

Håkansson, L., Westerlund, D., and Venge, P. (1987). A new method for the measurement of eosinophil migration. *J. Leukocyte Biol.* **42**:689-696.

Håkansson, L., Rak, S., Dahl, R., and Venge, P. (1989a). The formation of eosinophil and neutrophil chemotactic activity during a pollen season and after inhalation allergen challenge. *J. Allergy Clin. Immunol.* In press.

Håkansson, L., Carlson, M., Stålenheim, G., and Venge, P. (1989b). Migratory responses of eosinophil and neutrophil granulocytes from asthmatic patients. Submitted for publication.

Hällgren, R., Terent, A., and Venge, P. (1983). Eosinophil cationic protein (ECP) in the cerebrospinal fluid. *J. Neurol. Sci.* **58**:57-71.

Hällgren, R., Colombel, J. F., Dahl, R., Fredens, K., Kruse, A., Jacobsen, S., Venge, P., and Rambaud, J. C. (1989). Neutrophil and eosinophil involvement of the small bowel in patients with celiac disease and Crohn's disease. Studies on the secretion rate and immunohistochemical localization of granulocyte granule constituents in jejunum. *Am. J. Med.* **86**:56-64.

Hamblin, A. (1988). Lymphokines. In *In Focus.* Edited by D. Male. Oxford, Washington, IRL Press.

Harlin, S. L., Ansel, D. G., Lane, S. R., Myers, J., Kephart, G. M., and Gleich, G. J. (1988). A clinical and pathologic study of chronic sinusitis: the role of the eosinophil. *J. Allergy Clin. Immunol.* **81**:867-875.

Henderson, W. R., Chi, E. Y., and Klebanoff, S. J. (1980). Eosinophil peroxidase-induced mast cell secretion. *J. Exp. Med.* **152**:265-279.

Horn, H. R., Robin, E. D., Theodore, J., Van Kessel, A. (1975). Total eosinophil counts in the management of bronchial asthma. *N. Engl. J. Med.* **292**:1152-1155.

Huber, H. L., and Koessler, K. K. (1922). The pathology of bronchial asthma. *Arch. Intern. Med.* **30**:689.

Hubscher, T. T. (1975). Role of the eosinophil in the allergic reaction. II. Release of prostaglandins from human eosinophilic leukocytes. *J. Immunol.* **114**:1389-1393.

Jong, E. C., Mahmoud, A. A., and Klebanoff, S. J. (1981). Peroxidase-mediated toxicity of schistosomula of *Schistosoma mansoni*. *J. Immunol.* **126**:468-471.

Khalife, J., Capron, M., Cesbron, J. Y., Tai, P. C., Taelman, H., Prin, L., and Capron, A. (1986). Role of specific IgE antibodies in peroxidase (EPO) release from human eosinophils. *J. Immunol.* **137**:1659-1664.

Kierszenbaum, F., Villalta, F., and Tai, P. C. (1986). Role of inflammatory cells in Chagas' disease. III. Kinetics of human eosinophil activation upon interaction with parasites (*Trypanosoma cruzi*). *J. Immunol.* **136**: 662-666.

Lam, S., LeRiche, J., Phillips, D., and Chan-Yeung, M. (1987). Cellular and protein changes in bronchial lavage fluid after late asthmatic reaction in patients with red cedar asthma. *J. Allergy Clin. Immunol.* **80**: 44-50.

Lee, T. C., Lenihan, D. J., Malone, B., Roddy, L. L., Wasserman, S. I. (1984). Increased biosynthesis of platelet-activating factor in activated eosinophils. *J. Biol. Chem.* **259**:5526-5532.

Linder, A., Venge, P., and Deuschl, H. (1987). Eosinophil cationic protein and myeloperoxidase in nasal secretion as markers of inflammation in allergic rhinitis. *Allergy* **279**:385-391.

Mapp, C. E., Boschetto, P., Milani, G. F., Pivirotto, F., Tegazzin, V., Fabbri, L. M., and Zocca, E. (1987). Pathogenesis of late asthmatic reactions induced by exposure to isocyanates. *Clin. Respir. Physiol.* **23**: 583-586.

McLaren, D. J., McKean, J. R., Olsson, I., Venge, P., and Kay, A. B. (1981). Morphological studies on the killing of schistosomula of *Schistosoma mansoni* by human eosinophil and neutrophil cationic proteins in vitro. *Parasite Immunol.* **3**:359-373.

McLaren, D. J., Peterson, C. G. B., and Venge, P. (1984). *Schistosoma mansoni*: further studies of the interaction between schistosomula and granulocyte-derived cationic proteins in vitro. *Parasitology* **88**:491-503.

Metzger, W. J., Richerson, H. B., and Wasserman, S. I. (1986). Generation and partial characterization of eosinophil chemotactic activity and neutrophil chemotactic activity during early and late-phase asthmatic response. *J. Allergy Clin. Immunol.* **78**:282-290.

Mullarkey, M. F., Thomas, P. S., Hansen, J. A., Webb, D. R., and Nisperos, B. (1986). Association of aspirin-sensitive asthma with HLA-DQw2. *Am. Rev. Respir. Dis.* **133**:261-263.

Olsson, I., and Venge, P. (1974). Cationic proteins of human granulocytes. II. Separation of the cationic proteins of the granules of leukemic myeloid cells. *Blood* **44**:235-246.

Olsson, I., and Venge, P. (1979). The role of the eosinophil granulocyte in the inflammatory reaction. *Allergy* **34**:353-67.

Olsson, I., Venge, P., Spitznagel, J. K., and Lehrer, R. I. (1977). Arginine-rich cationic proteins of human eosinophil granules. Comparison of the constituents of eosinophilic and neutrophilic leukocytes. *Lab. Invest.* **36**:493-500.

Peterson, C. G. B., and Venge, P. (1983). Purification and characterization of a new cationic protein—eosinophil protein-x (EPX)—from granules of human eosinophils. *Immunology* **50**:19-26.

Peterson, C. G. B., and Venge, P. (1987). Interaction and complex-formation between the eosinophil cationic protein and alpha-2-macroglobulin. *Biochem. J.* **245**:781-787.

Peterson, C. G. B., Skoog, V., and Venge, P. (1986). Human eosinophil cationic proteins (ECP and EPX) and their suppressive effects on lymphocyte proliferation. *Immunobiology* **171**:1-13.

Peterson, C. G. B., Jörnvall, H., and Venge, P. (1988). Purification and characterization of eosinophil cationic protein from normal human eosinophils. *Eur. J. Haematol.* **40**:415-423.

Peterson, C. G. B., Garcia, R. C., Carlson, M. G. Ch., and Venge, P. (1989). Eosinophil cationic protein (ECP), eosinophil protein X (EPX) and eosinophil peroxidase (EPO): granule distribution and degranulation. Submitted for publication.

Pincus, S. H., Schooley, W. R., DiNapoli, A. M., and Broder, S. (1981). Metabolic heterogeneity of eosinophils from normal and hypereosinophilic patients. *Blood* **58**:1175-1181.

Rak, S., Håkansson, L., and Venge, P. (1987). Eosinophil chemotactic activity in allergic patients during the birch pollen season: the effect of immunotherapy. *Int. Arch. Allergy Appl. Immunol.* **82**:349-350.

Rak, S., Löwhagen, O., and Venge, P. (1988). The effect of immunotherapy on bronchial hyperresponsiveness and eosinophil cationic protein in pollen allergic patients. *J. Allergy Clin. Immunol.* In press.

Rak, S., Håkansson, L., and Venge, P. (1989a). Immunotherapy abrogates the generation of eosinophil and neutrophil chemotactic activity during pollen season. Submitted for publication.

Rak, S., Björnsson, A., Håkansson, L, Sörensson, S., and Venge, P. (1989b). Immunotherapy prevents eosinophil accumulation and production of eosinophil chemotactic activity in the lung of asthmatics during natural allergen challenge. Submitted for publication.

Riddle, J. M., and Barnhard, M. I. (1965). The eosinophil as a source for profibrinolysin in acute inflammation. *Blood* **25**:776-794.

Särnstrand, B., Westergren-Thorsson, G., Hernäs, J., Peterson, C., Venge, P., and Malmström, A. (1988). Eosinophil cationic protein and transforming growth factor-A stimulates synthesis of hyaluronan and proteoglycan in human lung fibroblast cultures. 5th International Colloquium on pulmonary fibrosis, Abstract.

Shaw, R. J., Cromwell, O., and Kay, A. B. (1984). Preferential generation of leukotriene C4 by human eosinophils. *Clin. Exp. Immunol.* **70**:716-722.

Slifman, N. R., Peterson, C. G. B., Gleich, G. J., Dunette, S. L., and Venge, P. (1989). Eosinophil-derived neurotoxin and eosinophilic protein-x: comparison of physiochemical, immunologic, and enzymatic properties. Submitted for publication.

Spry, C. J. F. (1988). *Eosinophils. A Comprehensive Review and Guide to the Scientific and Medical Literature.* Oxford/New York/Tokyo, Oxford University Press.

Tai, P. C., Spry, C. J. F., Peterson, C. G. B., Venge, P., and Olsson, I. (1984). Monoclonal antibodies distinguish between storage and secreted forms of eosinophil cationic protein. *Nature* **309**:182-184.

Taniguchi, N., Mita, H., Saito, H., Yui, Y., Kajita, T., and Shida, T. (1985). Increased generation of leukotriene C4 from eosinophils in asthmatic patients. *Allergy* **40**:571-573.

Taylor, K. J., and Luksza, A. R. (1987). Peripheral blood eosinophil counts and bronchial responsiveness. *Thorax* **42**:452-456.

Venge, P. (1985). The eosinophil in inflammation. In *Inflammation.* Edited by P. Venge and A. Lindbom. Stockhold, Almqvist & Wiksell Int., pp. 85-103.

Venge, P., and Peterson, C. G. B. (1989). Eosinophil biochemistry and killing mechanisms. In *Eosinophils in Asthma.* Edited by J. Morley. Orlando, FL, Academic Press.

Venge, P., Zetterström, O., Dahl, R., Roxin, L.-E., and Olsson, I. (1977). Low levels of eosinophil cationic proteins in patients with asthma. *Lancet* 373-376.

Venge, P., Dahl, R., Hällgren, R. (1979). Enhancement of factor XII dependent reactions by eosinophil cationic protein. *Thromb. Res.* **14**:641-649.

Venge, P., Dahl, R., and Håkansson, L. (1987). Heat-labile neutrophil chemotactic activity in asthmatics after allergen inhalation challenge. Relation to the late asthmatic reaction and effects of asthma medication. *J. Allergy Clin. Immunol.* **80**:679-688.

Venge, P., Dahl, R., Håkansson, L., and Peterson, C. (1982). Generation of heat-labile chemotactic activity in blood after inhalation challenge and its relationship to neutrophil and monocyte/macrophage turnover and activity. *Allergy* **37**:55-63.

Venge, P., Dahl, R., Fredens, K., Hällgren, R., and Peterson, C. (1983). Eosinophil cationic proteins (ECP and EPX) in health and disease. In

Immunobiology of the Eosinophil. Edited by T. Yoshida and M. Torisu. New York/Amsterdam/Oxford, Elsevier Publishing Co., pp. 163-179.

Venge, P., Dahl, R., and Peterson, C. G. B. (1988). Eosinophil granule proteins in serum after allergen challenge of asthmatic patients and the effects of anti-asthmatic medication. *Int. Arch. Allergy Appl. Immunol.* **87**:306-312.

Venge, P., Dahl, R., and Henriksen, J. (1989a). ECP in serum in exercise-induced asthma (EIA). Submitted for publication.

Venge, P., Henriksen, J., Dahl, R., and Håkansson, L. (1989b). Exercise-induced asthma and the generation of neutrophil chemotactic activity. Submitted for publication.

Verhagen, J., Bruynzeel, P. L. B., Koedam, J. A., Wassink, G. A., de Boer, M., Terpstra, G. K., Kreukniet, J., Veldink, G. A., and Vliegenthart, J. F. (1984). Specific leukotriene formation by purified human eosinophils and neutrophils. *FEBS Lett.* **168**:23-28.

Wardlaw, A. J., Moqbel, R., Cromwell, O., and Kay, A. B. (1986). Paf-acether—a potent chemotactic and chemokinetic factor for human eosinophils. *J. Clin. Invest.* **78**:1701-1706.

Wardlaw, A. J., Dunnette, S., Gleich, G. J., Collins, J. V., and Kay, A. B. (1988). Eosinophils and mast cells in bronchoalveolar lavage in subjects with mild asthma. Relationship to bronchial hyperreactivity. *Am. Rev. Respir. Dis.* **137**:62-69.

Wasmoen, T. L., Bell, M. P., Loegering, D. A., Gleich, G. J., Prendergast, F. G., and McKean, D. J. (1988). Biochemical and amino acid sequence analysis of human eosinophil granule major basic protein. *J. Biol. Chem.* **263**:12559-12563.

Weller, P. F., and Goetzl, E. J. (1980). The regulatory and effector roles of eosinophils. *Adv. Immunol.* **27**:339-371.

Weller, P. F., Goetzl, E. J., and Austen, K. F. (1980). Identification of human eosinophil lysophospholipase as the constituent of Charcot-Leyden crystals. *Proc. Natl. Acad. Sci. U.S.A.* **77**:7440-7443.

Winqvist, I., Olofsson, T., and Olsson, I. (1984). Mechanisms for eosinophil degranulation; release of the eosinophil cationic protein. *Immunology* **51**:1-8.

Yazdanbaksh, M., Tai, P. C., Spry, C. J., Gleich, G. J., and Roos, D. (1987). Synergism between eosinophil cationic protein and oxygen metabolites in killing of schistosomula of *Schistosoma mansoni. J. Immunol.* **138**:3443-3447.

Zabucchi, G., Menegazzi, R., Soranzo, M. R., and Patriarca, P. (1986). Uptake of human eosinophil peroxidase by human neutrophils. *Am. J. Pathol.* **124**:510-518.

19

Xanthines

ROMAIN PAUWELS

University Hospital
Ghent, Belgium

CARL G. A. PERSSON

University Hospital of Lund
and AB Draco
Lund, Sweden

Xanthines have been used for a very long time in the treatment of asthma and chronic obstructive pulmonary disorders (COPD). The development of sustained-release preparations of theophylline has increased the therapeutic use of this agent enormously. The arrival of other potent, easier to handle, therapeutic agents is causing a reassessment of the place of theophylline in the management of these diseases. This chapter will analyze critically the potential role of xanthines in the treatment of asthma and COPD. We will first discuss the actual therapeutic use of xanthines, mainly comparing its use with that of other therapeutic agents. We will then analyze our present knowledge about the xanthines' clinical and experimental pharmacology, highlighting pharmacological effects that may warrant further studies into the therapeutic application of xanthines. We end with a brief overview of potential modes of action.

I. Historical Background

It is now 200 years since William Withering (1786) placed "coffee made very strong" as the number one reliever of asthmatic symptoms. In his brief and brilliant piece on asthma, Withering does not produce a single additional comment about the use of coffee in this disease. It is, therefore, likely that earlier accounts of xanthines in asthma treatment can be found. Books on asthma remedies of the 17th and 18th century mention coffee, but not as a remedy (Persson, 1985). The pioneer in the field of treatment of asthma with xanthines was Henry Hyde Salter. Salter was an astute observer whose descriptions of asthma and its treatments are outstanding. From the complex therapeutic armamentarium of the 19th century, he selected strong coffee as the best remedy for his own asthma as well as for that of his many patients. His dose regimens must have given adequate amounts of caffein. As evidenced also by other workers, including Foucart, coffee should have been an essential drug for many patients in those prepharmacological days (Persson, 1985).

In the late 1800s and early 1900s, xanthines were obviously out of fashion. There is rarely any mention of them in the contemporary asthma literature. Furthermore, when caffeine was purified and synthesized, it did not become a drug for the treatment of asthma, and neither did theophylline. Around 1900, theophylline was much promoted as a diuretic agent. The lack of guidance concerning diuretic doses caused problems; most evident and serious were the seizures. In the early 1920s, a mixture of theophylline and theobromine was successfully used in asthma and evaluated in vitro on airway preparations. However, the emphasis was put on theobromine, which is much less potent than theophylline. The breakthrough for widespread use of xanthines came towards the end of the 1930s, when these drugs were reported to have a unique efficacy. Thus parenteral theophylline produced dramatic effects in patients with severe asthma for whom epinephrine was no longer effective.

The interest in intravenous (iv) and oral theophylline grew steadily. For a number of decades the use of this drug, its salts, and weakly active 7-derivatives rested a great deal on clinical impressions and evolving therapeutic tradition. In the early 1970s, when a range of new antiasthma drugs were being introduced (beta$_2$-agonists, cromoglycate, and inhaled glucocorticoids), the clinical scientific documentation of theophylline was not advanced and its role in therapy was questioned (in particular in Europe). The time lag between Europe and the United States concerning the introduction of novel drugs probably contributed to the fact that the pharmacokinetics and efficacy of theophylline became well studied in North America. The advent of long-acting oral formulations that allowed for twice-daily administration was an important development that contributed to making theophylline the most frequently prescribed antiasthma drug worldwide during the 1970s.

In the last few years there has been a resurgence of interest in the inflammatory aspects of asthma. This development is well founded in the clinical efficacy of glucocorticoids, which is evident also in mild and early asthma and in cases thought to be well controlled by other drugs. This changing concept is bringing inhaled glucocorticoids into the first line of treatment of asthma. Furthermore, long-acting (at least 12 h) inhalational beta-receptor agonist drugs are imminent on the therapeutic scene. Again, the role of xanthines in asthma treatment is questioned and this time on both sides of the Atlantic. This chapter will attempt to dissect facts about the clinical efficacy of xanthines in asthma. Indeed, the possibility that they are still indispensable drugs leads to questions about their target cells and subcellular modes of action. Perhaps xanthines should not even be labeled bronchodilators.

II. Clinical Use

A. Acute Severe Asthma

Both enprofylline and theophylline have been shown to cause bronchodilation in patients with reversible airway obstruction and have therefore been used in the treatment of acute severe asthma. The bronchodilating effect is related to the serum concentration of the drug (Racineux et al., 1981; Laursen et al., 1984). The relationship is, however, not linear and varies between individuals. Although the bronchodilating effect is observed shortly after intravenous administration, the maximal bronchodilating effect shows a considerable time lag after the serum concentration (Ishizaki et al., 1988). The development of selective beta$_2$-adrenergic agents has resulted in the preferential use of these sympathomimetics in an inhaled or intravenous form in the treatment of acute severe asthma. The concomitant use of intravenous xanthines has been questioned in view of the risk for serious side effects linked to an overdose of theophylline. A recent meta-analysis of 13 double-blind controlled studies on the value of adding theophylline to sympathomimetics in the treatment of acute asthma came to the conclusion that none of the studies published to date had sufficient power to give us a final answer to that question (Littenberg, 1988).

Enprofylline, a potent xanthine molecule without the risk for serious central nervous side effects, has been compared to high-dose inhaled terbutaline in a multicenter study in Australia involving 69 patients (Ruffin et al., 1988). The bronchodilating effect of intravenous enprofylline (2 mg/kg) was comparable to that of nebulized terbutaline (10 mg). The major side effects reported were tremor in the terbutaline-treated patients and nausea in the enprofylline-treated group. In another multicenter study carried out in Sweden and involving 176 patients, iv theophylline was given 1 h after administration of albuterol, either 5 μg/kg iv or 0.15 mg/kg by inhalation of nebulized drug. Theophylline produced significant (p < 0.001) further increase in peak expiratory flow values (Boe, 1988).

B. Chronic Asthma

Chronic treatment with oral sustained-release theophylline does, without any doubt, result in a significant improvement of symptoms and lung function in patients with chronic asthma (Weinberger, 1984). Even when the precaution of carefully titrating its initial administration is taken, about 10% of patients with asthma are unable to sustain chronic oral theophylline treatment. Chronic treatment with sustained-release enprofylline results likewise in a dosage-dependent improvement of symptoms and lung function in asthmatic patients who receive baseline therapy with inhaled beta-agonists (95%) plus inhaled glucocorticoids (77%). (Chapman et al., 1989). No one will deny the antiasthmatic effects of xanthines. The discussion will, however, start when one tries to determine the place of theophylline with respect to other treatment forms.

Joad et al. (1987) used a randomized, double-blind, double-dummy, crossover trial to compare slow-release theopylline with regularly inhaled salbutamol or a combination of the two. Each treatment regimen was administered for 1 month. All patients had been receiving regular theophylline treatment before the study. Eight of the 18 patients were receiving inhaled beclomethasone and one other patient received oral prednisone on an alternate-day basis. These treatments were maintained. The oral sustained release theophylline preparation was administered twice daily at a dosage that kept peak serum concentrations between 10 and 20 μg/ml. The beta$_2$-agonist salbutamol was administered as 2 puffs of 100 μg four times daily: on arising, at lunch, dinner, and bedtime. Chronic theophylline treatment either alone or in combination resulted in a significantly better control of the asthmatic symptoms and an increase in the number of days with no symptoms. The significantly higher frequency of nightime symptoms and lower morning peak expiratory flow rate (PEFR) attest to the shorter duration of action of inhaled salbutamol. A similar conclusion was reached in the study by Zwillich et al. (1989). The battle between sympathomimetics and xanthines is, however, not settled. The recent development of new, longer-acting inhaled sympathomimetics such as formoterol and salmeterol will undoubtedly lead to new comparative studies between the two groups of antiasthmatic drugs.

Chronic theophylline treatment has also been compared with chronic cromoglycate treatment (Hambleton et al., 1977; Edmunds et al., 1980; Furukawa et al., 1984). Most studies concluded that the two drugs are approximately equally effective in controlling symptoms in young patients with allergic asthma. The possibility that theophylline may cause slight learning disturbances caused some alarm and this question remains to be settled.

The development of topically active inhaled steroids has significantly altered the therapeutic approach to asthma in large parts of the world. They are without any doubt safer and frequently more effective than oral theophylline in the treatment of chronic asthma. The place of theophylline with respect to inhaled steroids remains to be determined. Two studies may illustrate the questions that remain.

Nassif et al. (1981) examined the value of continuing theophylline treatment in patients whose asthma was insufficiently controlled with theophylline alone and were put on maintenance therapy with inhaled beclomethasone diproprionate (BDP). Twenty-two patients were included in the study. Dosages of BDP ranged from 200 to 900 μg/day, with a mean dosage of 533 μg/day. In a double-blind randomized crossover trial, 1 month of continuous theophylline treatment was compared to 1 month of placebo. During the theophylline treatment period, the serum theophylline concentrations averaged 15.6 μg/ml. Asthmatic symptoms occurred less frequently and with less severity during treatment with theophylline and significantly more symptom-free days were observed during the theophylline treatment period (50 $\pm$ 7% vs. 71 $\pm$ 6%). Inhaled sympathomimetics were required twice as frequently during the period of placebo treatment. The data thus indicated that maintenance treatment with theophylline was beneficial for patients requiring inhaled BDP.

The second study that may contribute to the present discussion is that by Brenner et al. (1988). Concern about potential side effects of theophylline prompted Brenner et al. to investigate whether this drug could be eliminated from the multimedication regimen of a group of adolescents with very severe asthma. They all received alternate-day prednisone (10-30 mg) orally, inhaled beclomethasone dipropionate 100-200 μg four times a day, inhalations of nebulized beta$_2$-agonist and atropine four times a day, and inhaled cromoglycate 20 mg four times a day. The authors (and probably many others) were surprised to learn that elimination of theophylline was impossible in these patients. Despite marked further increases in the dosages of oral glucocorticoid and inhaled bronchodilators, patients' asthmatic condition underwent severe deterioration. Hence, none of the patients completed the intended placebo period of 4 weeks without use of theophylline. The observed deterioration also stopped recruitment of further patients to this trial, which involved only five subjects.

We may therefore conclude that the last word on chronic treatment with theophylline in asthma has not yet been said. It seems clear that in patients with severe asthma, theophylline will play a role in addition to high-dose inhaled steroids. At what dosage of inhaled steroids xanthines should be added is, in our view, dependent on the individual sensitivity for systemic effects of inhaled steroids and requires further investigation.

C. Chronic Obstructive Pulmonary Disorders

The role of theophylline in the treatment of COPD is another point of discussion. Most studies have looked at short-term symptomatic relief and very little attention has been given to any long-term effects, including the prognosis of these diseases and the further progression of airflow obstruction. Several studies demonstrate that theophylline may have favorable effects on spirometry, exercise performance, and the sensation of dyspnea in patients with COPD (Alexander et al., 1980; Jenne et al., 1984; Murciano et al., 1984; Taylor et al., 1985). A recently published study by Chrystyn and colleagues (1988) suggest that the major effect of theophylline on the pulmonary function of patients with COPD may be a decrease in the trapped gas volume. In a double-blind, randomized, crossover study in patients with COPD they compared the effect of placebo and three dose levels of theophylline. The effect on forced expiratory volume in 1s (FEV_1) and forced vital capacity (FVC) was minimal. A dose-dependent reduction of the trapped gas volume (the difference between total lung capacity measured by whole body plethysmography and that measured by helium dilution) and an increase in the slow vital capacity was observed, together with a decrease in dyspnea score and the use of a rescue-inhaler of sympathomimetics. These data would suggest that in patients with COPD the major pharmacological effect of theophylline may be situated at the level of the small airways. This would fit with the hypothesis that theophylline inhibits the airway inflammation present in the small airways of patients with COPD (Mullen et al., 1985).

Numerous studies have compared beta-agonists, anticholinergics, and theophylline in the treatment of COPD (Barclay et al., 1982; Filuk et al., 1985; Passamonte and Martinez, 1984). There is very little information available on whether theophylline can have additional effects beyond the results obtained with optimized dosages of inhaled beta-agonists and anticholinergics.

III. Clinical Pharmacology Studies

The bronchodilating and protective effects of theophylline on nocturnal asthma are well known (Barnes et al., 1982). The protective effect of theophylline on bronchial responsiveness is dependent both on the type of stimulus used in the assessment of the bronchial responsiveness and the severity of the asthma in the patients studied. Theophylline has been shown to inhibit in patients with mild asthma the airway responsiveness to histamine (Cartier et al., 1986), methacholine (Magnussen et al., 1987), exercise (Pollock et al., 1977), distilled water (Fabbri et al., 1986), and adenosine (Mann and Holgate, 1985). A study by Dutoit and co-workers (1987) failed to show any significant effect of 10 weeks of treatment with theophylline on the histamine responsiveness in a group of patients with severe asthma.

At least three studies have now demonstrated that theophylline inhibits the late asthmatic reaction following bronchial challenge with either an allergen or an occupational agent. The effect of theophylline on allergen-induced bronchoconstriction had not been extensively studied until quite recently; only the effect on the immediate bronchoconstriction had been investigated. Pauwels et al. (1985) studied the effect of theophylline and enprofylline on the allergen-induced immediate and late bronchoconstriction in nine asthmatic patients. The patients were challenged three times at weekly intervals with the same dosage of allergen. This dosage had previously been chosen as causing an immediate bronchoconstriction with an FEV_1 decrease between 20 and 50% of the prechallenge value. On the 3 treatment days FEV_1 and sGaw (specific airway conductance) were evaluated up to 6 h after challenge. The drugs were given intravenously. Placebo was given on the first occasion. Theophylline and enprofylline were administered on test days 2 and 3, with a double-blind, randomized, crossover technique. One hour before the allergen challenge, a loading dose was given during 60 min followed by a constant infusion over 6 h. The loading infusion was 7.2 mg/kg of theophylline of 2.7 mg/kg of enprofylline. The maintenance dosage was 74 mg/h and 71 mg/h, respectively. Theophylline and enprofylline both caused a minor initial bronchodilation. Theophylline and enprofylline slightly but significantly inhibited the immediate bronchoconstrictor reaction after allergen inhalation. Both drugs had a significant inhibitory effect on the late reaction. The mean plasma level of theophylline was 0, 10.8, 10.5, and 10.5 mg/L at 0, 1, 4, and 7 h after the start of the loading infusion. The corresponding mean plasma levels of enprofylline were 0, 2.6, 2.7, and 2.7 mg/L. The data thus showed that theophylline, at plasma levels considered therapeutic, inhibits both the immediate and the late bronchoconstrictory reaction after allergen challenge.

Mapp et al. (1987) investigated the effect of different antiasthmatic drugs on the immediate and late bronchoconstrictor reaction following challenge with toluene diisocyanate (TDI) in TDI-sensitive asthmatic patients. The drugs were administered for 1 week before the challenge. The last dose was administered a short time before the TDI exposure. Theophylline was administered at a dosage of 6.5 mg/kg of a slow-release preparation twice daily. The last dose of 10 mg/kg was taken 2 h before challenge. The bronchial response to TDI was evaluated and the bronchial responsiveness to methacholine was studied before and 8 h after the TDI challenge. Theophylline significantly inhibited the late reaction following TDI challenge but did not have a significant effect on the increase in methacholine responsiveness. The mean theophylline serum concentration in the six patients was 18 mg/L before and 20 mg/L 8 h after the TDI challenge.

The same group of investigators (Crescioli et al., 1988) recently confirmed the observation that theophylline inhibits both the immediate and late reaction following allergen challenge, but could again not demonstrate a significant inhibitory effect on the increase in methacholine responsiveness measured 8 h after the allergen challenge.

Animal studies are in accordance with the human observations. In a guinea pig model of allergen-induced bronchial reactions, Andersson et al. (1985) demonstrated that the intravenous injection of a low dose of theophylline immediately before the antigen challenge significantly inhibited the immediate bronchoconstriction and the late reaction. The late reaction in the guinea pig is characterized by the influx of neutrophils, eosinophils, and lymphocytes. Pretreatment with theophylline significantly reduced the neutrophilic airway inflammation. The intravenous injection of theophylline 90 min after the antigen-induced immediate bronchoconstriction also had an inhibitory effect on the late reaction. Similar findings were obtained in an allergic sheep model (Perruchoud et al., 1984). Theophylline at a serum concentration of 10 mg/L inhibited the late reaction after allergen challenge both when given before and after the allergen challenge.

IV. Mode of Action of Xanthines

A. Smooth Muscle Relaxation or Inhibition?

Smooth muscle relaxation was the first demonstrated airway action of the xanthines. Partly because of this, and in part due to a long-standing emphasis on the role of bronchoconstriction in asthma, the airway-relaxant effect of xanthines is generally considered their major therapeutic action. Xanthines do have interesting tracheobronchial relaxant characteristics, but these may not suffice to explain their clinical efficacy.

Xanthines relax airway smooth muscle in a manner that is relatively independent of which contractile agent has contributed to an increased tone. As demonstrated in animal and human airways in vitro, this general relaxation is independent of age, is without tachyphylaxis, and may be more effective (at large concentrations) than that induced by other bronchodilator drugs. From what is known about active concentrations in vitro, only a small bronchodilator action may be expected in vivo at therapeutic plasma levels of xanthines.

Another question that has been addressed in isolated airway experiments is whether the relaxant action of xanthines will protect against the effect of a contractile mediator. Thus, concentration-response to carbachol was evaluated in the presence and absence of relaxant concentrations of theophylline (40 and 80 μg/ml) and enprofylline (10 and 20 μg/ml) (Persson et al., 1988). The only interaction recorded was that the induced relaxation allowed carbachol to contract over a wider tension range. The concentration-response curves to carbachol were not shifted. Even the same absolute maximum tension as in controls was produced in the presence of the xanthines. The xanthines did not attenuate the initiation and development of a contractile effect. There was no prophylactic effect at the smooth muscle level. In asthmatic subjects, protection by xanthines against challenge with bronchoconstrictors has been recorded, but this protection has not corresponded to the degree of the initial xanthine-induced bronchodilation. Taken together, these in vitro and in vivo data suggest that protective actions of xanthines in asthma cannot be explained only on basis of airway smooth-muscle-relaxant effects of these drugs. The possibility remains that bronchodilatation in part explains their acute symptomatic effects in asthma.

B. Airway Anti-inflammatory Actions

A consistent sign of continued inflammatory processes in asthma and rhinitis is plasma exudation into the mucosa/submucosa and the airway lumen. Hence, by measuring plasma proteins and plasma-derived mediators in mucosal surface liquid, inflammation can be quantitated. In patients with allergic rhinitis, theophylline has been demonstrated to reduce nasal plasma exudation (Naclerio et al., 1986; Persson, 1988). Similar studies in asthmatic patients are now lacking, but there are other indices of tracheobronchial anti-inflammatory effects of theophylline and enprofylline in these patients (see above). Data obtained in guinea pig tracheobronchial mucosa confirm that xanthines reduce plasma exudation in a dose-dependent fashion and suggest that this action is in part directly on the endothelial barrier cells of the airway microvascular wall (Persson et al., 1988). In the complex mucosal inflammation that occurs during airway diseases, reduced plasma exudation could result from an effect at any level of the inflammatory process.

Several types of stationary and migrating cells of the airway may contribute to inflammation in asthma. Xanthines have been demonstrated to reduce the activity of basophils, macrophages, mast cells, platelets, and polymorphonuclear (PMN) leukocytes. In cooperation with other anti-inflammatory factors, xanthines exert particularly potent inhibitory effects. In 1971, Orange et al. demonstrated that 10^{-5} M of theophylline, if given together with isoprenaline, had pronounced inhibitory effects on the immunological release of mediators from human lung in vitro. Furthermore, at quite low concentrations, xanthines have significant inhibitory effects on the activity of platelets and PMN leukocytes if agents such as adenosine, prostacyclin, and isoproterenol are also present. A synergistic mechanism may thus contribute to the anti-inflammatory effects observed at therapeutic drug levels in vivo.

Consistent with this possibility, O'Neill et al. (1986) reported that human alveolar macrophages sampled from patients who took theophylline had considerably reduced activity (H_2O_2 release) compared with control cells. Kyong et al. (1982) found a reduced bactericidal capacity of PMN leukocytes obtained from patients receiving theophylline therapy. Recent in vitro work by Nielson et al. (1986) demonstrates that theophylline and enprofylline may be potent inhibitors of the activation of human PMN leukocytes, which suggests that synergistic interactions with other autacoids may not always be required for in vivo effects of xanthines on inflammatory cells.

The possibility that the anti-inflammatory effects of xanthines increase susceptibility to infections has been considered. The course of infections in obstructive airway disease may not be worsened by inhaled glucocorticoids, which have powerful anti-inflammatory effects. Hence, it is doubtful whether anti-inflammatory xanthines can increase the risk for airway infections.

In a rat model of endotoxin-induced airway hyperresponsiveness, theophylline reduced both influx of neutrophils and the associated responsiveness (Kips et al., 1989). Sensitized guinea pigs challenged with particulate antigen developed a late-phase reaction. Theophylline and enprofylline inhibited this response (Andersson et al., 1985) as well as the associated plasma leakage. These observations in animals are consistent with the view that functional anti-inflammatory effects of xanthines are involved in the therapeutic response to these drugs in asthma.

Inhibition of inflammatory cells may contribute to pulmonary effects of xanthines other than the antiasthma actions. Thus, theophylline reduces significantly bleomycin-induced airway inflammation and fibrosis in experimental animals (Lindenschmidt and Witschi, 1985). Theophylline and enprofylline also act prophylactically to reduce inflammatory stimulus-induced pulmonary edema (Persson et al., 1988). Another xanthine derivative, pentoxifylline, developed for the treatment of claudication has now been demonstrated to decrease endotoxin-induced neutrophil sequestration and protein-rich edema in canine lungs (Welsh et al., 1988).

Theophylline has been reported to increase the number and activity of "suppressor" T cells in asthma (Fink et al., 1987). Studies addressing the possibility that immunosuppressive effects of xanthines may play a role seem warranted.

C. A Nonairway Site of Antiasthma Action?

A variety of actions of xanthines outside the airways have been considered important for their clinical efficacy in asthma. In the 19th century, Salter rather convincingly emphasized a role for the CNS-stimulant action of coffee. He referred to the fact that another excitatory influence, sudden alarm, could instantaneously abolish asthmatic symptoms and that the opposite, a few hours of sleep, induces asthma. More recently it has been speculated that an urge for the vigilant actions may explain the popularity that theophylline has with many patients. Evidence in support of a CNS locus is now lacking. Indeed, a xanthine derivative without CNS-stimulant behavioral effects, enprofylline, has been demonstrated to be a more potent antiasthma drug and with no less efficacy than theophylline (Persson et al., 1988; Chapman et al., 1989).

Since the 1950s several attempts have been made to administer xanthines by the inhaled route. The lack of success in these trials, experienced also with more potent xanthines than theophylline, apparently favors an extra-airway site of action. Studies involving guinea pig airways and lungs indicate that topically applied theophylline distributes promptly, as sucrose does, in extracellular water and disappears very rapidly from airway tissue into pulmonary veins (Kroll et al., 1989). Hence, the high local concentration reached immediately after inhalation will not remain in the airway tissue for a sufficiently long period of time to reduce an asthmatic obstruction. A further complicating factor is the low potency of xanthines. By comparison, inhaled beta agonists bind to airway tissue and are about 1000 times more potent than the xanthines. Failure to induce acceptable effects via the inhalational route with the current xanthines is, therefore, compatible with an airway site for the clinically important antiasthma actions.

A catecholamine-releasing action has frequently been suggested to be important. It is clear from experimental findings that at least high doses of caffeine and theophylline can produce a release of epinephrine and norepinephrine from the adrenal medulla. However, actual observations in patients receiving theophylline are not consistent on this point and any rise in plasma epinephrine levels is not related in magnitude or time course to the antiasthma effect of theophylline (Andersson et al., 1984; Ishizaki et al., 1988). Moreover, a novel xanthine derivative, enprofylline, does not seem to share metabolic actions with theophylline (Andersson et al., 1984), but is nevertheless as efficaceous as this drug in acute and long-term treatment of asthma.

Theophylline is known to stimulate the heart and reduce pulmonary artery pressure, but the clinical relevance of these effects in asthma is unknown. A few years ago it was suggested that xanthines produced a highly important stimulant effect on diaphragmatic contractions. This action was found in dog experiments and was also reported in human patients. It received extensive attention and has now been critically examined in several laboratories. Today it must be concluded that there may be no such action of theophylline within reasonable plasma levels.

As long as the important mode of action of theophylline has not been defined, various even less well supported proposals will continue to attract interest. There is currently no proof of an important involvement of extra-airway actions in the therapeutic response to xanthines of asthmatic subjects.

D. Subcellular Mechanisms of Action

One obvious problem in a discussion about the subcellular mode of action of antiasthma xanthines is that the important target cells have not been identified. Even if the locus of action can be said to be the airways, the number of possible target cells is great. Another problem is that a biochemical mechanism is difficult to put into the context of cell function in vivo without unduly simplifying the immensely complex cellular and intercellular chemistry.

For a long time xanthines have been popular compounds in biological-biochemical research, which has been successful in attaching interesting mechanisms of action to them. This development has, in turn, increased the usefulness of xanthines as tools, making them some of the most frequently studied compounds in bioresearch. However, few studies have critically addressed the issue of whether the proposed mechanisms are critical for the therapeutic response in asthma. Perhaps none of the hitherto proposed mechanisms can explain the antiasthma efficacy. None of them has proven important enough to be of any guidance in finding new drugs for the treatment of asthma.

It is possible that xanthines and xanthiniums are active on the cell surface. Many different types of compounds have been examined as potential antagonists of xanthine-induced airway effects. No specific antagonism of the effects of xanthines has been obtained (Persson, 1986). Whereas presently there is no support for xanthines being receptor agonists, it has been known for over 30 years that theophylline is a potent adenosine receptor antagonist. In the last decade adenosine antagonism has attracted much interest because, based on circumstantial evidence, it has been advocated as an antiasthma mechanism. However, adenosine antagonism in the airways or elsewhere may not be relevant for the therapeutic action, mainly because a xanthine derivative, enprofylline, which is without adenosine antagonism, is more potent and as efficacious as theophylline in the treatment of asthma (Persson, 1986).

In 1957, the same year as Ther et al. demonstrated "Antagonismus zwischen Adenosine und Methylxanthine," Berthet et al. reported on experiments that seem to have been the first steps on the road to the discovery of cyclic 3', 5'-nucleotide-phosphodiesterase and its inhibition by xanthines. Since the 1960s, drug-oriented research in this field has been going on in several laboratories but still no phosphodiesterase-inhibiting antiasthma drugs have resulted. Old and new compounds with potent enzyme-inhibitory effects have been examined but with no success. More than 10 years ago Bergstrand and co-workers identified a number of isoenzymes in human lung and bronchi, but this advancement appeared to be of little help in explaining the airway actions of xanthines. There is currently renewed interest in the role of phosphodiesterase isoenzymes. Xanthines as well as other types of compounds aimed at asthma treatment continue to be studied for their ability to inhibit these enzymes.

Besides adenosine antagonism and phosphodiesterase inhibition, a large number of subcellular mechanisms has been proposed for the xanthines. These compounds are also included in increasingly detailed studies of cell membrane mechanisms involved in the regulation of cytosolic calcium concentration and other pathways of importance in the control of cell function. It can only be hoped that the current lines of research will reveal the crucial antiasthmatic mechanisms of the xanthines.

V. Conclusion

Theophylline is the most frequently used single drug in the treatment of asthma and its use is still rapidly increasing on a global basis. This development is amazing. However, recent studies with theophylline and enprofylline have demonstrated that long-term treatment with xanthines produces clinically significant effects in asthma. There is also a growing documentation, in particular in patients with severe and brittle asthma, of the possibility that xanthines may produce essential effects not readily mimicked by other drugs. Progress in research, partly sparked by the advent of enprofylline, has helped to focus on the importance of airway anti-inflammatory actions, and has taken attention away from bronchodilator and extrapulmonary aspects of the anti-asthma efficacy of xanthines. Enprofylline has also provided evidence against the importance of adenosine antagonism as a mode of action of antiasthma xanthines. Indeed, it is not possible to grade the importance of individual target cells for xanthines in asthmatic airways and, despite the enormous amount of data, the subcellular mechanism(s) of action of the antiasthma xanthines now remains speculative.

Discussion

Tattersfield: No one doubts that theophylline causes bronchodilatation. The question the clinician wants to answer is whether giving theophylline has a better or worse benefit/side effect ratio than other drugs such as inhaled steroids. Theophylline is used less often in the United Kingdom than in some countries because we believe there are more side effects or more risks than with many other drugs, and particularly the inhaled steroids. This is the question that these studies need to address.

Pauwels: Studies comparing effects of theophylline on asthmatic symptoms and side effects with that of other drugs have two methodological problems.

Some studies use patients who were already on theophylline and are therefore less sensitive to side effects. Other studies have involved patients who never took theophylline before. The careful titration of theophylline is often neglected in these studies, resulting in an unnecessary high number of caffeine-like side effects.

Leff: In COPD, theophylline reduced the volume of trapped gas. What is the mechanism?

Pauwels: The significant decrease in trapped gas volume suggests a major effect on small airways.

Barnes: Theophylline has no marked effect on bronchial reactivity, and perhaps this might be due to the lack of effect of "therapeutic concentrations" of theophylline on eosinophils.

Pauwels: Theophylline inhibits in vitro at high concentrations the activation of different cell types including mast cells, macrophages, polymorphonuclear cells, and platelets. The inhibitory effect is enhanced by the presence of small concentrations of sympathomimetics. The in vivo anti-inflammatory effects may be related either to an inhibition of the initially activated cells or to an inhibition of secondary activated and chemoattracted cells.

Schleimer: Along these lines it is important to remember that a phosphodiesterase (PDE) inhibitor such as theophylline is a much more effective inhibitor of mediator release in combination with an adenylate cyclase agonist. It may be that endogenous adenylate cyclase activators synergize with theophylline in vivo. The failure of theophylline to decrease bronchial hyperreactivity in vivo does not eliminate anti-inflammatory effects as important components of its action.

Woolcock: Clinically there are two groups of patients: those who do well on theophylline (usually those with severe disease) and those who do not like it. The cause of these two responses to theophylline is unknown and needs investigating. It is possible that some patients become "addicted" to the drug.

Pauwels: The present clinical experience and studies suggest that in patients with severe asthma, the addition of theophylline to other antiasthmatic drugs, including high doses of inhaled steroids, results in a beneficial effect on the asthmatic symptoms.

Tattersfield: Other studies have looked at the effect of theophylline on bronchial responsiveness and most have shown a small reduction in bronchial reactivity when it is given acutely.

Pauwels: Several studies have shown that short-term administration of theophylline has a protective effect on challenge with histamine, methacholine, exercise, or distilled water.

Karlsson: Xanthines seem to have little effect on bronchial responsiveness, which may or may not be related to an inflamed respiratory tract mucosa. Therefore, is anything known about the histological appearance of the bronchial mucosa, for example, from biopsies, during or after long-term treatment with xanthines?

Pauwels: Not to my knowledge.

Sertl: What is the effect of theophylline on the diaphragm?

Pauwels: The effect of theophylline on diaphragmatic contractility is a controversial subject. Different researchers come up with different answers. An apparent effect of theophylline on diaphragmatic contractility in patients with COPD may be explained by the decrease in trapped gas volume following theophylline treatment. Enprofylline has no effect on diaphragmatic contractility, yet it has comparable effects on the symptoms of asthmatic patients. Therefore, the clinical relevance of this questionable activity of theopylline may be very limited.

References

Alexander, M. R., Dull, W. L., and Kasik, J. E. (1980). Treatment of chronic obstructive pulmonary disease with orally administered theophylline. *JAMA* **244**:2286-2290.

Andersson, K. E., Johannesson, N., Karlberg, B., and Persson, C. G. A. (1984). Increase in plasma free fatty acids and natriuresis by xanthines may reflect adenosine antagonism. *Eur. J. Clin. Pharmacol.* **26**:33-38.

Andersson, P., Brange, C., Sonmark, B., Stahre, G., Erjeflt, I., Wieslander, E., and Person, C. G. A. (1985). Anti-anaphylactic and antiinflammatory effects of xanthines in the lung. In *Anti-Asthma Xanthines and Adenosine*. Edited by K. E. Andersson and C. G. A. Persson. Amsterdam, Excerpta Medica, pp. 187-192.

Barclay, J., Whiting, B., and Addis, G. J. (1982). The influence of theophylline on maximal response to salbutamol in severe chronic obstructive pulmonary disease. *Eur. J. Clin. Pharmacol.* **32**:389-393.

Barnes, P. J., Greening, A. P., Neville, L., Timmer, J., and Poole, G. W. (1982). Single-dose slow release aminophylline at night prevents nocturnal asthma. *Lancet* **1**:299-301.

Bergstrand, H. (1985). Xanthines as phosphodiesterase inhibitors. In: *Anti-asthma Xanthines and Adenosine*. Edited by K. E. Andersson and C. G. A. Persson. Amsterdam, Excerpta Medica, pp. 16-22.

Berthet, J., Sutherland, E. N., and Rall, T. W. (1957). The assay of glucagon and epinephrine with use of liver homogenates. *J. Biol. Chem.* **229**:351-355.

Boe, J. (1988). Swedish Society of Chest Medicine (1988). Salbutamol in acute asthma—a multicenter study. *Am. Rev. Respir. Dis.* **137**:36A.

Brenner, M., Berkowitz, R., Marshall, N., and Strunk, R. C. (1988). Need for theophylline in severe steroid-requiring asthmatics. *Clin. Allergy* **18**:143-150.

Cartier, A., Lemaire, I., L'Archeveque, J., Ghezzo, H., Martin, R. R., and Malo, J. L. (1986). Theophylline partially inhibits bronchoconstriction caused by inhaled histamine in subjects with asthma. *J. Allergy Clin. Immunol.* **77**:570-575.

Chapman, K. R., Bryant, D., Marlin, G. E., Mitchell, C., Ruffin, R., Inouye, T., Pedersen, B., Koskinen, S., Osen, S. S., Ringdal, N., Willey, R. F., Formgren, H., Persson, G., Kllen, A., and Ljungholm, K. (1989). A placebo-controlled dose-response study of enprofylline in the maintenance therapy of asthma. *Am. Rev. Respir. Dis.* **139**:688-693.

Chrystyn, H., Mulley, B. A., and Peake, M. D. (1988). Dose response relation to oral theophylline in severe chronic obstructive airways disease. *Br. Med. J.* **297**:1506-1510.

Crescioli, S., Spinazzi, A., Paleari, D., Pozzan, M., Mapp, C. E., and Fabbri, L. M. (1988). Theophylline inhibits early and late asthmatic reactions induced by allergens in atopic subjects with asthma. *Am. Rev. Respir. Dis.* **A35**.

Dutoit, J., Salome, C. M., and Woolcock, A. J. (1987). Inhaled corticosteroids reduce the severity of bronchial hyperresponsiveness in asthma but oral theophylline does not. *Am. Rev. Respir. Dis.* **136**:1174-1178.

Edmunds, A. T., Carswell, F., Robinson, P., and Hughes, A. O. (1980). Controlled trial of cromoglycate and slow-release aminophylline in perennial childhood asthma. *Br. Med. J.* **281**:842.

Fabbri, L. M., Allessandri, M. V., De Marzo, N., Zocca, E., and Paleari, D. (1986). Long-lasting protective effect of slow-release theophylline on asthma induced by ultrasonically nebulized distilled water. *Ann. Allergy* **56**:171-175.

Filuk, R. B., Easton, P. A., and Anthonisen, N. R. (1985). Responses to large doses of salbutamol and theophylline in patients with chronic obstructive pulmonary disease. *Am. Rev. Respir. Dis.* **132**:871-874.

Fink, G., Mittelman, M., Shohat, B., and Spitzer, S. A. (1987). Theophylline-induced alterations in cellular immunity in asthmatic patients. *Clin. Allergy* **17**:316-321.

Furukuwa, C. T., Shapiro, G. G., Bierman, W. C., Kraemer, M. J., Ward, D. J., and Pierson, W. E. (1984). A double-blind study comparing the effectiveness of cromolyn sodium and sustained-release theophylline in childhood asthma. *Pediatrics* **74**:453-459.

Hambleton, G., Weinberger, M., Taylor, J., Cavanaugh, M., Ginchansky, E., Godfrey, S., Tooley, M., Bell, T., and Greenberg, S. (1977). Comparison of cromoglycate (cromolyn) and theophylline in controlling symptoms of chronic asthma. *Lancet* 381-385.

Ishizaki, T., Minegishi, A., Morishita, M., Odajima, Y., Kanagawa, S., Nagai, T., and Yamaguchi, M. (1988). Plasma catecholamine concentrations during a 72-hour aminophylline infusion in children with acute asthma. *J. Allergy Clin. Immunol.* **82**:146-154.

Jenne, J. W. (1987). Physiology and pharmacodynamics of the xanthines. In *Drug Therapy for Asthma.* Edited by J. W. Jenne and S. Murphy. New York, Marcel Dekker, pp. 297-334.

Jenne, J. W., Siever, J. R., Druz, W. S., Solano, J. V., Cohen, S. M., and Sharp, J. T. (1984). The effect of maintenance theophylline therapy while standing and walking. *Am. Rev. Respir. Dis.* **130**:600-605.

Joad, J. P., Ahrens, R. C. Lindgren, S. D., and Weinberger, M. M. (1987). Relative efficacy of maintenance therapy with theophylline, inhaled albuterol, and the combination for chronic asthma. *J. Allergy Clin. Immunol.* **79**:78-75.

Kips, J., Pauwels, R., and Van Der Straeten, M. (1989). Effect of theophylline on the endotoxin-induced airway inflammation and bronchial hyperresponsiveness. *J. Allergy Clin. Immunol.* **83**:178 (Abst.).

Kröll, F., Karlsson, J. A., Nilsson, E., Ryrfeldt, A., and Persson, C. G. A. (1989). Rapid clearance of xanthines from airway and pulmonary tissues. *Am. Rev. Respir. Dis.* Submitted.

Kyong, C. U., Ponche, B. E., Fudenbergh, H. H., Glassman, A. B., and Mohrmann, M. E. (1982). Bactericidal capacity of polymorphonuclear leucocytes from patients receiving theophylline therapy. *J. Allergy Clin. Immunol.* **69**:444-449.

Laursen, L. C., Jonhannesson, N., Söndergaard, I., and Weeke, B. (1984). Maximally effective plasma concentrations of enprofylline and theophylline during constant infusion. *Br. J. Clin. Pharmacol.* **18**:591-595.

Lindenschmidt, R. C., and Witschi, H. P. (1985). Attenuation of pulmonary fibrosis in mice by aminophylline. *Biochem. Pharmacol.* **34**:4269-4273.

Littenberg, B. (1988). Aminophylline treatment in severe, acute asthma. *JAMA* **259**:1678-1684.

Magnussen, H., Reuss, G., and Jorres, R. (1987). Theophylline has a dose related effect on the airway response to inhaled histamine and methacholine in asthmatics. *Am. Rev. Respir. Dis.* **136**:1163-1167.

Mann, J. S., and Holgate, S. T. (1985). Specific antagonism of adenosine induced bronchoconstriction in asthma by oral theophylline. *Br. J. Clin Pharmacol.* **19**:85-92.

Mapp, C., Boshetto, P., Dal Veccho, L., Crescioli, S., De Marzo, N., Paleari, D., and Fabbri, L. M. (1987). Protective effect of antiasthma drugs on late asthmatic reactions and increased airway responsiveness induced by toluene diisocyanate in sensitized subjects. *Am. Rev. Respir. Dis.* **136**:1403-1407.

Mullen, J. B. M., Wright, J. L., Wiggs, B. R., Paré, P. D., and Hogg, J. C. (1985). Reassessment of inflammation of airways in chronic bronchitis. *Br. Med. J.* **291**:1235-1239.

Murciano, D., Aubier, M., Lecocguic, Y., and Pariente, R. (1984). Effects of theophylline on diaphragmatic strength and fatigue in patients with chronic obstructive pulmonary disease. *N. Engl. J. Med.* **311**:349-353.

Naclerio, R. M., Bartenfelder, D., Proud, D., Togias, A. G., Myers, D. A., Kagey Sobotka, A., Norman, P. S., and Lichtenstein, L. M. (1986). Theophylline reduces histamine release during pollen-induced rhinitis. *J. Allergy Clin. Immunol.* **78**:874-876.

Nassif, E. G., Weinberger, M., Thompson, R., and Huntley, W. (1981). The value of maintenance theophylline in steroid-dependent asthma. *N. Engl. J. Med.* **304**:71-75.

Nielson, C. P., Crowley, J. J., Cusak, B. J., and Vestal, R. E. (1986). Therapeutic concentrations of theophylline and enprofylline potentiate catecholamine effects and inhibit leukocyte activation. *J. Allergy Clin. Immunol.* **78**:660-667.

O'Niell, S. J., Sitar, D. S., Klass, D. J., Taraska, V. A., Kepron, W. A., and Mitenko, P. A. (1986). The pulmonary disposition of theophylline and its influence on human alveolar macrophage bactericidal function. *Am. Rev. Respir. Dis.* **134**:1225-1228.

Orange, R. P., Kaliner, M. A., Laraia, P. J., and Austen, K. F. (1971). Immunological release of histamine and slow reacting substance of anaphylaxis from human lung II. Influence of cellular levels of cyclic AMP. *Fed. Proc.* **30**:1725-1729.

Passamonte, P. M., and Martinez, A. J. (1984). Effect of inhaled atropine or metaproterenol in patients with chronic airway obstruction and therapeutic serum theophylline levels. *Chest* **85**:610-615.

Pauwels, R., Van Renterghem, D., Van Der Straeten, M., Johannesson, N., and Persson, C. G. A. (1985). The effect of theophylline and enprofylline on allergen-induced bronchoconstriction. *J. Allergy Clin. Immunol.* **76**:583-590.

Perruchoud, A. P., Yerger, L., and Abraham, W. (1984). Differential effects of aminophylline on the early and late antigen-induced bronchial obstruction in allergic sheep. *Respiration* **46**:44.

Persson, C. G. A. (1985). On the medical history of xanthines and other remedies for asthma. A tribute to H. H. Salter. *Thorax* **40**:881-886.

Persson, C. G. A. (1986). Development of safer xanthines for the treatment of obstructive airway disease. *J. Allergy Clin. Immunol.* **78**:817-824.

Persson, C. G. A. (1988). Xanthines as airway antiinflammatory drugs. *J. Allergy Clin. Immunol.* **81**:615-617.

Persson, C. G. A., Erjefält, I., Gustafsson, B. (1988). Xanthines—Symptomatic or prophylactic in asthma? In *Directions for New Anti-Asthma*

Drugs. Edited by S. R. O'Donnell and C. G. A Persson. Basel, Birkhauser, pp. 137-155.

Pollock, J., Kiechel, F., Cooper, D., and Weinberger, M. (1977). Relationship of serum theophylline concentration to inhibition of exercise-induced bronchospasm and comparison with cromolyn. *Pediatrics* **60**:840-844.

Racineux, J. L., Troussier, J., Turcant, Tuchais, E., and Allain, P. (1981). Comparison of bronchodilation effects of salbutamol and theophylline. *Bull. Eur. Physiopathol. Respir.* **17**:799-806.

Ruffin, R., Bryant, D., Burdon, J., Marlin, G., Mitchell, C., O'Hehir, R., Wilson, J., Woolcock, A., and Webb, S. (1988). Comparison of the effects of nebulized terbutaline with intravenous enprofylline in patients with acute asthma. *Chest* **93**:510-514.

Taylor, D. R., Buick, B., Kinney, C., Lowry, R. C., and McDevitt, D. G. (1985). The efficacy of orally administered theophylline, inhaled salbutamol, and a combination of the two as chronic therapy in the management of chronic bronchitis with reversible air-flow obstruction. *Am. Rev. Respir. Dis.* **131**:747-751.

Ther, L., Mashaweck, R., and Hergott, J. (1957). Antagonismus zwischen Adenosine und Methylxanthines am Reizleitungssystem des Herzens. *Arch. Exp. Pathol. Pharmacol.* **231**:586-595.

Weinberger, M. (1984). Pharmacology and therapeutic use of theophylline. *J. Allergy Clin. Immunol.* **73**:525-540.

Welsh, C. H., Lien, D., Worthen, G. S., and Veil, J. V. (1988). Pentoxifylline decreases endotoxin-induced pulmonary neutrophil sequestration and extravascular protein accumulatin in the dog. *Am. Rev. Respir. Dis.* **138**:1106-1114.

Withering, W. (1984). The spasmodic asthma. (Letter 1786). In *Modern Drug Use. An Inquiry into Historical Principles.* Edited by R. D. Mann. Lancaster, U. K., MTP Press, pp. 346-362.

Zwillich, C. W., Neagley, S. R., Cicutto, L., White, D. P., and Martin, R. J. (1989). Nocturnal asthma therapy. Inhaled bitolterol versus sustained-release theophylline. *Am. Rev. Respir. Dis.* **139**:470-474.

20

Beta Agonists

KAREL F. KERREBIJN

Erasmus University Hospital
Sophia Children's Hospital
Rotterdam, The Netherlands

I. Introduction

Beta-adrenergic drugs are increasingly used for the treatment of asthma in adults and children. Recently a number of excellent reviews have been published on their mechanisms of action, pharmacology, and effects and application in patients (Bousquet et al, 1988) Svedmyr and Löfdalhl, 1987; Jenne and Ahrens, 1987). Rather than repeat the contents of these reviews, this chapter will summarize and integrate recent information on beta-adrenergic agents in vitro and in vivo in humans and focus on their effect in mechanisms underlying asthma in relation to symptoms.

II. Structure

Beta-adrenergic agonists are phenylethylamine derivates. Their molecules have two distinct regions: a cathechol ring or a closely related group, which is important primarily for the potency and secondarily for selectivity, and an ethanolamine side chain, which confers selectivity and, to a lesser extent, potency. Selectivity refers to the comparative affinity of the drug for beta-1 and beta-2 receptors (Popa, 1984). However, beta agonists with a high efficacy at beta-2 receptors, which means that a maximum effect is obtained when only a small fraction of the receptors is occupied by the agonist, and a low efficacy at beta-1-receptors can show considerable functional beta-2 selectivity, even though their affinity for the receptor subtypes differs only marginally (Waldeck et al., 1988). The initial compounds were rapidly metabolized by catechol-O-methyltransferase and monoamine oxidase. Newly synthesized drugs are more or totally resistant to these enzymes, which results in an increase in the duration of their action. The selectivity and potency of the drugs vary with their structure (Svedmyr, 1985). Beta-2-selective drugs currently used most in Europe are fenoterol (Berotec), salbutamol (Ventolin), and terbutaline (Bricanyl). Newer agents are pirbuterol, clenbuterol, and procaterol, but their place has still to be established. In many European countries they have not yet been accepted by drug registration authorities. Long-acting beta-agonists for inhalation, such as salmeterol and formoterol, which have a bronchodilating effect that lasts for more than 12 h, are currently being tested in clinical trials (Ullman and Svedmyr, 1988a; Sybrecht, 1988).

The beta-2 selectivity of salmeterol has been shown to be similar to that of salbutamol (Ullman and Svedmyr, 1988a).

III. Modes of Administration

Beta-adrenergic drugs are available for inhalation or oral administration and as subcutaneous or intravenous suspension. For details, the reader is referred to work by Bousquet et al. (1988).

Advantages of inhaled over oral drug application are immediate effect, low dosage and flexible administration possible, easy establishment of dose-response relationship, and a low incidence of side effects. The dose-effect relationship can be monitored at home with daily peak flow measurements before and after drug inhaltion. The diurnal variation of peak flow (difference between morning and evening peak flow) and the increase after the administration of a bronchodilator are indicative of the severity of the disease process (Ryan et al., 1982).

Methods of administration are metered dose inhaler (MDI), MDI with auxiliary delivery systems, dry powder inhalation, and nebulizer suspension. For the MDI to be used correctly the canister must be activated at low lung volume, followed by a deep breath to total lung capacity (TLC) and breathhold for about 10 s, to allow sedimentation of inhaled particles (Newman, 1985). The MDI is not always used correctly, especially by small children. In such cases, a large holding chamber or spacer, interposed between the canister and the mouth, greatly facilitates lung deposition (Levison et al., 1985). The residence of the aerosol particles in the chamber makes a coordination between actuation of the canister and inhalation unnecessary and allows the patient to inhale slowly from the chamber. For children, a dry powder inhaler is sometimes easier to use than a MDI. It is as effective as a MDI with spacer. Dry powder inhalers have the advantage over spacers that they can be taken more easily.

A compressed air nebulizer can be applied in case of an acute attack of asthma, during which higher than usual amounts of drug are needed, or in patients who either are too young to inhale from a MDI with spacer or need high doses as maintenance treatment.

Oral administration is seldom indicated. It can be considered at bedtime to prevent attacks of cough and wheeze during the night. In general, however, no compelling reason exists for oral beta-agonists in patients who inhale adequately. Subcutaneous or intravenous administration is used during an acute attack, often in combination with an inhaled beta-2 agonist.

IV. Pharmacology

Asthma is characterized by airway inflammation, smooth muscle constriction, mucus hypersecretion, and increased vascular permeability.

Beta-adrenergic drugs relax human bronchial smooth muscle exclusively via beta-2-adrenergic receptors (Zaagsma et al, 1983). Beta-1 receptors play no role in the modulation of the contractile state of bronchial smooth muscle (Lofdahl and Svedmyr, 1982). Interaction of a beta-agonist with the beta-2 receptor, which is located on the outer surface of the cell membrane, activates adenylate cyclase. This process induces a multiple-step inactivation of the contractile process by cyclic AMP (Skidmore, 1984). Beta -2 agonists may reduce microvascular permeability and mucosal edema (Persson and Erjefält, 1988), inhibit cholinergic neurotransmission at the ganglionic level (Barnes, 1986), and may enhance mucociliary transport (Pavia et al., 1980), probably by increasing active ion transport and water secretion across human airway epithelium (Knowles et al., 1984). Whether this enhancement is of clinical relevance in patients with asthma is unknown (Wanner, 1988). Furthermore, the transport of albumin through the airway epithelium is strongly stimulated by beta-2 agonists (Widdicombe, 1989). Although beta-adrenergic stimulation depletes mucous cells in vitro, producing low fluid output containing high protein concentrations (Nadel, 1983), little is known about the effect of beta-2 agonists on mucus secretion in humans. No net effect was reported by Kaliner et al., (1988) in cultured human airways and nasal mucosa. From these actions, the smooth-muscle-relaxing effect is often considered to be the predominant mechanism (Tattersfield, 1983).

Beta-adrenergic drugs are very potent and, hence, administered at a low dose. This results in low plasma concentrations that are difficult to measure. Pharmacokinetic data are therefore limited. Most information is available for terbutaline and salbutamol. This has been reviewed by Jenne and Ahrens (1987). What is known about fenoterol has been evaulated by Svedmyr (1985).

A. Inhalation

Inhalation of a beta-2 agonist leads to rapid bronchodilatation despite barely measurable blood levels. If the agent is inhaled adequately, total lung deposition from a MDI is likely to be between 10 and 30% of the total output (Newman, 1985; Kim et al., 1987). Only few studies looked at the effect of auxiliary devices (Dolovich et al., 1983; Newman et al., 1984). They indicate that the total lung deposition is not improved with a small device, but that a substantial improvement may occur with large devices. These are especially helpful for patients who have incorrect inhalation tchnique. Oropharyngeal deposition decreased markedly with auxiliary devices, irrespective of their size. The duration of action of the currently available beta-2 agonists is relatively short (between 4 and 6 h and even shorter during acute periods of asthma).

Beta-receptors are present on airway smooth muscle, airway microvasculature, airway glands, and on airway epithelial cells from trachea to terminal bronchioles. Their density increases with decreasing airway size (Barnes, 1986). It seems likely that in patients with asthma not only the central but also the peripheral airways dilate after the inhalation of a beta-2 agonist (Paré et al., 1983). Inhaled drug is mainly deposited centrally, it seems however not only to exert a local effect but also to be absorbed and distributed throughout the bronchial tree from the central to the peripheral airways via the dense submucosal vascular network (Deffebach et al., 1987). Animal experiments have shown that the lungs contain far more unchanged drug than metabolites after intratracheal instillation, in contrast to what happens after oral administration. These data indicate that an inhaled beta-agonist has a far higher therapeutic ratio than when administered orally (Ryrfeld and Ramsey, 1984).

After local application of these agents, pharmacokinetics cannot be defined, but some approximations can be made. It has been calculated that after the inhalation of 500 μg terbutaline sulfate the amount of drug in the large conducting airways (up to generation 8) will be between 30 and 300 ng/cm^2, with its peak in the segmental bronchi. In the small conducting airways (generations 9-16) it will range from 1 to 30 ng/cm^2 (Newman, 1984). If we assume an average thickness of the periciliary fluid layer of 5-6 μm (Sleigh et al., 1988), the drug concentration in the fluid of the large airways will approximate 10^{-4}-10^{-3} M and in the smaller airways 10^{-5}-10^{-6} M. It will probably be less in the airway wall and submucosa, especially when there is mucus hypersecretion.

B. Oral Administration

The bioavailability of orally administered beta-agonists varies with the drug and is dependent on the absorption and the biotransformation in the gut mucosa and during the first liver passage immediately after absorption. Peak drug concentrations are achieved in 1-2 h. For terbutaline, the bioavailability of active drug in the nonfasting state is about 10%. It is slightly higher for salbutamol due to a better absorption and lower for fenoterol (Rominger and Harmer, 1986). This is, however, compensated by the fact that fenoterol has a higher bronchodilating potency than terbutaline and salbutamol. The variability in absorption and biotransformation is responsible for the variations in blood levels between individuals taking the same dosage.

At steady state taking 5 mg terbutaline 3 times daily for 13 days, the plasma concentration 12 h after the last dose was found to be half the peak level, which is about 5 ng/ml or 4×10^{-8} M. It declined thereafter, with a half-life of 20 h, indicating the slow unloading of drug from a large compartment in which equilibration is slow and steady state will only be reached after about 72 h.

According to Jenne and Ahrens (1987), similar circumstances are likely for salbutamol. The duration of action at equipotent bronchodilating doses of fenoterol seems to be the same as for terbutaline and salbutamol. Sustained-release tablets of terbutaline (Nyberg and Kennedy, 1984) and salbutamol (Powell et al., 1987) have recently been introduced that show a smoother but not a higher plasma concentration profile than the standard tablets. Furthermore, new prodrugs are currently being developed with a high lung uptake that have a prolonged duration of action and a reduced incidence of side effects (Svensson and Tunek, 1988).

The influence of various disease states on the pharmacokinetics of orally administered beta-agonists has not yet been studied.

C. Subcutaneous Administration

Subcutaneously administered terbutaline (0.5 mg) provides therapeutic levels (about 7 ng/ml) in minutes. Following the initial dose, subsequent doses should be given about every 3-4 h consistent with the approximate half-life in unequilibrated stages. It is likely that the same is true for salbutamol and fenterol.

D. Intravenous Infusions

Intravenous infusions of terbutaline or salbutamol can be used in a severe attack of asthma and as an alternative to inhalation. Terbutaline sulfate 250 μg results in a plasma peak level of about 10 ng/ml with a half-life of 1 h in the unequilibrated stage. Equilibration is slow, but once loading is achieved, the infusion rate must be markedly reduced to avoid toxic serum concentrations. Because routine monitoring of drug serum levels is not possible, drug monitoring is performed on cardiac rate.

Data on the effect of beta-agonists on mediator release from various cell types are scarce. In atopic individuals beta-agonists may decrease antigen induced histamine release from peripheral leukocytes in vitro up to about 50% with concentrations between 10^{-4} M and 10^{-5} M (Lichtenstein and Margolis, 1968; Mita and Shida, 1983; Marone et al., 1984). Cells involved are probably mainly basophils. Isoproterenol (10^{-6}-10^{-4} M) was found to be slightly more potent against leukotriene than against histamine release (Warner et al., 1988). Similar concentrations of beta-agonist also reduce the production of superoxide anion, beta-glucuronidase, and elastase from opsonized zymosan-activated (Busse and Sosman, 1984) and PMA or FMLP-activated (Neijens et al., 1989) granulocytes in vitro as well as oxygen radicals from guinea pig alveolar macrophages (Henricks et al., 1986). Isoprenaline did, however, not inhibit the release of thromboxane B_2, leukotrine B_4, N-acetylglucosaminidase, and superoxide anion from opsonized zymosan and IgE-activated macrophages (Fuller et al., 1988). No published data exist on the effect of beta-agonists on eosinophils in humans, which are a predominant cell type in asthma. It seems, however, unlikely that the sensitivity of eosinophils to beta-agonists differs greatly from that of other leukocytes. One study reported that salbutamol (10^{-5} and 10^{-9} M) did not inhibit superoxide anion production from opsonized zymosan and PMA-activated guinea pig eosinophils (Yukawa et al., 1988).

Beta-agonists also inhibit histamine release from passively sensitized human lung tissue fragments, which indicates an effect on the histamine release from mast cells. Concentrations of about 10^{-7}-10^{-10}M are reported to cause a 50% inhibition (Assem and Schild, 1969; Butchers, 1979; Mita and Shida, 1983; Petersson, 1984; Marone et al., 1984), but complete inhibition may only be obtained with concentrations as high as 10^{-5} M and there may be differences in inhibitory potency between beta-agonists (Subramanian, 1986). No data exist on the duration of the inhibitory effect of beta-agonists on cells.

These figures suggest that concentrations of an inhaled beta-agonist in the airways will be high enough to exert an antianalphylactic effect on mast cells. This explains in part the acute protective effect on the antigen-induced early asthmatic reaction and on exercise-induced asthma. It can, however, not be separated from the direct effect on smooth muscle and microvascular permeability. It seems unlikely that the drug concentration in the airway wall, especially of the more peripheral airways, will be high enough to suppress mediator release effectively from other cells than mast cells, such as macrophages, eosinophils, lymphocytes, and monocytes, which are either resident in the bronchi of patients with asthma (Holgate et al., 1989; Wardlaw et al., 1988) or appear during an acute increase of the inflammatory process (de Monchy et al., 1985). One study suggests otherwise, but these data remain to be confirmed (Perruchoud et al., 1984).

From these data it appears that beta-agonists are unlikely to affect airway inflammation, irrespective of their mode of administration.

The situation is different with regard to smooth muscle relaxation (Fig. 1). Not only the beta-2 receptor density but also the affinity of the relaxation by beta-agonists increases from central to peripheral airways (Zaagsma et al., 1983). In vitro concentration relaxation curves of bronchiolar preparations from nonasthmatic subjects showed a 80-90% relaxation of methacholine EC_{50}-induced contraction, with a concentration of 1-isoproterenol of

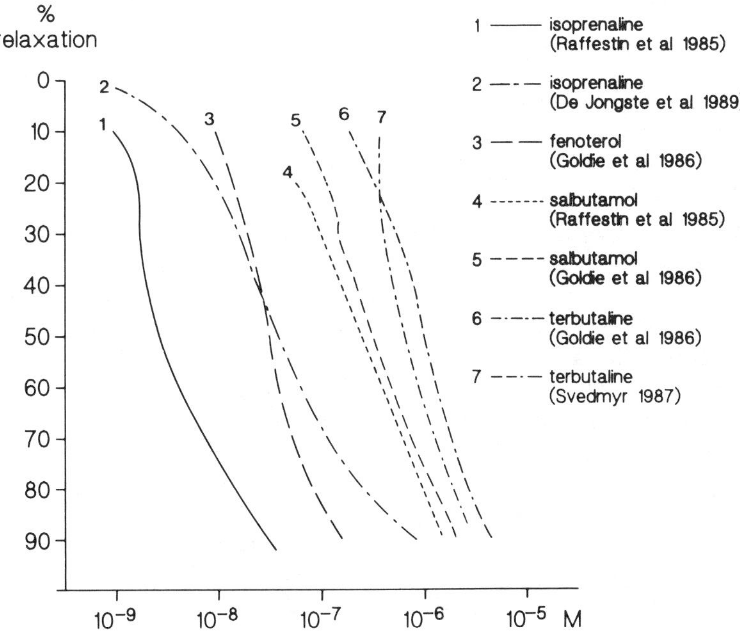

Figure 1   In vitro concentration-relaxation curves of human airway smooth muscle.

about 10^{-8} M in peripheral airways (de Jongste et al., 1989). Similar findings were published by Raffestin et al. (1985) based on tests after contraction with histamine. Goldie et al. (1984) and Svedmyr and Lofdahl (1987) reported the concentration of terbutaline needed to obtain a complete relaxation after carbachol EC_{50}-induced contraction to be about 10^{-7}-10^{-6} M. However, Finney et al. (1985) found that only 4 of 11 carbachol-contracted bronchiolar preparations relaxed with terbutaline in a concentration of about 5×10^{-5} M (not shown in Fig. 1 because of different starting point). Similar experiences have been reported by others (Guillot et al., 1984). For salbutamol, similar concentrations as for terbutaline are needed (Raffestin et al., 1985). Fenoterol appeared to be about four times less potent than isoprenaline on in vitro carbachol-induced contraction of bronchiolar preparations (Goldie et al., 1984). The mean relaxant potency of isoprenaline, terbutaline, and fenoterol was four to fivefold reduced in six bronchi from subjects with asthma who died during attacks and in one bronchus from an asthmatic subject who died because of coronary occlusion (Goldie et al., 1986). Bronchiolar strips from an asthmatic patient who underwent lung tissue resection while in a symptom-free period on maintenance treatment with inhaled beclomethasone relaxed normally to isoprenaline (de Jongste et al., 1987).

In a study on smooth muscle shortening and relaxation in intact airways, porcine tracheal rings achieved a maximum smooth muscle shortening of 44% with and 57% without cartilage, that is, the same contractile range as that used in relaxation experiments in vitro (James et al., 1987). Intact porcine tracheal rings, however, differ from the in vivo situation in that the transmural pressure is 0 and the surrounding connective and vascular tissue and nerve supply have been removed. Furthermore, beta-agonists may be less active in vitro than in vivo.

Diffusion of hydrophilic beta-agonists through the airway epithelium and subepithelial layer will reduce the drug concentration on the muscle and the vascular tissue (Jeppson et al., 1989). But even after a 100-fold reduction, concentrations will be high enough to exert relaxation in the relevant smooth muscle contractile range.

By taking these in vitro data together it can be concluded that the local beta-agonist concentration obtained after inhalation seems to be high enough to exert adequate smooth muscle relaxation. This is less clear with regard to orally or parenterally administered drug. In periods of disease activity, the drug concentration-relaxation curve will tend to shift to the right because of a diminished responsiveness of the beta-2 receptor system and an increase in functional antagonism of the cholinergic system. A number of studies has shown that plasma concentrations of terbutaline and improvement of airway calibre are related in patients with asthma but the effect is irreproducible and difficult to predict in individuals (Leferink, 1979; van den Berg et al.,

1980, 1984; Ripe et al., 1984). As we have seen, concentrations achieved after oral or parenteral administration amount to between 10^{-7} and 10^{-8} M. Based on in vitro relaxation data, these concentrations are too low to achieve adequate smooth muscle relaxation. However Leferink (1979) found that forced expiratory volume in 1s (FEV_1) in patients with asthma did not further improve when the plasma concentration of subcutaneously administered terbutaline was higher than about 10^{-8} M. Also, Fuglsang et al. (1989) reported that in about 6 of 10 children with asthma, maximum bronchodilatation after intravenous terbutaline was obtained at mean plasma concentrations of 3.6 $\times$ 10^{-8} M. In the first study, no details were presented. This makes it difficult to put the results in perspective with the in vitro findings. In the second study, FEV_1 had increased to 56-127% of predicted (mean, 96%) and MMEF to 27-104 percent of predicted (mean, 71%). In four subjects a plateau for FEV_1 and MMEF was not obtained.

These results suggest that in vitro concentration-relaxation curves of airway smooth muscle may have limited relevance for the in vivo situation. Olsson et al. (1979), who compared the relaxant potencies of orciprenaline, terbutaline, and fenoterol on in vitro contracted guinea pig trachea to the in vivo counteraction by these drugs of histamine-induced bronchial narrowing in the cat, found the in vitro potency for orciprenaline, terbutaline, and fenoterol to be lower than the in vivo potency. Whether in vitro and in vivo relaxant properties of beta-adrenergic drugs on human airway smooth muscle also differ is unknown. More data are needed before valid conclusions at this point can be drawn. In this respect, comparison of in vitro and in vivo relaxant properties of beta-agonists in humans is badly needed.

Interference of drugs with microvascular permeability has been reviewed recently by Persson and Svensjö (1985) and Persson and Erjefält (1988). In animal models, beta-2 agonists reduce inflammatory stimulus-induced leakage in a dose-dependent way. Svensjö and Roempke (1985) found that 10^{-6}-10^{-7} M terbutaline reduced macromolecular leakage in the hamster cheek pouch significantly. Also Erjefält and Persson (1985) found that concentrations of 10^{-7}-10^{-8} M terbutaline almost completely inhibited microvascular permeability of guinea pig trachea. No further diminishment was observed when the mucosa was injured. Salbutamol 20 μg/kg intravenously, which approximates the therapeutic dosage in humans, but also higher dosages (up to 320 μg/kg) failed, however, to inhibit platelet-activating factor (PAF)-induced microvascular leakage in guinea pig airways (Boschetto et al., 1989). Furthermore, 200 μg inhaled salbutamol only partially protected against PAF-induced bronchial obstruction in healthy nonasthmatic adults, possibly because of lack of inhibition of airway wall edema (Chung et al., 1989). Further data are needed on the effect of beta-2 agonists on vascular permeability in human airways, especially in view of the finding that beta-2 agonist plasma concentrations below the range in which in vitro smooth muscle relaxation takes place increase airway caliber and improve nocturnal symptoms. Only one study has been published on the concentration-response relation of a beta-2 agonist and secretion of airway mucus (Kyle et al., 1988). In ferret trachea in vitro, salbutamol (10^{-6}-10^{-3} M) had very little effect on mucus output but increased glycoprotein output dose-dependently two to threefold. Relatively high concentrations of salbutamol (2.10^{-5}-10^{-4} M) did not stimulate airway surface liquid flow but promoted the secretion of calcium and potassium and decreased pH in ferret trachea in vitro (Robinson et al., 1989).

In summary, airway concentrations achieved after inhalation of a beta-agonist are likely to be high enough for partial or complete inhibition of mediator release from mast cells and for smooth muscle relaxation. Whether beta-agonists will inhibit microvascular leakage in humans has not yet been established. Airway concentrations are probably not sufficient to inhibit mediator release from other inflammatory cells than mast cells. Plasma concentrations after oral or parenteral administration of beta-agonists in doses that can be tolerated are relatively low. More data are needed before the clinical effect of oral beta-agonists can be explained in terms of smooth muscle relaxation, reduction of microvascular leakage, or other mechanisms.

V. Effect on Bronchial Responsiveness to Histamine or Methacholine

Bronchial hyperresponsiveness (BHR) to histamine and methacholine is one of the prominent characteristics of asthma (see Chap. 2). Two kinds of studies on the effect of beta-agonists on BHR have been done:

1. During acute protection, when the dose-response curve is measured after smooth muscle relaxation, independent of prior treatment with a beta-agonist.

2. After long-term treatment with a beta-agonist for weeks or months. In these studies BHR was measured after a drug-free interval of 6-12 h.

After a single dose of beta-agonist, the dose-response curve to histamine or methacholine shifts to the right, resulting in an increase in the provocative dose (PD) or provocative concentration (PC) value from 1 to about 4 doubling doses. The effect is more pronounced after inhaled than after oral drug. It is dependent on the dose and the time interval between drug intake and the test. Few data exist on the duration of protection. Salome et al. (1983) found that this was shorter than 3 h in all subjects, whereas the improvement in FEV_1 was well maintained at 4 h in most subjects. Ahrens et al. (1984) and Joad et al. (1987) had similar findings.

Table 1 summarizes the results of acute protection studies after a single dose of a beta-agonist on the PD_{20} or $PC_{20}FEV_1$ to histamine or methacholine.

There is only a loose association between the degree of bronchodilatation and the shift of the dose-response curve. This might suggest that the underlying mechanisms are different. However, in patients with moderate or mild asthma the position of the dose-response curve to histamine and methacholine is largely independent of airway caliber (Yan et al., 1985; Ramsdale et al., 1985). Whether smooth muscle relaxation and protection by beta-agonists against bronchoconstrictor agents are both the result of inactivation of the smooth muscle contractile process has not yet been determined. The fact that the association between bronchodilatation with an anticholinergic drug (ipratropiumbromide) and inhibition of histamine-induced bronchoconstriction is less than that between a similar degree of bronchodilatation and inhibition after a beta-2 agonist (salbutamol) (Britton et al., 1988) suggests that smooth muscle relaxation is not the major determinant of change in airway responsiveness with bronchodilator drugs. This is supported by in vitro studies in which relaxation of guinea pig trachea with beta-agonists or xanthines did not affect the concentration-response relationship to carbachol (Persson, 1989 personal communication). The observations that BHR returns more rapidly towards baseline than FEV_1 indicates that the dose-effect relationship between bronchodilatation and protection may be different. This deserves further study, especially in view of the use of long-acting beta-agonists for inhalation. Only a few studies have been done on the effect of long-term administration of a beta-agonist on BHR to histamine or methacholine (Table 2). In none of these studies was a diminution of BHR shown. Kraan et al. (1985) and Kerrebijn et al. (1987) found a slight increase in BHR, but this was not the case in the studies by Peel and Gibson (9180) or Raes et al. (1989).

Tattersfield (1987) suggested that this "deterioration" might be caused by patient selection, because patients admitted had moderate to mild asthma and were in a stable condition with a greater chance of deterioration than of improvement. For obvious reasons, no placebo-treated control groups were used. However, the fact that patients characteristics in the studies by Kerrebijn and Raes were similar suggests that the slight deterioration of BHR in the first was due neither to patient selection nor to beta-agonist administration.

It can be concluded that although the currently available beta-2 agonists exert a significant acute protective effect on BHR to histamine or methacholine, this is of short duration. No improvement is seen after long-term administration. Chronic airway inflammation is considered to be a major determinant of BHR. It seems likely that the lack of effect of long-term administration of beta-agonists on BHR can be explained by the fact that the concentrations needed to exert an anti-inflammatory effect on many cell types involved in the inflammatory process are not achieved.

Table 1 Results of Acute Protection Studies

Author	Drug	Route/Dosage		Challenge	Interval Between drug Intake and Test (min)	Change in Mean PD_{20} or PC_{20}/FEV_1 in Doubling Doses
Casterline et al. (1976)	Salbutamol	Inhaled,	170 μg	Histamine	0	+3.6
Cockcroft et al. (1977)	Salbutamol	Oral,	4 mg	Histamine	60	+1.1
		Inhaled,	200 μg	Histamine	15	+3.6
Salome et al. (1981)	Fenoterol	Inhaled,	400 μg	Histamine	15	+2.4
		Oral,	5 mg	Histamine	90	+0.5
		Inhaled,	400 μg	Methacholine	15	+3.8
		Oral,	5 mg	Methacholine	90	+1.5
Bandouvakis et al. (1981)	Fenoterol	Inhaled,	800 μg	Histamine	45	+3
				Methacholine	45	+4
Chung et al. (1982)	Salbutamol	Inhaled,	200 μg	Histamine	30	+2.5
Salome et al. (1983)	Fenoterol	Inhaled,	100 μg	Histamine	15	+1.8
			200 μg	Histamine	15	+1.9
			400 μg	Histamine	15	+3.1
Chung and Snashall (1984)	Salbutamol	Inhaled,	200 μg	Methacholine	30	+3
Britton et al. (1988)	Salbutamol	Inhaled,	5 μg	Histamine	15	+0.3
			30 μg	Histamine	15	+1,1
			200 μg	Histamine	15	+1,5
			1000 μg	Histamine	15	+3.0

Table 2 Effect of Long-Term Administration on BHR to Histamine or Methacholine

Author (N)	Drug (Inhaled)	Dosage	Duration	Challenge	Interval Between Drug Intake and Test	Change in Mean PD_{20} or PC_{20}/FEV_1 in Doubling Doses
Peel and Gibson (1980) (8 adults)	Salbutamol	200 μg q. i. d.	4 weeks	Histamine	> 6 h 2 weeks	−0.25 −0.5
Kraan et al. (1985) (17 adults)	Terbutaline	500 μg q. i. d.	1 week 2 weeks	Methacholine	12-16 h	−0.8 −0.5
Kerrebijn et al. (1987) (7 children)	Terbutaline	500 μg t. i. d.	1 month 3 months 6 months	Methacholine	12 h	−0.9 −0.8 −0.8
Raes et al. (1989) (8 children)	Fenoterol		1 month 2 months 3 months 4 months	Histamine	12 h	+0.1 +0.2 +1.1 +1.9

VI. Clinical Effects

Beta-adrenergic drugs increase airway caliber in healthy subjects, in patients with asthma, and also in many patients with chronic obstructive lung disease (Postma et al., 1985). The magnitude of the effect is dependent on the severity of the airway obstruction, the underlying mechanisms, and the dose of agonist. In periods of increased disease activity, high doses of an inhaled beta-2 agonist may be needed for what is sometimes a limited degree of improvement, due to the smaller percentage of drug that is deposited in the airways because of the airway obstruction and subsequent difficulty in inhaling; the increased diffusion barrier between the airway mucosa and the beta-receptors on the vessel walls and smooth muscle; and the diminished responsiveness of the beta-2 receptors (Goldie et al., 1986).

It is important to realize that the response to bronchodilators can be expressed in various ways: in absolute terms, as a percentage of baseline, in relation to the difference between predicted and observed, and in percentage of predicted (Tashkin, 1987; Editorial, 1988). Especially in severely or mildly obstructed patients, bronchodilator responsiveness will vary greatly, depending on how it is defined. This is important to realize in studies on the effect of bronchodilator drugs and in studies on the outcome of chronic obstructive lung disease, if "reversibility" of bronchial obstruction is taken as an endpoint (Diener and Burrows, 1975; Traver et al., 1979; Postma et al., 1979; Kanner et al., 1979).

After the inhalation of a beta-2-adrenergic agonist, the increase in airway caliber in normal subjects is generally small (Watanabe et al., 1974) and may only become apparent when sensitive techniques for its measurement are used (Ekwo et al., 1983; Sourk and Nugent, 1983). In healthy persons, values obtained with forced expiratory maneuvers may even diminish, probably due to a decrease in airway wall stability after smooth muscle relaxation (Bouhuys and van de Woestijne, 1971). In wheezy infants, a nebulized beta-agonist may further impair expiratory flow by increasing airway wall compliance. If intrathoracic airway caliber is not coincidentally improved, the net effect may be little or no improvement in airway resistance or even a decline in expiratory flow rate during forced expiration (Prendiville et al., 1987).

The onset of bronchodilatation after inhalation follows within a few minutes. A maximum effect can be seen after about 20 min. The effect is sustained and may last up to 4-6 h, depending on the degree of baseline bronchoconstriction and the activity of the asthmatic process.

New compounds for inhalation therapy with a longer duration of action are currently being developed or in various stages of clinical trials. A recent study of salmeterol showed that more than half of the maximum bronchodilator effect remained after 12 h (Ullman and Svedmyr, 1988b).

After the administration of an inhaled beta-agonist, a dose-response relationship can be established. This is of clinical importance because, by means of a dose-response curve, the amount of drug can be determined that exerts optimal clinical benefit, for example, maximal bronchodilatation, maximal time course, minimal side effects.

Absorption of oral forms is dependent on the structure of the compound. The most widely used beta-2-selective adrenergic drugs (i.e., fenoterol, salbutamol, and terbutaline) seem to have similar potency and duration of action after oral use. Onset of action after oral administration is usually apparent after 1-2 h. The effect lasts for about 6 h.

Comparative data on newer beta-2 agonists such as pirbuterol and clenbuterol are scarce. Their place in the group of beta-2-selective compounds therefore remains to be established.

Sustained release (SR) oral beta-2 agonists such as SR terbutaline and SR salbutamol can be helpful in diminishing the symptoms of nocturnal asthma. Postma et al. (1986) reported that 5 mg SR terbutaline at 8 a.m. and 10 mg at 10 p.m. for 6 days suppressed plasma and urinary levels of epinephrine and prevented the nocturnal fall in FEV_1 in patients with chronic airflow obstruction. In another study it was found that SR terbutaline 7.5 mg twice daily improved mean morning peak expiratory flow with 20% and decreased nocturnal inhaler use in 9 patients with stable asthma but troublesome nocturnal wheeze or cough (Stewart et al., 1987). Plasma concentrations at 10 p.m. and 7 a.m. were 1.4×10^{-8}M, which is, as we have seen, lower than the concentrations needed for relaxation of smooth muscle in vitro. The reason may be that, apart from a possible difference in the in vitro and in vivo potency, other mechanisms than smooth muscle constriction, such as mucosal edema, play a role in nocturnal symptoms. SR salbutamol administered twice daily was reported at a number of meetings recently held in Europe to be effective in patients with asthma. Maessen and Smeets (1986) had good results with salbutamol SR 8 mg twice daily in patients with chronic obstructive lung disease. More data are, however, needed before the significance of SR beta-2 agonists for the treatment of asthma and obstructive lung disease can be established.

When different beta-2-agonists are inhaled, their clinical efficacy is similar despite differences in potency. This can be understood from the favorable concentration-relaxation relationship of inhaled drugs. Also orally administered beta-2 agonists exert a similar clinical effect. Differences in potency might be important after oral use because of the low plasma and tissue concentrations obtained but these appear to be compensated for by differences in bioavailability.

Responses to drugs and susceptibility to side effects can vary between patients for unexplained reasons (Madsen et al., 1979). It may therefore sometimes be necessary to change agents in order to find the one best suited for a particular patient.

As well as bronchodilatation, beta-adrenergic drugs have other effects. Several studies have shown that inhaled short-acting beta-agonists prevent the early, but not the late, asthmatic reaction after antigen challenge (Booij-Noord et al., 1970; Ruffin et al., 1978; Hegardt et al., 1981; Cockcroft and Murdock, 1987). As has been described earlier, this might be explained by the differences in drug concentration inhibiting histamine release from mast cells (which is considered to be the main mediator involved in the early asthmatic reaction), and drug concentration inhibiting cells involved in the late reaction. This is confirmed by a study of Howarth et al. (1985), who demonstrated that pretreatment with 200 μg inhaled salbutamol inhibited the allergen-induced early asthmatic reaction, together with increments in both plasma histamine and serum neutrophil chemotactic factor (NCA). A study by Venge et al. (1987) also demonstrated that single-dose pretreatment with 1250 μg inhaled terbutaline inhibited the generation of heat-labile NCA but was without effect on the late asthmatic reaction. Furthermore, the protective effect on smooth muscle and possibly vascular leakage will play a role. Prevention of the early but not of the late reaction also suggests that cells other than mast cells may be involved in initiating the late reaction, such as, for instance, macrophages (Tonnell et al., 1983) or T lymphocytes. Drug action has probably worn off at the time of the late asthmatic reaction. Preliminary data suggest that a long-acting beta-2 agonist may prevent the late asthmatic reaction (Palmquist et al., 1989), but further studies are needed to confirm this. In one study orally administered terbutaline (2.5 mg/h every 6 h for 36 h) has been reported to reduce sensitivity to inhaled grass or ragweed pollen and to decrease the plamsa histamine concentration and neutrophil chemotactic activity (Martin et al., 1980). The time interval between drug administration and allergen provocation was not given but since a steady state probably had not been reached after 36 h, it seems likely that it was short. More studies at this point are needed, in view of the development of oral SR formulations.

Inhaled beta-agonists also prevent the early asthmatic reaction after exercise (Anderson et al., 1979; König et al, 1984). No protection is obtained with regard to the late reaction after exercise (Kay, A. B., 1989, personal communication). The duration of the protection is 2-4 h (König et al., 1984; Kerrebijn et al., 1980), which is similar to that of the bronchodilatory action. In some studies, protection after oral administration was found (Morse et al., 1976; Eggleston et al., 1981a) but in another study it was not found after a dose that achieved significant bronchodilatation (Anderson et al., 1979). These findings, as well as those obtained by Eggleston et al. (1981b), who found bronchodilatation but no protection against exercise-induced asthma 1 h after inhaled isoproterenol, suggest that actions other than diminished smooth muscle constriction are involved in the prevention of bronchoconstriction after exercise by beta-agonists, for instance, inhibition of mediator release or diminished microvascular leakiness.

One of the hypotheses concerning the mechanism underlying exercise-induced asthma is respiratory heat loss, resulting in respiratory water loss (Anderson, 1985). Inhaled terbutaline was shown to inhibit bronchoconstriction dose-dependently due to isocapnic hyperventilation with cold air (O'Byrne et al., 1982). Other investigators found that a beta-agonist (metaproterenol) did not produce an all- or-none blockade to isocapnic hyperventilation with frigid air, but resulted in a parallel shift in the stimulus-response curve so that its protective effect could be overcome by increasing the stimulus (Rossing et al., 1982). In this study a fixed dose of agonist was given. In line with these findings were the results of Latimer et al. (1983), who concluded from their study on the protective effect of terbutaline and sodium cromoglycate on the response to respiratory heat loss that the combination of these drugs was more effective than either drug alone in the dosages given. These findings also suggest that protection by a beta-adrenergic agent against acute bronchial challenge is due to a combined effect on mediator release which is probably amplified by sodium cromoglycate, airway smooth muscle, and possibly microvascular leakage. Another hypothesis is that cooling of airway mucosa during exercise constricts the submucosal microvascular bed. Subsequent quick rewarming after discontinuation of exercise would cause vascular engorgement and edema (McFadden, 1987). Laitinen et al. (1987) found that 1.7×10^{-8} M salbutanol caused no vasoconstriction but a 25% reduction in tracheal vascular resistance in dogs. This observation makes it difficult to reconcile the protective effect of beta-agonists against exercise or cold air breathing with the hypothesis of McFadden.

In adults with asthma or chronic obstructive lung disease, provocation with a mist of distilled water often results in bronchoconstriction (Cheney and Butler, 1968; Booij-Noord et al., 1970). Subcutaneous epinephrine had only a minor protective effect (Booij-Noord et al., 1970), but inhaled salbutamol significantly reduced fog-induced bronchoconstriction (Allegra and Bianco, 1980; Pomari et al., 1984). Mediator release from mast cells also seems to be involved in this condition (Shaw et al., 1985). Furthermore, subcutaneous epinephrine and inhaled orciprenaline (Booij-Noord et al., 1970) as well as salbutamol (Koenig et al., 1987) protected against sulfur-dioxide-induced bronchoconstriction in subjects with asthma.

The importance of a possible facilitating effect of the bronchial epithelium in the mechanisms of action of inhaled beta-agonists has not yet been established. In rings of canine bronchi contracted with acetylcholine, removal of the epithelium reduced the relaxation induced by 5×10^{-5} and 10^{-4} M of the beta-2 agonist tulobuterol (Ruff et al., 1988). However, in human bronchial rings the reversal of the contractile response after acetylcholine was not significantly different between tissues with and without epithelium, although there was a tendency to a diminished relaxation in the bronchus without epithelium (Aizawa et al., 1988).

VII. Side Effects

A. Tachyphylaxis

Tachyphylaxis has been reviewed by Conolly et al. (1988) and Svedmyr (1989). It is the result of refractoriness of the beta-2 receptor to stimulation. Refractoriness involves a number of events, starting with receptor desensitization. Receptor desensitization is a two-step process involving a rapid diminishment of the affinity of the receptor for the agonist (i.e., reduction of the agonist-induced high-affinity state of the receptor) followed by uncoupling from adenylate cyclase. Thereafter, diminution of the number of receptors from the cell surface by internalization may take place. The first process occurs within a short period of time at low concentrations of agonist and is rapidly reversed as the agonist disappears. The second step occurs with more prolonged exposure to low or after shorter exposure to high concentrations and is reversed less rapidly.

Tachyphylaxis has been shown on human smooth muscle in vitro. Incubation with isoprenaline concentrations of 10^{-6}-10^{-4} M for 30-60 min reduced smooth muscle relaxation in a dose-dependent fashion (Davis and Conolly, 1980; Avner and Jenne, 1981; Guillot et al., 1984). Similar concentrations subsensitize lymphocytes (Kalisker et al., 1977). After administration of terbutaline 5 mg three times daily for 14 days (i.e., after the development of a steady state) the increase in c-AMP of mixed leukocytes diminished about threefold after incubation with a terbutaline concentration about ten thousand-fold that in plasma (10^{-4} M). Similar figures were found for isoprenaline. This effect had disappeared about a week after oral therapy had been discontinued (Bruynzeel et al., 1979). Also, Galant et al. (1980) and Tashkin et al. (1982) found that a similar dosage of terbutaline subsensitized beta-receptors on white blood cells but did not diminish the effect on symptoms, the acute bronchodilator response, or the protection against histamine-induced bronchoconstriction. This indicates that white blood cells are not a good model for beta-2 receptor tachyphylaxis of smooth muscle.

Results of in vitro studies of relaxant properties of airway smooth muscle from subjects who were treated with beta-adrenergic agents are conflicting. Svedmyr et al. (1976) showed normal dose-response curves for isoprenaline. Paterson et al. (1984) found that airways from asthmatic subjects treated with beta-2 agonists had reduced relaxant potency to isoprenaline in vitro.

Cerrina et al. (1986) reported, however, that bronchial smooth muscle preparations from subjects with stable asthma were less sensitive to isoprenaline than those from nonasthmatic subjects, although their patients had not received beta-2 agonists or steroids for at least 2 weeks before surgery. It is therefore difficult to conclude that drug-induced beta-2 receptor tachyphylaxis was the main factor responsible for the findings by Paterson et al. (1984). More data are needed before the role of treatment with beta-2 agonists in the diminished clinical responsiveness to these drugs in acute periods of asthma becomes clear (see sect. IV).

In vivo tachyphylaxis can be studied by assessing the bronchodilator response after the administration of a beta-2 agonist and by the degree of protection after bronchoconstrictor agents such as histamine or methacholine. Since bronchodilatation and protection are only loosely associated, these indicators may give different results.

For a review of clinical studies on beta-adrenergic tachyphylaxis and the complexities involved in these studies, the reader is referred to Conolly et al. (1988). Although the data from the clinical literature are also conflicting, most investigators agree that beta-2 agonists in the usual therapeutic dosages, even when administered for long periods, will not result in a clinically relevant reduction of baseline airway caliber or bronchodilator response in asthmatic patients. In view of the relatively short duration of action of inhaled beta-2 agonists, the most likely explanation is the limited period in which a drug concentration at the receptor level exists that is high enough to cause receptor uncoupling. The receptor can therefore recover before the next dose of drug is administered. This is supported by the observation of Svedmyr (1984), who noticed a slight tendency to tachyphylaxis after 3 weeks of treatment with a high dosage of inhaled salbutamol (2 mg three times daily). The same investigator reported, however, in a preliminary observation that the new long-acting inhaled beta-2 agonist salmeterol, which still has a significant bronchodilatatory action after 12 h, did not cause tachyphylaxis when given twice daily for 9 days (Ullman and Svedmyr, 1988b).

No diminution of the acute protective effect against histamine-induced bronchoconstriction was seen by most investigators after treatment with beta-2 agonists in moderate to high dosages for a period of 4 weeks (Peel and Gibson, 1980; Harvey and Tattersfield, 1982; Tashkin et al., 1982). But Vathenen et al. (1988) reported that treatment with terbutaline 750 μg three times daily for 2 weeks diminished the protection against histamine-induced bronchoconstriction and was followed by a rebound increase in bronchial responsiveness after cessation of treatment. They considered this indicative of beta-receptor tachyphylaxis. Patients were only studied for 24 h after terbutaline use was discontinued, so that it is unknown for how long these drug-induced changes were present. Although these findings need to be confirmed, they suggest that when high dosages of beta-agonists are stopped suddenly, patients may be more vulnerable to provocative stimuli. The time course of this increased vulnerability was not studied. In contrast to asthmatic subjects, administration of beta-agonists in the usual dosages to healthy individuals may result in tachyphylaxis to the bronchodilator effect (Holgate et al., 1977; Harvey and Tattersfield, 1982).

That tachyphylaxis after beta-agonist concentrations obtained in vivo is of limited degree is in accordance with the findings of Van der Heijden et al. (1984). These investigators showed that incubation of guinea pig tracheal smooth muscle with isoprenaline, terbutaline, fenoterol, and salbutamol in concentrations of 10^{-5} M for 30 min resulted in a shift to the right of the relaxant dose-response curve to isoprenaline of 0.3, 0.1, 0.4, and 0.7 decades, respectively. Comparable data were obtained with guinea pig lung parenchymal strips. The paper by Guillot et al. (1984) contains similar figures for isoprenaline on human smooth muscle, but Avner and Jenne (1981) observed a larger shift as well as a reduction in slope. Furthermore, Van der Heijden et al. (1984) found in the guinea pig that beta-receptors of cells that mediate antigen-induced release of mediators were more sensitive to tachyphylaxis than those mediating smooth muscle relaxation. Similar anecdotal findings after challenge with annual blue grass antigen were reported in humans by Tashkin et al. (1982). They observed in two patients a 10-15-fold decrease in acute protection by subcutaneously administered terbutaline against antigen-induced bronchoconstriction after 3-5 weeks of 5 mg oral terbutaline three times daily. Both subjects had a normal bronchodilatory response to terbutaline. Subsensitization of smooth muscle beta-receptors is therefore an unlikely explanation for this observation, but subsensitization of mast cell beta-receptors is a possibility. From clinical experience, little evidence exists that regular treatment with beta-agonists will reduce the protective effect against exercise-induced bronchoconstriction, although this was reported after treatment with a high dosage of oral salbutamol (6 mg for 4-20 weeks) by Gibson et al. (1978). No data exist on the tachyphylactic effect of beta-agonists on human mast cells or vascular tissue.

It is obvious from these data that plasma and airway concentrations after therapeutic dosages of a beta-agonist will be high enough to cause de(sub)sensitization of beta-receptors and possibly, in particular of those located on mast cells. It seems, however, that only high dosages may result in a clinically measurable tachyphylaxis of minor degree, which has no clinical significance.

B. Tremor

Striated muscle contains beta-2 receptors, which do not differ from those in bronchial smooth muscle (Löfdahl et al., 1984). Beta-2 agonists cause tremor by depression of slow contracting muscles (Svedmyr and Löfdahl, 1987). Muscle tremor is mainly seen in patients taking oral beta-2 agonists or after parenteral administration, in whom plasma drug concentrations are between 10^{-7} and 10^{-8} M. In these patients, tremor is often the dosage-limiting factor. After proper inhalation, no measurable plasma concentration is obtained. Therefore, tremor after inhalation of a beta-2 agonist often indicates a poor inhalation technique resulting a large drug deposition in the mouth and oropharynx and resorption into the general circulation, causing plasma concentrations high enough to give tremor. In such patients tremor often disappears after the use of a spacer (Lindgren and Carsson, 1982). In most patients on maintenance therapy with oral beta-2 agonists, tremor wears off within a few weeks because of receptor tachyphylaxis in striated muscle.

C. Cardiovascular Effects

Beta-2 agonists may induce tachycardia. Whether the main underlying mechanism is a direct stimulation of beta-2 receptors of cardiac muscle (Position Statement, 1985) or peripheral vasodilatation with reflex increase in heart rate (Svedmyr and Löfdahl, 1987) has not yet been resolved. Cardiac arrhythmia is rare and should not be considered a cause of cardiac death in subjects with asthma without heart disease or severe hypoxemia. Two studies reported an increased incidence of arrhythmias in patients who were treated with a combination of beta-agonists and theophylline (Laursen et al., 1985; Nicklas and Balzas, 1986). It has been suggested that hypokalemia caused by beta-2 agonists or theophylline gives rise to potentially fatal arrhythmias (Benatar, 1986). Because of the difference in plasma levels after different cardiovascular routes of administration, effects are more prevalent when given intravenously.

D. Hypoxemia

Inhaled beta-2 agonists may increase the intrapulmonary shunt transiently with a reduction in arterial oxygen tension (PaO_2) that rarely exceeds 1.33 kPa. This may affect oxygen saturation in patients with a baseline PaO_2 lower than 8-9 kPa. In severe attacks of asthma, beta-2 agonists should therefore be administered together with oxygen.

VIII. Summary and Conclusions

Beta-agonists are useful drugs for inducing bronchodilatation. They protect against acute challenges such as allergens, exercise, cold air breathing, mist, and air pollutants. They also exert an acute protective effect against inhalation with histamine or methacholine. They do not, however, diminish the late reaction after allergen inhalation or exercise, nor do they improve bronchial hyperresponsiveness to histamine or methacholine when administered for several weeks or months. Their potency is reduced during an acute asthmatic attack.

Beta-2-receptor-selective drugs are preferable over nonselective preparations. Concentrations achieved at the site of target organs are considerably higher when these agents are administered by the inhaled route than when given orally or parenterally. The duration of action of beta-2 agonists is 4-5 h, depending on the dosage given. Interesting new developments are long-acting inhaled beta-2 agonists, which seem to be effective for 12 h or more. Unless these agents are given in very high dosages, short-term and long-term side effects of beta-2 agonists of a magnitude that is clinically relevant, such as tachyphylaxis, tachycardia, cardiac arrhythmia, or transient reduction of arterial oxygen tension, are rare. Beta-2 agonists can therefore be considered safe drugs.

Many clinical effects of beta-agonists can be explained from the concentration-response relationship in vitro on target tissues. After inhalation, drug concentrations in the large conducting airways are probably high enough to result in relaxation of smooth muscle in the contractile range likely to be relevant in vivo. Concentrations after inhaled beta-agonists are also high enough to inhibit mast cell mediator release partly or completely, but not to affect macrophages, eosinophils, basophils, granulocytes, or T cells. This explains their acute inhibiting effect on inhalation of allergen and other substances and on exercise and their lack of effect on the late reaction after allergen inhalation and on the long-term modulation of bronchial hyperresponsiveness, which are closely related to airway inflammation.

Plasma concentrations after oral or parenterally administered beta-agonists are 1000-10,000-fold lower than those that may be obtained in the large airways after inhalation. Based on in vitro dose-relaxation curves of human airway smooth muscle, these concentrations would not be high enough to relax smooth muscle in vivo. The limited data from human studies in which plasma concentrations and airway caliber were compared indicate, however, that low plasma concentrations may achieve maximal bronchodilatation. This suggests a different dose-response relationship for beta-agonists in vitro and in vivo. Although a limited number of animal studies also indicate that the potency of beta-agonists may be higher in vivo than in vitro, more data, preferably from human studies, are needed to clarify this point. Data from in vitro animal studies on the effect of beta-agonists on the microvascular permeability are conflicting. No in vitro human data exist, but a recent in vivo study in humans suggested that a beta-2 agonist had not inhibited microvascular leakage after inhalation of PAF. Since microvascular leakage and airway edema may play an important role in the airway obstruction in asthma, the effect of drugs on microvascular leakage in animal and human models is an important area for future research. The same is true for mucus secretion and epithelial function, on which very little is known in terms of modulation by drugs.

What is the place of beta-adrenergic drugs in the treatment of asthma? No controversy exists about their use in periods of acute bronchial obstruction and for protection against the immediate reaction to inhaled agents and exercise. Their place as drugs of first choice in the maintenance treatment of chronic airway obstruction is less clear. Chronic airway obstruction in asthma, together with airway hyperresponsiveness, is maintained to a large extent by chronic airway inflammation. Anti-inflammatory drugs rather than beta-2 agonists, anticholinergics, or theophylline may therefore be more appropriate as the treatment of first choice in the maintenance therapy of chronic asthma. Only long-term clinical studies, which are currently being carried out in a number of centers, will answer this question. Furthermore, the place of newly developed long-acting inhaled and oral beta-2 agonists must be established.

Discussion

Kaliner: Our in vitro studies of beta-adrenergic effects on human lung mast cell degranulation in vitro demonstrated that 10^{-6}-10^{-7} M was required for effective inhibition. Thus, your suggested mast cell sensitivity to β-agonists is in error by 100-1000-fold. However, it may be that mast cells are more sensitive than other possible targets in treating asthma. As you know, cutaneous mast cells are not affected by oral beta-agonists (skin test reactions are normal).

Daniel:In determining the effects of beta agonists on various cellular systems, especially inflammatory cells, the data need to include evidence about which beta receptor subtype is involved and relate this to the agonists used and their concentrations.

Paré: Irrespective of β-agonists' effect on edema formation, airway wall thickening can have an important influence on the bronchodilatory effect of smooth-muscle-relaxing drugs. For a given amount of smooth muscle relaxation, there will be larger effect on airway caliber if the airway wall is thickened. Extensive changes in airway caliber can occur with relatively small amounts of smooth muscle relaxation in the presence of airway wall thickening.

Daniel: The immediate effect of beta-2 agonists is likely to be the result of smooth muscle relaxation.

Paré: I agree completely. Additional reduction of the mucosal thickness will even further diminish airflow limitation.

Fabbri: The inhibitory effect of β_2-agonists on microvascular leakage should be considered controversial, at the best. Boschetto et al. (*Am. Rev. Respir. Dis.* 1989) showed that epinephrine, but not salbutamol, inhibits PAF-induced microvascular leakage in guinea pigs.

Persson: We have demonstrated that i.v. or topical β-agonists reduce plasma exudation in mild topically induced airways inflammation, but with large doses of inflammatory mediators β-agonists may not reduce the plasma exudation response. The study by Boschetto et al. used near-shock intravenous dosages of PAF, which may have interacted with the intravenous sympathomimetic drugs at other sites than the airways. Furthermore, their technique of measuring "plasma leak" may not differentiate between the intravascular and extravascular plasma pool in the airway tissue (see text).

Widdicombe: You need high concentrations of β-agonists (? 10^{-5}) to promote gland secretion, and the output is very small. However an important target organ is the epithelium, where the concentration of inhaled β-agonists will be highest. The β-agonists promote secretion of ions, with water following, of albumin and of proteoglycans from the glycocalyx, all into the lumen.

Kerrebijn: Beta-agonists increase active ion transport and water secretion across human airway epithelium and may therefore contribute to dilution of sputum.

Sears: There is epidemiological evidence for increasing severity of asthma. Would you comment on the studies that have suggested that long-term use of β-agonists may not only have no protective effect on airway hyperresponsiveness but may also have an adverse effect in increasing airway hyperresponsiveness? What do you believe is the mechanism of such an effect?

Pauwels: I would like to ask Anne Tattersfield: What is the relevance of reported changes in reactivity occurring after treatment with β_2-agonists is stopped?

Tattersfield: The rebound increase in bronchial reactivity may be of no clinical significance but I do not think we can say that based on present evidence. In our study we unfortunately only evaluated the changes for 24 h after stopping treatment and it may not have been maximal then.

Can I ask about the plateau you describe with oral salbutamol? In most studies patients receiving oral beta agonists will show further bronchodilatation if they then inhale a beta agonist. My question is whether the plateau was a plateau to oral drugs only, and whether there was further capacity for bronchodilatation to occur.

Kerrebijn: In the study by Fuglsang et al. (1989), FEV_1 reached values near to 100% of predicted in the subjects who had a plateau.

Dahl: Inhaled beta-2 agonist given prior to an allergen challenge inhibits the early but not the late reaction. How does oral long-acting beta-2 agonist or the new inhaled long-acting beta-2-agonist influence the late reaction?

Pauwels: The lack of effect of sympathomimetics on the late asthmatic reaction following allergen challenge may be explained by the pharmacokinetic properties of these drugs. Long-acting sympathomimetics such as formoterol and salmeterol inhibit the late asthmatic reaction.

Fish: You state that inhaled beta-agonists inhibit early but not late reactions to allergen and that the drug works by inhibiting mast cells. If this is so, it implies that there is another primary effector cell involved in the early reaction. Would you elaborate on what you consider are candidates for this?

Kerrebijn: Possibly the macrophage.

Kay: Or the T cell.

There is a report showing that beta-agonists block the early phase of exercise-induced asthma (EIA) but not late-phase EIA (nor the concomitant elevation in NCA). On the other hand corticosteroids block late-phase (and NCA) but not immediate EIA.

References

Ahrens, R. C., Bonham, A. C., Maxwell, G. A., and Weinberger, M. M. (1984). A method for comparing peak intensity and duration of action of aerosolized bronchodilators using bronchoprovocation with methacholine. *Am. Rev. Respir. Dis.* **129**:903-906.

Aizawa, H., Miyazaki, N., Shigematsu, N., and Tomooka, M. (1988). A possible role of airway epithelium in modulating hyperresponsiveness. *Br. J. Pharmacol.* **93**:139-145.

Allegra, L., and Bianco, S. (1980). Non-specific bronchoreactivity obtained with an ultrasonic aerosol of distilled water. *Eur. J. Respir. Dis.* **61**(suppl. 106):41-49.

Anderson, S. D. (1985). Issues in exercise-induced asthma. *J. Allergy Clin. Immunol.* **76**:763-772.

Anderson, S. D., Seale, J. P., Ferris, L., Schoeffel, R., and Lindsay, D. A. (1979). An evaluation of pharmacotherapy for exercise-induced asthma. *J. Allergy Clin. Immunol.* **64**(part 2):612-624.

Anderson, S. D., Schoeffel, R. E., and Finney, M. (1983). Evaluation of ultrasonically nebulized solutions for provocation testing in patients with asthma. *Thorax* **38**:284-291.

Assem, E. S. K., and Schild, H. O. (1969). Inhibition by sympathomimetic amines of histamine release induced by antigen in passively sensitized human lung. *Nature* **224**:1028-1029.

Avner, B. P., and Jenne, J. W. (1981). Desensitization of isolated human bronchial smooth muscle to beta-receptor agonists. *J. Allergy Clin. Immunol.* **68**:51-57.

Bandouvakis, J., Cartier, A., Roberts, R., Ryan, G., and Hargreave, F. E. (1981). The effect of ipratropium and fenoterol on methacholine- and histamine-induced bronchoconstriction. *Br. J. Dis. Chest* **75**:295-305.

Barnes, P. (1986). Neural control of human airways in health and disease. State of the art. *Am. Rev. Respir. Dis.* **134**:1289-1314.

Benatar, S. R. (1986). Fatal asthma. *N. Engl. J. Med.* **314**:423-429.

Van den Berg, W., Feferink, J. G., Maes, R. A. A., Kreukniet, J., and Bruynzeel, P. L. B. (1980). Correlation between terbutaline serum concentrations, c-AMP plasma levels and lung function parameters. *Ann. Allergy* **44**:235-239.

Van den Berg, W., Leferink, J. G., Maes, R. A. A., Fokkens, J. K., Kreukniet, J., and Bruynzeel, P. L. B. (1984). The effects of oral and subcutaneous administration of terbutaline in asthmatic patients. *Eur. J. Respir. Dis.* **134**(suppl):181-193.

Booij-Noord, H., Orie, N. G. M., Berg, W. Chr., and de Vries, K. (1970). Results of provocation of human bronchial airways with allergic and non-allergic stimuli and of drug protection tests. In: *Bronchitis III.* Edited by N. G. M. Orie, and R. van der Lende. Assen, Royal Vangorcum, pp. 316-330.

Boschetto, P., Roberts, N. M., Rogers, D. F., and Barnes, P. L. (1989). Effect of antiasthma drugs on microvascular leakage in guinea pig airways. *Am. Rev. Respir. Dis.* **139**:416-421.

Bouhuys, A., and van de Woestijne, K. P. (1971). Mechanical consequences of airway smooth muscle relaxation. *J. Appl. Physiol.* **30**:670-675.

Bousquet, J., Clauzel, A. M., and Michel, F. B. (1988). Adrenergic agonists in asthma. In: *The Airways: Neural Control in Health and Disease, Lung Biology in Health and Disease,* vol. 33. Edited by M. A. Kaliner and P. Barnes. New York, Marcel Dekker, pp. 119-157.

Britton, J., Hanley, S. P., Garrett, H. V., Hadfield, J. W., and Tattersfield, A. E. (1988). Dose related effects of salbutamol and ipratropium bromide on airway calibre and reactivity in subjects with asthma. *Thorax* **43**:300-305.

Bruynzeel, P. L. B., van den Berg, W., Hamelink, M. L., van den Bogaard, W., Houben, L., and Kreukniet, J. (1979). Desensitization of the beta-adrenergic receptors on leucocytes after long-term oral use of a beta-sympathomimetic; its effect on the beta-adrenergic blockade hypothesis of Szentivanyi. *Ann. Allergy* **43**:150-159.

Busse, W. W., and Sosman, J. M. (1984). Isoproterenol inhibition of isolated human neutrophil function. *J. Allergy Clin. Immunol.* **73**:404-410.

Butchers, P. R., Fullerton, J. R., Skidmore, I. F., Thomson, L. E., Vardey, C. J., and Wheeldon, A. (1974). A comparison of the anti-anaphylactic activities of salbutamol and disodium-cromoglycate in the rat, the rat mast cell and in human lung tissue. *Br. J. Pharmacol.* **67**:23-32.

Casterline, C. L., Evans, R., and Ward, G. W. (1976). The effect of atropine and albuterol aerosols on the human bronchial response to histamine. *J. Allergy Clin. Immunol.* **58**:607-613.

Cerrina, J., Ladurie, M. L., Labat, C., Raffestin, B., Bayol, A., and Brink, C. (1986). Comparison of human bronchial smooth muscle responses to histamine in vivo with histamine and isoproterenol agonists in vitro. *Am. Rev. Respir. Dis.* **134**:57-61.

Cheney, F. W., and Butler, J. (1968). The effects of ultrasonically-produced aerosols on airway resistance in man. *Anesthesiology* **29**:1099-1106.

Chung, K. F., and Snashall, P. D. (1984). Methacholine dose-response curves in normal and asthmatic man: effect of starting conductance and pharmacological antagonism. *Clin. Sci.* **66**:665-673.

Chung, K. F., Morgan, B., Keyes, S. J., and Snashall, P. D. (1982). Histamine dose-response relationships in normal and asthmatic subjects. *Am. Rev. Respir. Dis.* **126**:849-854.

Chung, K. F., Dent, G., and Barnes, P. J. (1989). Effects of salbutamol on bronchoconstriction, bronchial hyperresponsiveness, and leucocyte responses induced by platelet activating factor in man. *Thorax* **44**:102-107.

Cockcroft, D. W., and Murdock, K. Y. (1987). Comparative effects of inhaled salbutamol, sodium cromoglycate, and beclomethasone dipropionate on allergen-induced early asthmatic responses, late asthmatic responses and increased bronchial responsiveness to histamine. *J. Allergy Clin. Immunol.* **79**:734-740.

Cockcroft, D. W., Killian, D. N., Mellon, J. J. A., and Hargreave, F. E. (1977). Protective effect of drugs on histamine-induced asthma. *Thorax* **32**:429-437.

Conolly, M. E., Jenne, J. W., Hui, K. K., and Borst, S. E. (1988). Beta-adrenergic tachyphylaxis (desensitization) and functional antagonism. In: *Drug Therapy for Asthma*. Edited by J. W. Jenne and S. Murphy. New York, Marcel Dekker, pp. 259-296.

Davis, C., and Conolly, M. E. (1980). Tachyphylaxis to beta-adrenoceptor agonists in human bronchial smooth muscle: studies in vitro. *Br. J. Clin. Pharmacol.* **40**:417-423.

Deffebach, M. E., Charan, N. B., Lakshminaryan, S., and Butler, J. (1987). The bronchial circulation. State of the art. *Am. Rev. Respir. Dis.* **135**:463-481.

De Jongste, J. C., Mons, H., Bonta, I. L., and Kerrebijn, K. F. (1987). In vitro responses of airways from an asthmatic patient. *Eur. J. Respir. Dis.* **71**:23-29.

De Jongste, J. C., Mons, H., Bonta, I. L., and Kerrebijn, K. F. (1989). Relaxation of human peripheral airway smooth muscle in vitro does not correlate with severity of chronic airflow limitation in vivo.*Pulm. Pharmacol.* **2**:75-79.

Diener, C. F., and Burrows, B. (1975). Further observations on the course and prognosis of chronic obstructive lung disease. *Am. Rev. Respir. Dis.* **111**:719-724.

Dolovich, M., Ruffin, R., Corr, D., and Newhouse, M. T. (1983). Clinical evaluation of a simple demand inhalation MDI aerosol delivery device. *Chest* **84**:36-41.

Editorial (1988). Airflow limitation-reversible or irreversible? *Lancet* **1**:26-27.

Eggleston, P. A., and Beasley, P. P. (1981a). Bronchodilation and inhibition of induced asthma by adrenergic agonists. *Clin. Pharmacol. Ther.* **29**: 505-510.

Eggleston, P. A., and Beasley, P. B., and Kindley, R. T. (1981b). The effects of oral doses of theophylline and fenoterol on exercise-induced asthma. *Chest* **79**:399-405.

Ekwo, E. E., Weinberger, M. M., Dusdieker, L. B., Huntley, W. H., Rodgers, P., and Maxwell, G. A. (1983). Airway responses to inhaled isoproterenol in normal children. *Am. Rev. Respir. Dis.* **127**:108-109.

Erjefält, I., A.-L., and Persson, C. G. A. (1985). Anti-asthma drugs and capsaicine-induced microvascular effects in lower airways. *Agents Actions* **16**:9-10.

Finney, M. J. B., Karlsson, J. A., and Persson, C. G. A. (1985). Effects of bronchoconstrictors and bronchodilators on a normal human small airway preparation. *Br. J. Pharmacol.* **85**:29-36.

Fuglsang, G., Pedersen, S., and Borgström, L. (1989). Dose-response relationships of intravenously administered terbutaline in children with asthma. *J. Pediatr.* **114**:315-320.

Fuller, R. W., O'Malley, G., Baker, A. J., and MacDermot, J. (1988). Human alveolar macrophage activation: inhibition by forskolin but not beta-adrenoceptor stimulation or phosphodiesterase inhibition. *Pulm. Pharmacol.* **1**:101-106.

Galant, S. P., Duriseti, L., Underwood, S., and Insel, P. A. (1980). Beta-adrenergic receptors of polymorph nuclear particulates in bronchial asthma. *J. Clin. Invest.* **65**:577-585.

Gibson, G. J., Greenacre, J. K., König, P., Conolly, M. E., and Pride, N. (1978). Use of exercise challenge to investigate possible tolerance to beta-adrenoceptor stimulation in asthma. *Br. J. Dis. Chest* **72**:199-206.

Goldie, R. G., Paterson, J. W., Spina, D., and Wale, J. L. (1984). Classification of β-adrenoceptors in human isolated bronchus. *Br. J. Pharmacol.* **81**:611-615.

Goldie, R. G., Spina, D., Henry, P. J., Lulich, K. M., and Paterson, J. W. (1986). In vitro responsiveness of human asthmatic bronchus to carbachol, histamine, β-adrenoceptor agonists and theophylline. *Br. J. Pharmacol.* **22**:669-676.

Guillot, C., Fornaris, M., Badier, M., and Orehek, J. (1984). Spontaneous and provoked resistance to isoproterenol in isolated human bronchi. *J. Allergy Clin. Immunol.* **74**:713-718.

Harvey, J. E., and Tattersfield, A. E. (1982). Airway response to salbutamol: effect of regular salbutamol inhalations in normal, atopic and asthmatic subjects. *Thorax* **37**:280-287.

Hegardt, B., Pauwels, R., and van der Straeten, M. (1981). Inhibitory effect of KW 2131, terbutaline, and DSCG on the immediate and late allergen-induced bronchoconstriction. *Allergy* **36**:115-122.

Van der Heijden, P. J. C. M., van Amsterdam, J. G. C., and Zaagsma, J. (1984). Desensitization of smooth muscle and mast cell beta-adrenoceptors in the airways of the guinea pig. *Eur. J. Respir. Dis.* **65**:suppl. 135:128-134.

Henricks, P. A., van Esch, B., and Nijkamp, F. P. (1986). Beta-agonists can depress oxidative metabolism of alveolar macrophages. *Agents Actions* **19**:353-354.

Holgate, S. T., Baldwin, C. J., and Tattersfield, A. E. (1977). Beta-adrenergic agonist resistance in normal human airways. *Lancet* **2**:375-377.

Holgate, S. T., Rosch, W., Roberts, A., and Beasly, R. V. (1989). Inflammation as the basis of asthma. In: *Bronchitis* IV. Edited by H. J. Sluiter and R. van der Lende. Assen, Vangorcum, pp. 163-171.

Howarth, P. H., Durham, S. R., Lee, T. H., Kay, A. B., Church, M. K., and Holgate, S. T. (1985). Influence of albuterol, cromolyn sodium and ipratropium bromide on the airway and circulating mediator responses to allergen bronchial provocation in asthma. *Am. Rev. Respir. Dis.* **132**:986-992.

James, A. L., Paré, P. D., Moreno, R. H., and Hogg, J. C. (1987). Quantitative measurement of smooth muscle shortening in isolated pig trachea. *J. Appl. Physiol.* **63**:1360-1365.

Jenne, J. W., and Ahrens, R. C. (1987). Pharmacokinetics of beta-adrenergic compounds. In: *Drug Therapy for Asthma; Research and Clinical Practice. Lung Biology in Health and Disease,* vol. 31. Edited by J. W. Jenne and S. Murphy. New York, Marcel Dekker, pp. 213-258.

Jeppson, A. B., Roos, C., Waldeck, B., and Widmark, E. (1989). Pharmacodynamic and pharmacokinetic aspects of the transport of bronchodilator drugs through the tracheal epithelium of the guinea pig. *Pharmacol. Toxicol.* **64**:58-63.

Joad, J. P., Ahrens, R. C., Lindgren, S., and Weinberger, M. M. (1987). Relative effiency of maintenance therapy with theophylline, inhaled albuterol and the combination for chronic asthma. *J. Allergy Clin. Immunol.* **79**:78-85.

Kaliner, M. A., Shelhamer, J. H., Borson, D. B., Patow, C. A., Maroni, Z., and Nadel, J. A. (1988). Respiratory mucus. In: *The Airways: Neural Control in Health and Disease.* Edited by M. A. Kaliner and P. J. Barnes. New York, Marcel Dekker, pp. 575-593.

Kalisker, A., Nelson, H. E., and Middletion, E., Jr. (1977). Drug induced changes of adenylate cyclase activity in cells from asthmatic and non-asthmatic subjects. *J. Allergy Clin. Immunol.* **60**:259-265.

Kanner, R. E., Renzetti, A. D., Klauber, M. R., Smith, C. B., and Golden, C. A. (1979). Variables associated with changes in spirometry in patients with obstructive lung diseases. *Am. J. Med.* **67**:44-50.

Kerrebijn, K. F., Neijens, H. J., and Wesselius, T. (1980). Vergleich des protektiven Wirkung eines Sympathomimetikums (Fenoterol), eines Parasympatholytikums (Oxitropium) und eines Mastzellenstabilisators (Dinatrium-Cromoglycat) auf das Anstrengungsasthma. In: *Interaktion von Vagus und Sympathikus bei Bronchialerkrankungen.* Edited by D. Nolte and A. Lichterfeld. Munchen/Wien/Baltimore, Urban and Schwartzenberg, pp. 129-134.

Kerrebijn, K. F., van Essen-Zandvliet, E. E. M., and Neijens, H. J. (1987). Effects of long-term treatment with inhaled corticosteroids and beta-agonists on the bronchial responsiveness in asthmatic children. *J. Allergy Clin. Immunol.* **79**:653-659.

Kim, C. S., Eldridge, M. E., and Sackner, M. A. (1987). Oropharyngeal deposition and delivery aspects of metered-dose inhaler aerosols. *Am. Rev. Respir. Dis.* **135**:157-164.

Knowles, M., Murray, G., Shallal, J., Askin, F., Ranga, V., Gatzy, J., and Boucher, R. (1984). Bioelectric properties and ion flow across exercised human bronchi. *J. Appl. Physiol.* **56**:868-877.

Koenig, J. Q., Marshall, S. G., Horike, M., Shapin, G. G., Furakawa, C. T., Bierman, C. W., and Piersson, W. E. (1987). The effects of albuterol on sulfur dioxide-induced bronchoconstriction in allergic adolescents. *J. Allergy Clin. Immunol.* **79**:54-58.

König, P., Hordvik, N. L., and Serby, C. W. (1984). Fenoterol in exercise-induced asthma. Effect of dose on efficacy and duration of action. *Chest* **85**:462-464.

Kraan, J., Kœter, G. H., van der Mark, Th. W., Sluiter, H. J., and de Vries, K. (1985). Changes in bronchial hyperreactivity induced by 4 weeks of treatment with anti-asthmatic drugs in patients with allergic asthma: a comparison between budesonide and terbutaline. *J. Allergy Clin. Immunol.* **76**:628-636.

Kyle, H., Widdicombe, J. G., and Wilffert, B. (1988). Comparison of mucus flow rate, radiolabelled glycoprotein output and smooth muscle contraction in the ferret trachea *in vitro*. *Br. J. Pharmacol.* **94**:293-298.

Laitinen, L. A., Laitinen, M. A., and Widdicombe, J. G. (1987). Dose-related effects of pharmacological mediators on tracheal vascular resistance in dogs. *Br. J. Pharmacol.* **92**:703-709.

Latimer, K. M., O'Byrne, P. J., Morris, M. M., Roberts, R., and Hargreave, F. E. (1983). Bronchoconstriction stimulated by airway cooling. *Am. Rev. Respir. Dis.* **128**:440-443.

Laursen, L. C., Tandorf, E., Gnospelius, Y., Gymose, E., and Weeke, B. (1985). Long term oral therapy of asthma with terbutaline and theophylline, alone and combined. *Eur. J. Respir. Dis.* **66**:82-90.

Leferink, J. G. (1979). Correlation of pharmacokinetics to lung function and tremor in asthmatic patients. Thesis, Utrecht, pp. 101-115.

Levison, H., Reilly, P. A., and Worsley, G. H. (1985). Spacing devices and metered dose inhalers in childhood asthma. *J. Pediatr.* **107**:662-668.

Lichtenstein, L. M., and Margolis, S. (1968). Histamine release in vitro: Inhibition by catecholamines and methylxanthines. *Science* **161**:902-903.

Lindgren, S. B., and Larsson, S. (1982). Inhalation of terbutaline sulphate through a conventional actuator or a pear-shaped tube: effect and side effect. *Eur. J. Respir. Dis.* **63**:504-509.

Löfdahl, C. G., and Svedmyr, N. (1982). Effects of prenolterol in asthmatic patients. *Eur. J. Clin. Pharmacol.* **23**:297-303.

Löfdahl, C. G., Svedmyr, K., Svedmyr, N., Andersson, P., Bengtsson, B., Olsson, O. A. T., and Waldeck, B. (1984). Comparison of beta-adrenoceptor stimulation in bronchial and skeletal muscle in experimental and clinical studies. *Eur. J. Respir. Dis.* **65**:suppl. 135:124-127.

Madsen, B. W., Tandon, M. K., and Paterson, J. H. (1979). Cross-over study of the efficacy of four beta-2-sympathomimetic bronchodilator aerosols. *Br. J. Pharmacol.* **8**:75-82.

Maessen, F. P. V., and Smeets, J. J. (1986). Comparison of a controlled-release tablet of salbutamol given twice daily with a standard tablet given four times daily in the management of chronic obstructive lung disease. *Eur. J. Clin. Pharmacol.* **31**:431-436.

Marone, G., Ambrosio, G., Bonaduce, D., Glenovese, A., Triggiani, M., and Condorelli, M. (1984). Inhibition of IgE-mediated histamine release from human basophils and mast cells by fenoterol. *Int. Arch. Allergy Appl. Immunol.* **74**:356-361.

Martin, G. L., Atkins, P. C., Dunsky, E. H., and Zweiman, B. (1980). Effects of theophylline, terbutaline, and prednisone on antigen-induced bronchospasm and mediator release. *J. Allergy Clin. Immunol.* **66**:204-212.

McFadden, E. R., Jr. (1987). Exercise-induced asthma. Assessment of current etiologic concepts. *Chest* **91**:151S-157S.

Mita, H., and Shida, T. (1983). Anti-allergic activity of formoterol, a new beta-adrenoceptor stimulant and salbutamol in human leucocytes and human lung tissue. *Allergy* **38**:547-553.

De Monchy, J. G. R., Kauffman, H. F., Venge, P., Kœter, G. H., Janssen, H. M., Sluiter, H. J., and de Vries, K. (1985). Bronchoalveolar eosinophilia during allergen-induced late asthmatic reaction. *Am. Rev. Respir. Dis.* **131**:373-376.

Morse, J. C., Jones, N. L., and Anderson, G. D. (1976). The effect of terbutaline in exercise-induced asthma. *Am. Rev. Respir. Dis.* **113**:89-92.

Nadel, J. (1983). Regulation of bronchial secretions. In: *Immunopharmacology of the lung. Lung Biology in Health and Disease,* vol. 19. Edited by H. H. Newball, New York, Marcel Dekker, pp. 109-139.

Newman, S. P. (1984). Therapeutic aerosols. In: *Aerosols and the Lung in Clinical and Experimental Aspects.* Edited by S. W. Clarke and D. Pavia. London, Butterworths, pp. 197-224.

Newman, S. P. (1985). Aerosol deposition considerations in inhalation therapy. *Chest* **88**(suppl):152S-160S.

Newman, S. P., Miller, A. B., Lennard-Jones, T. R., Moren, F., and Clarke, S. W. (1984). Improvement of pressurized aerosol deposition with Nebuhaler spacer device. *Thorax* **39**:935-941.

Neijens, H. J., Raatgeep, H. C., Degenhart, H. J., and Kerrebijn, K. F. (1989). Responses of neutrophilic granulocytes in vitro of asthmatic and healthy subjects and the degree of inhibition by several drugs. *Agents Actions* **26**:108-110.

Nicklas, R. A., and Balzas, T. (1986). Adverse effects of theophylline-beta agonist interactions. *J. Allergy Clin. Immunol.* **78**:806-811.

Nyberg, L., and Kennedy, B. M. (1984). Pharmacokinetics of terbutaline given in slow-release tablets. *Eur. J. Respir. Dis.* **65**(suppl. 134):119-139.

O'Byrne, P. M., Morris, M., Roberts, R., and Hargreave, F. E. (1982). Inhibition of the bronchial response to respiratory heat exchange by increasing doses of terbutaline sulphate. *Thorax* **37**:913-917.

Olsson, O. A. T., Swanberg, E., Svedinger, I., and Waldeck, B. (1979). Effect of beta-adrenoceptor agonists on airway smooth muscle and on slow-contracting skeletal muscle: *in vitro* and *in vivo* results compared. *Acta Pharmacol Toxicol.* **44**:272-276.

Palmquist, M., Balder, B., Löwhagen, O., Melander, B., Svedmyr, N., and Wählander, L. (1989). Late asthmatic reaction prevented by salbutamol and formoterol. *J. Allergy Clin. Immunol.* **83**:244 (abstr.)

Paré, P. D., Lawson, L. M., and Brooks, L. A. (1983). Patterns of response to inhaled bronchodilators in asthmatics. *Am. Rev. Respir. Dis.* **127**: 680-685.

Paterson, J. W., Lulich, K. M., and Goldie, R. G. (1984). Drug effects on beta-adrenoceptor function in asthma. In: *Beta-Adrenoceptors in Asthma.* Edited by J. Morley. London, Academic Press, pp. 245-268.

Pavia, D., Bateman, J. R. M., and Clarke, S. W. (1980). Deposition and clearance of inhaled particles. *Bull. Eur. Physiopathol. Respir.* **16**:335-366.

Peel, E. T., and Gibson, G. J. (1980). Effects of long-term inhaled salbutamol therapy on the provocation of asthma by histamine. *Am. Rev. Respir. Dis.* **121**:973-978.

Perruchoud, A. P., Yerger, L., Russio, E., Stevenson, J. S., and Abraham, W. M. (1984). Prevention of allergic late bronchial obstruction by metaproterenol. *Am. Rev. Respir. Dis.* **129**:A5.

Persson, C. G. A., and Erjefält, I., A.-L. (1988). Nonneural and neural regulation of plasma exsudation in airways. In: *Neural Regulation of the Airways in Health and Disease.* Edited by M. A. Kaliner and P. Barnes. New York, Marcel Dekker, pp. 523-549.

Persson, C. G. A., and Svensjö, E. (1985). Vascular responses and their suppression: drugs interfering with venular permeability. In: *Handbook of Inflammation.* Edited by I. L. Bonta, M. A. Bray, and M. J. Parnham. Amsterdam, Elsevier Science Publishers pp. 61-82.

Petersson, B. A. (1984). Sustained inhibition of antigen-induced histamine release from human lung by beta-2-adrenoceptor agonist terbutaline. *Allergy* **39**:351-357.

Pomari, C., Turco, P., and Trevisan, F. (1984). Multiparametrical approach to fog challenge-induced bronchial hyperreactivity in asthmatics, protective effects of salbutamol and salbutamol plus beclomethasone dipropionate. *Int. J. Clin. Pharmacol. Ther. Toxicol.* **22**:515-528.

Popa, V. (1984). Clinical pharmacology of adrenergic drugs. *J. Asthma* **21**: 183-207.

Position Statement (1985). Adverse effects and complications of treatment with beta-adrenergic agonist drugs. *J. Allergy Clin. Immunol.* **75**:443-449.

Postma, D. S., Burema, J., Gimeno, F., May, J. F., Smit, J. M., Steenhuis, E. J., van der Weele, L. Th., and Sluiter, H. J. (1979). Prognosis in severe chronic obstructive pulmonary disease. *Am. Rev. Respir. Dis.* **119**:357-367.

Postma, D. S., Gimeno, F., Van der Weele, Th., and Sluiter, H. J. (1985). Assessment of ventilatory variables in survival prediction of patients with chronic airflow obstruction: the importance of reversibility. *Eur. J. Respir. Dis.* **67**:360-368.

Postma, D. S., Kœter, G. H., Keyzer, J. J., and Meurs, H. (1986). Influence of slow-release terbutaline on the circadian variation of cathecholamines, histamine, and lung function in nonallergic patients with partly reversible airflow obstruction. *J. Allergy Clin. Immunol.* **77**:471-477.

Powell, M. L., Weinberger, M. M., Dowdy, Y., Gural, R., Symchowicz, S., and Patrick, J. E. (1987). Comparative steady state bioavailability of conventional and controlled-release formulations of albuterol. *Biopharm. Drug Dispos.* **8**:461-468.

Prendiville, A., Green, S., and Silverman, M. (1987). Paradoxical response to nebulized salbutamol in wheezy infants, assessed by partial expiratory flow-volume curves. *Thorax* **42**:86-91.

Raes, M. M. R., Mulder, P., and Kerrebijn, K. F. (1989). Long-term effect of ipratroprium bromide and fenoterol on the bronchial hyperresponsiveness in children with asthma. *J. Allergy Clin. Immun ol.* **84**:874-879.

Raffestin, B., Cerrina, J., Boullet, C., Labat, C., Benveniste, J., and Brink, C. (1985). Response and sensitivity of isolated human pulmonary muscle preparations to pharmacological agents. *J. Pharmacol. Exp. Ther.* **233**:186-194.

Ramsdale, E. H., Roberts, R. S., Morris, M. M., and Hargreave, F. E. (1985). Differences in responsiveness to hyperventilation and methacholine in asthma and chronic bronchitis. *Thorax* **40**:422-426.

Ripe, E., Hörnblad, Y., and Tegnér, K. (1984). Oral administration of terbutaline in asthmatic patients. *Eur. J. Respir. Dis.* **65**; suppl. 134:171-179.

Robinson, N. P., Kyle, H., Webber, S. E., and Widdicombe, J. G. (1989). Electrolyte and other chemical concentrations in the airway surface liquid and mucus secretion of the ferret trachea. *J. Appl. Physiol.* **66**:2129-2135.

Rominger, K. L., and Harmer, M. (1986). Neuere Ergebnisse zur Pharmakokinetik von Fenoterol. In: *Neueste Ergebnisse über Betamimetika.* Edited by H. Jung, H. Feudel, and C. Karl. Darmstadt, Steinkopff Verlag, pp. 5-12.

Rossing, T. H., Woodrow Weiss, J., Breslin, F. J., Ingram, Jr., R. H., and McFadden Jr., E. R. (1982). Effects of inhaled sympathomimetics on obstructive response to respiratory heat loss. *J. Appl. Physiol.* **52**:1119-1123.

Ruff, F., Zander, J. F., Edonte, Y., Santais, M. C., Flavahan, N. A., Verbeuren, T. J., and Vanhoutte, P. M. (1988). Beta-2-adrenergic responses to tulobuterol in airway smooth muscle, vascular smooth muscle and adrenergic nerves. *J. Pharmacol. Exp. Ther.* **244**:173-180.

Ruffin, R. E., Cockcroft, D. W., and Hargreave, F. E. (1978). A comparison of the protective effect of fenoterol and Sch 1000 on allergen-induced asthma. *J. Allergy Clin. Immunol.* **61**:42-47.

Ryan, G., Latimer, K. M., Dolovich, J., and Hargreave, F. E. (1982). Bronchial responsiveness to histamine: relationship to diurnal variation of peak flow, improvement after bronchodilator and airway calibre. *Thorax* **37**:423-429.

Ryrfeld, A., and Ramsey, C. H. (1984). Distribution of terbutaline. *Eur. J. Respir. Des.* **65**; suppl 134:63-73.

Salome, C. M., Schoeffel, R. E., and Woolcock, A. J. (1981). Effect of aerosol and oral fenoterol on histamine and methacholine challenge in asthmatic subjects. *Thorax* **36**:580-584.

Salome, C. M., Schoeffel, R. E., Yan, K., and Woolcock, A. J. (1983). Effect of aerosol fenoterol on the severity of bronchial hyperreactivity in patients with asthma. *Thorax* **38**:854-858.

Shaw, R. J., Anderson, S. D., Durham, S. R., Taylor, K. M., Schoeffel, R. E., Green, W. I., Torzillo, P., and Kay, A. B. (1985). Mediators of hypersensitivity and "fog"-induced asthma. *Allergy* **40**:48-57.

Skidmore, I. F. (1984). Drugs acting at adrenoceptors. In: *Development of Antiasthmatic Drugs.* Edited by D. R. Buckle and H. Smit. London, Hensworth, pp. 185-203.

Sleigh, M. A., Blake, J. R., and Liron, N. (1988). The propulsion of mucus by cilia. State of the art. *Am. Rev. Respir. Dis.* **137**:726-741.

Sourk, R. C., and Nugent, K. M. (1983). Bronchodilator testing: confidence intervals derived from placebo inhalations. *Am. Rev. Respir. Dis.* **128**:153-157.

Stewart, I. C., Rhind, G. B., Power, J. T., Flenley, D. C., and Douglas, N. J. (1987). Effect of sustained release terbutaline on symptoms and sleep quality in patients with nocturnal asthma. *Thorax* **42**:797-800.

Subramanian, N. (1986). Inhibition from immunological and nonimmunological histamine release from human basophils and lung mast cells by formoterol. *Drug Res.* **36**:502-504.

Svedmyr, N. (1984). Is beta-adrenoceptor sensitivity a limiting factor in asthma therapy? In: *Beta-Adrenoceptors in Asthma.* Edited by J. Morley. London, Academic Press, pp. 181-200.

Svedmyr, N. (1985). Fenoterol: a beta-2-adrenergic agonist for use in asthma. *Pharmacotherapy* **5**(3):109-126.

Svedmyr, N. (1990). Action of corticosteroids on beta-adrenergic receptors, clinical aspects. *Am. Rev. Respir. Dis.,* **141**:531-538.

Svedmyr, N., Larsson, S., and Thiringer, G. (1976). Development of "resistance" in beta-adrenergic receptors of asthmatic patients. *Chest* **69**:479-483.

Svedmyr, N., and Löfdahl, C. G. (1987). Physiology and pharmacodynamics of beta-adrenergic agonists. In: *Drug Therapy for Asthma; Research and Clinical Practice. Lung Biology in Health and Disease,* vol. 31. Edited by J. W. Jenne and S. Murphy. New York, Marcel Dekker, pp. 177-211.

Svensjö, E., and Roempke, K. (1985). Dose-related antipermeability effect of terbutaline and its inhibition by a selective β_2-receptor blocking agent. *Agents Actions* **16**:19-20.

Svensson, L. A., and Tunek, A. (1988). The design and bioactivation of presystemically stable prodrugs. *Drug Metab. Rev.* **19**:165-194.

Sybrecht, G. ed. (1988). *Formoterol—A New Long-Acting Bronchodilator* Toronto/Lewisting NY/Bern/Stuttgart, Hans Huber.

Tashkin, D. (1987). Measurement and significance of the bronchodilator response. In: *Drug Therapy for Asthma, Research and Clinical Practice.* Edited by J. W. Jenne and S. Murphy. New York, Marcel Dekker, pp. 535-613.

Tashkin, D. P., Conolly, M. E., Deutch, R. I., Hui, K. K., Littner, M., Scarpace, P., and Jabrass, I. (1982). Subsensitization of beta-adrenoceptors in airways and leucocytes of healthy and asthmatic subjects. *Am. Rev. Respir. Dis.* **125**:185-193.

Tattersfield, A. E. (1983). Autonomic bronchodilators. In: *Asthma.* Edited by T. J. H. Clark and S. Godfrey. London, Chapman and Hall, pp. 301-335.

Tattersfield, A. E. (1987). Effect of beta-agonists and anticholinergic drugs on bronchial reactivity. *Am. Rev. Respir. Dis.* **136**:S64-68.

Tonnell, A. B., Joseph, M., Gosset, Ph., Fournier, E., and Capron, A. (1983). Stimulation of alveolar macrophages in asthmatic patients after local provocation test. *Lancet* **i**:1406-1408.

Traver, G. A., Cline, M. G., and Burrows, B. (1979). Predictors of mortality in chronic obstructive pulmonary disease. *Am. Rev. Respir. dis.* **119**: 895-902.

Ullman, A., and Svedmyr, N. (1988a). Salmeterol, a new long acting inhaled β_2 adrenoreceptor agonist: comparison with salbutamol in adult asthmatic patients. *Thorax* **43**:674-678.

Ullman, A., and Svedmyr, N. (1988b). Inhaled salmeterol—a new beta-2-adrenoceptor agonist—gives sustained bronchodilatation in asthmatic patients without causing tachyphylaxis. *Am. Rev. Respir. Dis.* **137**:A32.

Vathenen, A. S., Knox, A. J., Higgins, B. G., Britton, J. R., and Tattersfield, A. E. (1988). Rebound increase in bronchial responsiveness after treatment with inhaled terbutaline. *Lancet* **1**:554-557.

Venge, P., Dahl, R., and Håkansson, L. (1987). Heat labile neutrophil chemotactic activity in subjects with asthma after allergen inhalation: Relation to the late asthmatic reaction and effects of asthma medication. *J. Allergy Clin. Immunol.* **80**:679-688.

Waldeck, B., Olsson, O. A. T., and Svensson, L.-A. (1988). New possibilities for the beta-adrenoceptor agonist bronchodilator drugs. *Agents Actions* (suppl)**23**:55-68.

Wanner, A. (1988). Autonomic control of mucociliary function. In: *The Airways. Neural Control in Health and Disease.* Edited by M. Kaliner and P. Barnes. New York, Marcel Dekker, pp. 551-574.

Wardlaw, A. J., Dunette, S., Gleich, G. J., Collins, J. V., and Kay, A. B. (1988). Eosinophils and mast cells in bronchoalveolar lavage in subjects with mild asthma. *Am. Rev. Respir. Dis.* **137**:62-69.

Warner, J. A., MacGlashan, D. W., Peters, S. P., Kagey-Sobotka, A., and Lichtenstein, L. M. (1988). The pharmacologic modulation of mediator release from human basophils. *J. Allergy Clin. Immunol.* **82**:432-438.

Watanabe, S., Renzetti, A., Begin, R., and Bigler, A. H. (1974). Airway responses to a bronchodilator aerosol. I. Normal human subjects. *Am. Rev. Respir. Dis.* **109**:530-537.

Widdicombe, J. G. (1989). Airway mucus. *Eur. Respir. J.* **2**:107-115.

Yan, K., Salome, C. M., and Woolcock, A. J. (1985). Prevalence and nature of bronchial hyperresponsiveness in subjects with chronic obstructive pulmonary disease. *Am. Rev. Respir. Dis.* **132**:25-29.

Yukawa, T., Chanez, P., Dent, G., Kroegel, C., Roberts, N. M., Chung, K. F., and Barnes, P. (1988). Bronchodilator agents do not inhibit oxygen free radical release from guinea pig eosinophils. *Am. Rev. Respir. Dis.* **137**:27A.

Zaagsma, J., van der Heijden, P. J. C. M., van der Schaar, M. W. G., and Bank, C. M. C. (1983). Comparison of functional beta-adrenoceptor heterogeneity in central and peripheral airway smooth muscle of guinea pig and man. *J. Recept. Res.* **3**:89-106.

21

Cromolyn Sodium and Nedocromil Sodium
Mast Cell Stabilizers, Neuromodulators, or
Anti-inflammatory Drugs?

MARTIN K. CHURCH, RICARDO POLOSA, and S. JANET RIMMER

Southhampton General Hospital
Southampton, England

I. Introduction

Cromolyn sodium has been on the market as an antiasthmatic drug for over
20 years, while nedocromil sodium has only been available for a short period
of time. The efficacy of these drugs in asthma has been the subject of
several reviews (Brogden et al., 1974; Murphy, 1987; Murphy and Kelly,
1987; Holgate, 1986; Gonzales and Brogden, 1987). In this chapter we consider the development and properties of these compounds and examine the
possible mechanisms by which they may be beneficial in asthma: mast cell
stabilization, effects on neuronal reflexes, and anti-inflammatory actions.
In the examples we use, we also consider how the drugs may be used as
pharmacological tools to explore disease mechanisms.

II. Development and Properties of Cromolyn Sodium and Nedocromil Sodium

A. Development

The range of drugs available for the treatment of asthma in the 1960s was
extremely limited compared to that available today. Bronchodilators in metered dose inhalers were the mainstay of treatment. However, these con-

tained the nonselective β-adrenoceptor stimulant isoproterenol or its longer-acting analogue, orciproterenol. The heavy reliance of asthmatic patients on these inhalers was accompanied by an increased death rate in patients with asthma, probably due to cardiovascular problems associated with their overuse (Inman and Adelson, 1969). Theophylline preparations were available, but the incidence of major side effects magnified by erratic absorption limited their use. Patients with more severe asthma had to rely on oral corticosteroids, since the inhaled form had not yet been developed.

Although medical opinion at that time agreed that asthma was a multifactorial disease, treatment and research were concentrating heavily on the early bronchoconstrictor phase of allergic asthma. The preoccupation with allergic asthma stemmed from the discovery of IgE in 1967 and the observations that levels of this reaginic antibody were raised in asthmatic subjects (Ishizaka and Ishizaka, 1967; Johansson, 1967). Thus drug developers targeted their prospective drugs against models of immediate hypersensitivity reactions in vivo and mast cell mediator release in vitro.

It was against this background that cromolyn sodium was discovered and marketed as a "mast-cell-stabilizing" drug. However, its development was not what would be considered to be typical, particularly by today's standards. Dr. Roger Altounyan believed that by chemical manipulation, the bronchodilator properties of the naturally occurring chromone isolated from the plant, *Amni visgna* (Anrep et al., 1947; Bagouri, 1949), could be separated from its vasodilator properties. Thus, chemical analogues were made and tested for toxicity in experimental models. The experimental model used to test for efficacy was anaphylactic bronchoconstriction induced in Dr. Altounyan by inhalation of pollen allergen (Altounyan, 1967; Cox, 1967). Only in subsequent studies were the effects of cromolyn sodium in models of immediate hypersensitivity, and on rodent and primate mast cells in particular, detailed (Cox et al., 1970).

If we bear in mind that many pharmaceutical companies had failed to develop a marketable analogue of cromolyn sodium using models of acute anaphylaxis in experimental animals (Church, 1978), the development of nedocromil sodium concentrated on its ability to reduce the inflammatory response in the lung (Auty, 1986). This has led to the introduction of a new antiasthmatic drug with many properties in common with cromolyn sodium and with potentially important activities in addition.

B. Pharmacokinetics

The direct relevance of pharmacokinetic studies to drug efficacy depends in part on the mechanism of action of the drug being examined. In the case of cromolyn sodium and nedocromil sodium, the drugs are thought to act primarily by a topical effect on inflammatory cells in the bronchial mucosa. Thus, the proportion of the dose administered that is detected in the circulation following inhalation may be considered to have diffused away from the site of action. However, only by such experiments can we glean information on how long cromolyn sodium and nedocromil sodium will remain in the lung and what problems are likely to ensue following its systemic absorption.

The physicochemical properties of cromolyn sodium and nedocromil sodium are similar, both being water-soluble salts of organic acids with pKa values between 2 and 3. Thus at physiological pH values both drugs are highly (>99%) ionized and consequently are poorly absorbed from the gastrointestinal tract (<4% of the dose administered) and do not readily cross the blood-brain or placental barriers (Walker, 1972; Neale et al., 1987). Furthermore, the inability of the drugs to penetrate cells and the lack of an extracellular route of metabolism results in their being excreted unchanged in the urine ($\sim$80%) and in the feces following biliary excretion ($\sim$20%) (Walker, 1972; Neale et al., 1987).

The earlier methods for the assay of cromolyn sodium, including radiometric measurement of ^{14}C-labeled drug (Walker, 1972) and the colorimetric assays (Moss et al., 1971) were not sensitive enough to allow the performance of definitive pharmacokinetic studies, which had to await the development of radioimmunoassays (Brown et al., 1983; Gardner et al., 1988). These studies have shown that SCG is rapidly absorbed through the lungs (Fuller and Collier, 1983). Quantitative data reported by Neale et al. (1986) suggest that of the 2.84 mg absorbed from a single 20 mg inhalation, approximately one-quarter was absorbed rapidly with a mean rate constant of 0.54/min; the remainder was absorbed more slowly with a rate constant of 0.0097/min. Nedocromil sodium showed a similar rapid two-compartment absorption profile, with approximately 6% of the total dose inhaled being observed in the circulation.

One feature common to many of the pharmacokinetic studies is the variability of drug absorption both between patients and within the same patient on repeated assessment (Neale et al., 1986; Richards et al., 1987). Since there appears to be a significant correlation between plasma drug levels and clinical efficacy (Patel et al., 1986; Yahev et al., 1988), it is important to understand the reasons for this variability. Richards et al. (1987, 1988) have addressed this question in detail by studying the absorption of cromolyn sodium under different conditions. In their first paper (Richards et al., 1987) they concluded that a major determinant in achieving high plasma levels with a Spinhaler was a high inspiratory flow rate. Also, they showed that the drug was well absorbed when delivered directly to a second-order bronchus. In their second paper (Richards et al., 1988) they showed that whereas broncho-constriction induced by methacholine dramatically increased the deposition of cromolyn sodium in the upper airways at the expense of the lower airways, the plasma concentrations were not significantly altered. This would suggest that the site of deposition of the drug within the lungs is less important than the total dose delivered, a factor that is controlled largely by inspiratory flow rates in experiments with the Spinhaler. Whether these criteria are specific for the Spinhaler or whether they may be extrapolated to the use of metered dose inhalers and nebulizers is not yet known.

Although it may seem anomalous that patients' responsiveness correlates with plasma levels for a drug that is purported to have a local action, this is not necessarily the case because both are likely to depend on delivery of the drug to the surface of the major bronchi. From the studies described, it would appear that efficient use of the inhalation device is a major determinant of bioavailability. However, studies by Neale et al. (1987) with nedocromil sodium showed that the systemic absorption of drug was reduced in patients with asthma, which suggests that either a physical ability to achieve high flow rates or physical barriers in the lung (e.g., bronchial mucus) prevent the drug from reaching its site of action or absorption.

C. Toxicity and Unwanted Effects

Cromolyn sodium and nedocromil sodium are essentially free from systemic toxicity. This is largely due to the extracellular nature of the drugs, the low systemic levels achieved following inhalation, and their rapid excretion in the unchanged form. Their high safety margin is supported by toxicity studies in experimental animals, which have shown both drugs to be free of toxicity in the wide variety of animal species examined (Cox et al., 1970; Edwards et al., 1985; Auty, 1986).

With cromolyn sodium, the major problem envisaged with its introduction was the potential irritant effect consequent upon the inhalation of a relatively large amount (20 mg) of drug powder into the lungs. Although this is a problem with occasional patients in whom it causes transient bronchospasm, it has not been as great a problem as was envisaged. In such patients, administration of a selective β_2-adrenoceptor agonist before cromolyn inhalation usually overcomes the problem. Very occasionally more serious side effects are reported. These include pulmonary eosinophilia (Lobel et al., 1974), pulmonary allergic granulomatosis (Burger et al., 1974), cardiac tamponade associated with peripheral eosinophilia (Slater, 1978), and even life-threatening anaphylaxis (Sheffer et al., 1975). Although the mechanisms of these responses are not clear, lymphocyte activation rather than an antibody-mediated response has been suggested (Sheffer et al., 1975).

Clinical experience with nedocromil sodium has shown that, like cromolyn sodium, it is well tolerated without unwanted effects in the vast majority of patients (Auty, 1986). A distinctive bitter taste and, to a lesser extent, headache and nausea have been reported (Gonzalez and Brogden, 1987).

III. Effects on Mast Cells

A. Biochemical Mechanisms

The majority of studies to determine the mechanisms by which antiallergic drugs inhibit mediator release have been performed using IgE-dependent mediator release from mast cells obtained from the peritoneal cavity of the rat. The stimulus dependency for demonstrating the inhibitory activity of cromolyn sodium activity is demonstrated by observations that mediator release induced by IgE-dependent mechanisms (Fullarton et al., 1973; Garland, 1973; Johnson and Van Hout, 1973), compound 48/80 (Garland, 1973; Orr et al., 1971), phospholipase A (Orr and Cox, 1969), polymyxin B (Orr, 1975), dextran plus phosphatidyl serine (Orr, 1975; Marshall, 1972), and low concentrations of calcium ionophore A23187 (Johnson and Bach, 1975) is inhibited whereas release induced by higher concentrations of A23187 (Foreman et al., 1977), substance P (Tasaka et al., 1986), and IgG-dependent mechanisms (Goose and Blair, 1969) is less readily inhibited. One characteristic of the effect of cromolyn sodium in rat mast cells is the rapid development of tachyphylaxis to its inhibitory effects (Sung, et al., 1977a,b). This phenomenon is also observed with other cromolyn-like antiallergic drugs including nedocromil sodium. Indeed, cross-tachyphylaxis with cromolyn sodium is often taken as an indication that a drug has a similar mechanism of action (Marshall et al., 1976). Although many attempts have been made to determine the mechanism(s) underlying these effects, we still have largely unproven theories rather than well-defined effects.

Because of its high ionization at physiological pH values, suggestions have been made that cromolyn sodium may exist in a lattice form in combination with divalent cations, particularly calcium, in the extracellular environment, thereby decreasing its availability for uptake into mast cells during mediator release (Cox, 1974). This theory of action is, however, unlikely since it does not explain the development of tachyphylaxis, the stimulus dependency of drug effects, or the differences in sensitivity of different mast cell populations to the inhibitory effects of these drugs. Furthermore, it does not explain the ability of cromolyn sodium to inhibit the release of histamine from rat mast cells induced by compound 48/80 in the absence of extracellular calcium (Pearce, 1982).

A second purported mechanism, which is unlikely to be relevant in whole cells, is the ability of antiallergic drugs to inhibit the actions of cyclic AMP phosphodiesterases. Cromolyn sodium and related compounds in high concentrations have been reported to be phosphodiesterase inhibitors in broken cell preparations (Roy and Warren, 1974; Tateson and Trist, 1976; Lavin et al., 1976). However, the acidic nature of cromolyn sodium and nedocromil sodium would preclude their entry into the cytoplasm of whole cells, a necessary prerequisite to such an effect. Furthermore, the characteristics of the actions of cromolyn sodium are quite distinct from those of methylxanthine inhibitors of phosphodiesterase (Church, 1985).

Since the effects of cromolyn sodium are essentially extracellular in nature, it is likely that its action would be at the cell surface, probably following its association with a membrane receptor. However, the search for such a receptor has proved to be difficult because cromolyn sodium is a notoriously poor ligand for affinity studies. Mazurek et al (1980) reported the existence of a specific binding site for cromolyn sodium on the membrane of rat basophil leukaemia cells (RBL-2H3). They suggested that this receptor is linked to a calcium gating mechanism (Mazurek et al., 1983). When reviewing these experiments, however, Pearce and Foreman (1988) indicated their reservations about the appropriateness of this model for several reasons, including a failure to be reproduced in patch clamping experiments in rat mast cells (Lindau and Fernandez, 1986), and because RBL-2H3 cells are relatively insensitive to the inhibitory effects of cromolyn sodium.

The observation that the inhibitory effect of cromolyn sodium and nedocromil sodium in rat mast cells is associated with the phosphorylation of a 78 kDa protein (Theoharides et al., 1980; Sieghart et al., 1981; Wells and Mann, 1983; Wells et al., 1986) provides a more likely mechanism. When rat mast cells are activated by antigen or compound 48/80 in the presence of ^{32}P, four proteins are phosphorylated (Sieghart et al., 1978; Wells and Mann, 1983). Three of these, with molecular weights of 42, 59, and 68 kDa, are phosphorylated within 10 s and are thought to be involved with the initiation of secretion. The fourth, a 78 kDa protein, is not evident for 30-60 s after challenge and is thought to be associated with termination of the secretory response. Exposure of cells to antiallergic drugs including cromolyn sodium and nedocromil sodium or to dibutyryl cyclic GMP causes phosphorylation of the 78 kDa protein in isolation. The observation that the decay of this protein parallels tachyphylaxis to cromolyn sodium (Theoharides et al., 1980; Wells and Mann, 1983) provides strong circumstantial evidence that it is responsible for the intracellular effects of antiallergic drugs in rat mast cells at least.

It has been suggested more recently that cromolyn sodium reduces mediator release from mast cells by inhibiting the actions of protein kinase C (Sagi-Eisenberg, 1985), an enzyme that requires calcium and phosphatidylserine for full expression of its activity (Kikkawa et al., 1982). The association of cromolyn sodium with protein kinase C stems from the observation that high extracellular levels of phosphatidylserine overcome the actions of the antiallergic drug (Garland and Mongar, 1974). Although there is no direct evidence for this theory in mast cells (Sagi-Eisenberg, 1985), it is supported by the preliminary observations of DeSouza and Findlay (1987). More direct evidence of an association between cromolyn sodium and protein kinase C stems from studies in the skin of the lizard *Anolis carolinensis* in which cromolyn sodium inhibits enhancement of melanosome dispersion by the phorbol ester, 12-0-tetradecanoylphorbol-13-acetate (TPA) (Lucas and Schuster, 1987). However, care must be used in interpreting these findings, since TPA also has other effects including inhibition of the hydrolysis of phosphoinositides (Watson and Lapetina, 1985; Orellana et al., 1985). The increasing volume of evidence linking the activity of cromolyn sodium and nedocromil sodium with protein kinase C and the observations of phosphorylation of a 78 kDa protein suggest that they must both play a role in the inhibitory effects of the drug. However, the relationship of these two processes is as yet unknown.

B. Mast Cell Heterogeneity

The recognized ability of antiallergic drugs to suppress mast cell mediator release has led to widespread research into the possible implications of mast cell heterogeneity in the responsiveness to drug therapy, since both interspecies and intraspecies differences have been observed.

Studies of rat mast cells have delineated two major subpopulations: mucosal mast cells and connective tissue mast cells. These subpopulations are clearly distinguishable by their respective size, number of secretory granules, content of histamine and 5-hydroxytryptamine, secretory characteristics, sensitivity to formaldehyde fixation, and staining with copper phthalocyanin dyes, the last two of which are considered to reflect differences in proteoglycan and protease content (Lee et al., 1985; Enerback, 1986; Woodbury and Miller, 1982). This heterogeneity is accompanied by differences in the responsiveness of the subpopulations to a number of secretory stimuli including neuropeptides (Shanahan et al., 1985; Foreman and Piotrowski, 1985); mast cells derived from connective tissues are responsive whereas those from the intestinal mucosa are not. These cells are also differentially inhibited by antiallergic drugs, both cromolyn sodium and nedocromil sodium being effective inhibitors of IgE-dependent mediator release from connective tissue mast cells derived from the peritoneal cavity (Fullarton et al., 1973; Garland, 1973; Johnson and Van Hout, 1975; Wells et al., 1986) and skin (Goose and Blair, 1969) but not from mast cells separated from the mucosal surface of the small intestine (Leung et al., 1984; Pearce et al., 1982).

In the mouse, cromolyn sodium is ineffective in inhibiting histamine release regardless of the type of antibody mediating the response (Miller,

1976) and more potent cromolyn-like drugs are only weakly effective even at high concentrations (Evans et al., 1974; Evans and Thomson, 1975; Miller and James, 1978). However, exposure of mouse bone-marrow-derived mast cells in culture to cromolyn sodium or nedocromil sodium for 4-7 days has been reported to inhibit IgE-dependent histamine release by 50% (Marquardt et al., 1978; Brodie et al., 1986). In the guinea pig, IgE-mediated anaphylaxis is partially inhibited by cromolyn sodium whereas IgG-dependent anaphylaxis is not (Taylor and Roitt, 1973; Carney, 1976; Andersson, 1980). The influence of mast cell heterogeneity in this species on the activity of antiallergic drugs is exemplified by the observations that brufolin, a compound with 300 times the activity of cromolyn sodium in rat PCA, inhibits anaphylactic bronchoconstriction and histamine release from guinea pig chopped lung but does not inhibit passive cutaneous anaphylaxis in guinea pig skin (Evans et al., 1974; Evans and Thomson, 1975). Studies in macaque monkeys have shown marked differences in the activity of the two drugs; mediator release from mast cells obtained from the lung by bronchoalveolar lavage (BAL) is inhibited by nedocromil sodium but not cromolyn sodium (Wells et al., 1986).

Human mast cells are also heterogeneous with respect to structure and function. The recent availability of monoclonal and polyclonal antibodies against human mast cell neutral proteases tryptase (Schwartz, 1985) and chymase (Schechter et al., 1986) has allowed human mast cells to be subclassified by their immunocytochemical characteristics. The mast cells of the lung and intestinal mucosa predominantly contain only tryptase and are dependent on T-cell factors for their maturation (Irani et al., 1986, 1987). In this respect, the tryptase-containing cells are analogous to mast cells derived from the intestinal mucosa of rodents. The mast cells of human skin and submucosal layers of the intestines contain both tryptase and chymase and do not appear to require T-lymphocyte products for their development (Irani et al., 1986, 1987), which suggests analogy with rodent connective-tissue-derived mast cells. Differences in sensitivity to formaldehyde fixation have also been used to differentiate between mast cell subtypes, but the results are not as clear or as reproducible as they are in rodent mast cells (Strobel et al., 1981; Pearce et al., 1982; Flint et al., 1985; Holgate et al., 1987). However, other aspects of rodent mast cell heterogeneity are not observed in human mast cells. For example, mast cells of the skin, lung, and intestines are similar in size and histamine content and contain the same characteristic crystalline secretory granules (Lagunoff, 1972; Orr, 1977; Caulfield et al., 1980; Fox et al., 1985; Church et al., 1982; Benyon et al., 1987; Rees et al., 1988).

To assess possible functional heterogeneity between different populations of human mast cells, we have examined the secretory response of cells dispersed from infant foreskin, adult breast skin, adenoids, tonsils, intestinal muscle, and the region of the intestine comprising both the mucosal surface and the immediate submucosal layers (Lowman et al., 1988a, Rees et al., 1988). These experiments showed that mast cells of all tissues released histamine in a concentration-related manner following IgE-dependent or calcium ionophore A23187 stimulation, whereas only mast cells from the skin released histamine in response to substance P, vasoactive intestinal peptide (VIP), somatostatin, morphine, poly-*L*-lysine, and the histamine-releasing substance, compound 48/80. These results indicate that unlike in rodent mast cells, the functional responsiveness of human mast cells is not correlated with protease content.

Human mast cells also show marked heterogeneity with respect to inhibition with antiallergic drugs. In human lung fragments, cromolyn sodium has only a partial and extremely variable inhibitory effect on IgE-dependent mediator release (Church and Young, 1983; Young and Church, 1983). Although cromolyn sodium shows a more consistent concentration-related inhibition of histamine release in dispersed lung mast cells, its effects are weak, particularly in comparison with the β-adrenoceptor agonist, albuterol (Church and Hiroi, 1987). Four other pertinent points may be gleaned from this study. First. human lung mast cells, like those of the rat, showed tachyphylaxis to the inhibitory effects of cromolyn sodium, the effect of the drug being negligible following 15 min preincubation with cells before challenge. Second, the efficacy of cromolyn sodium in suppressing histamine release was inversely related to the intensity of immunological stimulation and, consequently, to histamine release. Since the levels of immunological stimulation and consequential histamine in asthma release are low compared to in vitro tests (Howarth et al., 1985), it is likely that cromolyn sodium would be an effective inhibitor of mast cell mediator release in the clinical situation. Third, although cromolyn sodium at 1000 μM inhibited histamine release by only 25%, it inhibited the release of prostaglandin (PG) D_2 by 85%. This prostaglandin, which is derived only from mast cells (Church et al., 1982), is a potent bronchoconstrictor (Hardy et al., 1984) and induces the accumulation of secondary inflammatory cells (Soter et al., 1983). Fourth, three other cromolyn-like compounds, lodoxamide, traxanox, and RU31156, showed similar potencies to cromolyn sodium against human lung mast cells, whereas in rat passive cutaneous anaphylaxis, which is indicative of activity against rat connective tissue mast cells, their potencies differ markedly. Studies with nedocromil sodium have shown that although concentration-response curves are shifted 10-fold to the left, this drug has qualitatively similar effects to cromolyn sodium in that it is only a partial inhibitor of mediator release and exhibits tachyphylaxis (Leung et al., 1988).

In mast cells recovered from the lung by BAL, cromolyn sodium and nedocromil sodium appear to be more effective than against mast cells dispersed from human lung tissue by enzymatic digestion. Furthermore, there is not evidence of tachyphylaxis with prolonged incubation (Flint et al., 1985; Leung et al., 1988). This strongly suggests that BAL mast cells represent a separate subpopulation of human mast cells that are distinct from those located within the lung tissue.

A similar effect to that seen in BAL mast cells is seen with mast cells dispersed from human colon: extension of the preincubation time increases rather than decreases the inhibitory effects of cromolyn sodium (Church et al., 1989). It has also been reported that no tachyphylaxis to the inhibitory effects of cromolyn sodium is observed in human adenoidal mast cells (Schmutzler et al., 1985). In contrast, histamine release from dispersed human skin mast cells, like that from human basophils (Church et al., 1982), is insensitive to cromolyn sodium (Lowman et al., 1988b), and observation that is supported by the report that this drug does not inhibit mast cell degranulation or the wheal and flare response in vivo (Ting et al., 1983).

The use of antiallergic drugs such as cromolyn sodium and nedocromil sodium may, therefore, be used to explore mast cell heterogeneity. Conversely, the nature of a mast cell subtype will also influence the possible beneficial effects of drug treatment.

C. Clinical Evidence

The ability of both cromolyn sodium and nedocromil sodium to inhibit effectively the immediate bronchoconstrictor response following bronchial provocation of the airways with allergen indicates that the drugs are effective inhibitors of mast cell mediator release in the clinical environment. In support of this mechanism, two studies have shown inhibition by cromolyn sodium of increased circulating histamine and neutrophil chemotactic activity (NCA) following allergen challenge of patients with mild asthma (Atkins et al., 1978 Howarth et al., 1985). Similar results are obtained with β-adrenoceptor stimulants (Martin et al., 1980; Howarth et al., 1985). Single-dose studies have shown that cromolyn sodium and nedocromil sodium as well as inhibiting allergen-induced bronchoconstriction, also inhibit reactions induced by exercise (Davies, 1968; Bauer, 1986; Debelic, 1986), cold air (Breslin et al., 1980; del Bono et al., 1986; Rocchiccioli and Pickering, 1986), and ultrasonically nebulized distilled water (Robuschi et al., 1987), but not that induced by the smooth muscle contractile agonists histamine (Cushley and Holgate, 1985) and methacholine (Altounyan et al., 986b). Since mast cell stabilization is unlikely to be the sole beneficial mechanism in these responses, other mechanisms should be considered.

IV. Neuromodulatory Actions

The ability of cromolyn sodium and nedocromil sodium to inhibit the immediate bronchoconstrictor response to allergen challenge is likely to result from inhibition of the release of mast cell mediators. Inhibition of the late-phase asthmatic response and effects in reducing acquired bronchial hyperresponsiveness are likely to reflect an action on inflammatory cells. However, additional effects, particularly on nerve reflexes have been suggested.

The theory of an effect on nerve reflexes within the lung derives from experiments in dogs in which reflex-induced bronchoconstriction following stimulation of C-fiber sensory nerve endings with capsaicin was blocked by prophylactic treatment with cromolyn sodium (Dixon et al., 1980). Since C-fibers respond to chemical irritants rather than mechanical stimulation, their inhibition may be relevant to asthma induced by nonspecific irritation of the airways. Stimulation of the cough reflex by inhalation of citric acid in the dog has shown to be blocked by nedocromil sodium and codeine phosphate but not by cromolyn sodium, which suggests that nedocromil sodium suppresses sensory nerve reflex activity within the bronchial tree (Jackson, 1988). More recently, Jackson and Eady (1988) demonstrated that the early increase in bronchial hyperresponsiveness induced by sulfur dioxide exposure in anesthetized dogs, which may be due to activation of sensory nerve endings, is prevented by nedocromil sodium.

The possible antitussive effects of nedocromil sodium have also been examined in humans. An early clinical trial showed that nedocromil sodium, but not albuterol, reduced coughing in asthmatic patients (Chatterjee et al., 1986). In provocation studies in humans, cromolyn sodium and nedocromil sodium have been shown to protect against cough induced by ultrasonically nebulized distilled water and the C-fiber stimulants capsaicin and bradykinin (Lowry and Higgenbottam, 1988; Fuller et al., 1987). In contrast, cough induced by citric acid is not inhibited by nedocromil sodium (Lowry and Higgenbottam, 1988; Heyrman et al., 1987), which suggests that its beneficial effects are limited to specific neuronal pathways.

Further information about the possible actions of cromolyn sodium and nedocromil sodium on nervous reflexes may be gained by studying their effects on bronchoconstriction induced by provocants with an indirect effect on the airways. Adenosine and its more soluble precursor nucleotide, adenosine 5'-monophosphate (AMP), provokes bronchoconstriction when inhaled by asthmatic patients but not by normal subjects (Cushley et al., 1984). Since the response is prevented by the potent histamine H1 antagonist, terfenadine, the mechanism by which adenosine causes bronchoconstriction is thought to involve enhancement of the release of preformed mediators from mast cells (Rafferty et al., 1986; Marquardt et al., 1978). A neuronal component of the response has also been proposed from the observation that vagal blockade was inhibitory (Mann et al., 1984), a finding that is not supported by a more recent report (Okayama et al., 1986). Adenosine-induced bronchoconstriction is inhibited by both cromolyn sodium and nedocromil sodium, with nedocromil sodium being more effective in comparative trials (Cushley and Holgate, 1985; Altounyan et al., 1986b; Crimi et al., 1988). These results have been confirmed in a study in nonatopic patients with asthma in whom bronchoconstriction induced by AMP was prevented more effectively by nedocromil sodium than cromolyn sodium (Scott et al., 1988).

The bronchoconstrictor response to sulfur dioxide is also suggested to be mediated partly be neural mechanisms, since its effects are reduced by cholinergic antagonists (Nadel et al., 1965); in experimental animals it has been demonstrated to stimulate laryngeal afferent fibers (Boushey et al., 1974). This suggestion is supported by observations that bronchoconstriction induced by inhaled sodium metabisulfate, which leads to the local generation of sulfur dioxide in the airways, is partially abrogated by the cholinergic antagonist oxitropium but was unaffected by the H1 antagonist terfenadine (Chilvers et al., 1987; Dixon and Ind, 1988). Pretreatment of patients with cromolyn sodium or nedocromil sodium reduces the magnitude and duration of sulfur dioxide-induced bronchoconstriction (Harries et al., 1981; Dixon et al., 1987; Altounyan et al., 1986a). The last study demonstrated nedocromil sodium to be significantly more effective than cromolyn sodiium. Furthermore, the response to sodium metabisulfite is effectively inhibited by nedocromil sodium (Chilvers et al., 1987; Dixon and Ind, 1988). These results indicate that the inhibitory drugs have potents effects in vivo that are not dependent on their effects on mast cells.

Bradykinin, a nonapeptide that is generated by the action of plasma kallikrein on high-molecular-weight kininogen and causes vasodilation and increased capillary permiability, is also a potent bronchoconstrictor agent when inhaled by asthmatic subjects (Varonier and Panzani, 1968; Simonsson et al., 1973). The mechanism of action for bradykinin has been suggested to be a direct stimulation of neuronal reflexes in the airways (Kaufman et al., 1980; Barnes et al., 1986). In the dog, both bronchoconstriction (Kaufman et al., 1980) and increased mucus secretion (Davis et al., 1982) derive from the ability of bradykinin to stimulate afferent C-fibers to release neuropeptides including substance P, neurokinin A, and calcitonin gene-related peptide, all of which have purported bronchoconstrictor properties (Ueda et al., 1984; Geppetti et al., 1988). In humans, bradykinin-induced bronchoconstriction is prevented by prophylactic cromolyn sodium and nedocromil sodium (Dixon and Barnes, 1988). The observation that in a similarly designed study the selective histamine H1 antagonist terfenadine did not abrogate the response (Polosa and Holgate, 1988) suggests that drug effects are likely to involve mechanisms other than stabilization of mast cells. The theory that modulation of nerve reflexes may be at least partly responsible for the beneficial effects of antiallergic drugs is further supported by the observation that bronchoconstriction induced by inhalation of the sensory neuropeptides neurokinin A and substance P is prevented by nedocromil sodium (Joos et al., 1988; Crimi et al., 1988).

V. Anti-inflammatory Actions

A. Cellular Mechanisms

Because the late-phase asthmatic response to allergen challenge and the acquisition of increased bronchial responsiveness are thought to be related to the accumulation and activation of inflammatory cells, particularly eosinophils and neutrophils in the bronchial lumen (Metzger et al., 1986, de Monchy et al., 1985; Diaz et al., 1986), recent research has focused on the effects of antiasthmatic drugs on these cells.

Studies with human neutrophils have shown that expression of membrane receptors for complement (C3b) and IgG (Fc) and the enhanced killing of *Schistosomula* larvae induced by formyl-methionyl-leucyl-phenylalanine (FMLP) are markedly inhibited by both cromolyn sodium and nedocromil sodium (Moqbel et al., 1986a,b). Nedocromil sodium and cromolyn sodium have also been shown to inhibit activation of human neutrophils by platelet-activating factor (PAF) or zymosan-activated serum (Bruijnzeel et al., 1989a,b) and produce a small reduction in lysosome release from rabbit neutrophils induced by FMLP (Bradford and Rubin, 1986). Also, lysosome secretion induced by phorbol dibutyrate is inhibited by nedocromil sodium but not cromolyn sodium (Bradford and Rubin, 1986).

Like neutrophils, FMLP-induced receptor expression and schistosomula killing by human eosinophils are inhibited by cromolyn sodium and nedocromil sodium (Moqbel et al., 1986a,b). At high concentrations cromolyn sodium and nedocromil sodium have been reported to inhibit the release of eosinophil granule-associated peroxidase (EPO) and cationic protein (ECP) stimulated by incubation with sepharose C3b (Spry et al., 1986). Furthermore, LTC_4 release stimulated with either opsonized zymosan or calcium ionophore A23187 is inhibited in human eosinophils but not neutrophils (Bruijnzeel et al., 1989a,b). Nedocromil sodium also inhibits $Fc\epsilon R2$-mediated activation of rat monocytes or peritoneal macrophages (Joseph et al., 1986; Thorel et al., 1988a) and human monocytes or alveolar macrophages (Thorel et al., 1988b). In addition, nedocromil sodium variably reduces the release of

LTB$_4$ and 5-HETE stimulated by A23187 or opsonized zymosan from alveolar macrophages obtained by BAL from asthmatic patients (Godard et al., 1987).

Platelets may also be stimulated by interaction of allergen with a low-affinity FcϵR2 receptor to release cytotoxic mediators, an effect that is inhibited by nedocromil sodium (Thorel et al., 1988a,b). An interesting finding is that nedocromil sodium also inhibits in vitro or ex vivo aspirin-induced activation of platelets from aspirin-sensitive asthmatic patients, a feature not shared by cromolyn sodium (Thorel et al., 1987).

As with mast cells, attention is focusing on protein kinase C inhibition as a mechanism by which cromolyn sodium and nedocromil sodium modulate inflammatory cell function. Bruijnzeel et al. (1989a,b) suggested that the inhibition of cromolyn sodium and nedocromil sodium of activation of human neutrophils by PAF or zymosan-activated serum results from protein kinase C inhibition. Bradford and Rubin (1986) reported that both cromolyn sodium and nedocromil sodium produced a small reduction in lysosome release from rabbit neutrophils induced by FMLP, a chemotactic peptide that generates diacylglycerol and produces a rise in cytosolic calcium. However, when tested against phorbol dibutyrate, which activates only protein kinase C, only nedocromil sodium was active, which suggests that only this drug had a direct inhibitory effect on the enzyme.

B. Effects on the Late Asthmatic Response

The fall in airways function occurring 6-12 h after bronchial provocation, often referred to as the late or delayed asthmatic response, has been recognized for many years. However, the recent suggestions that it may be an important component of clinical asthma has focused attention on this somewhat enigmatic response. The progression of an early response to a late response is not ubiquitous. Indeed, isolated early responses and isolated late responses have been reported in addition to dual responses (Pepys, 1977). Under controlled laboratory conditions, 50-70% of patients challenged with specific allergen develop a late response following resolution of the immediate response (Booij Noord et al., 1972; Robertson et al., 1974; Pepys and Hutchcroft, 1975; Warner, 1976). Further late responses may occur with diminishing intensity over the following 2-3 days (Hargreave et al., 1974). Late asthmatic responses (LARs) are accompanied by an increase in bronchial responsiveness to nonspecific stimulation (Cartier et al., 1982). Although the mechanism of the LAR is not clear, it is associated with in influx of inflammatory cells into the airways. Examination of the cellular content of BAL fluid recovered from the lung in the late response shows increased numbers of both granular leukocytes and mononuclear cells, indicative of their migration from the blood vessels, through the bronchial tissues and into the bronchial lumen. Studies from several centers have shown an early accumulation of neutrophils followed later by a more persistent eosinophilia (Metzger et al., 1985; de Monchy et al., 1985; Diaz et al., 1986) and it has been suggested that recruitment of granulocytes, especially eosinophils, contributes to the functional abnormalities occuring in the airways (Durham and Kay, 1985). Activation of eosinophils for secretion is suggested from the loss of the central core of the granules when examined under the electron microscope, indicative of major basic protein (MBP) loss (Metzger et al., 1985), and increased levels of ECP in BAL fluid (de Monchy et al., 1985). Although macrophage numbers have not been reported to rise, evidence for macrophage activation by use of complement rosetting techniques has been presented (Diaz et al., 1986). Furthermore, studies by Gonzalez et al. (1986) have shown an increase in the ratio of helper to suppressor T lymphocytes in BAL fluid in the late response after allergen challenge.

Differences between the mechanisms of the early and late responses are demonstrated by the observations that prophylactic treatment with antiallergic drugs such as cromolyn sodium inhibits both phases. In contrast, similar treatment with β-adrenoceptor stimulant drugs such as albuterol inhibits only the early phase, while corticosteroid therapy inhibits only the late-phase response (Booij Noord et al., 1971; Hegardt et al., 1981; Cockcroft and Murdock, 1987).

The ability of cromolyn sodium administered before allergen challenge to inhibit the late-phase response is well established. A report that when cromolyn sodium is administered after the early response it did not inhibit the subsequent late response (Booij Noord et al., 1972) led to the hypothesis that these two events are intimately related. However, this is in conflict with the observations with β-adrenoceptor stimulants, in which suppression of demonstrable signs of the early response does not inhibit the subsequent late phase response (Hegardt et al., 1981; Cockcroft and Murdock, 1987). Furthermore, it has recently been reported that administration of SCG to asthmatic children 1 h before the expected onset of the LAR delays its occurrence and shortens its duration (Mattoli et al., 1987). This suggests that mechanisms other than mast cell stabilization are responsible for inhibition of the LAR. Possible mechanisms include its ability to reduce the accumulation of eosinophils in the lung (Diaz et al., 1984) and to inhibit activation of neutrophils, eosinophils, and macrophages (Moqbel et al., 1986; Joseph et al., 1986).

To investigate further the mechanisms of late responses that occur in the airways after exposure to allergen and the roles of antiasthmatic drugs in their inhibition, a number of animal models have been developed. These include models in the sheep (Abraham et al., 1983), rabbit (Shampain et al., 1983), squirrel monkey (Hamel et al., 1986), and guinea pig (Wieslander et al., 1985;

Iijima et al., 1987; Hutson et al., 1988a). With the use of these models, cromolyn sodium, nedocromil sodium, and β-adrenoceptor agonists have been shown to inhibit the early response whereas only cromolyn sodium and nedocromil sodium, given either before challenge or after the completion of the early response, inhibit the late response (Shampain et al., 1983; Abraham et al., 1983; Delehunt et al., 1984; Abraham et al., 1987). In our guinea pig model (Hutson et al., 1988a), inhalation of cromolyn sodium or nedocromil sodium 15 min before allergen challenge inhibited both the early- and late-phase responses, whereas albuterol inhibited only the early response. When inhaled 6 h after challenge (i.e., after completion of early response), cromolyn sodium and nedocromil sodium but not albuterol inhibited the 17 h late response and the further reduction in airways function observed at 72 h (Hutson et al., 1988b,c). These observations bring into question the relationship between the early and late responses. If the late response had been brought about as a direct consequence of the pathological events associated with the early response, (e.g., mast cell mediator release), albuterol would have been expected to have brought about a parallel inhibition of both phases of airflow limitation, whereas no inhibition of the late response should have been expected with administration of cromolyn sodium or nedocromil sodium after completion of an intact early response. The finding that this was not the case suggests that the development of the late-phase response, in the guinea pig at least, is not dependent on an intact early response.

In addition to causing limitations of airflow, allergen challenge of rabbits (Marsh et al., 1985), sheep (Abraham et al., 1987), and guinea pigs (Iijima et al., 1987; Hutson et al., 1988a) induces an influx of neutrophils followed by eosinophils into the bronchial lumen. In rabbits, the late response is abolished by depletion of granulocytes and restored by transfusion of granulocytes containing mainly neutrophils, suggesting a central role for the neutrophil in the LAR of this species (Murphy et al., 1986). However, Iijima et al. (1987) found no significant difference in neutrophil infiltration within the airway walls between guinea pigs showing late responses and those in which only an early response was demonstrable, which suggested that the neutrophil is not the cell that initiates the late response. A consistent finding in our guinea pig model is the temporal relationship between the late response and the accumulation of neutrophils in BAL fluid, both events peaking 17 h after challenge (Hutson et al., 1988a,b,c). Even though cromolyn sodium or nedocromil sodium inhaled 15 min before challenge caused a parallel inhibition of the late response and neutrophil accumulation in the lungs, three lines of evidence suggest that neutrophil influx is not responsible for the development of the late response. First, albuterol inhaled before challenge inhibited the neutrophil influx into the lung but did not reduce the late response measured at 17 h. Second, cromolyn sodium or nedocromil sodium administered after the completion of the early response inhibited the late response without altering the magnitude of the neutrophil influx. Third, pretreatment of animals with antineutrophil serum abolished the influx neutrophils into the lung without reducing the intensity of either the early or late responses (Hutson et al., 1990). The clear association of neutrophil influx with an intact early response suggests that the accumulation is stimulated by the mast-cell-associated high-molecular-weight neutrophil chemotactic factor (NCF) that has been shown to be released on allergen challenge of both guinea pig and human lung (Schenkel et al., 1982; O'Driscoll et la., 1983). Thus, although there is a temporal relationship between the late response and neutrophil influx, the use of antiallergic drugs to modulate the response has allowed us to conclude that these events are not functionally related in the guinea pig.

VI. Conclusions

By the use of specific examples, we have demonstrated that cromolyn sodium and nedocromil sodium have, in addition their ability to stabilize mast cells, profound anti-inflammatory properties in the lung and have effects consistent with modulation of neuronal reflexes that abrogate bronchoconstriction. All these actions would contribute to their beneficial effects in patients with asthma. Furthermore, we have illustrated that the use of cromolyn sodium and nedocromil sodium, in combination with other standard drugs with different mechanisms of action, can provide powerful pharmacological tools for the investigation of biological mechanisms and disease processes.

Discussion

Kaliner: Is cromolyn absorbed or does it only work on the epithelial surface?

Fuller: It is absorbed across the airway but not intestinal mucosa. We have measured the concentration of nedocromil in the lung and the concentration 1/2-1 h after inhalation is 10-100 nmol/L.

Kay: Is there cross-tachyphylaxis between cromolyn and nedocromil?

Church: Yes: nedocromil was selected through cross-tachyphylaxis with cromolyn in causing cardiovascular effects in dog. It is also cross-tachyphylactic in rat mast cells.

Sertl: Are there receptors for cromolyn?

Church: Pecht identified a specific binding site for cromolyn associated with calcium channels in rat basophil leukemia cells. However, these cells are largely unaffected by cromolyn, which throws some doubt on the relevance of this observation. Unfortunately, cromolyn and nedocromil are poor ligands for receptor studies.

Widdicombe: It is claimed that nedocromil is antitussive: does that tell us about its mode of action?

Church: It has been claimed that nedocromil but not cromolyn is antitussive but reports are so far conflicting.

Schleimer: Cromolyn causes the phosphorylation of a 78 kDa protein in rat mast cells and this correlates with inhibition of mediator release. Has this been pursued and what is known of the function of this protein?

Church: Such studies have not been done on human mast cells to my knowledge.

O'Byrne: You showed that cromolyn inhibits the late response after inhaled allergen in guinea pigs. Does it inhibit eosinophil influx?

Church: There is evidence of eosinophil degranulation in the late response, but we do not know the effects of cromolyn on this yet.

References

Abraham, W. M., Delehunt, J. C., Yerger, L., and Marchette, B. (1983). Characterization of a late phase pulmonary response following antigen challenge in allergic sheep. *Am. Rev. Respir. dis.* **128**:839-844.

Abraham, W. M., Stevenson, J. S., Chapman, G. A., Tallent, M. W., and Jackowski, J. (1987). The effect of nedocromil sodium and cromolyn sodium on antigen-induced responses in allergic sheep in vivo and in vitro. *Chest* **92**:913-917.

Altounyan, R. E. C. (1967). Inhibition of experimental asthma by a new compound—disodium cromoglycate, "Intal." *Acta Allergol.* **22**:487.

Altounyan, R. E. C., Cole, M., and Lee, T. B. (1986a). Inhibition of sulphur dioxide induced bronchoconstriction by nedocromil sodium and sodium cromoglycate in non-asthmatic atopic subjects. *Eur. J. Respir. Dis.* **69** (Suppl 147):274-276.

Altounyan, R. E. C., Lee, T. B., Rocchiccioli, K. M. S., and Shaw, C. L. (1986b). A comparison of the inhibitory effects of nedocromil sodium and sodium cromoglycate on adenosine monophosphate-induced bronchoconstriction in atopic subjects. *Eur. J. Respir. Dis.* **69** (Suppl. 147): 277-279.

Andersson, P. (1980). Antigen-induced bronchial anaphylaxis in actively sensitized guinea-pigs. Antianaphylactic effects of sodium cromoglycate and aminophylline. *Br. J. Pharmacol.* **69**:467-472.

Anrep, G. V., Barsoum, G. S., Kenawy, M. R., and Misrahy, G. (1947). Therapeutic uses of khellin. *Lancet* **1**:557-558.

Atkins, P. C., Norman, M. E., and Zweiman, B. (1978). Antigen-induced neutrophil chemotactic activity in man: correlation with bronchospasm and inhibition by disodium cromoglycate. *J. Allergy Clin. Immunol.* **62**:149-155.

Auty, R. M. (1986). The clinical development of a new agent for the treatment of airway inflammation, nedocromil sodium (Tilade). *Eur. J. Respir. Dis.* **69** (Suppl 147):120-131.

Bagouri, M. M. (1949). The coronary vasodilator action of the crystalline principles of *Ammi visnaga*. *J. Pharm. Pharmacol.* **1**:177-180.

Barnes, P. J. (1986). Asthma as an axon reflex. *Lancet* **2**:242-245.

Bauer, C. P. (1986). The protective effect of nedocromil sodium in exercise-induced asthma. *Eur. J. Respir. Dis.* **69** (Suppl 147):252-254.

Benyon, R. C., Lowman, M. A., and Church, M. K. (1987). Human skin mast cells: their dispersion, purification and secretory characterization. *J. Immunol.* **138**:861-867.

Booij Noord, H., Orie, N. G. M., and de Vries, K. (1971). Immediate and late bronchial obstructive reactions to inhalation of house dust and protective effects of disodium and cromoglycate and prednisolone. *J. Allergy Clin. Immunol.* **48**:344-354.

Booij Noord, H., de Vries, K., Sluiter, H. J., and Orie, N. G. M. (1972). Late bronchial obstructive reaction to experimental inhalation of house dust mite extract. *Clin. Allergy* **2**:43-61.

Boushey, H. A., Richardson, P. S., Widdicombe, J. G., and Wise, J. C. M. (1974). The response of laryngeal afferent fibres in mechanical and chemical stimuli. *J. Physiol.* **240**:153-175.

Bradford, P. G., and Rubin, R. P. (1986). The differential effects of nedocromil sodium and sodium cromoglycate on the secretory response or rabbit peritoneal neutrophils. *Eur. J. Respir. Dis.* **69** (Suppl. 147):238-240.

Breslin, F. J., McFadden, E. R., and Ingram, R. H. (1980). The effects of cromolyn sodium on the airway response to hypernoea and cold air in asthma. *Am. Rev. Respir. Dis.* **122**:11-16.

Brodie, D., Marquardt, D., and Wasserman, S. (1986). Effect of nedocromil sodium and sodium cromoglycate on connective tissue and bone marrow derived mast cells: acute and chronic studies. *Eur. J. Respir. Dis.* **69** (Suppl. 147):196-198.

Brogden, R. N., Speight, T. M., and Avery, G. S. (1974). Sodium cromoglycate (cromolyn sodium): a review of its mode of action, pharmacology, therapeutic efficacy and use. I. Asthma. *Drugs* **7**:164-282.

Brown, K., Gardner, J. J., Lockley, W. J. S., Preston, J. R., and Wilkinson, D. J. (1983). Radioimmunoassay for sodium cromoglycate in human plasma. *Ann. Clin. Biochem.* **20**:31-36.

Bruijnzeel, P. L. B., Hamelink, M. L., and Kok, P. T. M. (1989a). Nedocromil sodium inhibits the A23187- and opsonized zymosan-induced leukcotriene formation by human eosinophils but not by human neutrophils. *Br. J. Pharmacol.* **96**:631-636.

Bruijnzeel, P. L. B., Waainga, R. A. J., and Kok, P. T. M. (1989b). Inhibition of platelet activating factor and zymosan activated serum induced chemotaxis to human neutrophils by nedocromil sodium, BN 52021 and sodium cromoglycate. *Br. J. Pharmacol.* In Press.

Burger, L. W., Kass, I., and Schenken, J. R. (1974). Pulmonary allergic granulomatosis: a possible drug reaction in a patient receiving cromolyn sodium. *Chest* **66**:83-84.

Carney, I. F. (1976). IgE-mediated anaphylactic bronchoconstriction in the guinea pig and effect of DSCG. *Int. Arch. Allergy Appl. Immunol.* **50**: 322-328.

Cartier, A., Thomson, N. C., Frith, P. A., Roberts, R., and Hargreave, F. E. (1982). Allergen-induced increase in bronchial responsiveness to histamine: relationship to the late asthmatic response and change in airway calibre. *J. Allergy Clin. Immunol.* **70**:170-177.

Caulfield, J. P., Lewis, R. A., Hein, A., and Austen, K. F. (1980). Secretion of dissociated human pulmonary mast cells: evidence for solubilization of granule contents before discharge. *J. Cell. Biol.* **85**:299-311.

Chatterjee, P. C., Fyans, P. G., and Chatterjee, S. S. (1986). A trial comparing nedocromil sodium (Tilade) and placebo in the management of perennial bronchial asthma. *Eur. J. Respir. Dis.* **69** (Suppl. 147):314-316.

Chilvers, E. R., Dixon, C. M. S., and Ind, P. W. (1987). Mechanism of metabisulphate-induced bronchoconstriction in atopic non-asthmatic subjects. *Thorax* **42**:745-746.

Church, M. K. (1978). Cromoglycate-like anti-allergic drugs. *Drugs Today* **14**:281-341.

Church, M. K. (1982). The role of basophils in asthma: 1; Sodium cromoglycate on histamine release and content. *Clin. Allergy* **12**:223-228.

Church, M. K. (1985). The biochemical basis of pulmonary and anti-allergic drugs. In *Pulmonary and Anti-Allergic Drugs*. Edited by J. P. Devlin. New York, Wiley, pp. 43-121.

Church, M. K., and Hiroi, J. (1987). Inhibition of IgE-dependent histamine release from human dispersed lung mast cells by anti-allergic drugs and salbutamol. *Br. J. Pharmacol.* **90**:421-429.

Church, M. K., and Young, K. D. (1983). The characteristics of inhibition of histamine release from human lung fragments by sodium cromoglycate, salbutamol and chlorpromazine. *Br. J. Pharmacol.* **78**:671-679.

Church, M. K., Pao, G. J.-K., and Holgate, S. T. (1982). Characterization of histamine secretion from dispersed human lung mast cells: effects of anti-IgE, calcium ionophore A23187, compound 48/80 and basic polypeptides. *J. Immunol.* **129**:2116-2121.

Church, M. K., Benyon, R. C., Rees, P. H., Lowman, M. A., Campbell, A. M., Robinson, C., and Holgate, S. T. (1989). Functional heterogeneity of human mast cells. In *Mast Cell and Basophil Differentiation and Function in Health and Disease.* Edited by S. J. Galli and K. F. Austen. New York: Raven Press, pp. 161-170.

Cockcroft, D. W., and Murdock, K. Y. (1987). Comparative effects of inhaled salbutamol, sodium cromoglycate, and beclomethasone dipropionate on allergen-induced early asthmatic responses, late asthmatic responses, increased bronchial responsiveness to histamine. *J. Allergy Clin. Immunol.* **79**:734-740.

Cox, J. S. G. (1967). Disodium cromoglycate (FPL 670, Intal): a specific inhibitor of reaginic antibody-antigen mechanisms. *Nature* **216**:1328-1329.

Cox, J. S. G. (1974). Biological and clinical studies with Intal. *Abst. Am. Chem. Soc.* **167**:24.

Cox, J. S. G., Beach, J. E., and Blair, A. M. J. N. (1970). Disodium cromoglycate (Intal). *Adv. Drug. Res.* **5**:115-196.

Crimi, N., Palermo, F., Oliveri, R., Cacopardo, B., Vancheri, C., and Mistretta, A. (1986). Adenosine-induced bronchoconstriction: comparison between nedocromil and sodium cromoglycate. *Eur. J. Respir. Dis.* **69** (Suppl 147):258-262.

Crimi, N., Palermo, F., Oliveri, R., Palermo, B., Vancheri, C., Polosa, R., and Mistretta, A. (1988). Effect of nedocromil sodium on bronchospasm induced by inhalation of substance P in asthmatic subjects. *Clin. Allergy* **18**:375-382.

Cushley, M. J., and Holgate, S. T. (1985). Adenosine induced bronchoconstriction in asthma: role of mast cell mediator release. *J. Allergy Clin. Immunol.* **75**:272-278.

Cushley, M. J., Tattersfield, A. E., and Holgate, S. T. (1984). Adenosine induced bronchoconstriction in asthma: antagonism by inhaled theophylline. *Am. Rev. Respir. Dis.* **129**:380-384.

Davies, S. E. (1968). Effect of disodium cromoglycate on exercise induced asthma. *Br. Med. J.* **3**:593-594.

Davis, B., Roberts, A. M., Coleridge, H. M., and Coleridge, J. C. G. (1982). Reflex tracheal gland secretion evoked by stimulation of bronchial C-fibres in dogs. *J. Appl. Physiol.* **53**:985-991.

de Monchy, J. G. R., Kauffman, H. F., Venge, P., Koeter, G. H., Jansen, H. M., Sluiter, H. J., and de Vries, K. (1985). Broncho-alveolar eosinophilia during allergen-induced late asthmatic reactions. *Am. Rev. Respir. Dis.* **131**:373-376.

Debelic, M. (1986). Nedocromil sodium and exercise-induced asthma in adolescents. *Eur. J. Respir. Dis.* **69** (Suppl 147):266-267.

del Bono, L., Dente, F. L., Patalano, F., and del Bono, N. (1986). Protective effect of nedocromil sodium and sodium cromoglycate on bronchospasm induced by cold air. *Eur. J. Respir. Dis.* **69** (Suppl 147):268-270.

Delehunt, J. C., Perruchoud, A. P., Yerger, L., Marchette, B., Stevenson, J. S., and Abraham, W. M. (1984). The role of slow reacting substance of anaphylaxis in the late bronchial response after allergen challenge in allergic sheep. *Am. Rev. Respir. Dis.* **130**:748-754.

DeSouza, R. N., and Findlay, J. B. C. Cited in Kay, A. B. (1987). The mode of action of anti-allergic drugs. Report of a meeting of the Section of Clinical Immunology and Allergy, Royal Society of Medicine, London, February 1986. *Clin. Allergy* **17**:153-164.

Diaz, P., Gonzalez, C., Galleguillos, F., Ancic, P., and Kay, A. B. (1986). Eosinophils and macrophages in bronchial mucus and bronchoalveolar lavage during allergen-induced late-phase asthmatic reactions [Abstract]. *J. Allergy Clin. Immunol.* **77**(Suppl):244.

Dixon, C. M. S., and Barnes, P. J. (1988). Bradykinin induced bronchoconstriction: inhibition by nedocromil and cromoglycate. *Thorax* **43**:225.

Dixon, C. M. S., and Ind, P. W. (1988). Metabisulphite induced bronchoconstriction does not involve mast cells. *Thorax* **43**:226-227.

Dixon, M., Jackson, D. M., and Richards, I. M. (1980). The action of sodium cromoglycate on "C" fibre endings in the dog lung. *Br. J. Pharmacol.* **70**:11-13.

Dixon, C. M. S., Fuller, R. W., and Barnes, P. J. (1987). Effect of nedocromil sodium on sulphur dioxide induced bronchoconstriction. *Thorax* **42**:462-465.

Durham, S. R., and Kay, A. B. (1985). Eosinophils, bronchial hyperreactivity and late-phase asthmatic reactions. *Clin. Allergy* **15**:411-418.

Edwards, A. M., Auty, R. M., Clarke, A. J., and Orr, T. S. C. (1985). Nedocromil sodium: a new modulator of inflammation for the treatment of asthma. *J. Allergy Clin. Immunol.* **75**:199.

Enerback, L. (1986). Mast cell heterogeneity: the evolution of the concept of a specific mucosal mast cell. In *Mast Cell Differentiation and Heterogeneity*. Edited by A. D. Befus, J. Bienenstock, and J. A. Denburg. New York: Raven Press, pp. 1-26.

Evans, D. P., and Thomson, D. S. (1975). Inhibition of immediate hypersensitivity reactions in laboratory animals by a phenanthroline salt (ICI-74917). *Br. J. Pharmacol.* **53**:409-418.

Evans, D. P., Gilman, D. J., Thomson, D. S., and Waring, W. S. (1974). Inhibition of allergic reactions by a novel phenanthroline, ICI-74917. *Nature* **250**:592-593.

Flint, K. C., Leung, K. B. P., Pearce, F. L., Hudspith, B. N., Brostoff, J., and Johnson, N. Mc. I. (1985). Human mast cells recovered from bronchoalveolar lavage: their morphology, histamine release and effects of sodium cromoglycate. *Clin. Sci.* **68**:427-432.

Foreman, J. C., and Piotrowski, W. (1985). Some effects of substance P antagonists on mast cells. In: *Tachykinin Antagonists.* Edited by R. Hakanson and F. Sundler. Amsterdam, Elsevier, pp. 405-412.

Foreman, J. C., Hallett, M. B., and Mongar, J. L. (1977). Site of action of the antiallergic drugs cromoglycate and doxantrazole. *Br. J. Pharmacol.* **59**:473-474.

Fox, C. C., Dvorak, A. M., Peters, S. P., Kagey-Sobotka, A., and Lichtenstein, L. M. (1985). Isolation and characterization of human intestinal mucosal mast cells. *J. Immunol.* **135**:483-491.

Fullarton, J., Martin, L. E., and Vardey, C. J. (1973). Studies on the inhibition of cellular anaphylaxis. *Int. Arch. Allergy Appl. Immunol.* **45**: 84-86.

Fuller, R. W., and Collier, J. G. (1983). The pharmacokinetic assessment of disodium cromoglycate. *J. Pharm. Pharmacol.* **33**:744-745.

Fuller, R. W., Dixon, C. M. S., Cuss, F. M. C., and Barnes, P. J. (1987). Bradykinin-induced bronchoconstriction in humans. Mode of action. *Am. Rev. Respir. Dis.* **135**:176-180.

Gardner, J. J., Preston, J. R., Gilbert, C. M., Wilkinson, D. W., Lockley, W. J. S., and Brown, K. (1988). Radioimmunoassay for nedocromil sodium. *J. Pharm. Biomed. Anal.* **6**:285-297.

Garland, L. G. (1973). Effect of cromoglycate on anaphylactic histamine release from rat peritoneal mast cells. *Br. J. Pharmacol.* **49**:128-130.

Garland, L. G., and Mongar, J. L. (1974). Inhibition by cromoglycate of histamine release from rat peritoneal mast cells induced by mixtures of dextran, phosphatidylserine and calcium ions. *Br. J. Pharmacol.* **50**: 137-143.

Geppetti, P., Maggi, C. A., Peretti, F., Frilli, S., and Manzini, S. (1988). Similtaneous release by bradykinin of substance P and calcitonin gene related peptideimmunoreactivities from capsaicin sensitive structures in guinea-pig heart. *Br. J. Pharmacol.* **94**:288-290.

Godard, P., Chavis, C., Daures, J. P., Crastes de Paulet, A., Michel, F. B., and Damon, M. (1987). Leukotriene B4 and 5-HETE release by alveolar macrophages in asthmatic patients: inhibition by nedocromil sodium. *Am. Rev. Respir. Dis.* **135**:A318.

Gonzalez, J. P., and Brogden, R. N. (1987). Nedocromil sodium: a preliminary review of its pharmacodynamic and pharmacokinetic properties, and therapeutic efficacy in the treatment of reversible obstructive airways disease. *Drugs* **34**(5):560-577.

Goose, J., and Blair, A. M. J. N. (1969). Passive cutaneous anaphylaxis in the rat induced by two homologous reagin-like antibody sera and its specific inhibition with disodium cromoglycate. *Immunology* **16**:749-760.

Hamel, R., McFarlane, C. S., and Ford-Hutchinson, A. W. (1986). Late pulmonary responses induced by *Ascaris* allergen in conscious squirrel monkeys. *J. Appl. Physiol.* **61**:2081-2087.

Hardy, C. C., Robinson, C., Tattersfield, A. E., and Holgate, S. T. (1984). The bronchoconstrictor effect of inhaled prostaglandin D2 in normal and asthmatic men. *N. Engl. J. Med.* **311**:209-213.

Hargreave, F. E., Dolovich, J., Robertson, D. G., and Kerigan, A. T. (1974). The late asthmatic responses. *Can. Med. Assoc. J.* **110**:415-421.

Harries, M. G., Parkes, P. E. G., Lessof, M. H., and Orr, T. S. C. (1981). Role of bronchial irritant receptors in asthma. *Lancet* **1**:5-6.

Hegardt, B., Pauwels, R., and van der Straeten, M. (1981). Inhibitory effect of KWD 2131, terbutaline, and DSCG on the immediate and late allergen-induced bronchoconstriction. *Allergy* **36**:115-122.

Heyrman, R., De Backer, W., Willemen, M., Bogaerts, M., and Vermeire, P. (1987). Effect of nedocromil sodium on citric acid induced cough in asthmatic subjects. *Bull. Eur. Physiopathol. Respir.* **23** (Suppl. 12):411s.

Holgate, S. T. (1986). Clinical evaluation of nedocromil sodium in the treatment of asthma. *Eur. J. Respir. Dis.* **69** (Suppl. 147):149-159.

Holgate, S. T., Rafferty, P., Beasley, R., Robinson, C., Hovell, C. J., Curzen, N. P., and Church, M. K. (1987). In vitro and in vivo studies on mast cells of human skin and airways. In: *Allergy and Inflammation.* Edited by A. B. Kay. London: Academic Press, pp. 29-52.

Howarth, P. H., Durham, S. R., Lee, T. H., Kay, A. B., Church, M. K., and Holgate, S. T. (1985). Influence of albuterol, cromolyn sodium and ipratropium bromide on the airway and circulating mediator responses to antigen bronchial provocation in asthma. *Am. Rev. Respir. Dis.* **132**:986-992.

Hutson, P. A., Church, M. K., Clay, T. P., Miller, P., and Holgate, S. T. (1988a). Early and late phase bronchoconstriction following allergen challenge of nonanaesthetized guinea pigs: I. The association of disordered airway physiology to leucocyte infiltration. *Am. Rev. Respir. Dis.* **137**:548-557.

Hutson, P. A., Holgate, S. T., and Church, M. K. (1988c). Inhibition by nedocromolyn sodium and albuterol on early and late phase bronchoconstriction and airway leukocyte infiltration following allergen challenge of non-anaesthetized guinea-pigs. *Am. Rev. Respir. Dis.* **138**:1157-1163.

Huston, P. A., Holgate, S. T., and Church, M. K. (1988c). Inhibition by nedocromil sodium of early and late bronchoconstriction and airways cellular infiltration provoked by ovalbumin in conscious sensitized guinea pigs. *Br. J. Pharmacol.* **94**:6-8.

Hutson, P. A., Sanjar, S., Kings, M., Holgate, S. T., and Church, M. K. (1990). Evidence that neutrophils do not participate in the late phase airways response provoked by ovalbumin inhalation in conscious sensitized guinea-pigs. *Am. Rev. Respir. Dis.* **141**:535-539.

Iijima, H., Ishii, M., Yamauchi, K., Chao, C. L., Kimura, K., Shimura, S., Shindoh, Y., Inoue, H., Mue, S., and Takishima, T. (1987). Broncho-alveolar lavage and histologic characterization of late asthmatic response in guinea pigs. *Am. Rev. Respir. Dis.* **136**:922-929.

Inman, W. H. W., and Adelson, A. M. (1969). Rise and fall of asthma mortality in England and Wales in relation to the use of pressurised aerosols. *Lancet* **2**:279-285.

Irani, A. A., Schechter, N. M., Craig, S., DeBlois, G., and Schwartz, L. B. (1986). Two types of human mast cells that have distinct neutral protease compositions. *Proc. Natl. Acad. Sci. U.S.A.* **83**:4464-4468.

Irani, A. A., Craig, S. S., DeBlois, G., Elson, C. O., Schechter, N. M., and Schwartz, L. B. (1987). Deficiency of the tryptase-positive chymase-negative mast cell type in gastrointestinal mucosa of patients with defective T-lymphocyte function. *J. Immunol.* **138**:4381-4386.

Ishizaka, K., and Ishizaka, T. (1967). Identification of gamma-E antibodies as a carrier of reaginic activity. *J. Immunol.* **99**:1187-1198.

Jackson, D. M. (1988). The effects of nedocromil sodium, sodium cromoglycate and codeine phosphate on citric acid-induced cough in dogs. *Br. J. Pharmacol.* **93**:609-612.

Jackson, D. M., and Eady, R. P. (1988). Acute transient SO2-induced airway hyperreactivity: effects of nedocromil sodium. *J. Appl. Physiol.* **65**(3):1119-1124.

Johansson, S. G. O. (1967). Raised levels of a new immunoglobulin class (IgND) in asthma. *Lancet* **2**:951-953.

Johnson, H. G., and Bach, M. K. (1975). Prevention of calcium ionophore-induced release of histamine in rat mast cells by disodium cromoglycate. *J. Immunol.* **114**:514-516.

Johnson, H. G., and Van Hout, C. A. (1973). The enhanced efficacy of disodium cromoglycate (DSCG) in DSCG predosed rats. *Proc. Soc. Exp. Biol. Med.* **143**:427-429.

Joos, G. S., Pauwels, R. A., and Van Der Straeten, M. E. (1988). The effect of nedocromil sodium on the bronchoconstrictor effect of neurokinin A in asthmatics. *J. Allergy Clin. Immunol.* **81**:276.

Joseph, M., Capron, A., Thorel, T., and Tonnel, A. B. (1986). Nedocromil sodium inhibits IgE-dependent activation of rat macrophages and platelets as measured by schistosome killing, chemiluminescence and enzyme release. *Eur. J. Respir. Dis.* **69** (Suppl 147):220-222.

Kaufman, M. P., Coleridge, H. M., Coleridge, J. C. G., and Baker, D. G. (1980). Bradykinin stimulates afferent vagal C-fibers in intrapulmonary airways of dogs. *J. Appl. Physiol.* **48**:511-517.

Kikkawa, U., Takai, Y., Minakuchi, R., Inohara, S., and Nishizuka, Y. (1982). Calcium-activated, phospholipid-dependent protein kinase from rat brain: subcellular distribution, purification and properties. *J. Biol. Chem.* **257**:13341-13348.

Lagunoff, D. (1972). Contributions of electron microscopy to the study of mast cells. *J. Invest. Dermatol.* **58**:296-311.

Lavin, N., Rachelefsky, G. S., and Kaplan, S. A. (1976). An action of disodium cromoglycate: inhibition of cyclic 3', 5'-AMP phosphodiesterase. *J. Allergy Clin. Immunol.* **57**:80-88.

Lee, T. D. G., Swieter, M., Bienenstock, J., and Befus, A. D. (1985). Heterogeneity in mast cell populations. *Clin. Immunol. Rev.* **4**:143-199.

Leung, K. B. P., Barrett, K. E., and Pearce, F. L. (1984). Differential effects of anti-allergic compounds on peritoneal mast cells of the rat mouse and hamster. *Agents Actions* **14**:461-467.

Leung, K. B. P., Flint, K. C., Brostoff, J., Hudspith, B. N., Johnson, N. Mc. I., Lau, H. Y. A., Liu, W. L., and Pearce, F. L. (1988). Effects of sodium cromoglycate and nedocromil sodium on histamine secretion from human lung mast cells. *Thorax* **43**:756-761.

Lindau, M., and Fernandez, J. M. (1986). IgE-mediated degranulation of rat mast cells does not require opening of ion channels. *Nature (Lond)* **319**:150.

Lobel, H., Machtey, I., and Eldin, M. Y. (1974). Pulmonary infiltrates with eosinophilia in an asthmatic patient treated with disodium cromoglycate. *Lancet* **2**:1032.

Lowman, M. A., Rees, P. H., Benyon, R. C., and Church, M. K. (1988a). Human mast cell heterogeneity: histamine release from mast cells dispersed from skin, lung, adenoids, tonsils and intestinal mucosa in response to IgE-dependent and non-immunological stimuli. *J. Allergy Clin. Immunol.* **81**:590-597.

Lowman, M. A., Benyon, R. C., and Church, M. K. (1988b). Human skin mast cells: effects of salbutamol and sodium cromoglycate on histamine release induced by anti-IgE and substance P. *Skin Pharmacol.* **1**:63-64.

Lowry, R. H., and Higenbottam, T. W. (1988). Antitussive effect of nedocromil sodium on chemically induced cough. *Thorax* **43**:256.

Lucas, A. M., and Schuster, S. (1987). Cromolyn inhibition of protein kinase C activity. *Biochem. Pharmacol.* **36**:562-565.

Mann, J. S., Cushley, M. J., and Holgate, S. T. (1984). Effect of vagal blockade on adenosine induced bronchoconstriction in asthma [abstract]. *Thorax* **39**:230-231.

Marquardt, D. L., Parker, C. W., and Sullivan, T. J. (1978). Potentiation of mast cell mediator release by adenosine. *J. Immunol.* **120**:871-878.

Marquardt, D. L., Walker, L. L., and Wasserman, S. I. (1986). Cromolyn inhibition of mediator release in mast cells derived from bone marrow. *Am. Rev. Respir. Dis.* **133**:1105-1109.

Marsh, W. R., Irvin, C. G., Murphy, K. R., Behrens, L., and Larsen, G. L. (1985). Increases in airway hyperreactivity to histamine and inflammatory cells in bronchoalveolar lavage after the late asthmatic reaction in an animal model. *Am. Rev. Respir. Dis.* **131**:875-879.

Marshall, P. W., Thomson, D. S., and Evans, D. P. (1976). The mechanism of tachyphylaxis to ICI 74,917 and disodium cromoglycate. *Int. Arch. Allergy Appl. Immunol.* **51**:274-283.

Marshall, R. (1972). Protective effect of disodium cromoglycate on rat peritoneal mast cells. *Thorax* **27**:38-43.

Martin, G. L., Atkins, P. C., Dunsky, E. H., and Zwieman, B. (1980). Effects of theophylline, terbutaline and prednisolone on antigen-induced bronchospasm and mediator release. *J. Allergy Clin. Immunol.* **66**:204-212.

Mattoli, S., Foresi, A., Corbo, G. M., Polidori, G., and Ciappi, G. (1987). Effects of two doses of cromolyn on allergen-induced late asthmatic response and increased responsiveness. *J. Allergy Clin. Immunol.* **79**: 747-754.

Mazurek, N., Berger, G., and Pecht, I. (1980). A binding site on mast cells and basophils for the antiallergic drug cromolyn. *Nature* **286**:722-723.

Mazurek, N., Baskin, P., Loyter, A., and Pecht, I. (1983). Restoration of the calcium influx and degranulation capacity of variant RBL-2H3 cells upon implantation of isolated cromolyn binding protein. *Proc. Natl. Acad. Sci. U.S.A.* **80**:6014-6018.

Metzger, W. J., Richerson, H. B., Worden, K., Monick, M., and Hunninghake, G. W. (1986). Bronchoalveolar lavage of allergic asthmatic patients following allergen provocation. *Chest* **89**:477-483.

Miller, P. (1976). Pinnal anaphylaxis in the mouse (PhD. thesis). London, Council for National Academic Awards, pp. 127-132.

Miller, P., and James, G. W. L. (1978). Inhibition of immediate hypersensitivity reactions by a novel xanthone, RU-31,156. *Arch. Int. Pharmacodyn. Ther.* **231**:328-339.

Moqbel, R., Walsh, G. M., Macdonald, A. J., and Kay, A. B. (1986a). Effect of disodium cromoglycate on activation of human eosinophils and neutrophils following reversed (anti-IgE) anaphylaxis. *Clin. Allergy* **16**:73-83.

Moqbel, R., Walsh, G. M., and Kay, A. B. (1986b). Inhibition of human granulocyte activation by nedocromil sodium. *Eur. J. Respir. Dis.* **69** (Suppl 147):227-229.

Moss, G. F., Jones, K. M., Ritchie, J. T., and Cox, J. S. G. (1971). Plasma levels and urinary excretion of disodium cromoglycate after inhalation by human volunteers. *Toxicol. Appl. Pharmacol.* **20**:147-156.

Murphy, K. R., Wilson, M. C., Charles, G. I., Laurie, S. G., Marsh, W. R., Haslett, C., Henson, P. M., and Larsen, G. L. (1986). The requirement for polymorphonuclear leukocytes in the late asthmatic response and heightened airways reactivity in an animal model. *Am. Rev. Respir. Dis.* **134**:62-68.

Murphy, S. (1987). Cromolyn sodium. In *Drug Therapy for Asthma: Research and Clinical Practice.* Edited by J. Jenne and S. Murphy. New York: Marcel Dekker, pp. 669-717.

Murphy, S., and Kelly, H. W. (1987). Cromolyn sodium: a review of mechanisms and clinical use. *Drug Intell. Clin. Pharm.* **21**:22-35.

Nadel, J. A., Salem, H., Tamplin, B., and Tokiwa, Y. (1965). Mechanism of sulphur dioxide induced bronchoconstriction in normal and asthmatic man. *J. Appl. Physiol.* **20**:164-167.

Neale, M. G., Brown, K., Hodder, R. W., and Auty, R. M. (1986). The pharmacokinetics of sodium cromoglycate in man after intravenous and inhalation administration. *Br. J. Clin. Pharmacol.* **22**:373-382.

Neale, M. G., Brown, K., Foulds, R. A., Lal, S., Morris, D. A., and Thomas, D. (1987). The pharmacokinetics of nedocromil sodium, a new drug for the treatment of reversible obstructive airways disease, in human volunteers and patients with reversible obstructive airways disease. *Br. J. Clin. Pharmacol.* **24**:493-501.

O'Driscoll, B. R. C., Lee, T. H., Cromwell, O., and Kay, A. B. (1983). Immunologic release of neutrophil chemotactic activity from human lung tissue. *J. Allergy Clin. Immunol.* **72**:695-701.

Okayama, M., Ma, J. Y., Hataoka, I., Kimura, K., Iijima, H., Inoue, H., and Takishima, T. (1986). Role of vagal nerve activity on adenosine-induced bronchoconstriction in asthma. *Am. Rev. Respir. Dis.* **133**(Suppl): A93.

Orellana, S. A., Solski, P. A., and Brown, J. H. (1985). Phorbol ester inhibits phosphoinositide hydrolysis and calcium mobilization in cultured astrocytoma cells. *J. Biol. Chem.* **260**:5236-5239.

Orr, T. S. C. (1975). Recent developments concerning the mast cell and the mode of action of disodium cromoglycate. *Acta Allergol.* **12**(suppl.):13-29

Orr, T. S. C. (1977). Fine structure of the mast cell with special reference to human cells. *Scand. J. Respir. Dis.* **98**(Suppl):1-7.

Orr, T. S. C., and Cox, J. S. G. (1969). Disodium cromoglycate, an inhibition of mast cell degranulation and histamine release induced by phospholipase A. *Nature* **233**:197-198.

Orr, T. S. C., Hall, D. E., Gwilliam, J. M., and Cox, J. S. G. (1971). Effect of disodium cromoglycate on the release of histamine and degranulation of mast cells induced by compound 48/80. *Life Sci.* **10**:805-812.

Patel, K. R., Tullett, W. M., Neale, M. G., Wall, R. T., and Tan, K. M. (1986). Plasma concentrations of sodium cromoglycate given by nebulization and metered dose inhalers in patients with exercise induced asthma: relationship to protective effect. *Br. J. Clin. Pharmacol.* **21**:231-233.

Pearce, F. L. (1982). Calcium and histamine secretion from mast cells. *Progr. Med. Chem.* **19**:59-109.

Pearce, F. L., and Foreman, J. C. (1988). Cromolyn. In: *Allergy, Principles and Practice*, 3rd ed. Edited by E. Middleton, C. E. Reed, E. F. Ellis, N. F. Adkinson, and J. W. Yunginger. St. Louis: C. V. Mosby, pp. 766-781.

Pearce, F. L., Befus, A. D., Gauldie, J., and Bienenstock, J. (1982). Mucosal mast cells. II. Effects of anti-allergic compounds on histamine secretion by isolated intestinal mast cells. *J. Immunol.* **128**:2481-2486.

Pepys, J. (1977). Clinical and therapeutic significance of patterns of allergic reactions of the lung to extrinsic agents. *Am. Rev. Respir. Dis.* **116**:573-588.

Pepys, J., and Hutchcroft, B. J. (1975). Bronchial provocation tests in etiologic diagnosis and analysis of asthma. *Am. Rev. Respir. Dis.* **112**:829-859.

Polosa, R., and Holgate, S. T. (1988). Bradykinin induced bronchoconstriction: inhibition by terfenadine. *Thorax* **43**:864.

Rafferty, P., Beasley, C. R., and Holgate, S. T. (1986). The inhibitory effect of terfenadine on bronchoconstriction induced by adenosine monophosphate and allergen. *Thorax* **41**:734.

Rees, P. H., Hillier, K., and Church, M. K. (1988). The secretory characteristics of mast cells isolated from human large intestinal mucosa and muscle. *Immunology* **65**:437-442.

Richards, R., Dickson, C. R., Renwick, A. G., Lewis, R. A., and Holgate, S. T. (1987). The effect of inspiratory effort on the plasma pharmacokinetics of cromolyn sodium. *J. Pharmacol. Exp. Ther.* **241**:1028.

Richards, R., Haas, A., Simpson, S., Britten, A., Renwick, A. G., and Holgate, S. T. (1988). Effect of methacholine induced bronchoconstriction on the pulmonary distribution and plasma pharmacokinetics of inhaled sodium cromoglycate in subjects with normal and hyperreactive airways. *Thorax* **43**:611-616.

Robertson, D. G., Kerigan, A. T., Hargreave, F. E., Chalmers, R., and Dolovich, J. (1974). Late asthmatic responses induced by ragweed pollen antigen. *J. Allergy Clin. Immunol.* **54**:244-254.

Robuschi, M., Vaghi, A., Simone, P., and Bianco, S. (1987). Prevention of fog-induced bronchospasm by nedocromil sodium. *Clin. Allergy* **17**: 69-74.

Rocchiccioli, K., and Pickering, C. A. C. (1986). A double-blind crossover study to compare the effects of nedocromil sodium (4 mg) and placebo given by pressurized aerosol in cold air bronchial challenge in asthmatic patients: a preliminary report. *Eur. J. Respir. Dis.* **69** (Suppl. 147):292-293.

Roy, A. C., and Warren, B. T. (1974). Inhibition of cAMP phosphodiesterase by disodium cromoglycate. *Biochem. Pharmacol.* **23**:917-920.

Sagi-Eisenberg, R. (1985). Possible role for a calcium-activated, phospholipid-dependent protein kinase in mode of action of DSCG. *Trends Pharmacol. Sci.* **6**:198-200.

Schechter, N. M., Choi, J. K., Slavin, D. A., Deresienski, D. T., Sayama, S., Dong, G., Lavaker, R. M., Proud, D., and Lazarus, G. S. (1986). Identification of a chymotrypsin-like proteinase from human mast cells. *J. Immunol.* **137**:962-970.

Schenkel, E., Atkins, P. C., Yost, R., and Zweiman, B. (1982). Antigen-induced neutrophil chemotactic activity from sensitized lung. *J. Allergy Clin. Immunol.* **70**:321-325.

Schmutzler, W., Delmich, K., Eichelberg, D., Gluck, S., Greven, T., Jurgensen, H., and Riesener, K. P. (1985). The human adenoidal mast cell. Susceptibility to different secretagogues and secretion inhibitors. *Int. Arch. Allergy Appl. Immunol.* **77**:177-178.

Schwartz, L. B. (1985). Monoclonal antibodies against human mast cell tryptase demonstrate shared antigenic sites on subunits of tryptase and selective localization of the enzyme to mast cells. *J. Immunol.* **134**:526-531.

Scott, V. L., Phillips, G. D., Richards, R., and Holgate, S. T. (1988). Inhibition of AMP induced bronchoconstriction in non-atopic asthma by sodium cromoglycate and nedocromil sodium. *Thorax* **43**:225-226.

Shampain, M. P., Behrens, B. L., Larsen, G. L., and Henson, P. M. (1983). An animal model of late pulmonary responses to *Alternaria* challenge. *Am. Rev. Respir. Dis.* **126**:493-498.

Shanahan, F., Denburg, J. A., Fox, J., Bienenstock, J., and Befus, D. (1985). Mast cell heterogeneity: effects of neuroenteric peptides on histamine release. *J. Immunol.* **135**:1331-1337.

Sheffer, A. L., Rocklin, R. E., and Goetzl, E. J. (1975). Immunologic components of hypersensitivity reactions to cromolyn sodium. *N. Engl. J. Med.* **293**:1220-1224.

Sieghart, W., Theoharides, T. C., Alper, S. E., Douglas, W. W., and Greengard, P. (1978). Calcium-dependent protein phosphorylation during secretion by exocytosis in the mast cell. *Nature* **275**:329-331.

Sieghart, W., Theoharides, T. C., Douglas, W. W., and Greengard, P. (1981). Phosphorylation of a single mast cell protein in response to drugs that inhibit secretion. *Biochem. Pharmacol.* **30**:2737-2738.

Simonsson, B. G., Skoogh, B. E., Bergh, N. P., Anderson, R., and Svedmyr, N. (1973). In vivo and in vitro effect of bradykinin on bronchial motor tone in normal subjects and in patients with airway obstruction. *Respiration* **30**:378-378.

Slater, E. E. (1978). Cardiac tamponade and peripheral eosinophilia in a patient receiving cromolyn sodium. *Chest* **73**:878-879.

Soter, N. A., Lewis, R. A., Corey, E. J., and Austen, K. F. (1983). Local effects of synthetic leukotrienes (LTC4, LTD4, LTE4 and LTB4) in human skin. *J. Invest. Dermatol.* **80**:115-119.

Spry, C. J. F., Kumaraswami, V., and Tai, P. C. (1986). The effect of nedocromil sodium on secretion from human eosinophils. *Eur. J. Respir. Dis.* **69** (Suppl 147):241-243.

Strobel, S., Miller, H. R. P., and Ferguson, A. (1981). Human intestinal mucosal mast cells: evaluation of fixation and staining techniques. *J. Clin. Pathol.* **34**:851-858.

Sung, C. P., Saunders, H. L., Krell, R. D., and Chakrin, L. W. (1977a). Studies on the mechanism of tachyphylaxis to disodium cromoglycate. *Int. Arch. Allergy Appl. Immunol.* **55**:374-384.

Sung, C. P., Saunders, H. L., Lenhardt, E., and Chakrin, L. W. (1977b). Further studies on the tachyphylaxis to disodium cromoglycate: the effects of concentration and temperature. *Int. Arch. Allergy Appl. Immunol.* **55**:385-394.

Tasaka, K., Mio, M., and Okamoto, M. (1986). Intracellular calcium release induced by histamine releasers and its inhibition by antiallergic drugs. *Ann. Allergy* **56**:464-469.

Tateson, J. E., and Trist (1976). Inhibition of adenosine 3'5'-cyclic monophosphate phosphodiesterase by potential anti-allergic compounds. *Life Sci.* **18**:153-162.

Taylor, W. A., and Roitt, I. M. (1973). Effect of disodium cromoglycate on various types of anaphylactic reactions in the guinea pig. *Int. Arch. Allergy Appl. Immunol.* **45**:795-807.

Theoharides, T. C., Seighart, W., Greengard, P., and Douglas, W. W. (1980). Antiallergic drug cromolyn may inhibit secretion by regulating phosphorylation of a mast cell protein. *Science* **207**:80-82.

Thorel, T., Ameisen, J. C., Joseph, M., Vorng, H., Tonnel, A. B., Marquette, C. H., and Capron, A. (1987). Preventative effect of nedocromil sodium on the abnormal response to aspirin of platelets from aspirin-sensitive asthmatics. *Am. Rev. Respir. Dis.* **135**:A398.

Thorel, T., Joseph, M., Tsicipoulos, A., Tonnel, A. B., and Capron, A. (1988a). Inhibition by nedocromil sodium of IgE-mediated activation of human mononuclear phagocytes and platelets in allergy. *Int. Arch. Allergy Appl. Immunol.* **85**:232-237.

Thorel, T., Joseph, M., Vorng, H., and Capron, A. (1988b). Regulation of IgE-dependent antiparasite functions of rat macrophages and platelets by nedocromil sodium. *Int. Arch. Allergy Appl. Immunol.* **85**:227-231.

Ting, S., Zweiman, B., and Lavker, R. M. (1983). Cromolyn does not modulate human allergic skin reactions in vivo. *J. Allergy Clin. Immunol.* **71**:12-17.

Ueda, N., Maramatsu, I., and Fijiwara, M. (1984). Capsaicin and bradykinin induced substance P-ergic responses in the iris sphincter muscle of the rabbit. *J. Pharmacol. Exp. Ther.* **230**:469-473.

Varonier, M. S., and Panzani, R. (1968). The effects of inhalations of bradykinin on healthy and atopic children. *Int. Arch. Allergy* **34**:293-296.

Walker, S. R. (1972). The fate of [14C] disodium cromoglycate in man. *J. Pharm. Pharmacol.* **24**:525-531.

Warner, J. O. (1976). Significance of late reactions after bronchial challenge with house dust mite. *Arch. Dis. Child* **51**:905-911.

Watson, S. P., and Lapetina, E. G. (1985). 1,2 Diacylglycerol and phorbol esters inhibit agonist-induced formation of inositol phosphates in human platelets: possible implications for negative feedback regulation of inositol phospholipid hydrolysis. *Proc. Natl. Acad. Sci. U.S.A.* **82**:2623-2626.

Wells, E., and Mann, J. (1983). Phosphorylation of a mast cell protein in response to treatment with anti-allergic compounds. Implications for the mode of action of sodium cromoglycate. *Biochem. Pharmacol.* **32**:837-842.

Wells, E., Jackson, C. G., Harper, S. T., Mann, J., and Eady, R. P. (1986). Characterization of primate bronchoalveolar mast cells. II. Inhibition of histamine, LTC4, and PGD2 release from primate bronchoalveolar mast cells and a comparison with rat peritoneal mast cells. *J. Immunol.* **137**:3941-3945.

Wieslander, E., Andersson, P., Linden, M., Axelsson, B., Kallstrom, L., Brasttsand, R., and Paulsson, I. (1985). Importance of particulate antigen for the induction of dual bronchial reaction in guinea-pigs. *Agents Actions* **16**:37-38.

Woodbury, R. G., and Miller, H. R. P. (1982). Quantitative analysis of mucosal mast cell protease in the intestine of *Nippostrongylus*-infected rats. *Immunology* **46**:487-495.

Yahev, Y., Dany, S., Katznelson, D., and Farfel, Z. (1988). Sodium cromoglycate in asthma: correlation between response and serum concentrations. *Arch. Dis. Child* **63**:592-597.

Young, K. D., and Church, M. K. (1983). Passive anaphylaxis in human lung fragments as a model for testing anti-allergic drugs: its variability and constraints. *Int. Arch. Allergy Appl. Immunol.* **70**:138-142.

22

Role of Allergens in Asthma and Airway Hyperresponsiveness
Relevance to Immunotherapy
and Allergen Avoidance

THOMAS A.E. PLATTS-MILLS, SUSAN M. POLLART, MARTIN D. CHAPMAN, and CHRISTINA M. LUCZYNSKA

University of Virginia Medical Center,
Charlottesville, Virginia

In 1873 Charles Blackley (1959) reported the use of pollen extracts to demonstrate immediate hypersensitivity to grass pollen in the skin and noses of patients with hay fever. In the same book he described (his own) positive bronchial responses to inhaled particles, including fungal spores. Over the next half century positive wheal and flare skin tests were demonstrated in relation to a variety of different diseases. In particular, sensitivity to extracts of house dust was found to be very common among patients with asthma (Kern, 1921). At that time and for 40 years afterwards the constituents of house dust were not well understood, and it was difficult to establish the relevance of the skin reactions. Since 1964 it has become increasingly clear that immediate skin sensitivity is due to specific antibodies of the IgE isotype and that in most parts of the world the dominant "unseen" sources of antigens in house dust are dust mites of the genus *Dermatophagoides* (Voorhorst et al., 1967; Ishizaka et al., 1967).

In early studies on pollen there was considerable confusion about whether skin reactions were due to pollen toxin or whether this was an example of "supersensitivity without immunity." The problem arose because none of the in vitro techniques available for examining immunity at that time could detect specific antibodies to pollen in sera from patients with hay fever. The initial studies on immunotherapy were reported by Noon in 1911, who, at least in part, thought he was raising immunity against pollen toxin. It is now clear that the main allergenic proteins from pollen, dust mites, or cat dander are not toxic, that patients who become allergic have made specific immune response to these proteins, and that, in general, nonallergic individuals are nonresponders. Individuals who are allergic to pollen or dust mite have made specific T-cell responses, and have produced antibodies of IgG and IgA isotypes as well as IgE antibodies to proteins from these sources (Platts-Mills, 1979, 1982; Rawle et al., 1984).

Immunotherapy was strongly recommended for patients with asthma by early enthusiasts who were brave about reactions. At that time there was clearly much less pharmacological treatment available (Spivacke and Grove, 1925). In the early experiments on immunotherapy for asthma, many different allergens or mixtures of allergens were used. House dust was and still is a common constituent of immunotherapy mixtures. It is very difficult to interpret any of those results because there was no standardization of the extracts, and it is impossible to know now what the extracts contained. The first reliable standardization of extracts came with the measurement of *Amb a* I from ragweed (previously termed antigen E) in the late 1960s (reviewed by Norman, 1980). The experiments carried out then on immunotherapy of seasonal rhinitis established that the treated patients improved, and that higher doses work better than lower doses. A cumulative dose of at least 50 μg of the major allergen appeared to be necessary for effective treatment. Following the discovery of house dust mites and the development of techniques to culture them, it became possible to purify and measure mite allergens in house dust (Chapman and Platts-Mills, 1980; Tovey et al., 1981a). In studies on the immunotherapy of perennial rhinitis it appeared that a similar dose of mite allergen (i.e., ~ 50 μg cumulative dose) was necessary for effective treatment. When dust mite extracts were used for immunotherapy of asthma, the results were not consistent (see Graft and Valentine, 1985). Many variables could influence the therapeutic responses to immunotherapy. These include the level of exposure at home, nonspecific reactivity, and bronchial obstruction at the time of the injection, as well as the level of immediate hypersensitivity. Since it has only recently become possible to measure exposure to allergens at home, it is perhaps not surprising that many answers about the criteria for and the effectiveness of immunotherapy for perennial asthma are not available. In considering the mechanism of immunotherapy in the 1990s the question is going to be which aspect of the immune response does the treatment alter. Indeed, many studies are now underway to attempt to produce fragments of allergen molecules that will alter T-cell responses without or with minimal effect on B cells.

Awareness of dust mites in house dust has dramatically increased our understanding of this source of allergen exposure (see Voorhorst et al., 1969; Fain et al., 1989). This lead to increased interest in procedures for reducing exposure to indoor allergens. Initial enthusiastic reports on the benefits of dust mite avoidance measures were followed by negative results of controlled trials (Sarsfield et al., 1974; Burr et al., 1980; Korsgaard, 1982). However, with more effective and more aggressive measures, success has been achieved (Murray and Ferguson, 1983; Walshaw and Evans, 1986; Mitchell et al., 1989). Nonetheless, it is still difficult to define a regimen for the whole house that will consistently reduce exposure sufficiently to reduce symptoms of asthma.

Most of the early studies on skin testing in patients with asthma simply reported a high prevalence of positive skin tests among clinic patients. However, there are now sufficient epidemiological studies to be certain that immediate hypersensitivity to dust mites, cats, grass pollen, cockroach allergen, and others can be a major risk factor for asthma. The initial studies on large numbers of English schoolchildren by Morrisson Smith and his colleagues showed a very strong correlation between asthma and positive skin tests to dust mites (Smith et al., 1969). A similar association between mite allergy and asthma has been found in population samples of children in Australia and New Zealand (Green et al., 1986; Sears et al., 1989, see Chapter 1). Furthermore, in a prospective study of 80 children with 1 atopic parent, the association between mite allergy and asthma was clear at 5 years of age and is now very strong at age 12 (Rowntree et al., 1985; Sporik et al., 1990). Epidemiological surveys are more difficult in adults, but Burrows and his colleagues found a very strong correlation between total IgE, positive skin tests, and new-onset asthma in young adults (Burrows et al., 1989). Furthermore, in two recent studies on adults presenting to emergency rooms, IgE antibodies were shown to be a major risk factor for asthma. In Virginia, IgE antibodies to mites, cats, cockroach, and pollen were each significantly related to asthma in adults ≤ 50 years old (Fig. 1; Pollart et al., 1989a), while in northern California during the grass pollen season IgE antibody to rye grass pollen was the single dominant risk factor (Pollart et al., 1988). Thus, there is no serious doubt that IgE antibodies (ab) to allergens, predominantly those in houses, can be a risk factor for chronic and acute asthma. At present the epidemiological evidence about asthma relates to a small number of inhalant allergens; however, many different inhaled pollens, animal danders, or fungi may be important in individual cases. In addition, some patients with "intrinsic" asthma who have no IgE antibodies to inhalants are highly allergic to the dermatophytes, yeasts, and aspergilli that colonize them (Ward et al., 1989).

This chapter will focus on several aspects of the relationship between allergens and asthma, in particular those areas in which specific quantitative

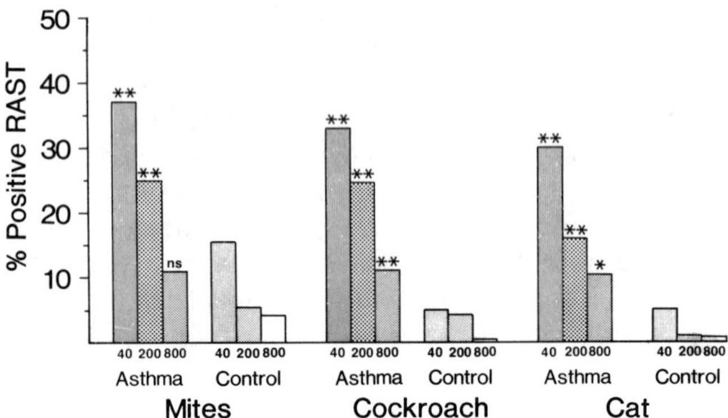

Figure 1   Prevalence of IgE antibodies to three indoor allergens in sera from 68 patients with acute asthma and 81 controls aged < 50 years old. Values under the bars are RAST units/ml (units are ~ 0.1 ng IgE antibody). The difference between patients and controls was highly significant for each allergen (** = p < 0.005). Cockroach and cat allergy were independent, since none of the patients had ⩾ 200 units IgE antibody to both allergens (from Pollart et al., 1989a, by permission of *J. Allergy Clin. Immunol.*).

assays of allergens have already helped to improve our understanding of the role of allergens.

I. Techniques for Measuring Allergens

The levels of natural exposure to inhaled allergens are very low: $< 1\mu g$ and often around 10 ng/m³ of inhaled air. The levels of allergen in floor dust range from 10 ng to approximately 200 μg/g of dust. Thus, any technique for measuring exposure must be capable of measuring a few nanograms of protein. Two techniques are well established for comparing the overall potency of extracts: radioallergosorbent testing (RAST) inhibition and skin testing. However, both these techniques are relatively imprecise, slow, and neither can be standardized relative to an absolute measurement. The alternative is to measure a single representative protein using some form of radioimmunoassay (RIA). Conventional inhibition RIA requires a supply of purified antigen and monospecific polyclonal antiserum, which may be difficult to maintain. Monoclonal antibodies (mAb) solve many problems; they can be selected for the specificity required; their specificity is permanent and does not have to be reestablished with each new batch of reagent; and they can be produced in very large quantities relatively cheaply (Chapman et al., 1984; De Groot et al., 1988; Horn and Lind, 1987; Esch and Klapper, 1989). The easiest way to use mAb to measure protein is in a two site immunometric assay (Fig. 2) using mAb directed at separate sites on a given allergen molecule (Chapman et al., 1987; Luczynska et al., 1989). The second mAb is either enzyme labeled or radiolabeled. It is also possible to use a single mAb on the plate and conventional antiserum to detect bound antigen. These assays can be sensitive down to 0.2 ng protein and can be completed in 4 h. They are already being used for research in many different centers and could be used as part of routine practice. Standardization of assays for specific proteins can be carried out using national or international standards (Ford et al., 1985). Perhaps most important is that the results can be given in absolute values (μg), because in several cases the proteins have been purified and can be weighed accurately. In addition, sequencing of allergens, particularly those from dust mites, is now progressing rapidly (Chua et al., 1988). At present, the most relevant standards for asthma are the WHO International Standard for *D. pteronyssinus*, which is considered to contain 12.5μg *Der p* I and the U.S. national standard for cat allergen, which contains 4 Food and Drug Administration (FDA) units of the major cat allergen *Fel d* I, which is 16 μg *Fel d* I (Leiterman and Ohman, 1984; Chapman et al., 1988). International standards are currently being developed for *D. farinae*, cat, and *Alternaria*.

Measurement of a single allergen does not measure total potency but will provide a reasonable guide to potency, provided that the protein measured is representative and that its concentration bears a consistent relationship to other proteins from a particular source. At present, accurate measure-

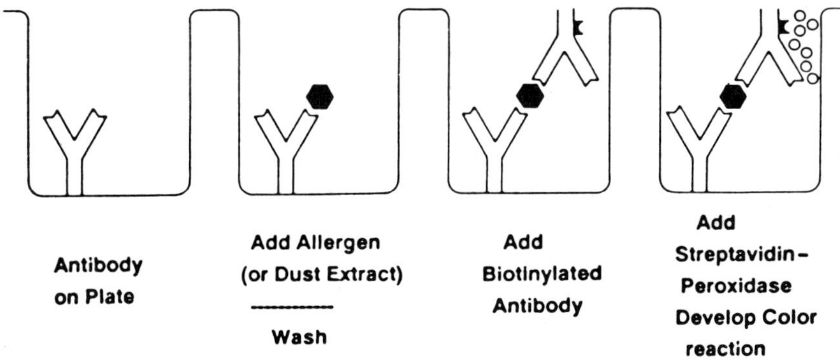

Figure 2 Two-site enzyme immunoassay for allergen in house dust samples. The assay can be carried out with conventional polyclonal antibodies or monoclonal antibodies. The use of monoclonal antibodies requires two separate epitopes on the molecule. For details of assays and relevant monoclonal antibodies see Luczynska et al., 1989; Chapman et al., 1987, 1988; Pollart et al., 1989b.

ments of mite, cat, grass pollen, and ragweed pollen allergens can be made. Quantitative measurements of allergens from other sources such as cockroach or *Alternaria* can be made, but the absolute quantities are not established. Many techniques can give reliable measurements of individual allergens; these include inhibition RIA, radial immunodiffusion, and rocket immunoelectrophoresis. In general, these techniques are slower and/or less sensitive than two-site immunometric assays using mAb.

II. Bronchial Reactivity and Allergen Exposure

The first clear statement that allergen exposure could be an important cause of bronchial reactivity came from Dr. Roger Altounyan (Altouyan, 1970). He reported that patients with grass pollen hay fever developed increased bronchial reactivity to histamine during the grass pollen season and that this reactivity gradually resolved after the season. This observation has been confirmed for other pollens (Boulet et al., 1983). In addition, Hargreave and his colleagues demonstrated that bronchial challenge with allergen could lead to increases in reactivity to histamine lasting days or even weeks (Cartier et al., 1982; Cockcroft et al., 1977). For mite-allergic patients, the "season" is not sufficiently well-defined to allow us to observe changes of this kind. However, it was found that removing mite-allergic patients from their houses could lead to decreases in nonspecific bronchial reactivity. These results have been seen in high-altitude sanatoria in Davos, Switzerland, and in the French mountains (Kerrebijn, 1970; Vervloet et al., 1982; Charpin et al., 1988). Both of these sanatoria have been shown to be essentially mite free. In addition, we found that five of seven mite-allergic patients in London who stayed away from their houses and lived in "allergen-free" hospital rooms for 6 weeks to 6 months had significant decreases in nonspecific bronchial reactivity (Platts-Mills et al., 1982). Since that time there have been many experiments on changes in "bronchial reactivity" following antigen exposure, however, many of them have been short-term experiments in which the patients have either not fully recovered baseline forced expiratory volume in 1 s (FEV_1) or have had episodes of bronchoconstriction within hours. In our experiments, in those at Davos, and the studies by Dr. Hargreave and his colleagues in Hamilton, changes in histamine reactivity occurred against constant baseline FEV_1. A striking feature of all these experiments is that normalization or significant decrease in bronchial reactivity has always taken weeks or months.

III. Natural Exposure to Inhaled Allergens

Exposure to inhaled allergens can induce an acute attack of bronchoconstriction and/or contribute to bronchial inflammation and nonspecific bronchial reactivity (Fig. 3). The actual allergen inhaled is that small fraction of floor dust that becomes airborne or becomes adjacent to the mouth or nose (i.e., on blankets, pillows, or upholstered furniture). To understand the quantitites that enter the lung, it is essential to measure both the airborne quantities and their particle size. Since the airborne levels are very low, it is clear that particle sizing will only be possible using very sensitive assays or high-volume sampling (Platts-Mills et al., 1989; Swanson et al., 1989). The problem with high-volume samplers is that when they are used in an enclosed space they will disturb the room air, repeatedly sample the same air, or if exhausted out of the room, will create an influx of air from outside the room. Several different devices have been used to analyze particle sizes: Anderson samplers, cascade impactor, and liquid impinger. Each is a method of measuring terminal velocity. Air is sucked through progressively smaller orifices so that progressively smaller particles impact on a solid surface (or impinge on a liquid surface) at each stage (Solomon and Mathews, 1978). Results have been obtained for many different indoor allergens, but the most consistent results have been obtained for airborne dust mite and airborne cat allergens. Using a cascade impactor and an inhibition RIA for the dust mite allergen *Der p* I, we reported that mite allergen only became airborne during disturbance and that >90% of the allergen was associated with particles >10μm in diameter (Tovey et al., 1981a,b). Direct examination of the particles carrying allergen showed them to be mite fecal particles. Subsequent studies using an Anderson sampler

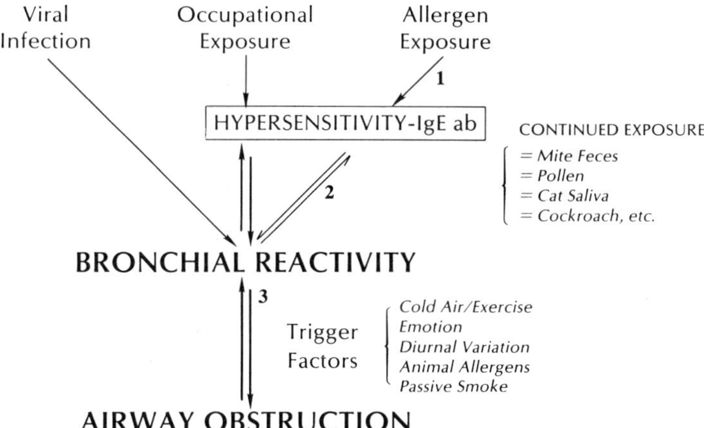

Figure 3 Exposure to allergens can play three different roles in asthma: (1) as a cause of sensitization of IgE antibody production, which may take years; (2) as a contributing cause of bronchial reactivity, which may take weeks and is at least in part reversible; (3) as a trigger of acute attacks. For the first two of these the response is influenced by both heredity and the quantity of exposure. Triggering of acute attacks (3) is only likely to occur if a large number of small allergen particles becomes airborne.

and RAST inhibition confirmed that a large proportion of the airborne mite allergen was on particles >5 μm in diameter and that most of this allergen fell within a few hours (Swanson et al., 1985; Platts-Mills et al., 1986a). Results from Japan have recently suggested that group II allergens also become airborne on large particles, even though these allergens are present in higher concentrations in whole body mite extracts (Yasueda et al., 1989; Heymann et al., 1989).

Airborne cat allergen in houses has been measured using basophil histamine release and RAST inhibition (Findlay et al., 1983a,b; Swanson, et al., 1985). The results suggested that the allergen was present on both small- (<4 μm) diameter and large particles, and that at least part of the cat allergen remained airborne for long periods of time. Van Metre and his colleagues (1986) also reported measurements of airborne *Fel d* I in an experimental room. However, they found that it took a large fan to increase airborne allergen sufficiently to provoke bronchial reactions in patients. We have recently reported a series of experiments using a two-site monoclonal antibody-based assay for cat allergen *Fel d* I. These experiments used two different samplers and evaluated levels before, during, and after disturbance. The results showed that in many houses a significant proportion of cat allergen (mean, 26%) is airborne on very small particles (i.e., <2 μm diameter). These particles, in keeping with their sizes, tend to remain airborne and will accumulate if the ventilation rate is *low* (Luczynska et al., 1990a). During disturbance, the quantity of cat allergen airborne on these small particles can reach levels as high as 40 ng *Fel d* I/m^3.

The more sensitive assay for *Fel d* I has also allowed a series of experiments looking at the effects of vacuum cleaners and air filters on airborne cat allergen. These experiments have identified major differences between types of vacuum cleaners and some very striking variables in filter performance (Luczynska et al., 1990b). All vacuum cleaners increase airborne allergen by disturbing dust in front of or around them. In addition, many vacuum cleaners allow considerable quantities of dust to come through the bag. However, some of the vacuum cleaners promoted as especially suitable for reducing airborne allergen levels also allow allergen to escape. One water-trap type of vacuum cleaner produced a fine cloud of small droplets that carry large quantities of airborne allergen. By contrast, high efficiency particulate air (HEPA) or HEPA-type filters on vacuum cleaners will almost completely prevent any allergen from being passed through the filter.

Cockroach and mouse allergens have been measured in the air of houses in New York (Swanson et al., 1985). At present, it is difficult to compare the levels with those of cat or dust mite because these other allergens have been measured in arbitrary units or in nanograms of protein (rather than nanograms of a specific allergen). Measurements of airborne rat urinary allergen in animal houses have found high levels of the protein alpha$_2$ U-globulin associated with particles of a mean size 7 μm diameter, which is significantly less than the size of mite fecal particles but larger than the small particles carrying cat allergen (Table 1).

A. Relevance of Particle Size to the Symptoms of Asthma

Are these differences in the size of naturally occurring particles relevant to the symptoms of asthma? Cat-allergic patients often report the acute onset of bronchospasm on entering a house with a cat in it. Similar rapid asthmatic responses can occur when rat-allergic individuals enter an animal facility. By contrast, it is very unusual for mite-allergic individuals to react rapidly on entering a house known to have high levels of mite allergen in the floor dust. We have studied houses in which the quantity and particle size of airborne cat allergen are similar to that necessary to cause bronchial provocation using nebulized allergen extract. If the air in a house contains 40 ng/m^3

Table 1 Particle Size of Some Common Airborne Allergens: Relationship to the Estimated Quantity of Allergen per Particle

	Dust mite (*Der p* I)	Rat (2 μm globulin)	Cat (*Fel d* I)	Bronchial Provocation
Diameter (μm)[a]	20	7.0	2.0	2.0
Maximum allergen per particle	~0.2ng	~0.002ng	~0.2pg	<0.01pg
Number of particles to deliver 10 ng	~50	≥5,000	≥50,000	≥10^6
Deposition in the lung (%)[c]	5	~35	~40	~40

[a]The diameters given are mean values for mite (Tovey et al., 1981a) and rat (Platts-Mills et al., 1986a). The particle size given for cat allergen is that of the small particles that may represent 50% of the airborne allergen in some "airtight" houses (Luczynska et al., 1990a).

[b]The quantity of allergen in droplets used for bronchial provocation assumes that the extract used contains 10 μg/ml of the dominant allergen. The values for mite fecal particles and pollen grains have been calculated (Tovey et al., 1981b; Marsh, 1975). The values for allergen content on rat or cat airborne particles assume maximum concentration of 10 mg allergen/cm^3.

[c]Values for deposition in the lung are estimates based on published reports (Task Group on Lung Dynamics, 1966; Svartengren et al., 1987).

of particles $<2\mu$m diameter, it would take an adult $\sim$15 min to inhale 10 ng *Fel d* I. Previous studies have estimated that a sensitive patient will respond with a 20% fall in FEV_1 to $\sim$8 ng *Fel d* I given over a 2 min period (Taylor et al., 1978; Van Metre et al., 1986). In a mite-infested house with $\geqslant$40 μg *Der p* I/g of floor dust, levels of airborne allergen during disturbance may reach 30ng/m^3; however, less than 5% of this allergen is associated with small particles. Without disturbance, very little mite allergen becomes airborne, so it is not surprising that mite-allergic patients do not report acute symptoms on entering "mite-infested" houses. The question is what effect exposure to a relatively *small number* of large particles has on the lung (Table 1). We have estimated that natural exposure to mite fecal particles may be to as few as 200 (i.e., $\sim$40ng *Der p* I)/day. Of this number we would expect 5-10% to enter the lung during quiet breathing. During forced inspiration the proportion of large particles entering the lung will decrease. Particles greater than 5 or 10 μm diameter are sometimes referred to as "nonrespirable"—as if they did not enter the lung. However, the term *nonrespirable* was meant to apply to the alveoli or respiratory bronchioles. The most careful studies on inhalation of particles via the mouth into the human lung have consistently shown that a proportion of larger particles do enter the bronchi (Svartengren et al., 1987; Task Group on Lung Dynamics, 1966). Although the percentage of large particles that enters the trachea is low, even with particles as large as 15 μm diameter, 5-10% will enter the large or medium airways. It is certain that very few (i.e. <0.1%) particles $>5\mu$m diameter will reach the peripheral lung, however the inflammation in asthma does not generally affect the peripheral lung. The impact of large particles (in a restricted number) on the bronchi would be expected to be very different from that of a large number of small particles carrying the same quantity of allergen. If a patient inhales $\geqslant10^6$ droplets using bronchial provocation or during natural exposure to cat allergen, mast cell triggering would be expected to occur in many different bronchi. This could trigger symptoms and a measurable fall in FEV_1, but the local concentration in each bronchus might be insufficient to produce further inflammatory events. By contrast, the *local* concentration (and quantity) of allergen at the site of arrival of a mite fecal particle or pollen grain would be at least 1000-fold higher, and a series of inflammatory events would be expected at that restricted site (Fig. 4). The likely sequence following natural exposure to dust mite allergens is a series of immediate, late, and prolonged inflammatory events occurring at restricted sites. These events would not be expected to trigger a diffuse increase in airway resistance and might not be appreciated by the patient. The impact of these local events on the lung will then depend on how long the changes persist. If the local inflammation and associated irritability healed quickly, the effects would not accumulate. On the other hand, if the "inflammation" persisted for weeks, as is

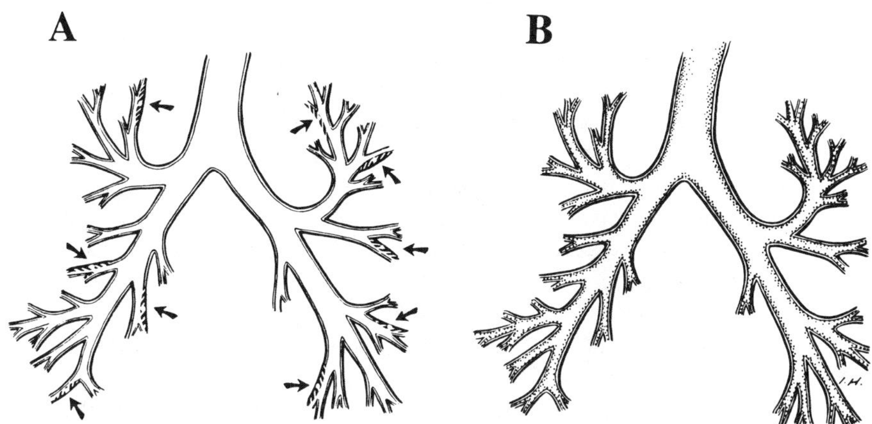

Figure 4 Exposure of the lungs to allergens. (A) Natural exposure to a relatively few (i.e., 10-100) mite fecal particles, pollen grains, or large fungal spores per day. Each of these particles ($>10\mu$m diameter) carries a *large* quantity of allergen (~0.2 ng) and would cause a local inflammatory response. However, because of the small number there might be no significant fall in FEV_1 or symptoms at the time of exposure. (B) Bronchial provocation with nebulized extract or exposure to animal allergens (e.g., cat or rat) may represent as many as 10^6-10^8 droplets inhaled within 10 min. Each droplet contains a very small quantity of allergen (<0.001 pg), so that mast cell triggering could occur with or without subsequent epithelial inflammation or damage. Because of the large number of particles, the airway response would be diffuse, giving rise to symptoms and a measurable fall in FEV_1.

suggested by the results following bronchial provocation (Cartier et al., 1982), the local irritable foci could accumulate to a level at which the whole lung was reactive, that is, had bronchial hyperreactivity (BHR). Without an understanding of the mechanism of bronchial irritability, it is not possible to explain the factors that lead to "healing." However, as outlined elsewhere in this volume, it is likely that mast cells, T lymphocytes, and eosinophils are all involved in the local inflammation that follows deposition of a mite fecal particle, pollen grain, or similar particle carrying proteins to which the exposed individual has IgE antibodies.

B. Specific Levels of Allergen Exposure Associated with Asthma

To study the relationship between allergen exposure and asthma, it is essential to use measurements that are simple, can be standardized between laboratories, can be maintained over a period of years, and preferably are in absolute rather than arbitrary units. Although airborne allergen is inhaled, the techniques currently available for measuring airborne allergen are too complex for widespread use. At a recent international workshop it was concluded that dust samples obtained from bedding, carpets, furniture, and other items were the most reliable way of assessing mite exposure (Platts-Mills and de Weck, 1988). In addition, it was recommended that results should be expressed as the quantity of a defined allergen per gram of dust. This was decided because of the great difficulty in standardizing collection procedures, which are highly dependent on the performance of the vacuum cleaner used. For indoors allergens the only data that can be analyzed in assessing the levels of allergen that are a risk for asthma are expressed as mites/g of dust or μg *Der p* I/g of dust. For pollen, the situation is different because a simple airborne count of pollen grains can be taken as a reasonable assessment of exposure for all individuals within an area. However, even with pollen indoor exposure may be important. More complicated problems arise with assessing exposure to other allergens, especially the fungi (see below).

C. Exposure to Mites and Mite Allergens as a Risk Factor for Asthma

In 1964 Voorhorst and colleagues observed that dust obtained from the houses of mite-allergic patients who had symptoms often contained ≥500 mites per gram of dust. A formal epidemiological study from Denmark comparing the houses of mite-allergic asthmatic patients and random control patients concluded that the presence of >100 mites/dust in the houses was a sevenfold risk factor for asthma (Korsgaard, 1983a). That study reported a surprisingly low level of mites in the houses of the control subjects. This raises an important issue: within an area exposure to an allergen could be uniformly high, uniformly low, or variable. If all houses in an area have high levels of mites, we would not expect to find major differences between the houses of patients with asthma and those without. In that case the key question would be whether the individual developed an IgE antibody response. However, one would expect that within an area where "all" houses had high levels of mite allergen, the prevalence of IgE antibodies to mite would be higher. This would be comparable to the situation within an area of high pollen exposure, where genetic factors rather than differences in exposure play the major role in deciding which patients develop hay fever (Marsh, 1975, 1986). In England we did not see differences between house comparable to those reported from Denmark; however, in the United States many houses have very low numbers of mites (i.e., ≤10/g dust).

A very dramatic situation has recently developed in Papua New Guinea, where asthma developed as a new disease in a group of villages. The prevalence of the disease apparently rose from ~0.7% to 7% and the timing correlated with the introduction of blankets that many of the villagers wrapped round their heads at night (Dowse et al., 1985). Examining the villagers huts revealed no mattresses, no carpets, no furniture, and very few mites except in the blankets. Almost all the villagers who developed asthma were found to have positive skin tests to mite extract and serum IgE antibodies to mites. The mean number of mites in dust collected from the blankets was ~1,300/g dust. Thus, it seems clear that exposure to this level of mites was sufficient both to induce IgE antibody responses in a proportion of the population and to induce symptomatic (often severe) asthma in some of the allergic individuals. More recently, Woolcock and her colleagues have studied skin tests to mites, bronchial reactivity, and the number of mites in the houses of schoolchildren in Australia. The results showed very striking differences between the Belmont suburb of Sydney, which is coastal and humid, and the inland town of Wagga-Wagga, which is dry. In Sydney there was a very strong correlation between positive skin tests to mites and bronchial hyperreactivity. In keeping with this, most dust samples from Belmont contained ⩾100 mites/g dust (Green et al., 1986; Peat et al., 1989). By contrast, in Wagga-Wagga the mite levels were generally less than 100/g dust and although there were some children with positive skin tests to mites, these did not correlate with asthma symptoms or BHR. The results again suggest that exposure to 100 mites/g of dust was a risk factor for both IgE antibody formation and the development of BHR in children (Table 2).

As discussed previously, mite counts are difficult to standardize and therefore not suitable for widespread or routine clinical use. However, it is possible to make a reasonable correlation between mite allergen and mite numbers (Platts-Mills et al., 1986c; Van Bronswijk et al., 1989). One hundred mites have been found to be equivalent to 2μg group I mite allergen and 500 mites are equivalent to 10μg. Several studies have now been published in which it is possible to equate a particular level of mite allergen in dust with severity, prevalence, or improvement in asthma. Studies in England, Atlanta, Charlottesville, Baltimore, and Sao Paulo have all found that most mite-allergic patients presenting with symptomatic asthma have greater than $2\,\mu$g group I mite allergen/g of dust in their houses (Table 2) (Smith et al., 1985; Platts-Mills et al., 1982, 1986b; Arruda et al., 1989; Wood et al., 1989b). By contrast, dust collected from the houses of patients in northern California who presented with "grass pollen asthma" generally contain low levels of group I mite allergen (i.e., $<2\,\mu$g/g) (Pollart et al., 1988). On the basis of studies on houses of asthmatic children in Baltimore Wood et al. (1989b) calculated that a group I mite allergen level of 1.9 μg/g dust was a significant risk factor for mite allergy. Similarly, Dr. Wahn and his group have reported

Table 2 Studies in Which a Specific Level of Mites or Mite Allergen Has Been Recognized as a Risk Factor for Asthma

Nature of Study	Site	Number of Mites/g dust[a]	Authors
Dust mites			
Symptomatic asthma	Netherlands	≥500	Voorhorst et al., 1969
Clinic asthma in adults	Denmark	>100	Korsgaard, 1983a
New onset of asthma in adults	Papua New Guinea	~1,300	Dowse et al., 1985
Bronchial reactivity in schoolchildren	Australia	>100	Green et al., 1986 Peat et al., 1989
Reduction in bronchial reactivity	Switzerland/ Netherlands	<20	Kerrebijn, 1970
Reduction in bronchial reactivity	France	<20	Vervloet et al., 1982
Mite allergen		*μg Group I Mite Allergen/g dust[b]*	
Development of IgE and asthma	Poole, U.K.	≥5	Rowntree et al., 1985 Sporik et al., 1989
Exacerbations of asthma	Virginia	>10	Platts-Mills et al., 1986b
Presentation with symptomatic asthma			
Mite-allergic children	Atlanta, GA	>10	Smith et al., 1985
	Berlin	>6.4	Chur et al., 1988
	Baltimore	1.9	Wood et al., 1989b
	Sao Paulo, Brazil	>10	Arruda et al., 1989
Reversal of BHR	London, U.K.	13.4 → <0.2[c]	Platts-Mills et al., 1982

[a]Mites counted and identified microscopically after separation.
[b]Mites allergen *Der p* I or group I or antigen P_1 equivalent measured by RIA or two-site immunometric assay.
[c]Mean level in the patients homes was 13.4 μg/g dust and in the hospital room was <0.2 μg/g.

that mite-allergic children presenting for treatment of asthma were significantly more likely to have >2 μg group I allergen/g of house dust than comparable asthmatic children who were not allergic to mite allergens (Chur et al., 1988).

D. Levels of Cat Allergens and Other Allergens

Symptoms of seasonal hay fever correlate well with the onset of pollination of the relevant plants. In addition, in many areas a particular pollen count is recognized that will cause "all" the patients with hay fever in that area to have symptoms. However, there are relatively few areas of the world where there are sufficient cases of asthma associated with pollen season to allow us to reach conclusions about the level of pollen exposure that is a risk factor for asthma. In addition, a simple correlation with outdoor pollen count may not be expected since pollen enters houses and pollen allergens may rise to high levels in house dust (Platts-Mills et al., 1986b). In northern California there is a very sharp pollen season that causes an annual epidemic of asthma at Travis Air Force Base hospital. In that area it is possible to specify the pollen count that will increase the number of patients entering the hospital emergency room with asthma (Fig. 5) (Pollart, et al., 1988). These patients

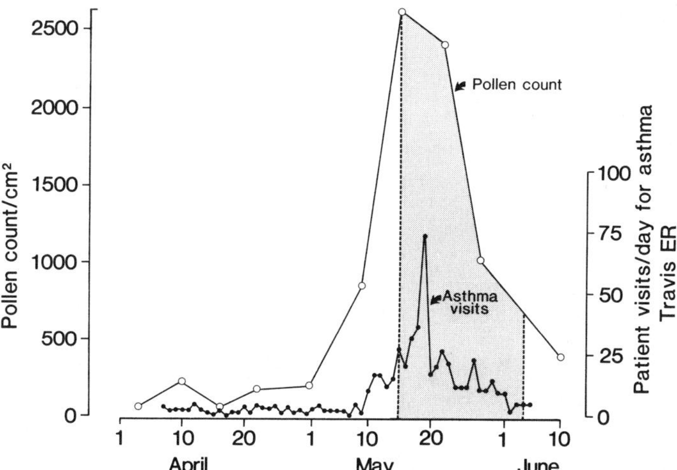

Figure 5 Relationship between pollen count and acute admissions due to asthma at Travis Air Force Base in northern California; 54 of 59 patients with acute asthma entering this hospital during the shaded period had high levels (>200 RAST units) of IgE antibodies to rye grass pollen; by contrast only 6 of 59 controls had similar levels. Analysis of these values suggests that >90% of acute asthma episodes during this period are related to sensitivity to rye grass pollen (reprinted from Pollart et al., 1988, by permission of *J. Allergy Clin. Immunol.*).

(where studied) had high levels of grass pollen allergen in their houses; the levels were estimated to be $\geqslant$10 μg *Lol p* I/g of dust in 13 of 15 houses (Lol p I is the major allergen from rye grass *Lolium perene*).

Cat allergen (*Fel d* I) levels in house dust have been measured by several groups. In general, patients who are selectively allergic to cat dander are aware of symptoms in houses that do not have a cat. Houses with a cat routinely have $\geqslant$ 4 FDA units of *Fel d* I/g of dust (i.e., $>$16μg *Fel d* I/g). Houses without a cat vary in their content of cat allergen from $\leqslant$ 0.1 μg to $\sim$ 10μg *Fel d* I/g (Ohman and Lorusso, 1987; Wood et al., 1989a; Chapman et al., 1988). The source of cat allergen in a house without a cat is not entirely clear, but allergen carried on clothing from one house to another is a significant source. The levels of cat allergen found in houses with a cat are a risk factor for IgE antibody responses, increased bronchial reactivity, and symptomatic asthma. It is not clear whether the levels found in some houses without a cat (i.e., 0.1-1μg *Fel d* I/g dust) are relevant or not. Some individuals have positive skin tests to cat dander extracts although they deny that they have lived in a house with a cat. It is not possible to say whether these patients were sensitized by occasional exposure to houses with cats or by prolonged exposure to low levels in their own house. It has also not been resolved whether the low levels of cat allergen found in houses without a cat can contribute to chronic symptoms of asthma even if they do not cause acute symptoms.

There is very little known about specific levels of other allergens such as fungi, cockroaches, dog dander, pet guinea pigs, and others. This is because there are usually only occasional patients who have these allergens as a dominant or sole sensitivity and because in most cases there have not been simple enough techniques for measuring exposure. *Alternaria* spores can give rise to "epidemics" of asthma in the upper midwest with a significant number of severe or fatal cases (O'Hallaren et al., 1986, 1988). These episodes are generally associated with very high counts of *Alternaria* spores. It is likely that many different fungi contribute to asthma and that most patients are sensitive to several different species. This makes it very difficult to define any specific threshold level. Cockroach allergy is certainly a risk factor for asthma and in some houses cockroach allergen appears to be the dominant foreign protein in dust (Pollart et al., 1989b). However, no data would allow definition of a specific number of cockroaches or of cockroach allergen that should be regarded as a risk for asthma.

IV. Allergen Avoidance

Attempts to reduce exposure to house dust as a method of treating asthma were applied on an occasional basis prior to this century. After the introduction of skin testing, dust avoidance became part of normal practice simply on the grounds that it was logical for patients who were allergic to dust to reduce their exposure. The view that house dust avoidance would be beneficial was supported by consistent reports that asthmatic patients improved when they were taken into hospitals or sanatoria. Because of the experience of Dutch patients who improved in Switzerland, Dr. Storm van Leeuwn developed a "climate chamber" to treat asthma. The chamber was a dust-free room in which clean air was taken down a long pipe from 60 feet up. He reported that three-quarters of asthmatic patients improved when in the chamber (Storm van Leeuwen, 1927). The techniques for reducing dust in houses did not improve until the discovery of dust mites in the mid-1960s. The first studies attempting to reduce mites in houses reported successful results (Sarsfield et al., 1974). Following that, two controlled studies reported negative results. However, each of those studies actually demonstrated that the measures routinely recommended to patients did not reduce exposure to mite allergens (Burr et al., 1980; Korsgaard, 1982). Indeed, the conclusion of those studies was that it is difficult to reduce mite levels in a house.

In the last 8 years three studies have achieved more successful results. The first, by Murray and Ferguson (1983), found improved symptoms and reduced bronchial reactivity in children whose bedrooms were changed to resemble a hospital room: no carpets, covered mattress, regular hot washing of all bed clothes, and removal of all sundries from the bedroom. Walshaw and Evans (1986) reported significant improvement with a regimen that was similarly aggressive in changing the patients' bedrooms. Mitchell and his colleagues (1989) used pirimiphos methyl to treat carpets as well as aggressive mite control in bedrooms. In that study the improvement in the treated patients was very striking. However, the placebo effect of treating carpets with the solvent was marked as well; in fact, mite allergen levels fell in the houses of the "control" patients. Over the whole group there was a significant correlation between reduction in mite allergen level and improvement in symptoms.

The objective of an avoidance study can be seen in several ways: to ask whether these measures should be part of normal treatment; to define which procedures are effective; and/or to define the quantitative change in allergen exposure necessary to produce a significant benefit. With most published studies it is not possible to define the change in allergen level that occurred. However, one study suggested that a reduction of 80% or to below 1μg *Der p* I/g of dust would be effective (Mitchell et al., 1989). In our earlier study on patients in hospital rooms, the mean level of allergen at home was 13.4 μg *Der p* I/g of house dust, while the hospital room had a mean level of ≤ 0.2 μg *Der p* I/g (Platts-Mills et al., 1982). This represents a reduction of 98%, which from current results would be very difficult to achieve in a house. However, it seems reasonable to propose that procedures should aim for a 90% reduction of exposure and that the levels achieved should be below 1 μg group I mite allergen/g of house dust.

A. Techniques for Allergen Avoidance

Mites

Bedrooms are the most important source of mite allergen exposure and the first site to focus on in avoidance. Patients spend long periods of time in their bedrooms and are usually willing to make changes to them; in addition, the appropriate measures are better defined. The mattress should be encased in plastic or some other nonpermeable material. Vacuum cleaning of mattresses will remove surface dust but makes no effect on the number of live mites, and is too laborious to be useful (Carswell et al., 1982). All bedding should be washed in hot water on a weekly basis. Cool washing does not kill mites and cool wash detergents do not harm mites. The actual temperature required to kill mites is not well defined, but 135 °F or 60 °C has been recommended. Hot drying is less effective; it has been estimated that it would take 2 h of hot drying to kill mites. Pillows are very important to treat because of their proximity to the head; they can be treated either by regular hot washing of artificial fiber or by encasing them. Encasing pillows (as with mattresses) may cause problems because the plastic is uncomfortable or causes sweating. This can be handled either by using double pillow cases or a mattress pad, or by using better-quality encasings. Mattress pads must also be washed in hot water. Water beds pose a special problem if they have padding incorporated into the bed that cannot be washed. Again, encasing the whole water bed may be the best answer. Removal of books, toys, and anything that allows accumulation of dust is obvious. Soft toys must be washable; stuffed animals suitable for hot washing have recently been introduced. Bedroom carpets are a problem because they can become heavily infested and also because they tend to reinfest the bedding. The only reliable procedure is to replace the carpet with a polished floor, either vinyl or wood.

In the remainder of the house there are multiple sites at which mite growth can occur; however, there are two major problems: carpets and upholstered furniture. The main determinants of mite growth are temperature and humidity (Voorhorst et al., 1969; Platts-Mills et al., 1986b; Arlian et al., 1982). This means that both growth patterns and control strategies are very different in different climatic areas or different forms of housing. In Denmark, Korsgaard (1983b) has shown that simply opening windows for 2 h per day will reduce absolute indoor humidity below the level of 8g/kg that is optimal for mite growth (see Fig. 6). This was because the major source of humidity in

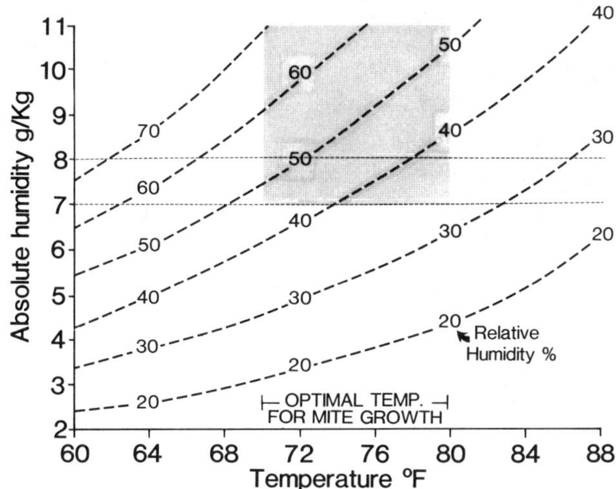

Figure 6 Optimal conditions for mite growth are a temperature between 70° and 80 °F and absolute humidity greater than 8 k/kg. The temperature that houses are maintained at with central heating, together with the effects of decreasing ventilation, have brought many houses close to these optimal conditions.

those houses was the inhabitants. In the north central area of the United States and Canada, houses can only maintain humidity if they are airtight. By contrast, in the southeast or the Gulf coast of the United States, mean outdoor absolute humidity is often as high as 13 g/kg in the summer (Platts-Mills et al., 1986b). Under those conditions humidity can only be controlled by air conditioning. The alternative way to reduce mite growth in humid summers is the traditional method of putting carpets into storage from May to October. It is possible to identify a series of changes in houses that have occurred over the last 40 years and that have probably increased dust mite growth in houses (Table 3). Carpets are a particular problem if they are laid on an unventilated floor (i.e., concrete slab in a basement). These carpets remain damp and it is not unusual to find >100 μg group I mite allergen/g (= >1000 mites/g dust) in dust obtained from them. Indeed, we consider that it would be wise to introduce building legislation that prohibits "permanent" fitting of carpets to unventillated floors.

Sofas and other upholstered furniture represent a "massive" nest for mites to flourish in. Indeed our results showed the highest levels of mite allergen in dust from sofas and the least seasonal variation (Fig. 7). The implication is that sofas, because of their depth of padding, take many months to

Table 3 Design Changes in Houses and Household Management that Have Improved the Environment for Dust Mites

Central heating: by maintaining temperatures over 65 °F in all rooms has increased mite growth in carpets, sofas, and beddings

Wall-to-wall carpets (in combination with vacuum cleaners) have established a permanent habitat for mites that cannot be cleaned without a chemical

Tight houses: many modern houses have very low air exchange (e.g., $\leqslant 0.3$ air changes per hour), which allows persistance of high indoor humidity.

Cool wash detergents have made it possible to wash sheets and bed covers at temperatures that do not kill mites

Source: Modified from *Parade* Magazine, Feb. 12th, 1989.

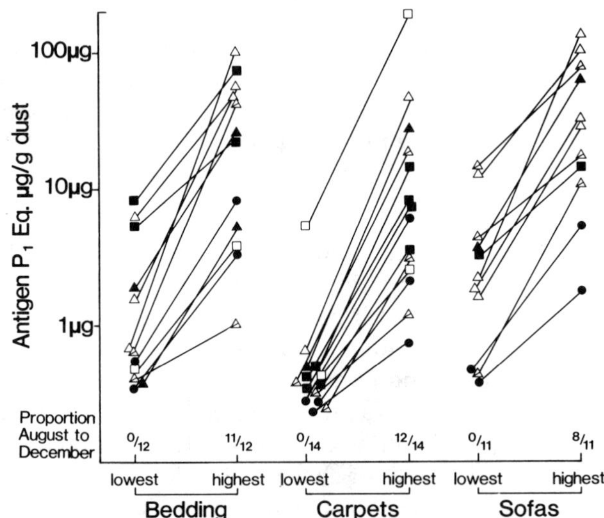

Figure 7 Seasonal variation in the quantity of group I mite allergen (here labeled as Antigen P_1 eq./g dust) in samples obtained monthly from 12 houses in Virginia. The maximum levels were generally (31 of 37 sites) seen between August and December, while the lowest levels never occurred at this time of year and were generally between February and May. At many sites the levels of allergen in dust changed by over 10-fold; however, in one carpet and one bed the level was less than $1\mu g/g$ all year, and in two sofas levels remained $> 10\mu g/g$ all year (reprinted from Platts-Mills et al., 1986b, by permission of *J. Allergy Clin. Immunol.*).

dry out and remain a good environment for mite growth. Prolonged release of mite fecal pellets from the upholstery could account for persistance of allergen. However, the evidence from studies using the acaricide pirimiphos methyl was that levels of allergen fell rapidly once mites were killed (Mitchell et al., 1985). Thus, it seems more likely that sofas represent a humid haven for persistent mite growth rather than a reservoir of mite allergen.

In the past few years there has been an upsurge of interest in chemical means of controlling mite growth or mite allergens (Table 4). Many chemicals were identified as acaricides in the early 1970s but a suitable chemical or application procedure was not developed for household use. The most promising acaricides are pirimiphos methyl and benzyl benzoate (Mitchell et al., 1985; Heller-Haupt and Busvine, 1974; Dietemann et al., 1989; Lau et al., 1989) while tannic acid has been shown to be a highly effective method of denaturing mite allergens (Green, 1984; Miller et al., 1989). The most effective way of using these chemicals has not yet been determined, but it seems increasingly likely that one chemical or another will become part of mite control. At present, it seems that the key sites for which acaricides would be helpful are carpets and sofas outside bedrooms.

In conclusion, several good studies indicate that aggressive mite avoidance measures can be helpful in the treatment of asthma. With increasing

Table 4 Low-Toxicity Chemicals Used in Controlling Mites and Mite Allergens

Chemical	Action	Other Uses
Pirimiphos methyl	Acaricide	Control of storage mites on grain in United States and elsewhere
Benzyl benzoate[a,b]	Acaricide	Scabies treatment
Natamycin	Antifungal (indirect effect on mites)	Food preservative (cheese, etc.)
Tannic acid[c]	Protein-denaturing agent	Traditional for tanning, treating burns, etc.
Liquid nitrogen[d]	Kills mites	Cryopreservative, etc.

[a]A complex mixture of 1% tannic acid and a derivative of benzyl benzoate is marketed in Australia as "benzyl tannate," combining acaricidal and antigen-denaturing effects.
[b]Benzyl Benzoate is marketed in Europe and the United States in the form of a moist powder.
[c]Tannic acid is currently marketed in the United States as a 3% solution.
[d]See Dorward et al., 1988.

understanding of mite biology, and better techniques for monitoring, these avoidance measures are continuing to improve. Using a combination of physical measures (i.e., encasement, washing, and carpet removal), humidity control, and chemicals, it now seems possible to design avoidance regimens that will consistently reduce mite exposure by 90%.

Cats and Airborne Cat Allergen

Removing cats from the house is a reliable but surprisingly slow method of reducing cat allergen. Levels generally fall progressively but may take 3 months or more to reach levels seen in houses without cats (Wood et al., 1989a). Using aggressive cleaning such as removing carpets, washing walls, and changing furniture, it is possible to clean a house quickly after removal of the cat. A partial measure is to keep cats outside or in restricted parts of the house. From recent results measuring cat allergen on clothing, it is clear that cat allergen is carried in large quantities around a house so that restricting the cat to one room can only be partially effective. There still remain approximately 2 million cat-allergic patients in the United States (1/3 of the cat-allergic individuals) who choose to live with a cat and are resistant, if not hostile, to any talk of removing the cat. As discussed in an earlier section, it is now clear that in most houses with a cat there is a large reservoir of cat allergen in carpets and soft furnishings (Ohman and Lorusso, 1987; Luczynska et al., 1989b; Wood et al., 1989a). Furthermore, since a significant proportion of cat allergen is airborne on small particles that tend to remain airborne, air filtration may have a role. Our own studies in houses found that airborne cat allergen levels correlated better with the quantity of soft furnishings than with the number of cats. Preliminary results suggested that airborne cat allergen can be reduced by a combination of air filtration and cleaning or removing furnishings. Air filters will only be effective if the air coming out of them does not disturb more allergen. However, a HEPA filter air cleaner placed on a steam-cleaned carpet or polished floor can reduce airborne cat allergen by 80 or 90%. Thus, there may be sensible advice that can be given to a cat-allergic patient who insists on living in a house with a cat.

The contrast between cat allergen and mite allergen is illustrated very well by this advice. Any form of water cleaning of carpets will in general produce an increase in mite growth. Similarly, there is little chance that air filtration will affect levels of airborne mite allergen, because the particles are only transiently airborne. Thus, the advice given to patients should reflect the source of allergen, the biological nature of the allergen, and the particle size on which it becomes airborne.

B. Control of Other Allergens

Although many different allergens may contribute to house dust, only limited information is available about most of them because simple techniques are not available for measuring them. For cockroach, it is obvious that killing roaches is a relevant objective, but it is not simple and there are no data available on the effectiveness of insecticides in reducing cockroach allergen levels. Although it is clear that many asthmatic patients are allergic to fungi that grow indoors, it is not clear what should be done. Obvious measures, such as washing surfaces with a chlorine bleach or removing articles that can become contaminated, should be recommended. In addition, basements are usually contaminated with fungi. Allergic patients should not work or live in basements because basements can grow both fungi and mites. The optimal conditions for growing mites are also excellent for growing fungi. On the other hand, fungi can grow over a much wider range of conditions. Thus fungi will flourish at much colder temperatures, while in humid and hot conditions fungi often overgrow mite cultures. Furthermore, fungi can grow on flat surfaces such as walls and shower curtains where mites cannot survive. It will be difficult to make further progress in understanding avoidance measures for fungi without simpler methods to monitor the measures taken.

V. Immunotherapy for Asthma

Immunotherapy (or desensitization) treatment was initially introduced for patients with hay fever, but it was rapidly extended to patients with other diseases associated with immediate hypersensitivity (Noon, 1911). Many of the early proponents and many allergists today consider that regular injections of allergen are very effective in the treatment of some patients with asthma. Indeed some authors considered that immunotherapy was more effective for asthma than for hay fever (Cooke, 1918; Rackemann and Lamsa, 1965). However, desensitization treatment for asthma remains controversial. There are several reasons why immunotherapy for perennial asthma should pose greater problems than the treatment of seasonal hay fever or seasonal asthma. In 1923 Spivacke and Grove described their experience with a difficult asthmatic patient who had repeated episodes of anaphylaxis following injections before tolerating the treatment and responding well to injections of house dust. Of course today it is impossible to define what was in the extract of house dust that they used, but the propensity of asthmatic patients to have anaphylactic reactions, including severe bronchospasm, is well recognized. Indeed, taking histories from venom-allergic patients suggests that lower airway obstruction is an uncommon feature of anaphylaxis unless the patient already has asthma. Severe anaphylaxis following injections of potent allergen extracts remains a major problem (Committee on Safety of Medicine, 1986; Lewis and Thompson, 1989; Lockey et al., 1987). There is little doubt that use of potent mite extracts in mite-allergic asthmatic patients has been overrepresented in the most severe reactions. One reason why immunotherapy for asthma is difficult may be the perennial nature of exposure. This problem was spelled out by Herxheimer and Prior in 1952, reporting a series of attempts to achieve desensitization by repeated inhalations of allergen. They reported that progressive desensitization could be achieved, but that if high-dose natural exposure occurred (to house dust) the patient would become "hypersensitized" again. This may well be the earliest description of allergen exposure causing increased nonspecific reactivity. The message, however, was that it is very difficult to desensitize a patient who is concurrently exposed to high doses of the relevant allergen. Thus, there are two separate problems: first, patients with perennial asthma are hyperreactive, and therefore, prone to have more severe reactions; and second, repeated natural exposure to the relevant allergen (most often dust mites) makes it more difficult to achieve effective desensitization. Indeed, there may be levels of natural exposure that are so high that they make it impossible to achieve desensitization.

A. Reported Studies on Immunotherapy for Asthma

Only a limited number of controlled studies on immunotherapy for asthma have been published. Although the results have generally been successful, that has certainly not been true in all cases (see Graft and Valentine, 1985). The first successful study using a defined extract was reported by Frankland and Augustin in 1954. The study used grass extract and reported successful reduction in asthma symptoms during the pollen season. Reid et al. (1986) likewise reported successful reduction of grass pollen-related asthma symptoms using grass extract in northern California. Several successful studies have been reported using house dust or mixtures for immunotherapy. Two studies were carried out with well-defined mite extract but with very different preparations of the allergen. The first used aqueous mite extract in a form that is known to give rise to 10-fold increases in IgG antibody (D'Souza et al., 1973; Platts-Mills and Chapman, 1987). In the second study the mite allergen had been denatured with gluteraldehyde and absorbed to tyrosine (Warner et al., 1978). This formulation produced a significant clinical improvement, with marked reduction in late reactions following bronchial provocation but little or no increase in serum IgG antibodies (Turner et al., 1984). Successful results have also been reported with immunotherapy for asthma caused by exposure to cats (Taylor et al., 1978; Van Metre et al., 1988). In each case improvement was judged by response to bronchial provocation rather than by symptoms.

Several studies have now reported that immunotherapy can reduce late reactions in the skin and bronchi. It was therefore logical to ask whether there would be a progressive fall in nonspecific BHR. However, the published data have not been encouraging since at least three studies have reported *increased* nonspecific BHR during immunotherapy (Murray et al., 1985; Formgren et al.,

1985; Rak et al., 1988). There are no controlled studies documenting *decreased* nonspecific bronchial reactivity following immunotherapy. Given the successful reported results, this may seem surprising. However, two factors may contribute: many studies use bronchial challenge to define the patient population, which may serve to increase reactivity; and most studies have not continued long enough. Clinical experience suggests that the patients who really do well on immunotherapy continue to improve over a period of several years.

B. Conclusions Regarding Immunotherapy

At present, it is very difficult to reach firm conclusions about the effectiveness or the role of allergen-specific immunotherapy for asthma. The efficacy studies leave little doubt that it can be beneficial in some cases, but in general are not sufficiently well controlled to define which patients benefit. Most of the good studies on the mechanism of response relate to seasonal rhinitis rather than asthma (Norman, 1980). It has not been established that clinical improvement in patients with asthma is related to changes in serum IgE or IgG antibody, T-cell responses, nonspecific reactivity, or any other defined parameter of the immune response.

There are several variables in making any decision about the therapeutic role of immunotherapy. Perhaps the two clearest are, first, the increasing use of inhaled anti-inflammatory medicines (e.g., local steroids or cromolyn) and, second, allergen exposure. Given the clear evidence that either avoidance measures or anti-inflammatory treatment can benefit patients with asthma, it is going to be increasingly difficult to carry out controlled studies of immunotherapy for asthma. Given the known propensity of asthmatic patients to react badly to allergen injections, it is essential that all such treatment should be supervised by a physician who is experienced with the use of immunotherapy. Finally, our own limited experience and the older literature suggest that allergen exposure is an important variable both in the response to immunotherapy and in the tendency to have systemic reactions. Thus, we would strongly recommend that aggressive avoidance measures in the home precede immunotherapy. The questions now is whether the combination of local steroids/or cromolyn and well-designed avoidance measures will leave a major role for immunotherapy in patients with asthma.

VI. Conclusions

Despite an apparently impressive list of new medicines available for the treatment of asthma, neither the morbidity nor the mortality of the disease have decreased. Thus, it is appropriate to readdress the causes of perennial asthma and to consider possible ways in which causative factors might have become worse. Since the original descriptions of an association between house dust sensitivity and asthma, a wealth of epidemiological evidence has shown that mite sensitivity is an important risk factor for asthma. This relates both to population studies and to case-control studies on patients with acute asthma or clinic patients. The conclusion is that mite allergy is not only a risk factor for asthma but also, in many areas of the world, appears to explain a major proportion of asthma in children and young adults. Other allergens contribute to asthma including cat, cockroach, grass pollen, and fungi, but the dust mite is dominant in many areas and it seems reasonable to ask whether some of the apparent increase in the disease could be explained by changes in houses.

Increasing understanding of mite biology combined with an ability to measure mite allergens has allowed much better analysis of what happens in houses. Fitted carpets, central heating, cool wash detergents, and decreased ventilation have all served to improve conditions for mite growth. Whether conditions have also improved for fungal growth or cockroach growth is not clear, although some high-efficiency houses or mobile homes become overtly moldy. Cats have not multiplied more freely, but the small particles on which cat allergen becomes airborne will increase in houses with poor air exchange. Studies on airborne allergens remain difficult because of the very small quantities involved and are not yet suitable for either routine monitoring of exposure or for defining standards. However, airborne studies have identified major differences in the form in which different allergens become airborne. Mite allergen is predominantly airborne on large particles, probably fecal, which are comparable in size to pollen grains and would only be inhaled in small numbers. By contrast, cat allergen is airborne in particles of many different sizes including a significant proportion of particles $<2.0\ \mu$m in diameter (i.e., comparable in size to the droplets produced by a nebulizer). Under some circumstances these small particles can reach levels in houses comparable to those that will produce bronchial provocation (i.e., very large numbers inhaled). Thus, it is possible that airborne mite fecal pellets represent an ideal form of exposure to produce focal inflammation in the lung and increased BHR *without* overt episodes of acute bronchospasm. Since cat allergen is airborne on large particles as well as small particles, it is possible that the small number of large particles contribute to BHR, while the large number of small particles gives rise to acute episodes of bronchospasm.

Several different studies have reported a level of mites or mite allergens in houses that is a risk factor for the development of IgE antibodies, bronchial reactivity, or symptomatic asthma. These studies have led to the proposal of standards for indoor mite allergen levels, based on floor, bedding, or furniture samples. It now seems clear that some level of mite, cat, cockroach, or other allergens in houses is indeed a risk factor for sensitization and also for the development of asthma. However, the real test of these risk levels would be to demonstrate that reducing exposure can consistently reduce the symptoms of asthma *or* the prevalence of sensitization. The goal of reducing exposure has often been dismissed as impossible. However, the knowledge of mite habitat and growth conditions has improved the approach to bedrooms and a variety of new chemical approaches to carpets and furniture suggest that mite allergen exposure can be reduced. Understanding cat exposure has likewise shown that airborne levels of cat allergen can be reduced as much as 10-fold even with a cat in the house. There is now a real possibility of designing studies on allergen avoidance at home that will be able to duplicate the effects that can be achieved in "climate chambers," high-altitude sanatoria, or allergen-free rooms.

That allergens contribute to asthma is not in doubt; what has been in doubt is how that knowledge contributes to treatment. Over the last 10 years several major developments have altered the equation. First, it appears likely that changes in the way we live have contributed both to mite growth and increased morbidity of asthma. Second, it has become possible to measure house dust and define specific levels that should be regarded as a risk factor for asthma. Finally, we are now in a position to design vigorous measures that can consistently reduce exposure by 10-fold or greater. Given the enormous, worldwide prevalence of asthma, it seems inevitable that controlling exposure to protein allergens in houses will become part of normal management and possibly a major public health concern.

Discussion

Tattersfield: If I understand you correctly, you are suggesting that asthma prevalence and severity may be correlated with allergen levels. However, to make this hypothesis, you should determine the relationship in varied areas rather than correlating the variables only among your own regional asthma patients.

Platts-Mills: Such correlations have been determined, and in separate studies have been shown to correlate closely with asthma prevalence and severity. In New Guinea, introduction of wool blankets, which became infested with mites, was associated with an increase in prevalence of asthma from 0.7% to 7%. High-altitude villages in the south of France have a low incidence of asthma in association with reduced number of dust mites. Emergency room visits for asthma in inland California are closely associated with the grass pollen season. The incidence of asthma in South Africa is directly associated with the prevalence of dust mites. Thus, these data support our hypothesis.

Sears: The data from Dunedin indicate that risk associated with house dust mite or cat sensitivity was seven or fivefold higher, respectively, than the remainder of the population. Thus, sensitivity to these antigens introduced a greatly increased risk of developing asthma.

Leff: What about immunotherapy and asthma?

Platts-Mills: There is no question that immunotherapy is effective for rhinitis. Current data also indicate effectiveness of cat and dog immunotherapy in asthmatic patients sensitive only to these antigens.

Pauwels: Are there studies comparing the degree of allergen exposure and the development of either rhinitis or asthma?

Platts-Mills: Overall, it appears that higher levels of IgE are found in asthmatic persons. However, apparently equally allergic individuals may develop either rhinitis, asthma, or eczema.

Pauwels: Is there a relationship between age, sensitization, and symptom development?

Platts-Mills: I believe that older patients are at less risk for the development of asthma and that they have lower IgE levels. In the case of adults, if they become exposed to potent antigens, such as mite allergens, they can develop new IgE responses and develop asthma.

Kerribijn: You suggested that central heating enhances the levels of mites in the home. However, central heating can lower the humidity, and that should reduce mite numbers.

Platts-Mills: You are correct, if the heating is associated with increased dryness. However, the usual case is warmer air in a moist house (such as in London), and increased mite exposure.

Fish: Would you care to speculate as to why some allergic individuals develop asthma and others rhinitis?

Platts-Mills: The simple answer is that we do not know. It is possible that factors such as the number of allergenic particles that enter the lung might be important. The rate at which allergic inflammation in the airways heals might also be important. However, the bottom line is that we do not know.

Hargreave: The risk factors you have defined for the development of asthma are the same as have been determined for the development of late asthmatic responses and increased airway hyperactivity.

Platts-Mills: That is an interesting point. It seems accurate that the patients with the highest levels of IgE are at increased risk of asthma as well as developing LPR.

O'Byrne: Do we actually know if patients with rhinitis have normal lungs on pathological examination?

Platts-Mills: We know that most patients with rhinitis have normal airway reactivity, but we do not know the microscopic appearance of their lungs.

Acknowledgment

This work was supported by N.I.H. grant no. A1-20565.

References

Altounyan, R. E. C. (1970). Changes in histamine and atropine responsiveness as a guide to diagnosis and evaluation of therapy in obstructive airways disease. In: *Disodium Chromoglycate in Allergic Airways Disease*. Edited by J. Pepys and A. W. Frankland. London, Butterworth, pp. 47-53.

Arlian, L. G., Bernstein, I. L., and Gallagher, J. S. (1982). The prevalence of house dust mites *Dermatophagoides* spp., and associated environmental conditions in homes in Ohio. *J. Allergy Clin. Immunol.* **69**:527-532.

Arruda, K., Baggio, D., Rizzo, M. C., Platts-Mills, T. A. E., Chapman, M. D., and Naspitz, C. K. (1989). Exposure of dust mite allergic asthmatic patients to mite allergens in Sao Paulo, Brazil. In preparation.

Blackley, C. H. (1959). *Experimental Research in the Causes and Nature of Catarrhus Aestivus (Hay Fever or Hay Asthma)*. London, Dawson Publishing Co. (reprinted from Bailliere Tindall & Cox, 1873), pp. 57-58.

Boulet, L.-P., Cartier, A., Thomson, N. C., and Hargreave, F. E. (1983). Asthma and increases in nonallergic bronchial responsiveness from seasonal pollen exposure. *J. Allergy Clin. Immunol.* **71**:399-406.

Burr, M. L., Dean, B. V., Merritt, T. S., Neale, E., St-Leger, A. S., and Verrier-Jones, E. R. (1980). The effects of anti-mite measures on children with mite sensitive asthma. A controlled trial. *Thorax* **35**:506.

Burrows, B., Martinez, F. D., Halonen, M., Barbee, R. A., and Cline, M. G. (1989). Association of asthma with serum IgE levels and skin test reactivity to allergens. *N. Eng. J. MEd.* **320**:271-276.

Carswell, F., Robinson, D. W., and Oliver, J. (1982). House dust mite in Bristol. *Clin. Allergy* **12**:533-545.

Cartier, A., Thomson, N. C., Frith, P. A., Roberts, M., and Hargreave, F. E. (1982). Allergen-induced increase in bronchial responsiveness to histamine: relationship to the late asthmatic response and change in airway caliber. *J. Allergy Clin. Immunol.* **70**:170-178.

Chapman, M. D., and Platts-Mills, T. A. E. (1980). Purification and characterization of the major allergen from *Dermatophagoides pteronyssinus*—antigen P_1. *J. Immunol.* **125**:587-592.

Chapman, M. D., Sutherland, W. M., and Platts-Mills, T. A. E. (1984). Recognition of two *Dermatophagoides pteronyssinus*-specific epitopes on antigen P_1 using monoclonal antibodies: binding to each epitope can be inhibited by sera from dust mite-allergic patients. *J. Immunol.* **133**: 2488-2495.

Chapman, M. D., Heymann, P. W., Wilkins, S. R., Brown, M. B., and Platts-Mills, T. A. E. (1987). Monoclonal immunoassays for the major dust mite (*Dermatophagoides*) allergens, *Der p* I and *Der f* I, and quantitative analysis of the allergen content of mite and house dust extracts. *J. Allergy Clin. Immunol.* **80**:184-194.

Chapman, M. D., Aalberse, R. C., Brown, M. J., and Platts-Mills, T. A. E. (1988). Monoclonal antibodies to the major feline allergen *Fel d* I. II. Single step affinity purification of *Fel d* I, N-terminal sequence analysis, and development of a sensitive two-site immunoassay to assess *Fel d* I exposure. *J. Immunol.* **140**:812-818.

Charpin, D., Kleisbauer, J. P., Lanteaume, A., Vervloet, D., and Charpin, J. (1988). Asthma and allergy to house dust mites in patients living in high altitude. *Chest* **93**:758-766.

Chua, J., Stewart, G. A., Thomas, W. R., Simpson, R. J., Dilworth, R. J., Plozza, T. M., and Turner, K. J. (1988). Sequence analysis of cDNA coding for a major house dust mite allergen, *Der p* I. *J. Exp. Med.* **167**: 175-182.

Chur, V., Falkenhorst, G., Heremannsdorfer, P., Lau, S., and Wahn, U. (1988). Studies on the influence of mite allergen exposure on sensitization and bronchial hyperreactivity of atopic children. *N. Eng. Reg. Allergy Proc.* **9**:295.

Cockcroft, D. W., Ruffin, R. E., Dolovitch, J., and Hargreave, F. E. (1977). Allergen induced increase in non-allergic bronchial reactivity. *Clin. Allergy* **7**:503-513.

Committee on Safety of Medicine (1986). Desensitizing vaccines. *Br. Med. J.* **293**:948.

Cooke, R. A. (1918). Hay fever and asthma: the uses and limitations of desensitization. *N.Y. State J. Med.* **107**:577.

De Groot, H., van Swieten, P., van Leeuwan, J., Lind, P., and Aalberse, R. C. (1988). Monoclonal antibodies to the major feline allergen *Fel d* I. I. Biologic activity of affinity-purified *Fel d* I and of *Fel d* I-depleted extracts. *J. Allergy Clin. Immunol.* **82**:778-786.

Dietemann, A., Hoyet, C., Bessot, J. C., de Blay, F., and Pauli, G. (1989). Effects of acaricide application on mite allergen levels and on symptoms of *Dermatophagoides pteronyssinus* (D.pt) allergic asthmatic patients. *J. Allergy Clin. Immunol.* (abstract) **83**:1:263.

Dorward, A. J., Colloff, M. J., MacKay, N. S., McSharry, C., and Thomson, N. C. (1988). Effect of house dust mite avoidance measures on adult atopic asthma. *Thorax* **43**:98-105.

Dowse, G. K., Turner, K. J., Stewart, G. A., Alpers, M. P., and Woolcock, A. J. (1985). The association between *Dermatophagoides* mites and the increasing prevalence of asthma in village communities within the Papua New Guinea Highlands. *J. Allergy Clin. Immunol.* **75**:75.

Esch, R. E., and Klapper, D. G. (1989). Identification and localization of allergenic determinants on grass group I antigens using monoclonal antibodies. *J. Immunol.* **142**:179-184.

Fain, A., Guerin, B., and Hart, B. J. (1989). *Acariens et Allergies.* Varennes en Argonne, France, Allerbio.

Findlay, S., Stosky, E., Lietermann, K., Hemady, Z., and Ohman, J. (1983a). Airborne cat-associated allergens. *J. Allergy Clin. Immunol.* **71**:160.

Findlay, S., Stosky, E., Lietermann, K., Hemady, Z., and Ohman, J. L. (1983b). Allergens detected in association with airborne particles capable of penetrating into the peripheral lung. *Am. Rev. Respir. Dis.* **128**:1008-1012.

Ford, A. W., Rawle, F. C., Lind, P., Spieksma, F. Th. M., Lowenstein, H., and Platts-Mills, T. A. E. (1985). Standardization of *Dermatophagoides pteronyssinus*: assessment of potency and allergen content in ten coded extracts. *Int. Arch. Allergy Appl. Immunol.* **76**:58-67.

Formgren, H., Dreborg, S., Kober, A., Lanner, A., and Olofson, E. (1985). A controlled trial of immunotherapy with Pharmalgen, *D farinae* mite extract. *Ann. Allergy* **55**(2):312.

Frankland, A. W., and Augustin, R. (1954). Prophylaxis of summer hay fever and asthma: controlled trial comparing crude grass pollen extracts with isolated main component. *Lancet* **1**:1055.

Graft, D. F., and Valentine, M. D. (1985). Immunotherapy. In *Allergy*. Edited by A. Kaplan. New York, Churchill Livingstone, pp. 679-692.

Green, W. F. (1984). Abolition of allergens by tannic acid. *Lancet* **2**:160.

Green, W. R., Woolcock, A. J., Stuckey, M., Sedgwick, C., and Leeder, S. R. (1986). House dust mites and skin tests in different Australian localities. *Aust. N.Z. J. Med.* **16**:639.

Heller-Haupt, A., and Busvine, J. R. (1974). Tests of acaricides against house dust mites. *J. Med. Entomol.* **2**:551-558.

Herxheimer, H., and Prior, F. N. (1952). Further observations on induced asthma and bronchial hyposensitization. *Int. Arch. Allergy* **3**:189.

Heymann, P. W., Chapman, M. D., Aalberse, R. C., Fox, J. W., and Platts-Mills, T. A. E. (1989). Antigenic and structural analysis of Group II allergens (*Derf* II and *Derp* II) from house dust mites (Dermatophagoides spp). *J. Allergy Clin. Immunol.* **83**:1055-1067.

Horn, N., and Lind, P. (1987). Selection and characterization of monoclonal antibodies against a major allergen in *D. Pteronyssinus*: species-specific and common epitopes in three *Dermatophagoides* species. *Int. Arch. Allergy Appl. Immunol.* **83**:404-409.

Ishizaka, K., Ishizaka, T., and Hornbrook, M. M. (1967). Allergen binding activity of nE, yG and yA, antibodies in sera from atopic patients. *in vitro* measurements of reaginic antibody. *J. Immunol.* **98**:490.

Kern, R. A. (1921). Dust sensitization in bronchial asthma. *Med. Clin. North Am.* **5**:751.

Kerrebijn, K. F. (1970). Endogenous factors in childhood CNSLD: methodological aspects in population studies. In *Bronchitis III*. Edited by N. G. M. Orie and R., van der Lende. Assen, The Netherlands, Royal Vangorcum, pp. 38-48.

Korsgaard, J. (1982). Preventative measures in house dust allergy. *Am. Rev. Respir. Dis.* **125**:80.

Korsgaard, J. (1983a). Mite asthma and residency: a case control study on the impact of exposure to house-dust mites in dwellings. *Am. Rev. Respir. Dis.* **128**:231-235.

Korsgaard, J. (1983b). House dust mites and absolute indoor humidity. *Allergy* **38**:85-92.

Lau, S., Rusche, A., Weber, A., Bischoff, E., and Wahn, U. (1989). Short term efficacy of benzylbenzoate on mite allergen concentrations in house dust. *J. Allergy Clin. Immunol.* (abstract) **83**:1:263.

Leiterman, K., and Ohman, J. L. (1984). Cat allergen 1: biochemical, antigenic and allergenic properties. *J. Allergy Clin. Immunol.* **74**:147-153.

Lewis, M. A., and Thompson, R. A. (Chairman) (1989). Current status of allergen immunotherapy. Report of a WHO International Union of Immunological Societies Working Group Report. *Lancet* **1**:259-261.

Lockey, R. F., Benedict, L. M., Turkeltaub, P. C., and Bukantz, S. C. (1987). Fatalities from immunotherapy (IT) and skin testing (ST). *J. Allergy Clin. Immunol.* **79**:660-677.

Luczynska, C. M., Arruda, L. K., Platts-Mills, T. A. E., Miller, J. D., Lopez, M., and Chapman, M. D. (1989). A two-site monoclonal antibody ELISA for the quantitation of the major *Dermatophagoides* spp. allergens, *Der p* I and *Der f* I. *J. Immunol. Methods* **118**:227-235.

Luczynska, C. M., Li, Y., Chapman, M. D., and Platts-Mills, T. A. E. (1990a). Airborne concentrations and particle size distribution of allergen derived from domestic cats (*Felis domesticus*): measurements using cascade impactor, liquid impinger and a two site monoclonal antibody assay for *Fel d* I. *Am. Rev. Respir. Dis.* **141**:361-367.

Luczynska, C. M., Chapman, M. D., and Platts-Mills, T. A. E. (1990b). Airborne levels and particle size distribution of cat allergen (*Fel d* I) following use of vacuum cleaners and room air cleaners. In preparation.

Marsh, D. G. (1975). Allergens and the genetics of allergy. In *The Antigens*, vol. III. Edited by M. Sela. New York, Academic Press, pp. 271-360.

Marsh, D. G. (1986). Defining human immune response finger prints toward ultrapure allergens. In *Proceedings of the XII International Congress of Allergology and Clinical Immunology*. St. Louis, C. V. Mosby, pp. 2426-2480.

Miller, J. D., Miller, A., Luczynska, C., Rose, G., and Platts-Mills, T. A. E. (1989). Effect of tannic acid spray on dust mite antigen levels in carpets. *J. Allergy Clin. Immunol.* (abstract) **83**:(1):262.

Mitchell, E. B., Wilkins, S. R., Deighton, J. M., and Platts-Mills, T. A. E. (1985). Reduction of house dust allergen levels in the home: use of acaricide pirimphos-methyl. *Clin. Allergy* **15**:235-240.

Mitchell, E. B., *et al.* (1989). Controlled trial of mite avoidance in the management of asthma: use of the acaricide pirimiphos methyl. In preparation.

Murray, A. B., and Ferguson, A. C. (1983). Dust-free bedrooms in the treatment of asthmatic children with house dust mite allergy: a controlled trial. *Pediatrics* **71**:418.

Murray, A. B., Ferguson, A. C., and Morrison, B. J. (1985). Nonallergic bronchial reactivity in asthmatic children decreases with age and increases with mite immunotherapy. *Ann Allergy* **54**:541-544.

Noon, L. (1911). Prophylactic innoculation for hay fever. *Lancet* **1**:1572.

Norman, P. S. (1980). An overview of immunotherapy: implications for the future. *J. Allergy Clin. Immunol.* **65**:87.

O'Hallaren, M. T., Sachs, M. I., Yunginger, J. W., O'Connell, E. J., and Wynn, S. R. (1986). Alternaria sensitivity as a possible risk factor for respiratory arrest in children with asthma. *J. Allergy Clin. Immunol.* **77**:199 (abs).

O'Hallaren, M. T., Sachs, M. I., O'Connell, E. J., and Yunginger, J. (1988). Allergen exposure as a possible precipitating factor for respiratory arrest in young adults with asthma. *J. Allergy Clin. Immunol.* **81**:246 (abs).

Ohman, J. L., and Lorusso, J. R. (1987). Cat allergen content of commercial house dust extracts: comparison with dust extracts from cat-containing environment. *J. Allergy Clin. Immunol.* **79**:955-959.

Peat, J. K., Salome, C. M., Sedgwick, C. J., Kerrebijn, J., and Woolcock, A. J. (1989). A prospecitve study of bronchial hyperresponsiveness and respiratory symptoms in a population of Australian schoolchildren. *Clin. Exp. Allergy* **19**:299-306.

Platts-Mills, T. A. E. (1979). Local production of IgG, IgA, and IgE antibodies in grass pollen hay fever. *J. Immunol.* **122**:2218-2225.

Platts-Mills, T. A. E. (1982). Type I or immediate hypersensitivity. In *Clinical Aspects of Immunology,* 4th ed. Edited by P. J. Lachmann and D. K. Peters. Oxford, Blackford, pp. 579-686.

Platts-Mills, T. A. E., and Chapman, M. D. (1987). Dust mites: immunology, allergic disease, and environmental control. *J. Allergy Clin. Immunol.* **80**:755-775.

Platts-Mills, T. A. E., and de Weck, A. L. (1988). Dust mite allergens and asthma—a world wide problem. Report of an International Workshop, Bad Kreuznach, F. R. G., September 1987. *Bull WHO*, 66:(6), and *J. Allergy Clin. Immunol.* **83**:416-427.

Platts-Mills, T. A. E., Tovey, E. R., Mitchell, E. B., Moszoro, H., Nock, P., and Wilkins, S. R. (1982). Reduction of bronchial hyperreactivity during prolonged allergen avoidance. *Lancet* **2**:675.

Platts-Mills, T. A. E., Heymann, P. W., Longbottom, J. L., and Wilkins, S. R. (1986a). Airborne allergens associated with asthma: particle sizes carrying dust mite and rat allergens measured with a cascade impactor. *J. Allergy Clin. Immunol.* **77**:850-857.

Platts-Mills, T. A. E., Hayden, M. L., Chapman, M. D., and Wilkins, S. R. (1986b). Seasonal variation in dust mite and grass pollen allergens in dust from the houses of patients with asthma. *J. Allergy Clin. Immunol.* **79**:781-791.

Platts-Mills, T. A. E., Heymann, P. W., Chapman, M. D., Hayden, M. L., and Wilkins, S. R. (1986c). Cross-reacting and species-specific determinants on a major allergen from *Dermatophagoides pteronyssinus* and *D. farinae*: development of a radioimmunoassay for antigen P_1 equivalent in house dust and dust mite extracts. *J. Allergy Clin. Immunol.* **78**:398-407.

Platts-Mills, T. A. E., Chapman, M. D., Heymann, P. W., and Luczynska, C. M. (1989). Measurements of airborne allergen using immunoassays. In *Immunology and Allergy Clinics of North America*. Edited by W. Solomon. Philadelphia, W. B. Saunders, 9:2.

Pollart, S. M., Reid, M., Brown, M., Kwasnicki, M., Fling, J., Chapman, M. D., and Platts-Mills, T. A. E. (1988). Epidemiology of emergency room asthma in northern California: association with IgE antibody to rye grass pollen. *J. Allergy Clin. Immunol.* **82**:224.

Pollart, S. M., Chapman, M. D., Fiocco, G. P., Rose, G., and Platts-Mills, T. A. E. (1989a). Epidemiology of acute asthma: IgE antibodies to common inhalant allergens as a risk factor for emergency room visits. *J. Allergy Clin. Immunol.* **83**:875-880.

Pollart, S. M., Platts-Mills, T. A. E., and Chapman, M. D. (1989b). Identification, quantitation and purification of cockroach (CR) allergens using monoclonal antibodies (mAb). *J. Allergy Clin. Immunol.* (abs.) **83**:293.

Rackemann, F. M., and Lamsa, T. (1965). The natural history of ragweed hay fever. *J. Allergy Clin. Immunol.* **36**:258.

Rak, S., Lowhagen, O., and Venge, P. (1988). The effect of immunotherapy on bronchial hyperresponsiveness and eosinophil cationic protein in pollen allergic patients. *J. Allergy Clin. Immunol.* **82**:470-480.

Rawle, F. C., Mitchell, E. B., and Platts-Mills, T. A. E. (1984). T. cell responses to the major allergen from the house dust mite *Dermatophagoides pteronyssinus* antigen P_1: comparison of patients with asthma, atopic dermatitis, and perennial rhinitis. *J. Immunol.* **133**:195-201.

Reid, M. J., Moss, R. B., Hsu, Y. P., Kwasnicki, J. M., Commerford, T. M., and Nelson, B. L. (1986). Seasonal asthma in northern California: allergic causes and efficacy of immunotherapy. *J. Allergy Clin. Immunol.* **78**: 590.

Rowntree, S., Cogswell, J. J., Platts-Mills, T. A. E., and Mitchell, E. B. (1985). The development of IgE and IgG antibodies to food and inhalant allergens in children at risk of allergic disease. *Arch Dis. Child.* **60**:727-735.

Sarsfield, J. K., Gowland, G., Toy, R., and Normal, A. L. (1974). Mite-sensitive asthma of childhood: trial of avoidance measures. *Arch. Dis. Child.* **49**:711-716.

Sears, M. R., Herbison, G. P., Holdaway, M. D., Hewitt, C. J., Flannery, E. M., and Silva, P. A. (1989). The relative risks of sensitivity to grass pollen, house-dust mite, and cat dander in the development of childhood asthma. *Clin. Exp. Allergy* **19**:419-424.

Smith, J. M., Disney, M. E., Williams, J. P., and Goels, Z. A. (1969). Clinical significance of skin reactions to mite extracts in children with asthma. *Br. Med. J.* **2**:723-726.

Smith, T. F., Kelly, L. B., Heymann, P. W., Wilkins, S. R., and Platts-Mills, T. A. E. (1985). Natural exposure and serum antibodies to house dust mite of mite-allergic children with asthma in Atlanta. *J. Allergy Clin. Immunol.* **76**:782-788.

Solomon, W. R., and Mathews, K. P. (1978). Aerobiology and inhalant allergens. In *Allergy: Principles and Practice.* Edited by E. Middleton, C. E. Reed, and E. F. Ellis. St. Louis, C. V. Mosby, pp. 899-956.

D'Souza, M. F., Pepys, J., Wells, I. D., Tai, E., Palmer, F., Overell, B. G., McGrath, I. T., and Megson, M. (1973). Hyposensitization with *Dermatophagoides pteronyssinus* in house dust allergy. A controlled study of clinical and immunological effects. *Clin. Allergy* **3**:177.

Spivacke, C. A., and Grove, E. F. (1925). Studies in hypersensitiveness XIV: a study of the atopen in house dust. *J. Immunol.* **10**:465.

Sporik, R., Holgate, S., Platts-Mills, T. A. E., Cogswell, J. (1989). Prospective study of the development of IgE antibodies and asthma in 70 children in Poole, Dorset, from birth to age 12. In preparation.

Storm van Leeuwen, W. (1927). Asthma and tuberculosis in relation to "climate allergens." *Br. Med. J.* **2**:344-347.

Svartengren, M., Falk, R., Linnman, L., Philipson, K., and Camner, P. (1987). Deposition of large particles in human lung. *Exp. Lung Res.* **12**:75-88.

Swanson, M. C., Agarwal, M. K., and Reed, C. E. (1985). An immunochemical approach to indoor aeroallergen quantitation with a new volumetric air sampler: studies with mite, roach, cat, mouse, and guinea pig antigens. *J. Allergy Clin. Immunol.* **76**:724-729.

Swanson, M. C., Campbell, A. R., Klauck, P. C., and Reed, C. E. (1989). Correlations between levels of mite and cat allergens in settled and airborne dust. *J. Allergy Clin. Immunol.* **83**:776-783.

Task Group on Lung Dynamics (1966). Deposition and retention models for internal dosimetry of the human respiratory tract. *Health Phys.* **12**: 173-207.

Taylor, W. W., Ohman, J. L., and Lowell, F. C. (1978). Immunotherapy in cat-induced asthma. Double blind trial with evaluation of bronchial response to cat allergen and histamine. *J. Allergy Clin. Immunol.* **61**: 283-287.

Tovey, E. R., Chapman, M. D., Wells, C. W., and Platts-Mills, T. A. E. (1981a). The distribution of dust mite allergen in the houses of patients with asthma. *Am. Rev. Respir. Dis.* **124**:630-635.

Tovey, E. R., Chapman, M. D., and Platts-Mills, T. A. E. (1981b). Mite faeces are a major source of house dust allergens. *Nature* **289**:592-593.

Turner, M. W., Yalcin, L., Soothill, J. F., Price, J. F., Warner, J. O., Hey, E. N., Chapman, M. D., and Platts-Mills, T. A. E. (1984). In vitro investigations in asthmatic children undergoing hyposensitization with tyrosine-absorbed *Dermatophagoides pteronyssinus* antigen. *Clin. Allergy* **14**:221-231.

Van Bronswijk, J. E. M. H., Bischoff, E., Schirmacher, W., and Kniest, F. M. (1989). Evaluating mite (*Acari*) allergenicity of house dust by guanine quantification. *J. Med. Entomol.* **26**:55-59.

Van Metre, T. E., Marsh, D. G., Adkinson, N. F., Fish, J. E., Kagey-Sobotka, A., Norman, P. S., Radden, E. B., and Rosenberg, G. K. (1986). Dose of cat (*Felis domesticus*) allergen 1 (*Fel d* I) that induces asthma. *J. Allergy Clin. Immunol.* **78**:62-75.

Van Metre, T. E., March, D. G., and Adkinson, N. F. (1988). Immunotherapy for cat asthma. *J. Allergy Clin. Immunol.* **82**:1055-1068.

Vervloet, D., Penaud, A., Razzouk, H., Arnaud, A., Boutin, C., and Charpin, J. (1982). Altitude and dust mites. *J. Allergy Clin. Immunol.* **69**: 290-296.

Voorhorst, R., Spieksma, F. Th. M., Varenkamp, H., Leupen, M. J., and Lyklema, A. W. (1967). The house dust mite (*Dermatophagoides pteronyssinus*) and the allergens it produces: identify with the house dust allergen. *J. Allergy* **39**:325.

Voorhorst, R., Spieksma, F. Th. M., and Varenkamp. N. (1969). *House Dust Atopy and the House Dust Mite Dermatophagoides pteronyssinus* (Troussart, 1897). Leiden, Stafleu's Scienfic Pub. Co.

Walshaw, M. J., and Evans, C. C. (1986). Allergen avoidance in house dust mite-sensitive adult asthma. *Q. J. Med.* **58**:199-215.

Ward, G. W., Karlsson, G., Rose, G., and Platts-Mills, T. A. E. (1989). Trichophyton asthma: specific sensitization of the bronchi and upper airways to a dermatophyte antigen. *Lancet* **1**:259-262.

Warner, J. O., Price, J. F., Soothill, J. F., and Hey, E. N. (1978). Controlled trial of hyposensitization to *Dermatophagoides pteronyssinus* in children with asthma. *Lancet* **2**:912-915.

Wood, R. A., Chapman, M. D., Adkinson, N. F., and Eggleston, P. A. (1989a). The effect of cat removal on *Fel d* I content in household dust samples. *J. Allergy Clin. Immunol.* **83**:730-734.

Wood, R. A., Eggleston, P. A., Mudd, K. E., and Adkinson, N. F. (1989b). Indoor allergen levels as a risk factor for allergic sensitization. *J. Allergy Clin. Immunol.* (abstract) **83**(1):199.

Yasueda, H., Mita, H., Yui, Y., and Shida, T. (1989). Comparative analysis of physiochemical properties of the two major allergens from *Dermatophagoides pteronyssinus* and *D. farinae*. *Int. Arch. Allergy Appl. Immunol.* **62**:000.

23

Clinical Responses to Corticosteroids

ANN J. WOOLCOCK and CHRISTINE R. JENKINS

Royal Prince Alfred Hospital
Sydney, New South Wales, Australia

Corticosteroids (CS) have been used in the treatment of asthma for the last 40 years. This chapter discusses the properties of the commonly used CS and what has been learned from their clinical and experimental use. The actions of systemic and inhaled forms are discussed in relation to their effects on acute attacks, their use in long-term management, and their effects on experimental bronchoconstriction. Some of the important unanswered questions are listed and the conclusions about the nature of asthma that can be drawn from the known effects of CS are summarized.

Asthma is a disease of the airways that causes them to narrow too easily and too much in response to a wide variety of provoking stimuli that have no effect in normal people. The disease is characterized by a specific form of asthmatic inflammation that has been described in previous chapters. In discussing treatment with CS, the disease "asthma" is differentiated from episodes of airway narrowing or "attacks of airway narrowing" that may be either acute or subacute. In this chapter, the term systemic CS refers to both oral and intravenous forms.

I. Early Use of Corticosteroids in the Treatment of Asthma

It is now 40 years since CS were first shown to be effective in the management of asthma (Carryer et al., 1950; Randolph and Rollins, 1950). In the 1950s both intravenous hydrocortisone (Burrage and Irwin, 1955) and oral prednisone (Barach et al., 1955) were shown to reduce symptoms in patients with chronic asthma. However, it soon became clear that, although these drugs were very effective in controlling the symptoms caused by airway narrowing, prolonged use resulted in an unacceptable level of side effects. This led to the synthesis of methylprednisolone, cortisone, dexamethasone, and triamcinolone, but none appeared to have an advantage over prednisolone. In the early 1970s, inhaled forms with a high topical to systemic ratio became widely available. These drugs have been shown to be effective in reducing the severity of symptoms, in improving lung function, and in allowing reduction in the dosages of oral CS. Nonetheless, in some countries controversy still surrounds the use of inhaled CS as an alternative to oral drugs in children with moderately severe asthma (Wyatt et al., 1978; Vaz et al., 1982).

II. Pharmacology of Commonly Used Corticosteroids

Table 1 shows the relative anti-inflammatory and glucocorticoid actions of eight commonly used corticosteroids (Michealides, 1981; Haynes and Murad, 1985, 1986; Johansson et al., 1982; Schleimer et al., 1981). Their anti-inflammatory action is expressed relative to hydrocortisone and based on a skin vasoconstriction model (Place, 1970). Mineralocorticoid action is expressed as sodium-retaining potency. The plasma half-life and the duration of hypothalamic-pituitary-adrenal (HPA) axis suppression are shown. The relative potency for the inhibition of histamine release from basophils has been studied (Schleimer et al., 1981) for some of the drugs and appears to be best for dexamethasone.

Neither beclomethasone nor budesonide is inactivated in the lung, and both drugs reach the circulation after inhalation by crossing airway mucosal surfaces (Brattsand et al., 1987; Johansson et al., 1982). They are rapidly absorbed and have systemic effects when given in high dosages (Smith and Hodson, 1983; Toogood et al., 1988). The swallowed portion of inhaled CS is metabolized in the first bypass of the liver and does not have measurable systemic activity (Brattsand et al., 1987). The plasma concentrations of systemic CS required to affect the function of airway epithelial cells are unknown. However, prednisolone is poorly excreted into the alveoli compared to methylprednisolone (Braude and Rebuck, 1983).

Table 1 Relative Topical and Systemic Potency of Some Commonly Used Corticosteroids

Drug	Anti-inflammatory Potency[a]	Equivalent Dose (mg)	Na-Retaining Potency	Approx. Plasma T1/2 (min)	Duration of HPA Suppression (days)
Hydrocortisone	1.0	20	+ +	90	1.25-1.5
Prednisone	4.0	5	+	60	1.25-1.5
Prednisolone	4.0	5	+	200	1.25-1.5
Methylprednisolone	5.0	4	0	180	1.25-1.5
Dexamethasone	20-30	0.75	0	200	2.75
Triamcinolone acetonide	5.0	4	0	>300	2.25
Betamethasone	20-30	0.6	0	7300	3.25
Bidomethasone diproprionate	300	1.0	0	-	-
Budesonide	600	1.0	0	168	-

[a]All drugs are considered relative to hydrocortisone.

Topically active CS were first studied in vivo in a skin vasoconstriction model (Place, 1970), which has since become widely used to assess the anti-inflammatory potency of CS. There is a good correlation between the ability of a drug to induce vasoconstriction in normal human skin and the ability to produce improvement in inflammatory skin disorders. Although the anti-inflammatory potency of budesonide and beclomethasone has been extensively studied in the rat and guinea pig (Kallstrom et al., 1987; Brattsand et al., 1987), neither model closely mimics human asthma, and it has been difficult to differentiate between local and systemic effects of inhaled CS in these studies. At present, therefore, there is no totally satisfactory model to demonstrate topical CS potency in the human airway.

The systemic effects of topical CS can be assessed by their effect on plasma cortisol in humans or by thymus involution in animals. Harris (1975) found beclomethasone diproprionate to be about 500 times more topically potent than dexamethasone but, when given intravenously, equipotent in causing adrenal suppression. Budesonide, a nonhalogenated glucocorticosteroid with a high topical to systemic ratio, has been shown to be slightly more potent than beclomethasone in the skin vasoconstriction model and to have less systemic potency (Johansson et al., 1982). However, most clinical studies that have compared the drugs suggest that they have equal efficacy, although budesonide may produce marginally less adrenal suppression (Field et al., 1982; Ebden et al., 1986). Both triamcinolone and flunisolide are used as aerosols in the treatment of asthma but, in the limited number of comparative studies performed, superior clinical eficacy has not been demonstrated (Bernstein et al., 1982; Shapiro et al., 1981).

III. Clinical Effects of Systemic Corticosteroids

A. Acute Attacks

Are Systemic CS Needed in the Treatment of Acute Exacerbations of Asthma?

Studies in hospital emergency departments have provided evidence for the efficacy of CS in patients with acute attacks (Fanta et al., 1982; Fiel et al., 1983; Littenburg et al., 1986; Storr et al., 1982, 1987; Pierson et al., 1974; Harris et al., 1987). These studies, summarized in Table 2, show that CS terminate exacerbations more rapidly than adequate bronchodilator therapy alone. There are, however, no precise guidelines for the type, dosage, and route of administration. While some studies suggest that the addition of CS to bronchodilator therapy in the management of acute attacks of asthma does not affect outcome (McFadden et al., 1976; Kattan et al., 1980), these studies were limited by either small patient numbers, short assessment periods, or subjective measurement of response.

Which CS for the Management of Acute Attacks?

In a comparison of intravenous hydrocortisone, methylprednisolone, and dexamethasone in steroid-dependent patients, no significant differences in improvement in forced expiratory volume in 1 s (FEV1) during acute exacerbations were evident at 24 h (Sue et al., 1986). The authors concluded, on the basis of cost, longer dose intervals, and reduced sodium-retaining capacity, that methylprednisolone is the treatment of choice for acute exacerbations of asthma. A comparative study of betamethasone, hydrocortisone, and dexamethasone in children showed equal efficacy when resolution of airway obstruction and improvement in arterial hypoxaemia were assessed (Pierson et al., 1974).

What Dosage and What Route of CS Administration?

Table 3 summarizes some of the studies that have investigated the dosages of CS in the management of acute attacks. Daily dosages higher than the equivalent of 80 mg of methylprednisolone seem to have little added advantage in reducing the reversal time. In spite of this evidence, higher dosages are commonly used, probably because physicians hope to achieve an optimal concentration in the airways and high dosages appear to have few side effects in the short term.

B. Treatment of Asthma

What is the Place for Oral CS in the Maintenance Treatment of Patients with Asthma?

Before the introduction of inhaled CS, oral forms were widely used in patients with severe asthma. No guidelines for dosage and forms were available and the dosages used were apparently based on symptoms or lung function measurements. Apart from a study by Tiffeneau and Dunoyer (1956) using hydrocortisone, the effect of steroids on the severity of asthma, as reflected by measurements of bronchial hyperreactivity (BHR), was not tested until 1979 (Wolfe et al., 1979). No effect was found in either study. Since then, oral CS have been shown to produce improvement in BHR only when they are used in high dosages.

Studies that have examined the effect of systemic forms of CS on BHR are shown in Table 4. Two studies (Wolfe et al., 1979; Mattoli et al., 1985), one in which prednisone 40 mg was given daily for 5 days and the other in

Table 2 Controlled Trials of CS Management of Acute Exacerbations of Asthma

Reference	No. Subjects	Description of Subjects	Drug	Dosage	Route	Observation Period	Placebo	Outcome
Kattan et al., 1980	19	Inadequate response to bronchodilator	HCq6h	7 mg/kg	IVI	36 h	NO: control group	No significant benefit on CS
McFadden et al., 1976	38	Mean FEV_1 27% predicted	HC	0.25, 0.5, or 1.0 g stat	IVI	6 h	YES	No statistical differences in outcome
Littenberg and Gluck, 1986	97	Mean FEV_1 40% predicted	MFP	125 mg	IVI	Mean 4 h	YES	↑ FEV_1, symptoms↓ sig ↓ hospital admissions
Fanta et al., 1982	20	Mean FEV_1 25% predicted	HC	2 mg/kg bolus then 0.5 mg/kg/h	IVI	24 h	YES	Sig ↑ FEV_1 ↑ recovery rate

Fiel et al., 1983	76	Mean PEFR 160 L/min	MP	4 mg/kg then 64 mg/day	IV bolus oral	7-10 days	YES	Sig ↓ symptoms, ↓ relapse rate
Storr et al., 1987	140	Children	PRED	30 mg or 60 mg[a]	oral single dose	36 h	YES	↓ Relapse rate ↓ length of stay
Harris et al., 1987	41	Children with severe obstruction	PRED	60 mg or 80 mg/day for 1 week	oral	14 days	YES	↑ Response rate, ↑ PEF
Pierson et al., 1974	45	Mean FEV_1 30% predicted, children	HC, DXM, or BM	See reference	IVI	24 h	YES	↓ Arterial hypoxaemia on CS

HC, hydrocortisone; MP, methylprednisolone; PRED, prednisolone; DXM, dexamethasone; BM, betamethasone; IVI, intravenous infusion.
[a]Dosage based on weight.

Table 3 Comparisons of Dosage in Studies of CS in Management of Acute Exacerbations of Asthma

Reference	No. Subjects	Description of Subjects	Drug	Duration	Dosage (Daily)	Route	Observation Period	Outcome
McFadden et al., 1976	38	Mean FEV$_1$ 27% predicted	HC	1 dose	0.25g, 0.5g, 1.0g	IV single dose only	6 h	No significant differences
Britton et al., 1976	26	Mean FEV$_1$ <0.5L	HC	8-10 days	36, 61, 175 mg/kg	IVI	8-10 days	No significant differences
Raimondi et al., 1986	40	Mean FEV$_1$ <0.6L	HC	5 days	20 mg/kg or 1.5mg/kg q6h	IVI	5 days	No significant differences
Tanaka et al., 1982	10	Mean FEV$_1$ ≤0.8L	MP	7 days	20mg or 125 mg q6h	IVI	10 days	No significant differences
Haskell et al., 1983	25	Mean FEV$_1$ 26% predicted	MP	3 days	15 mg, 40 mg q6h, 125 mg	IVI	72 h	FEV$_1$ improvement greater and quicker in high and moderate-dose group

HC, hydrocortisone; MP, methylprednisolone; IVI, intravenous infusion.

Table 4 Summary of Effects of Systemic Corticosteroids on Sensitivity to Histamine and Methacholine

Reference	Total No. Subjects	No. Improved >One doubling Concentration	Description	Drug	Dosage (Daily)	Duration	Mean Initial PC20 (mg/ml) or PD20 (μmol)	Mean FINAL PC20 (mg/ml) or PD20 (μmol)
Tiffeneau and Dunoyer, 1956	24	0	FEV_1 0.7-1.7L	HC	40-80mg	4-10 days	see reference	
Wolfe et al., 1979	5	0	Not stated	PRED	40 mg	5 days	10.2	8.34
Mattoli et al., 1985	12	0	Mean FEV_1 86% predicted	MP	1 mg/kg IVI	Single dose	0.41	0.38
	6	0		MP	32 mg	8 days	0.41	0.44
Bhagat and Grunstein, 1985	12	3	Mean FEV_1 84% predicted	MP	32 mg	Total dose	1.5	2.5[a]
		4		MP	128 mg	Total dose	1.5	2.8[a]
Israel et al., 1984	10	2	Children; mean FEV_1 84% predicted	PRED	60 mg	1 week	1.47	2.04
Wilmsmeier et al., 1986	12	Not stated	Not stated	PRED	15 mg	2 weeks	0.13	0.27
Jenkins and Woolcock, 1988	18	4	Mean FEV_1 56% predicted	PRED	12.5 mg	3 weeks	0.56	0.59

HC, hydrocortisone; MP, methylprednisolone; PRED, prednisone.
[a]Approximate PD20s from cumulative doses given.

which methylprednisolone was given for 8 days showed no change in BHR. High dosages of oral or intravenous corticosteroids can shift the dose-response curves to a small extent (Israel et al., 1984; Bhagat and Grunstein, 1985). These data, together with data that show that inhaled CS can lead to a marked improvement in BHR, suggest that there is probably no place for daily oral CS in the long-term treatment of newly diagnosed patients in whom the aim is to return airway function to normal. This is discussed further below.

What is the Best Regimen in Patients Who Need Oral CS to Stay Free from Acute Attacks?

Single morning doses of oral CS cause less adrenal suppression than more frequent dosing (Ackerman and Nolan, 1968), as does the use of steroids with a short serum half-life, such as prednisone. Alternate-day administration, used widely in the United States, reduces HPA axis suppression and does not compromise control in patients with stable symptoms, but it is unsatisfactory in many patients with "unstable" symptoms (Fauci, 1978; Toogood et al., 1984a; Toogood, 1987). Alternate-day therapy has been a mainstay of asthma management in children with severe disease in the United Stated, where debate continues over the relative merits of high-dosage inhaled CS and alternate day oral CS (Wyatt et al., 1978; Nassif et al., 1987). In adults in whom larger doses of inhaled CS can be given before important systemic effects are evident, there is little doubt that the inhaled forms are the treatment of choice. In a comparative crossover study, 800 or 1600 μg of budesonide was superior to 15, 30, and 60 mg of prednisone daily in improving lung function and symptoms (Toogood, 1987). There was no difference in the degree of adrenal supression as measured by morning cortisol levels. However, low-dose alternate day oral CS therapy may be indicated if compliance or proficiency with aerosol inhalation is poor (Toogood et al., 1984a).

Thus, overall, it appears that the only place for oral CS is in patients receiving low dosages who, for any reason including severe disease, cannot be transferred to treatment via the inhaled route.

C. Corticosteroid Resistance

A few asthmatic subjects appear not to benefit from CS treatment either symptomatically or with objective changes in lung function. In a clinical study (Carmichael et al., 1981), the CS-resistant patients were found to have a longer history of asthma, were older, had more nocturnal wheezing, and more dipping of morning PEF values. They also had more severe BHR, as measured by methacholine, than the CS-sensitive patients. In subsequent studies (Kay et al., 1981; Wyllie et al., 1986) it has been shown that monocytes from CS-resistant patients have reduced sensitivity to CS in vitro, particularly at low CS concentrations. It is unclear whether diminished CS responsiveness in monocytes is a function of previous CS treatment or whether intrinsic defects predate treatment. However, basophils from CS-treated patients are less sensitive to the inhibiting effects of dexamethasone on histamine release than those from untreated patients (Lampl et al., 1985). Several other explanations for apparent resistance to CS during acute attacks have been suggested, including reduced bioavailability of prednisone, accelerated plasma cortisol clearance, steroid resistance at the intracellular steroid receptor level, and physical factors such as inspissated secretions.

IV. Clinical Effects of Inhaled Corticosteroids

A. Treatment of Asthma (Decreasing Airway Inflammation)

Reduction of Oral CS Requirement

Early studies on beclomethasone dipropionate (BDP) were unanimous in confirming its effectiveness in reducing the dosage of oral CS required to control symptoms and maintain lung function (Cameron et al., 1973; British Thoracic and Tuberculosis Association, 1976; Brompton Hospital/MRC Collaborative trial, 1979). In these studies, in which daily dosages of 400 μg were used and subsequent studies, which demonstrated a dose-related effect (Costello and Clark, 1974; Toogood et al., 1977a,b), suggest that the rates of oral steroid withdrawal would have been higher had larger dosages been given. A recent study comparing daily dosages of 800 and 2000 μg BDP in oral CS-1 (OCS) dependent patients found that the higher dosage was significantly better in facilitating reduction of the oral CS dose while maintaining symptom control and lung function (Tarlo et al., 1988).

Predictors of Response to Inhaled CS.

Although higher IgE levels, better resting lung function, greater acute bronchodilator reversibility, and younger age have been shown to be associated with a beneficial response to beclomethasone (Vandenberg et al., 1975; Cooper and Grant, 1977), the most consistent predictor of oral CS reduction is the previous maintenance dosage. Patients on lower dosages were more likely to cease use of oral steroids altogether (Brompton Hospital/MRC Collaborative trial, 1979; Vandenberg et al., 1975; Gwynn and Smith, 1974).

Toogood et al. (1977a,b, 1982) demonstrated that increasing the dosage of inhaled CS can have beneficial effects, and they attempted to find an index to predict improvement. No suitable index was found, although there was less improvement in those known to have little acute reversibility in airway obstruction, although this did not preclude improvement in symptoms.

Effect of Dosage

The effectiveness of inhaled CS is related to the dosage in most patients with asthma (Johansson et al., 1982; Costello and Clark, 1974; Toogood et al., 1977a,b). One early study failed to find any benefit from beclomethasone 1600 μg compared to 400 μg daily, but the patients studied probably had irreversible airway damage associated with long-standing airway obstruction (Gaddie et al., 1973). Costello and Clark (1974) subsequently showed a significant improvement in FEV1 in patients when the dosage of beclomethasone was increased from 400 to 1000 μg daily. Toogood et al. (1982) showed a linear increase in PEF when increasing the dosage of budesonide from 400 to 1600 μg daily. Laursen et al. (1986), in a year-long study of oral CS-dependent patients, found that 1600 μg compared to 400 μg of budesonide had a greater prednisone-sparing effect, allowed a greater reduction in inhaled bronchodilator use, and produced greater improvements in mean values of PEF. These results have been confirmed in a recent study that compared 800 and 2000 μg of beclomethasone daily in patients dependent on oral CS. Both dosages permitted a reduction in oral CS, but this effect was greater in patients receiving the higher dosage (Tarlo et al., 1988).

In a study of patients not dependent on oral CS, 25, 100, and 400 μg daily of budesonide have been shown to achieve dose-dependent increases in PEF (Johansson and Dahl, 1988). In addition, it is now clear that twice daily doses are just as effective as 6 hourly doses in controlling symptoms in patients with stable asthma (Toogood et al., 1982), and this dosage schedule may help to increase compliance.

Effect on Bronchial Hyperresponsiveness

The principal findings of studies of the effects of inhaled CS (ICS) on BHR are summarized in Table 5. In conventional dosages of less than 1 mg daily, ICS reduces the severity of BHR to histamine and methacholine. This possibility was first suggested by a retrospective study of 35 adult asthmatic patients in whom histamine provocation tests were carried out on two occasions at least 10 months apart (Juniper et al., 1982). There was no change in the severity of BHR in those patients taking salbutamol alone, while a slight improvement occurred in those taking BDP (100-400 μg daily). Another study of 14 patients taking an average daily dosage of 400-600 μg of BDP for between 1 and 5 months showed a similar change (Clarke, 1982).

The improvement in BHR does not appear to be dependent on, or a result of, change in airway caliber. There is some evidence for a relationship between dosage of ICS and improvement in BHR (Kraan et al., 1985). In addition, one study has shown that change in BHR during inhaled CS therapy is time-dependent (Kraan et al., 1988). In all of these studies the magnitude of the

Table 5 Summary of Effects of Inhaled Steroids on Airway Sensitivity to Histamine and Methacholine[a]

Reference	Drug	No. Patients	Daily Dosage (mg)	Duration	Mean Initial PD20/PC20	Mean Final PD20/PC20	Individual Minimum Change[b]	Individual Maximum Change[b]	Comments
Juniper et al., 1982	BDP	35	100-400	10-30 months	0.5	1.23	0.6	4.0	Retrospective
Clarke, 1982	BDP	14	400-1200	1-5 months	9.75	33.6	0	4.0	Nonstandard HIT
Kraan et al., 1985	BUD	17	400	2 weeks	4.3	7.2	NS	NS	No individual data after treatment given
				4 weeks	4.3	9.5	NS	NS	BUD compared to terbutaline
Kraan et al., 1988	BUD	15	200	2 weeks	0.90	1.21	0.5	3.5	
				8 weeks	0.90	1.55	0.7	5.6	
		15	800	2 weeks	0.91	1.84	0.9	6.0	
				8 weeks	0.91	2.74	1.2	8.5	
Easton, 1985	BDP	7	400	4 months	1.16	2.73	0.88	13.0	Given values in paper logarithmically transformed
Dutoit et al., 1987	BDP	14	800	4 weeks	0.09	0.63	1.4	12.8	
				10 weeks	0.09	0.74	1.1	36.0	
Ryan et al., 1985	BDP	10	400	4 weeks	0.61	0.77	0.60	2.3	
Ostergaard and Pedersen, 1986	BUD	13	400	4 weeks	0.08	0.13	NS	NS	Children
				8 weeks	0.08	0.11	NS	NS	BUD compared to SCG
Kerribijn et al., 1987	BUD	12	600	6 months	1.52	2.01	0.81	15.2	Time-related effect
Jenkins and Woolcock, 1988	BDP	18	1200	3 weeks	0.38	1.01	0.6	10.0	BDP compared prednisone
Wilmsmeier et al., 1986	BDP	12	1000	2 weeks	0.13	0.27	NS	NS	BDP compared to prednisone

NS, individual values not stated; HIT, histamine inhalation test; SCG, sodium cromoglycate.
[a]Only includes papers in which individual data are given.
[b]Ratio of PD_{20} or PC_{20} after treatment/before treatment.

change in BHR is similar for comparable dosages of inhaled CS with a two-
to threefold change in the provoking concentration (PC20) or dose (PD20)
causing a 20% decrease in FEV1 on dosages between 400 and 800 μg daily.
In most studies, some patients improved very little while others returned to
normal airway responsiveness. As yet it has not been possible to identify
this group of responders on the basis of history or clinical findings. In a long-
term study of beclomethasone and "tight control" of daily flow readings,
Woolcock and colleagues, (1988) showed that it is possible to reduce the
severity of BHR markedly, but that many months of treatment are needed
(Fig. 1).

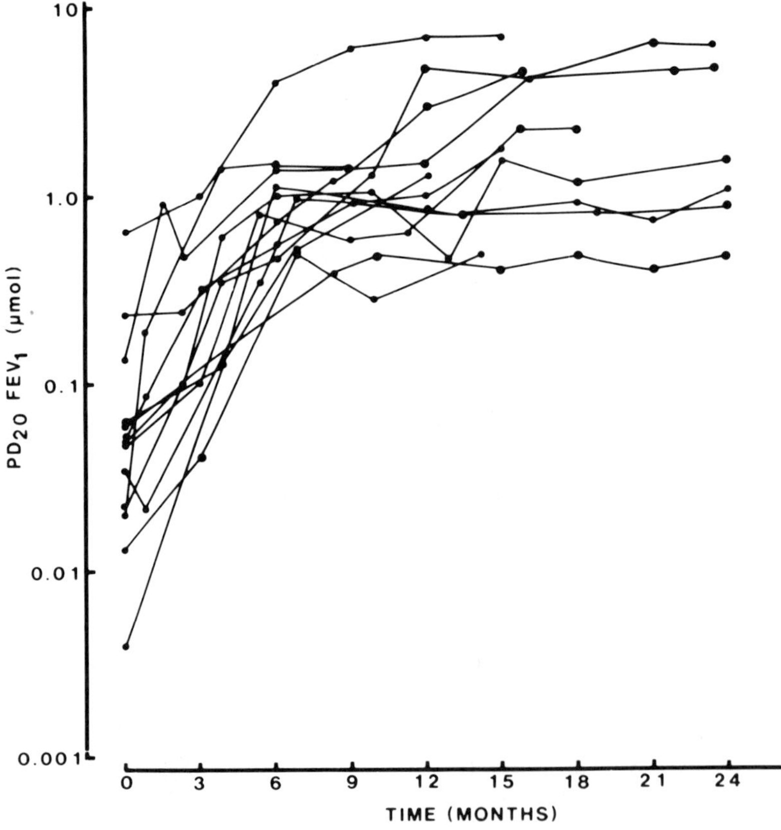

Figure 1   Improvement in the severity of BHR, measured as the PD_{20} FEV_1 to histamine in 12 patients with moderate and severe BHR treated with inhaled beclomethasone
and "tight control" of daily lung function. Maximal improvement took from 5 to 12
months.

Only two studies have compared the effect of inhaled and oral corticosteroids on BHR. In comparing BDP 1000 μg daily with prednisone 15 mg daily for 2 weeks, Wilsmeier et al. (1986) showed that PC20 improved in patients receiving BDP but not prednisone, despite better improvement of peak flows while receiving OCS. Jenkins and Woolcock (1988) showed a significant improvement in PD20 in patients taking BDP 1200 μg daily for 3 weeks but no change in PD20 in the same patients taking prednisone 12.5 mg daily for the same period. Both medications produced significant improvements in airflow rates and in diurnal variation, which suggest that ICS produce changes in BHR that are not merely a result of improvement in lung function. Although it is not possible to determine the equipotent dosages of OCS and ICS, it is clear from these and other studies that at conventional therapeutic dosages, ICS can reduce BHR to a much greater extent than OCS.

Place of ICS in the Management of Acute Attacks

There appear to have been no trials in which inhaled CS were added to oral or intravenous CS in patients with acute attacks. In Australia it is common practice to cease use of inhaled CS temporarily in the treatment of acute attacks. Since inhaled CS are so effective in reducing the severity of the disease in the long term (Woolcock et al., 1988), there seems little point in ceasing their use during acute attacks.

However, insufficient dosages reaching the airways during acute attacks, as illustrated in Figure 2, may limit their effectiveness. A topical steroid

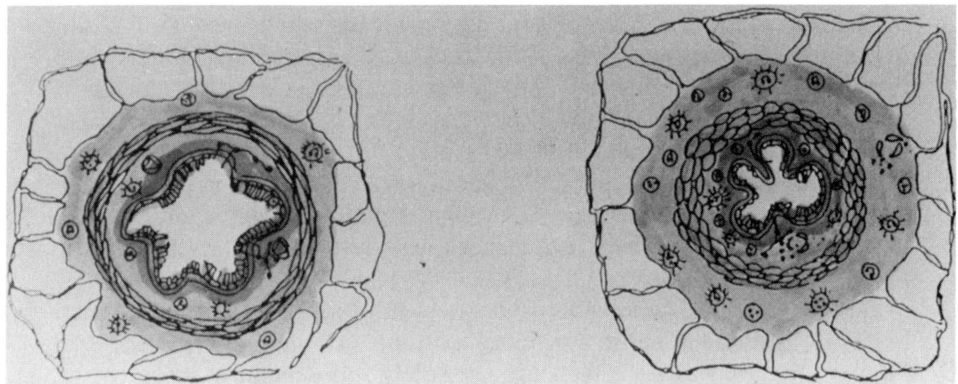

Figure 2 Representations of an asthmatic small airway in cross-section between and during an attack. The light shading suggests the area of wall reached by adequate concentrations of systemically administered CS, the dark shading indicates the area that inhaled CS probably reach. During an attack, the inhaled form may be ineffective because it does not penetrate sufficiently.

that can be effectively nebulized may solve this problem but is, as yet, unavailable.

V. Experimental Effects of Corticosteroids in Humans

A. Effects on the Early and Late Asthmatic Responses

It is commonly stated that both oral and inhaled forms block the late asthmatic response (LAR) but do not modify the early asthmatic response (EAR) (Booij-Noord et al., 1971; Pepys et al., 1974). However some studies (Burge, 1982; Dahl et al., 1982) suggest that with longer treatment it is possible to demonstrate an effect of oral CS on the EAR. Prednisone does not always reduce the EAR, even after prolonged pretreatment (Booij-Noord et al., 1971; Pipkorn et al., 1986). Dose dependency for the effects of oral and inhaled steroids on the EAR has not been studied systematically, although comparisons between dosages suggest a dose-dependent effect (Burge, 1982; Dahl et al., 1982; Pipkorn et al., 1986; Burge et al., 1982). These studies are summarized in Table 6. In toluene diisocyanate (TDI)-induced asthma, both ICS (Mapp et al., 1987) and OCS (Boschetto et al., 1987; Fabbri et al., 1985) have been shown to inhibit the LAR and the associated inflammatory response, and prior administration of BD—1000 μg daily for 1 week also prevents the increase in BHR following TDI exposure (Mapp et al., 1987). It is likely that ICS act on mucosal inflammatory cells to inhibit the release of mediators and chemotactic factors rather than by modifying the behavior of circulating leukocytes, as OCS are thought to do (Martin et al., 1980).

Studies with allergens indicate that CS can modify both the EAR and the LAR if administered for several days prior to a challenge (Booij-Noord et al., 1971; Van der Star et al., 1976; Cockcroft and Murdock, 1987). Modifying the EAR may not be as important as modifying the LAR, which is associated with an increase in BHR (Cartier et al., 1982; Cockcroft and Murdock 1987; Durham et al., 1988). The ability of inhaled CS (Pepys et al., 1974; Van der Star, 1976) and OCS (Booij-Noord et al., 1971) to inhibit LAR and the associated increase in BHR suggests that this may be an important mechanism by which inhaled CS reduce the severity of BHR over longer periods of time.

However, since beneficial responses to inhaled CS also occur in nonallergic subjects and in persons with occupational asthma (Fabbri et al., 1985; Lam et al., 1987), these effects are not solely IgE-dependent.

B. Effects on Inflammatory Cells

Although CS do not directly inhibit mast cell degranulation in vitro, they have been shown to blunt the late response induced by anti-IgE and mast cell granules (Schleimer et al., 1981). This suggests that CS can interfere with the inflammatory events following mast cell degranulation (Oertel and Kaliner, 1981). In the nose, ICS reduce mast cell histamine content, possibly by reducing histamine synthesis. In vitro, they also inhibit neutrophil aggregation, lysosomal enzyme release, and superoxide generation (Goldstein et al., 1976; Clark et al., 1979), which effects may indirectly lead to a reduction in eosinophil accumulation in sites of airway inflammation. Eosinopenia and reduced localization of eosinophils have been demonstrated in subjects with acute cutaneous wheal and flare reactions after 1 week of steroid medication (Slott and Zweiman, 1975). Most importantly, prednisone consistently produces reduced eosinophil chemotaxis and endothelial adherence (Clarke et al., 1979), thus having a direct effect on eosinophil behavior, which might contribute to reduced epithelial damage and to attenuation of the increase in BHR resulting from this.

Epithelial damage has been shown to be associated with increased BHR (Laitinen et al., 1985; Seltzer et al., 1986; Flavahan et al., 1988) and, of the several cells implicated in this, the eosinophil may be the most important. Major basic protein (MBP) and eosinophil cationic protein (ECP) are present in bronchoalveolar lavage (BAL) fluid from patients with asthma who develop LAR (De Monchy et al., 1985) and have been shown to destroy epithelial cells in vitro (Frigas et al., 1980, 1981). Budesonide can inhibit the release of eosinophil cytotoxic proteins (Venge, 1984). This is a possible mechanism by which inhaled CS might prevent epithelial damage and the development of BHR.

C. Effects in the Nose

A different effect for topical and systemic steroids has also been demonstrated in patients with allergic rhinitis. Pipkorn et al. (1986) showed that prednisone reduced both nasal symptoms and mediator release after allergen challenge, but did not modify the EAR even after 1 week of pretreatment. By contrast, topical flunisolide (Pipkorn et al., 1987) also reduced the EAR and increased the threshold dosage for a positive response (the dosage required for a double or greater increase in mediators above baseline) to antigen. A more important finding was that premedication with the topical steroid prevented the increased sensitivity following rechallenge, a phenomenon not observed with prednisone in the previous study. These findings are in keeping with observations of steroid effects on BHR in the lower airways. Inhibition of the LAR and inflammatory response by both inhaled and oral CS in studies of nasal allergen challenge indicate that the beneficial effects of CS on lung function and on the severity of BHR are a result of their anti-inflammatory actions.

Table 6 Effect of CS Treatment on Bronchial Provocation Tests/Allergen Exposure

Reference	Stimulus	Drug	Dosage	Duration	EAR Effect	LAR Effect	Comment
Booij-Noord et al., 1971	Allergen	Prednisone	15-20 mg daily	9-16 days	None	Abolished	
Boschetto et al., 1987	TDI	Prednisone	50 mg daily	3 days	None	Abolished	Prevented BHR
Martin et al., 1980	Allergen	Prednisone	40 mg daily	7 days	73% blocking index	Abolished	
Fabbri et al., 1985	TDI	Prednisone	50 mg daily	3 days	None	Abolished	LAR and increase in BHR prevented by prednisone
Sotomayor et al., 1984	Natural Allergen Exposure	MP	16 mg daily	7 days		Reversed seasonal, increase in BHR	
Pepys et al., 1974	Mostly Chemical Sensitizers n = 3 allergen	BDP	200 mg	30 min before and q3h during BPT	None	Inhibited	

Mapp et al., 1987	TDI	BDP	1000 μg twice daily	7 days	None	Abolished
Cockcroft and Murdock, 1987	Allergen	BDP	200 μg	10 min before BPT	Slight reduction	Abolished
Dahl et al., 1982	Allergen	BUD	1000 μg	12 and 4 h before BPT	No change	Abolished
Dahl et al., 1982	Allergen	BUD	1000 μg daily	7 days	Reduced, not abolished	Abolished
Dahl et al., 1982	Allergen	BUD	1000 μg	4 weeks	Inhibited	Abolished
Burge, 1982	Allergen	BDP	400 μg daily	7 days	Blocked in 40% subjects	Blocked in 82% subjects
Burge et al., 1982	Allergen	BDP	800 μg daily	7 days	Blocked in 60% subjects	Abolished

D. Effects in Seasonal Asthma

In a study designed to examine one of the mechanisms of action of oral CS on BHR, Sotomayor et al. (1984) demonstrated that 16 mg of methylprednisolone daily for 1 week could reverse the allergen-induced increase in BHR that occurs during the grass pollen season. These changes were statistically significant, but small compared with the more substantial changes in BHR documented after therapy with ICS.

VI. Side Effects of Corticosteroids

The side effects of oral CS are well known and have been reviewed extensively (David et al., 1970; Seale and Compton, 1986). Their inevitable development and disabling nature have been the major stimuli for the development of topically active CS with minimal systemic activity. However, inhaled CS also have side effects because they are absorbed into the systemic circulation (Johansson et al., 1982; Brattsand et al., 1987) and both BDP and budesonide have weakly active metabolites after undergoing biotransformation in the liver (Martin et al., 1974; Andersson et al., 1982). Depression of morning cortisol levels can occur in adults taking more than 1500 μg, but this is probably not clinically important for most patients. Other systemic side effects have been reported rarely (Reid et al., 1986; Allen et al., 1988; Clark, 1972) and it is still uncertain whether high-dosage ICS cause alterations in calcium metabolism and osteoporosis. (Toogood et al., 1988). In children, adrenal suppression can occur at dosages under 800 μg daily, although the clinical significance of this is uncertain. (Nassif et al., 1987). The relationship of total daily dosage of inhaled CS to body weight may be important in children, in whom slowing of growth may occur when receiving dosages under 1 mg daily. Individual susceptibility probably plays a major role in the expression of side effects, and variability of aerosol deposition might also contribute to this.

Local side effects often contribute to lack of patient compliance. The prevalence of candidiasis is strongly related to total daily dosage of ICS (Toogood et al., 1977a, 1984b) and can be reduced by lowering the frequency of administration as well as the total number of puffs per day (Toogood et al., 1980). Use of a pear-shaped cone spacer (Toogood et al., 1981) or Aerochamber (Salzman and Pyszczynski, 1988) also reduces the incidence of oropharyngeal side effects in patients receiving ICS. Oral colonization with *Candida* species has been reported in up to 70% patients taking beclomethasone dipropionate (Cayton et al., 1974). Clinical thrush only affects about 15% (Toogood et al., 1980). Hoarseness is a more frequent side effect, affecting up to 30% of patients in some studies (Toogood et al., 1981, 1984b). Although it is not related to candidiasis, it will improve with the same measures, particularly a reduction in frequency and the use of a spacer (Toogood et al., 1984c).

VII. Questions that Remain Unanswered

A. Systemic Corticosteroids in Acute Attacks

1. What is the minimum effective dosage of SCS that optimizes the special rate of recovery and minimizes relapse rates?

2. What schedule is best for tapering the dosage of SCS after recovery from an acute attack?

3. Which drug is most effective in patients recovering from acute attacks?

4. In view of the studies indicating that high dosages of SCS can ameliorate BHR, should the outcome of therapy with SCS be the reduction of BHR rather than simply improvement in airway obstruction?

B. Inhaled Corticosteroids

1. What dosages produce the greatest and most rapid improvement in BHR in patients with asthma of varying severity?

2. For how long and with what dosages can the improvement be maintained?

3. Are patients with recent onset of the disease more likely to achieve normal responsiveness than those with long-standing disease?

4. What histological features of airway inflammation improve with ICS therapy?

5. Does the institution of high-dosages ICS, together with SCS, at the onset of an acute exacerbation, result in more rapid return to normal lung function?

C. Experimental Use of Corticosteroids

1. What is the minimal dosage of CS required to inhibit the allergen-induced LAR?

2. Is inhibition of the EAR an important contributing factor in the reduction of BHR, or a result of it?

3. Why do some subjects completely lose their BHR after short periods of treatment with ICS?

VIII. Conclusions

The effectiveness of CS in treating acute attacks and long-term asthma support the concept that asthma is an inflammatory disease with acute exacerbations.

There is a dose-related improvement in asthma severity and BHR resulting from both ICS and SCS, but the improvement in BHR is not just a function of improved resting lung function. The ICS, at currently used dosages, have a greater effect on BHR than do SCS.

The superior effect of ICS on BHR may result from their intrinsically high topical activity or from the concentration of the drug in the epithelial and subepithelial regions.

The more satisfactory effects of SCS in treating acute exacerbations of asthma may be due to the failure of the ICS to penetrate the airways once edema has occurred. It is possible that if higher concentrations of ICS could be delivered to the airways in acute attacks, they would be as effective as SCS.

CS probably influence the LAR by interfering with the consequences of mediator release, preventing the recruitment and activation of acute inflammatory cells that promote ongoing airway inflammation and the associated increase in BHR.

Although premedication with ICS for a week can modify the EAR, this may be a function of improved nonspecific BHR.

The facts that CS do not cure asthma and that relapses occur after time without treatment with them indicate that these drugs are playing only a suppressing role.

The reduction of vascular leak is probably one of the major anti-inflammatory effects of CS.

Discussion

Daniel: Presumably inhaled steroids cannot reach the peribronchial region, which may be "untethered" in asthma. How can you explain their effects on reactivity if this is the case?

Woolcock: We do not know how far into the airway wall inhaled steroids can penetrate, nor do we know how much inflammation exists outside the muscle in most asthmatic patients.

Kerrebijn: Inhaled drugs may be absorbed into the bronchial circulation and taken to the peripheral airways, which could explain their anti-inflammatroy effect in the entire bronchial tree.

Woolcock: This has certainly been shown for cromolyn, but not yet for steroids.

Barnes: The condition of many patients, especially with intrinsic asthma, may be controlled on a critical dosage of oral steroids (e.g., prednisolone 9 mg daily) but if the dosage is reduced minimally (e.g., to 8 mg), asthma often goes out of control. It is difficult to understand this in terms of pharmacology, since it implies that some critical cell is suppressed and only minimal reduction in receptor occupancy allows inflammation to flare up.

Woolcock: It is a common observation in patients, but I cannot explain it.

Sybrecht: Lundgren et al. (*Eur. J. Respir. Dis.* 1988) have presented morphological data from patients before and after 10 years' treatment with beclomethasone. Inflammation was reduced but BHR was not.

Woolcock: We do not know the cause of BHR: there are at least three distinct possibilities.

Fabbri: Do inhaled steroids reverse BHR if given after allergen?

Kerrebijn: In a study we have just completed we found that inhaled budesonide (200 μg three times daily), started approximately 16 h after allergen challenge did prevent the increase in BHR 72 h after challenge.

Tattersfield: The changes in BHR after 4 months in your study are much greater than in placebo-controlled trials: do you think this is due to other aspects of management in addition to steroids?

Woolcock: To achieve these improvements (10-100-fold over 6-24 months) you need inhaled steroids plus "tight control."

Hargreave: One explanation for the small effect of steroids on BHR in placebo-controlled studies is the selection of subjects. Most have mild and stable asthma in which inflammation and the effects of steroids would be expected to be less.

References

Ackerman, G. L., and Nolan, C. M. (1968). Adrenocortical responsiveness after alternate day corticosteroid therapy. *N. Engl. J. Med.* **278**:405-409.

Allen, M. B., Ray, S., Dhillon, B., Cullen, R., and Leitch, A. G. (1988). Do steroid aerosols cause cataracts in asthmatic patients? *Thorax* **43**: 845-846.

Andersson, P., Edsbacker, S., and Ryrfeldt, A. (1982). In vitro biotransformation of budesonide, triamcinolone acetonide and hydrocortisone in liver and skin from man, rat and hairless mouse. *J. Steroid Biochem.* **16**:787-796.

Barach, A. L., Bickerman, H. A., and Beck, G. J. (1955). Clinical and physiological studies on the use of metacortandracin in respiratory disease. 1. Bronchial asthma. *Dis. Chest* **27**:515-522.

Bernstein, I. L., Chervinsky, P., and Falliers, C. J. (1982). Efficacy and safety of triamcinolone acetonide aerosol in chronic asthma. *Chest* **81**:20-26.

Bhagat, R., and Grunstein, M. (1985). Effect of corticosteroids on bronchial responsiveness to methacholine in asthmatic children. *Am. Rev. Respir. Dis.* **131**:902-906.

Booij-Noord, H., Orie, N. G. M., and de Vries, K. (1971). Immediate and late bronchial obstructive reactions to inhalation of house dust and protective effects of disodium cromoglycate and prednisolone. *J. Allergy Clin. Immunol.* **48**:344-354.

Boschetto, P., Fabbri, L. M., Zocca, E., Milani, G., Pivirotto, F., Dal Vecchio, A., Plebani, M., and Mapp, C. E. (1987). Prednisone inhibits late asthmatic reactions and airway inflammation induced by toluene diisocyanate in sensitized subjects. *J. Allergy Clin. Immunol.* **80**:261-267.

Brattsand, R., Andersson, P. T., Edsbacker, S., and Ryrfeldt, A. (1987). Development of glucocorticosteroids with lung selectivity. In *Advances in the Use of Inhaled Corticosteroids*. Edited by R. Ellul-Micaleff, W. K. Lam, and J. H. Toogood. Amsterdam, Excerpta Medica, pp. 60-85.

Braude, A. C., and Rebuck, A. S. (1983). Prednisone and methylprednisolone disposition in the lung. *Lancet* **2**:995-997.

British Thoracic and Tuberculosis Association (1976). A controlled trial of inhaled corticosteroids in patients receiving prednisone tablets for asthma. *Br. J. Dis. Chest* **70**:95-102.

Britton, M. G., Collins, J. V., Brown, D., Fairhurst, N. P. A., and Lambert, R. G. (1976). High-dose corticosteroids in severe acute asthma. *Br. Med. J.* **2**:73-74.

Brompton Hospital/MRC Collaborative Trial (1979). Double blind trial comparing two dosage schedules of beclomethasone dipropionate aerosol with a placebo in chronic bronchial asthma. *Br. J. Dis. Chest* **73**:121-132.

Burge, P. S. The effects of corticosteroids on the immediate asthmatic reaction. (1982). *Eur. J. Respir. Dis.* **63** (Suppl. 122):163-166.

Burge, P. S., Efthimiou, J., Turner-Warwick, M., and Nelmes, P. T. J. (1982). Double-blind trials of inhaled beclomethasone dipropionate and floucortin butyl ester in allergen-induced immediate and late asthmatic reactions. *Clin. Allergy* **12**:523-531.

Burrage, W. S., and Irwin, J. W. (1985). Hydrocortisone in the therapy of asthma. *Ann. N.Y. Acad. Sci.* **66**:37-41.

Cameron, S. J., Cooper, E. J., Crompton, E. J., Hoare, M. V., and Grant, I. W. B. (1973). Substitution of beclomethasone aerosol for oval prednisolone in the treatment of chronic asthma. *Br. Med. J.* **4**:205-207.

Carmichael, J., Paterson, I. C., Diaz, P., Crompton, G. K., Kay, A. B., and Grant, I. W. B. (1981). Corticosteroid resistance in chronic asthma. *Br. Med. J.* **282**:1419-1422.

Carryer, H. M., Prickman, L. E., and Maytum, C. K. (1950). Effects of cortisone on bronchial asthma and hayfever occurring in subjects sensitive to ragweed pollen. *Proc. Mayo Clin.* **25**:282-287.

Cartier, A., Thompson, N. C., Frith, P. A., Roberts, R., and Hargreave, F. E. (1982). Allergen-induced increase in bronchial responsiveness to histamine: relationship to the late asthmatic response and change in airway calibre. *J. Allergy Clin. Immunol.* **70**:170-177.

Cayton, R. M., Soutar, C. A., Stanford, C. S., Turner, G. C., and Nunn, A. J. (1974). Double-blind trial comparing two dosage schedules of beclomethasone dipropionate aerosol in the treatment of chronic bronchial asthma. *Lancet* **2**:303-306.

Clarke, P. S. (1982). The effect of beclomethasone dipropionate on bronchial hyperreactivity. *J. Asthma* **19**:91-93.

Clark, R. A., Gallin, J. I., and Fauci, A. S. (1979). Effects of in vivo prednisone on in vitro eosinophil and neutrophil adherence and chemotaxis. *Blood* **53**:633-641.

Clark, T. J. H. (1972). Effect of beclomethasone dipropionate delivered by aerosol in patients with asthma. *Lancet* **1**:1361-1365.

Cockcroft, D. W., and Murdock, K. Y. (1987). Comparative effects of inhaled salbutamol, sodium cromoglycate, and beclomethasone dipropionate on allergen induced early asthmatic responses, late asthmatic responses and increased bronchial responsiveness to histamine. *J. Allergy Clin. Immunol.* **79**:734-470.

Cooper, E. J., and Grant, I. W. B. (1977). Beclomethasone dipropionate aerosol in treatment of chronic asthma. *Q. J. Med.* **183**:295-308.

Costello, J. F., and Clark, T. J. H. (1974). Response of patients receiving high dose beclomethasone dipropionate. *Thorax* **29**:571-573.

Dahl, R., Henriksen, J. M., and Johansson, S. A. (1982). Importance of duration of treatment with inhaled budesonide on the immediate and late bronchial reaction. *Eur. J. Respir. Dis.* **63** (Supp 122):167-175.

David, D. S., Greico, M. H., and Cushman, P. (1970). Adrenal glucocorticoids after 20 years: a review of their clinically relevant consequences. *J. Chron. Dis.* **22**:637-711.

De Monchy, J. G. R., Kauffman, H. F., Venge, P., Koeter, G. H., Jansen, H. M., Sluiter, H. J., and De Vries, K. (1985). Bronchoalveolar eosinophilia during allergen-induced late asthmatic reactions. *Am. Rev. Respir. Dis.* **131**:373-376.

Durham, S. R., Craddock, C. F., Cookson, W. O., and Benson, M. K. (1988). Increases in airway responsiveness to histamine precede allergen-induced late asthmatic responses. *J. Allergy Clin. Immunol.* **82**:764-770.

Dutoit, J. I., Salome, C. M., and Woolcock, A. J. (1987). Inhaled corticosteroids reduce the severity of bronchial hyperresponsiveness but oral theophylline does not. *Am. Rev. Respir. Dis.* **136**:1174-1178.

Easton, J. G. (1985). Effect of an inhaled corticosteroid on methacholine airway reactivity. *J. Allergy Clin. Immunol.* **67**:388-393.

Ebden, P., Jenkins, A., Houston, G., and Davies, B. H. (1986). Comparison of two high dose corticosteroid aerosol treatments, beclomethasone dipropionate (1500 mcg/day) and budesonide (1600 mcg/day) for chronic asthma. *Thorax* **41**:869-874.

Ellis, E. F. (1988). Adverse effects of corticosteroid therapy. *J. Allergy Clin. Immunol.* **80**:515-517.

Fabbri, L. M., Chiesura-Corona, P., Dal Vecchio, L., Di Giacomo, G. R., Zocca, E., De Marzo, N., Maestrelli, P., and Mapp, C. E. (1985). Prednisone inhibits late asthmatic reactions and the associated increase in airway responsiveness induced by toluene diisocyanate in sensitized subjects. *Am. Rev. Respir. Dis.* **132**:1010-1014.

Fanta, C. H., Rossing, T. H., and McFadden, E. R. (1982). Glucocorticoids in acute asthma: a critical controlled trial. *Am. Rev. Respir. Dis.* **125** (Suppl):94.

Fauci, A. S. (1978). Alternate-day corticosteroid therapy. *Am. J. Med.* **64**: 729-731.

Fiel, S. B., Swartz, M. A., Glanz, K., and Francis, M. E. (1983). Efficacy of short-term corticosteroid therapy in outpatient treatment of acute bronchial asthma. *Am. J. Med.* **75**:259-262.

Field, H. V., Jenkinson, P. M. A., Frame, M. H., and Warner, J. O. (1982). Asthma treatment with a new corticosteroid aerosol, Budesonide, administered twice daily by spacer inhaler. *Arch. Dis. Child.* **57**:864-866.

Flavahan, N. A., Slifman, N. R., Gleich, G. J., and Vanhoutte, P. (1988). Human eosinophil major basic protein causes hyperreactivity of respiratory smooth muscle. Role of the epithelium. *Am. Rev. Respir. Dis.* **138**:685-688.

Frigas, E., Loegering, D. A., and Gleich, G. J. (1980). Cytotoxic effects of the guinea pig eosinophil major basic protein on tracheal epithelium. *Lab. Invest.* **42**:35.

Frigas, E., Loegering, D. A., Solley, G. O., Farrow, G. M., and Gleich, G. J. (1981). Elevated levels of the eosinophil granule major basic protein in the sputum of patients with bronchial asthma. *Mayo Clin. Proc.* **56**:345.

Gaddie, J., Reid, I. W., Skinner, C., Petrie, G. R., Sinclair, D. J. M., and Palmer, K. N. V. (1973). Aerosol beclomethasone dipropionate: a dose-response study in chronic bronchial asthma. *Lancet* **3**:280-281.

Goldstein, L. M., Ross, D., Weisman, G., and Kaplan, H. G. (1976). Influence of corticosteroids on human polymorphonuclear leucocyte function in vitro. Reduction of lysosomal enzyme release and superoxide production. *Inflammation* **1**:305-308.

Gwynn, C. M., and Smith, J. M. (1974). A 1-year follow-up of children and adolescents receiving regular beclomethasone dipropionate. *Clin. Allergy* **4**:325-327.

Harris, D. M. (1975). Some properties of beclomethasone dipropionate and related steroids in man. *Postgrad. Med. J.* **51** (Suppl 4):20-25.

Harris, J. B., Weinberger, M. M., Nassif, E., Smith, G., Milavetz, G., and Stillerman, A. (1987). Early intervention with short courses of prednisone to prevent progression of asthma in ambulatory patients incompletely responsive to bronchodilators. *J. Pediatr.* **110**:627-633.

Haskell, R. J., Wong, B. M., and Hansen, J. E. (1983). A double-blind randomized clinical trial of methylprednisolone in status asthmaticus. *Arch. Intern. Med.* **143**:1324-1327.

Haynes, R. C., and Murad, F. (1985). Adrenocorticotropic hormone; adrenocortical steroids and their synthetic analogues; inhibitors of adrenocortical steroid biosynthesis. In *The Pharmacologic Basis of Therapeutics*, 7th edition. Edited by A. G. Goodman, L. S. Gilman, T. W. Rall, and F. Murad. New York, Macmillan, pp. 1472-1506.

Israel, R., Poe, R. H., Wicks, C. M., and Greenblatt, D. W. (1984). The protective effect of methylprednisolone on carbachol-induced bronchospasm. *Am. Rev. Respir. Dis.* **130**:1019-1022.

Jenkins, C. R., and Woolcock, A. J. (1988). A comparative study of the effect of prednisone and beclomethasone dipropionate on airway responsiveness in asthma. *Thorax* **43**:378-384.

Johansson, S. A., and Dahl, R. (1988). A double-blind dose-response study of budesonide by inhalation in patients with bronchial asthma. *Allergy* **43**:173-178.

Johansson, S. A., Andersson, K. E., Brattsand, R., Gruvstad, E., and Hedner, P. (1982). Topical and systemic glucocorticoid potencies of budesonide and beclomethasone dipropionate in man. *Eur. J. Clin. Pharmacol.* **22**:523-529.

Juniper, E. F., Frith, P. A., and Hargreave, F. E. (1982). Long-term stability of bronchial responsiveness to histamine. *Thorax* **37**:288-291.

Kallstrom, L., Brattsand, R., Lovgren, U., Svensjo, E., and Roempke, K. (1987). A rat model for testing anti-inflammatory action in lung and the effect of glucocorticoids in this model. In *Advances in the Use of Inhaled Corticosteroids*. Edited by R. Ellul-Micaleff, Lam, W. K., Toogood, J. H. pp. 60-85. Excerpta Medica.

Kattan, M., Gurwitz, D., and Levison, H. (1980). Corticosteroids in status asthmaticus. *J. Pediatr.* **96**:596-599.

Kay, A. B., Diaz, P., Carmicheal, J., and Grant, I. W. B. (1981). Corticosteroid resistant chronic asthma and monocyte receptors. *Clin. Exp. Immunol.* **44**:576-580.

Kerrebijn, K. F., van Essen-Zandvliet, E. E. M., and Neijens, H. J. (1987). Effect of long-term treatment with inhaled corticosteroids and beta-agonists on the bronchial responsiveness in children with asthma. *J. Allergy Clin. Immunol.* **79**:653-659.

Kraan, J., Koeter, G. H., Mark, T. W., Sluiter, M. D., and de Vries, K. (1985). Changes in bronchial hyperreactivity induced by four weeks treatment with anti-asthmatic drugs in patients with allergic asthma: a comparison between budesonide and terbutaline. *J. Allergy Clin. Immunol.* **76**:628-636.

Kraan, J., Koeter, G. H., van der Mark, T. H., Boorsma, M., Kukler, J., Sluiter, H. J., and de Vries, K. (1988). Dosage and time effects of inhaled budesonide on bronchial hyperreactivity. *Am. Rev. Respir. Dis.* **137**: 44-48.

Laitinen, L. A., Heino, M., Laitinen, A., Kava, T., and Haahtela, T. (1985). Damage of the airway epithelium and bronchial reactivity in patients with asthma. *Am. Rev. Respir. Dis.* **131**:599-606.

Lam, S., LeRiche, J., Phillips, D., and Chan-Yeung, M. (1987). Cellular and protein changes in bronchial lavage fluid after late asthmatic reaction in patients with red cedar asthma. *J. Allergy Clin. Immunol.* **80**: 44-50.

Lampl, K. L., Lichtenstein, L. M., and Schleimer, R. P. (1985). In vitro resistance to dexamethasone of basophils from patients receiving long-term steroid therapy. *Am. Rev. Respir. Dis.* **132**:1015-1018.

Laursen, L, Taudorf, E., and Weeke, B. (1986). High dose inhaled budesonide in treatment of severe steroid dependent asthma. *Eur. J. Respir. Dis.* **68**:19-28.

Littenberg, B., and Gluck, E. H. (1986). A controlled trial of methylprednisolone in the emergency room treatment of acute asthma. *N. Engl. J. Med.* **314**:150-152.

Littlewood, J. M., Johnson, A. W., Edwards, P. A., and Littlewood, A. E. (1988). Growth retardation in asthmatic children treated with inhaled beclomethasone dipropionate. *Lancet* **1**:115-116.

Mapp, C., Boschetto, P., Dal Vecchio, L., Crescioli, S., De Marzo, N., Paleari, D., and Fabbri, L. M. (1987). Protective effect of antiasthma drugs on late asthmatic reactions and increased airway responsiveness induced by toluene diisocyanate in sensitized subjects. *Am. Rev. Respir. Dis.* **136**: 1403-1407.

Martin, G. L., Atkins, P. C., Dunsky, E. H., and Zweiman, B. (1980). Effects of theophylline, terbutaline and prednisone on antigen-induced bronchospasm and mediator release. *J. Allergy Clin. Immunol.* **66**:204-212.

Martin, L. E., Tanner, R. J. N., Clark, T. J. H., and Cochrane, G. M. (1974). Absorption and metabolism of orally administered beclomethasone dipropionate. *Clin. Pharmacol. Ther.* **15**:267-275.

Mattoli, S., Rosati, G., Flaminio, M., and Ciappi, G. (1985). The immediate and short-term effects of corticosteroids on cholinergic hyperreactivity and pulmonary function in subjects with well-controlled asthma. *J. Allergy Clin. Immunol.* **76**:214-222.

McFadden, E. R., Kiser, R., deGroot, W. J., Holmes, B., Kiker, R., and Viser, G. (1976). A controlled study of the effects of single doses of hydrocortisone on the resolution of acute attacks of asthma. *Am. J. Med.* **60**:52-57.

Michealides, D. N. (1981). Equivalent potency of corticosteroid preparations used in reversible obstruction. *Immunol. Allergy Pract.* **3**:36-40.

Nassif, E., Weinberger, M., Sherman, B., and Brown, K. (1987). Extrapulmonary effects of maintenance corticosteroid therapy with alternate-day prednisone and inhaled beclomethasone in children with chronic asthma. *J. Allergy Clin. Immunol.* **80**:518-529.

Oertel, H., and Kaliner, M. (1981). The biological activity of mast cell granules in rat skin: effects of adrenocorticosteroids on late phase inflammatory responses induced by mast cell granules. *J. Allergy Clin. Immunol.* **68**:238-245.

Ostergaard, P. A., and Pedersen, S. (1986). The effect of inhaled sodium cromoglycate and budesonide on bronchial responsiveness to histamine and exercise in asthmatic children: a clinical comparison. In *Glucocorticosteroids in Childhood Asthma*. Edited by S. Godfrey. Proceeding of a Symposium in Budapest, pp. 55-65.

Pauwels, R. (1986). Mode of action of corticosteroids in asthma and rhinitis. *Clin. Allergy* **16**:281-288.

Pepys, J., Davies, R. J., Breslin, A. B. X., Hendrick, D. J., and Hutchcroft, B. J. (1974). The effects of inhaled beclomethasone dipropionate (Becotide) and sodium cromoglycate on asthmatic reactions to provocation tests. *Clin. Allergy* **4**:13-27.

Pierson, W. E., Bierman, C. W., and Kelley, V. C. (1974). A double-blind trial of corticosteroid therapy in status asthmaticus. *Pediatrics* **54**:282-289.

Pipkorn, U., and Enerback, L. (1987). Nasal mucosal mast cells and histamine in hay Fever. Effect of topical glucocorticoid treatment. *Int. Arch. Allergy Appl. Immunol.* **84**:123-128.

Pipkorn, U., Proud, D., Lichtenstein, L. M., Schleimer, R. P., Peters, S. P., Adkinson, N. F., Kagey-Sabotka, A., Norman, P. S., and Naclerio, R. M. (1986). Effect of short-term systemic glucocorticoid treatment on human nasal mediator release after antigen challenge. *J. Allergy Clin. Immunol.* **77**:180 (Suppl).

Pipkorn, U., Proud, D., Lichtenstein, L., Kagey-Sabotka, A., Norman, P. S., and Naclerio, R. M. (1987). Inhibition of mediator release in allergic rhinitis by pretreatment with topical glucocorticosteroids. *N. Engl. J. Med.* **316**:1506-1510.

Place, V. A. (1970). Precise evaluation of topically applied corticosteroid potency. *Arch. Dermatol.* **101**:531-537.

Raimondi, A. C., Figueroa-Casas, J. C., and Roncoroni, A. J. (1986). Comparison between high and moderate doses of hydrocortisone in the treatment of status asthmaticus. *Chest* **89**:832-835.

Randolph, T. G., and Rollins, J. P. (1950). Effect of cortisone on bronchial asthma. *J. Allergy* **21**:288-291.

Reid, D. M., Nicoll, J. J., Smith, M. A., Higgins, B., Tothill, P., and Nuki, G. (1986). Corticosteroids and bone mass in asthma: comparisons with rheumatoid arthritis and polymyalgia rheumatica. *Br. Med. J.* **293**:1463-1466.

Ryan, G., Latimer, K. M., Juniper, E. F., Roberts, R. S., and Hargreave, F. E. (1985). Effect of beclomethasone dipropionate on bronchial responsiveness to histamine in controlled nonsteroid-dependent asthma. *J. Allergy Clin. Immunol.* **75**:25-30.

Salzman, G. A., and Pyszczynski, D. R. (1988). Oropharyngeal candidiasis in patients treated with beclomethasone dipropionate delivered by metered-dose inhaler alone and with Aerochamber. *J. Allergy Clin. Immunol.* **81**:424-428.

Schleimer, R. P., Lichtenstein, L. M., and Gillespie, E. (1981). Inhibition of basophil histamine release by anti-inflammatory steroids. *Nature* **292**:454-455.

Seale, J. P., and Compton, M. R. (1986). Side-effects of corticosteroid agents. *Med. J. Aust.* **144**:139-142.

Seltzer, J., Bigby, B. G., Stulbarg, M., Holtzman, M. J., Nadel, J. A., Ueki, I. F., Leikauf, G. D., Goetzel, E. J., and Boushey, H. A. (1986). O3-induced change in bronchial reactivity to methacholine and airway inflammation in humans. *J. Appl. Physiol.* **60**:1321-1326.

Shapiro, G. G., Izu, A. E., Furukawa, C. T., Pierson, W. E., and Bierman, C. W. (1981). Short term, double blind evaluation of flunisolide aerosol for steroid dependent asthmatic children and adolescents. *Chest* **80**: 671-675.

Slott, R. I., and Zweiman, B. (1975). Histologic studies of human skin test responses to ragweed and compound 48/80. *J. Allergy Clin. Immunol.* **55**:232-237.

Smith, M. J., and Hodson, M. E. (1983). Effects of longterm inhaled high dose beclomethasone dipropionate on adrenal function. *Thorax* **38**:676-681.

Sotomayor, H., Badier, M., Vervolet, D., and Orehek, J. (1984). Seasonal increase of carbachol airway responsiveness in patients allergic to grass pollen. Reversal by corticosteroids. *Am. Rev. Respir. Dis.* **130**:56-58.

Storr, J. G., Barry, W., Barrell, E., Lenney, W., and Hatcher, G. (1987). Effect of a single oral dose of prednisolone in acute childhood asthma. *Lancet* **1**:879-882.

Sue, M. A., Kwong, F. K., and Klaustermeyer, W. B. (1986). A comparison of intravenous hydrocortisone, methylprednisolone and dexamethasone in acute bronchial asthma. *Ann. Allergy* **56**:406-409.

Tanaka, R. M., Santiago, S. M., Kuhn, G. J., Williams, R. E., and Klaustermeyer, W. B. (1982). Intravenous methylprednisolone in adults in status asthmaticus. *Chest* **82**:438-440.

Tarlo, S. M., Broder, I., Davies, G. M., Leznoff, A., Mintz, S., and Corey, P. N. (1988). Six month, double-blind, controlled trial of high dose, concentrated beclomethasone dipropionate in the treatment of severe chronic asthma. *Chest* **5**:998-1002.

Tiffeneau, R., and Dunoyer, P. (1956). Action de la cortisone sur l'hypersensibilite cholinergique pulmonaire de l'asthmatique. *Presse Med.* **64**: 719-721.

Toogood, J. H., Lefcoe, N. M., Haines, D. S. M., Jennings, B. A., Errington, N., Baksh, L., and Chuang, L. (1977a). A graded dose assessment of the efficacy of beclomethasone dipropionate aerosol for severe chronic asthma. *J. Allergy Clin. Immunol.* **59**:298-308.

Toogood, J. H., Baskerville, J., Errington, N., Chuang, L., and Lefcoe, N. (1977b). Determinants of the response to beclomethasone aerosol at various dosage levels: a multiple regression analysis to identify clinically useful predictors. *J. Allergy Clin. Immunol.* **60**:367-376.

Toogood, J. H., Jennings, B., Greenway, R. W., and Chuang, L. (1980). Candidiasis and dysphonia complicating beclomethasone treatment of asthma. *J. Allergy Clin. Immunol.* **65**:145-153.

Toogood, J. H., Jennings, B., Baskerville, J., and Newhouse, M. (1981). Assessment of a device for reducing oropharyngeal complications during beclomethasone treatment of asthma. *Am. Rev. Respir. Dis.* **123**:113.

Toogood, J. H., Baskerville, J. C., Jennings, B., Lefcoe, N. M., and Johansson, S. A. (1982). Influence of dosing frequency and schedule on the response of chronic asthmatics to the aerosol steroid, budesonide. *J. Allergy Clin. Immunol.* **70**:288-298.

Toogood, J. H., Jennings, B., Baskerville, J., and Lefcoe, N. M. (1984a). Personal observations on the use of inhaled corticosteroid drugs for chronic asthma. *Eur. J. Respir. Dis.* **65**:321-338.

Toogood, J. H., Jennings, B., Baskerville, J., Anderson, J., and Johansson, S. A. (1984b). Dosing regimen of budesonide and occurrence of oropharyngeal complications. *Eur. J. Respir. Dis.* **65**:35-44.

Toogood, J. H., Baskerville, J., Jennings, B., Lefcoe, N. M., and Johansson, S-A. (1984c). Use of spacers to facilitate inhaled corticosteroid treatment of asthma. *Am. Rev. Respir. Dis.* **129**:723-729.

Toogood, J. H. (1987). Comparisons between inhaled and oral corticosteroids in patients with chronic asthma. In *Advances in the Use of Inhaled Corticosteroids*. Edited by R. Ellul-Micaleff, W. K. Lam, and J. H. Toogood. Amsterdam, Excerpta Medica, pp. 140-149.

Toogood, J. H., Crilly, R. G., Jones, G., Nadeau, J., and Wells, G. A. (1988). Effect of high-dose inhaled beclomethasone on calcium and phosphate metabolism and the risk of osteoporosis. *Am. Rev. Respir. Dis.* **138**: 57-61.

Van der Star, J. G., Berg, W. C., Steenhuis, E., and de Vries, K. (1976). The effect of beclomethasone dipropionate aerosol on bronchial obstruction after the inhalation of house dust. *Ned. Tijdschr. Geneeskd.* **120**:1928-1932.

Vandenberg, R., Tovey, E., Love, I., Russell, P., Tidmarsh, J., Wilson, P., and Geddes, B. (1975). A trial of a new inhalational steroid preparation in treatment of steroid dependent chronic asthmatics. *Med. J. Aust.* **1**:189-191.

Vaz, R., Senior, B., Morris, M., and Binkiewicz, A. (1982). Adrenal effects of beclomethasone inhalation therapy in asthmatic children. *J. Pediatr.* **100**:660-662.

Venge, P. (1985). Eosinophil and neutrophil granulocytes in asthma. In *Glucocorticosteroids, Inflammation and Bronchial Hyperreactivity*. Edited by J. C. Hogg, R. Ellul-Micaleff, and R. Brattsand. Basel, Excerpta Medica, pp. 21-37.

Wardlaw, A. J., Dunnette, S., Gleich, G. J., Collins, J. V., and Kay, A. B. (1988). Eosinophils and mast cells in bronchoalveolar lavage in subjects with mild asthma. Relationship to bronchial reactivity. *Am. Rev. Respir. Dis.* **137**:62-69.

Weller, F. R., Weller, H. H., Kallenberg, C. G. M., The, T. H., and Orie, N. G. M. (1986). Sensitivity to hydrocortisone is relevant factor in the immunoendocrine relationship. *J. Allergy Clin. Immunol.* **78**:423-30.

Wilmsmeier, W., Wagner, T. O. F., and Sybrecht, G. W. (1986). Effect of inhaled versus oral steroids on symptoms, bronchial hyperreactivity and adrenal function in asthmatic patients. *Bull. Eur. Physiopathol.* **22**:91.

Wolfe, J. D., Rosenthal, R. R., Bleecker, E., Laube, B., Norman, P. S., and Permutt, S. (1979). The effect of corticosteroids on cholinergic hyperreactivity. *J. Allergy Clin. Immunol.* **63**:162.

Woolcock, A. J., Yan, K., and Salome, C. M. (1988). Effect of therapy on bronchial hyperresponsiveness in the long-term management of asthma. **18**:165-176.

Wyatt, R., Waschek, J., Weinberger, M., and Sherman, B. (1978). Effects of inhaled beclomethasone dipropionate and alternate day prednisone on pituitary-adrenal function in children with chronic asthma. *N. Engl. J. Med.* **299**:1387-1392.

Wyllie, A. H., Pozansky, M. C., and Gordon, A. C. H. (1986). Glucocorticoid-resistant asthma: evidence for a defect in mononuclear cells. In *Asthma. Clinical Pharmacology and Therapeutic Progress.* Edited by A. B. Kay. Oxford, Blackwell Scientific Publications, pp. 306-314.

24

Glucocorticoids
Experimental Approaches

RALPH BRATTSAND

AB Draco,
Lund, Sweden

ULF PIPKORN

University Hospital of Lund
Lund, Sweden

I. Introduction

Glucocorticoids (GCS) have a multiplicity of physiological and pharmacological actions (for reviews, see Ellul-Micallef, 1987; Schleimer et al., 1989), and it is currently difficult to pinpoint which actions are the most essential for their antiasthmatic efficacy. Probably their unique efficacy depends on a combination of several mechanisms, leading to a broad anti-inflammatory activity. Before one starts to discuss any therapeutic implication of GCS, it is important to bear in mind that GCS are naturally occurring hormones that have important physiological roles in normal human homeostasis (Addison, 1855; Baxter and Rousseau, 1979). When GCS are administered with a pharmacological aim, it should be noted that the desired but also the unwanted effects are mostly exaggerations of their normal physiological functions, even if certain effects of the drugs never are reached with endogenously released GCS. It has been proposed that one major physiological functions of GCS is to modulate the response to stress (Munch et al., 1984). One role may be to protect tissues outside a localized inflammation or infection to toxic host-defense mechanisms of the body. To exert such protection in the systemic circulation the evolution has given GCS the ability to induce various acute as well as protracted anti-inflammatory activities. The hypothesis of the stress response as a feedback system aimed at triggering endogenous anti-inflammatory actions (Fig. 1) is supported by new findings showing that even sub-pyrogenic dosages of interleukin I (IL-1) can induce adrenocorticotrophic hormone (ACTH) and cortisol secretion (Besedovsky et al., 1986). Other experiments have shown that administration of IL-1 can protect against carrageenan-induced edema via such enhanced GCS secretion (Nakamura et al., 1988). As well as this stress-induced triggering of anti-inflammatory activity, the normal physiological GCS levels (with their diurnal variation) attenuate inflammation. An exaggerated response to inflammatory stimuli is easily demonstrated in adrenalectomized rats (Flower et al., 1986; Laue et al., 1988; Brattsand et al., unpublished data).

Crucial points to discuss are the dose at target site and the duration of treatment required to induce the various types of anti-inflammatory action.

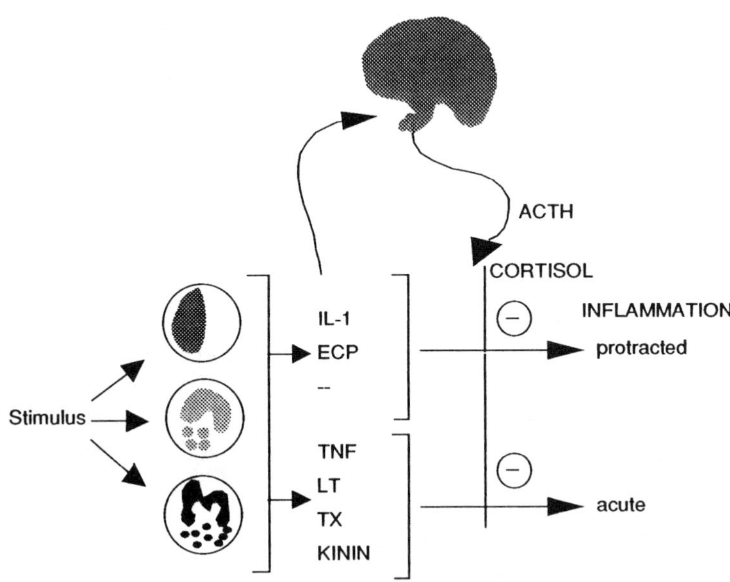

Figure 1 The stress response: an anti-inflammatory feedback system. Even in sub-pyrogenic doses IL-1 can (Besedovsky et al., 1986) trigger ACTH release and, by that, enhanced cortisol production. TNF may also have this ability. The physiological purpose of this feedback system is probably to protect tissues outside a local inflammation site from toxic host defense mechanisms. To exert protection of that kind, evolution has given glucocorticosteroids the ability to trigger several types of anti-inflammatory actions against both acute as well as protracted inflammation.

These points are well suited for experimental approaches. Regarding duration, the time period during which the GCS needs to be present in surplus around the target cell (here called *trigger time*) and the latency time (time from GCS deposition to appearance of biological effects) must be differentiated. Protracted trigger and latency times can sometimes be examined in vitro works but frequently in vivo studies are required. Long treatment periods are often discussed for induction of unwanted effects such as atropy and reduction of growth (Munch et al., 1984), but should be equally stressed for induction of certain desirable effects. For example, the lack of induction of dermal atrophy and of inhibitory effects on allergen-induced immediate wheal and flare responses by short-term glucocorticoid treatment is well known (Poothullil et al., 1976; Talbot et al., 1987). On the other hand, long-term local dermal GCS therapy with potent preparations will induce dermal atrophy (Stefanovic, 1972) as well as a strong reduction in the wheal and flare responses in the skin (Pipkorn et al., 1989a).

This review will discuss experimental approaches to clarifying the underlying mechanisms for the therapeutic efficacy of GCS in asthma. Since the main clinical improvement of GCS therapy during the last years has been reached through inhaled GCS, special emphasis will be devoted to the action and mechanisms induced by such drugs.

II. Main Pathophysiological Mechanisms in Asthma as Seen in a Challenge Setting

The main thrust during recent years has been to stress asthma as an inflammatory disease of the lower airways characterized by the presence of, for example, eosinophils rather than as a spasmodic disease (Hargreave et al., 1986; Kay, 1986; Wardlaw et al., 1988). A similar trend has emerged in the discussion of the pathophysiology of allergic rhinitis, which could then be considered to constitute an inflammatory disease of the upper airways, also characterized by the presence of eosinophils (Bascom et al., 1988; Naclerio et al., 1987). With this in mind, it should be relevant to draw conclusions about mode of action of such an anti-inflammatory drug as GCS on basic expressions of mucosal inflammation, regardless of whether these are based on findings obtained in the lower or upper airways. The human upper airways allow accessibility to repeated in vivo samplings of cells, secretion, and measurements of various vascular parameters such as blood flow and plasma leakage, which are not obtainable in the lower airway (Naclerio et al., 1984; Holmberg et al., 1988; Pipkorn and Karlsson, 1988; Svensson et al., 1989). Furthermore, the same individual can be studied in a symptom-free and a symptomatic state, such as in normal seasonal hay fever (Pipkorn et al., 1989b; Andersson et al., 1989c), and nasal allergen challenge experiments can be done easily and in a safe way in humans (Pipkorn et al., 1988b). Based on such experiments, there are several pieces of relevant upper airway data included in the present review. Similar experimental data are not yet available from the lower airways.

GCS can, in theory, act on every step involved in the pathogenesis of allergic mucosa, whether it occurs in the lower airways, as asthma, or in the upper airways, as in rhinitis. Well aware that challenge experiments cannot mimic the complete disease of asthma, we will nevertheless look upon the various putative pathogenetic aspects as seen in a laboratory allergen challenge setting. In such experiments an initial trigger leads to mediator release, giving rise to an initial response and often to a protracted late inflammatory phase, with features such as obstruction or symptoms, change in airway reactivity, and an influx of inflammatory cells (Fig. 2).

A. Immediate Response

GCS might interfere with mechanisms leading to the presence and degree of sensitization of mediator cells as well as with those cells involved in the establishment of contact between these and the offending allergen. The contact between the antigen and the trigger cells loaded with IgE on its surface leads to the release of proinflammatory mediators, which can act directly on

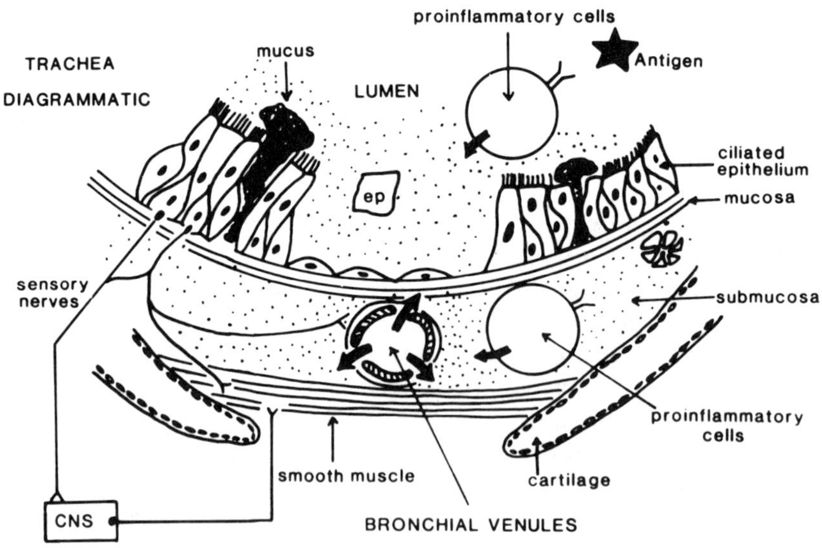

Figure 2 Diagrammatic presentation of bronchial mucosa and submucosa as target area for GCS therapy in asthma. ep, Sloughed epithelium (from O'Donnell, 1988).

the target organs and indirectly by inducing neural reflexes. As part of the pathogenesis, the airways may also have a constitutional or acquired "habitual" change in responsiveness to mediators (Altounyan, 1970; Hartley and Walters, 1982). This may well be a result of a prolonged inflammatory state and in this review this is differentiated from the rapid change in responsiveness seen after a single allergen exposure, a phenomenon that has been termed *priming* (Connell, 1969). The initial signs and symptoms produced by the mediators released would then be considered the immediate response in an allergen challenge model. As well as a decrease in "habitual hyperreactivity" (Easton, 1981; Ryan et al., 1985) seen after long-term therapy, the GCS were previously considered to lack any inhibitory effect on the immediate response to allergen in a challenge situation (Booij-Nord et al., 1972; Pepys and Hutchcroft, 1975; Martin et al., 1980). This notion was mainly based on studies using rather short-term treatments with oral steroids prior to the allergen challenge. There is, however, accumulating evidence showing that GCS have an inhibitory effect on the immediate allergic response as well. This effect becomes apparent after prolonged treatment with topical GCS. The GCS-induced inhibition of the immediate response is most rapidly induced in experimental challenges of the upper airways, in which 1 week of topical GCS treatment induced a 40-50% reduction in the signs and symptoms of the immediate response (Vilsviik et al., 1975; Okuda and Senba, 1980; Pipkorn, 1982a; Pipkorn et al., 1987c) (see Fig. 5). Similar effects of prolonged treatment with topical GCS have been obtained in the lower airways (Dahl and Johansson, 1982; Burge, 1982) as well as in the skin (Andersson and Pipkorn, 1987; Pipkorn et al., 1989a).

B. Expressions of Postallergen Mucosal Inflammatory Response

The immediate response is often followed by a protracted inflammatory response. The two responses may exhibit a biphasic pattern (Booij-Nord et al., 1972) but, depending on the variable measured, a more continuous protracted response pattern is also evident (Hammarlund et al., 1989). The protracted inflammatory reaction may include a local accumulation of inflammatory cells, specifically the eosinophil in the tissue that has been experimentally exposed to the allergen (deMonchy et al., 1985; Bascom et al., 1988; Solley et al., 1976). Similar kinetics of eosinophilic infiltration have been demonstrated following natural allergen exposure in patients with allergic mucosal disease (Pipkorn et al., 1988b). The allergen challenge-induced late decrease in forced expiratory volume (FEV) in the lower airways is often referred to as the "late phase response" (Booij-Nord et al., 1972). In order not to confound this term with other expressions of the post-allergen inflammatory response one should at each instance clarify what is meant when the term *late phase response* is used and perhaps avoid it as a general term of just one part of a reaction. Another important expression of the postallergen inflammatory response is a change in responsiveness to exposure to specific as well as unspecific stimuli (Connell, 1969; Cockcroft et al., 1987; Naclerio et al., 1987; Pipkorn et al., 1987b,c; Andersson et al., 1989a,b). This change occurs in actual disease, as is clearly demonstrated in patients with seasonal allergic disease, whether in the upper and lower airways (Sotomayor et al., 1984; Konno et al., 1981). From a pathogenetic point of view, the enhanced responsiveness could be considered a vicious circle. As will be described below, the seasonally altered responsiveness is susceptible to GCS treatment (Sotomayor et al., 1984; Borum et al., 1983).

III. Basic Subcellular Mechanisms of GCS Activity

A. GCS Receptors

It is generally considered that most effects of GCS are secondary to stimulation of specific GCS receptors (GCS-R), which are present in most cell types including lung tissue. For overviews on GCS-R, see work by Baxter and Rousseau (1979), Wikström et al. (1987), and Brönnegård (1988). The main concepts of the receptor theory on steroid hormone action are shown in Figure 3. Due to their lipophilic character, endogenous as well as synthetic GCS penetrate freely into the cell cytoplasm, where they can interact with the specific

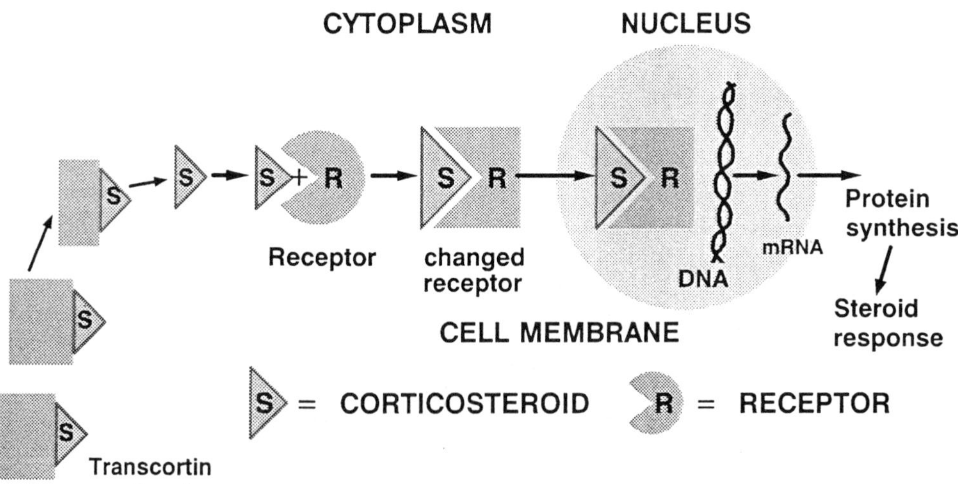

Figure 3 Model for the basic subcellular mechanism of GCS action.

GCS-R. It has not been hitherto possible to differentiate the GCS-R into subtypes in the normal cells of the body. The binding of a GCS agonist leads to a conformational change so that the DNA-binding site of GCS-R can bind to DNA and activate transcription. The complex binds to 5'-sequences of target genes upstream of the site of initiation of transcription (Brönnegård, 1988). At these sites the complex acts as a transcriptional enhancer. However, there are examples also of negative regulations, for example, the down-regulation of mRNA-formation for the GCS-R by the hormone itself (homologous regulation) and for IL-1. A moderate downregulation of the number of GCS-R seems to occur within some hours after the start of intense GCS treatment.

The prerequisite of receptor coupling for the induction of GCS activity is strongly supported by studies with different steroid structures (Baxter and Rousseau, 1979). Figure 4 demonstrates within a series of nine GCS agonists of different potency a close positive correlation (r = 0.98) between their affinity to the rat GCS-R (given as relative binding affinity) and their topical anti-inflammatory potency in vivo (given as relative potency). This suggests that the affinity to the GCS receptor can predict the intrinsic GCS activity at the application site. However, this prompt method of estimating GCS potency must be complemented with a check that the steroid is an agonist leading to

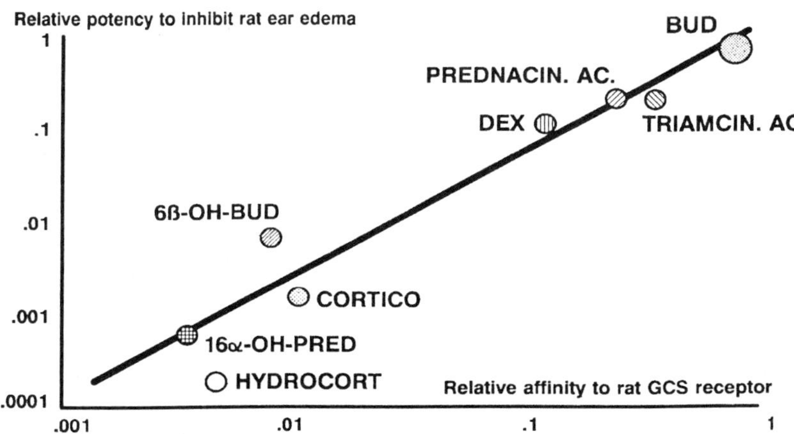

Figure 4 Correlation between the relative binding affinity to rat GCS receptor (determined in vitro) and the topical anti-inflammatory potency in the rat ear edema model (determined in vivo). Bud, budesonide; Prednacin.ac., prednacinolone acetonide; Triamcin.ac., triamcinolone acetonide; Dex, dexamethasone; cortico, corticosterone; 16α-OH-Pred, 16α-OH-prednisolone; Hydrocort., hydrocortisone (adapted from Dahlberg et al., 1984; Brattsand et al., 1987).

functional GCS activity. Some steroid structures can bind to the GCS-R in such a manner that the complex does not function in the subsequent steps (e.g., the GCS antagonist RU 38486). With such antagonists it has been demonstrated that the antiedema efficacy of dexamethasone in the carrageenan pleurisy, paw, and peritonitis models are all mediated over GCS-R (Tsurufuji et al., 1980; Peers et al., 1988; Hirschmann et al., 1988). Also the inhibiting effect of GCS on leukocyte infiltration and on generation of PGE_2, LTB_4 and lyso-PAF was reversed by RU 38486 (Peers et al., 1988; Laue et al., 1988).

B. Time-Sequence Studies of Receptor Mechanism

Trigger Time

Time sequence studies in isolated cells have shown that the coupling to the cytoplasmic GCS-R happens within seconds (Fahey et al., 1981), the activation of this complex takes 30-60 s, and the subsequent nuclear binding less than 10 s. This means that already within a few minutes there may be a production of mRNA (Fahey et al., 1981). which can then propagate the response further to the ribosomes (Fig. 3). The half-life of the mRNA for the main GCS-induced proteins is not known, but as an example it can be mentioned that the mRNA for the GCS-R itself has a half-life of a few hours. Hence for triggering a cellular action, the critical time for presence of GCS may be only minutes. For some types of GCS actions this is also supported by functional studies. Crabtree et al. (1979) have reported that cortisol needed to be present just for the first 5 min to trigger reduced glucose uptake and subsequent cell lysis in thymocytes. A short trigger time is also sufficient for the vascular antipermeability effect of GCS (Svensjö and Roempke, 1985; Miller-Larsson and Brattsand, 1990). On the other hand, induction of some other GCS actions (e.g., reduced lymphocyte proliferation [Axelsson, B., unpublished data], reduced TNF production [Waage and Bakke, 1988] requires continuous GCS contact for a much longer period than just a few minutes.

Latency Time

The full mechanism sequence outlined in Figure 3 (including new protein synthesis) normally requires a latency time of 1 to several hours until biological activity appears. However, for some actions a shorter latency time can be demonstrated, probably due to the presence of a preformed pool of proteins mediating the activity (see below). Thus Blackwell et al. (1980) showed that in rat leukocytes there is a lipocortin pool, which can be released within 30 min after GCS induction. However, this release also seems to be receptor mediated. After this rapid release there is a prolonged latency time until new lipocortin has been synthesized and can be secreted (Carnuccio et al., 1981).

C. GCS-Induced Proteins as Mediators of Biological Activity

Because the anti-inflammatory action of GCS is blocked by inhibitors of RNA and protein synthesis (Tsurufuji et al., 1980; Fahey et al., 1981) it is generally agreed that this action depends on the induction of new proteins or peptides. Regarding the number of protein species induced, Voris and Young (1981) found in thymocytes that the synthesis of six to eight proteins was reinforced in the presence of GCS. For some proteins the reinforcement was evident within 15-30 min, while the concentration of others was enhanced first after several hours. Table 1 summarizes the properties of some proteins proposed to be mediators of the anti-inflammatory action of GCS.

Lipocortins and Lipocortinlike Proteins

Sequence analyses show that the lipocortins belong to a large family of calcium- and phospholipid-binding proteins. The main biochemical activity proposed for the lipocortins is their ability to block phospholipase A_2 and by that the formation of arachidonic acid metabolites. Human lipocortin I is reported to

Table 1 Proteins Proposed to Mediate Anti-Inflammatory Activity of GCS

Protein	Physiochemical properties	Biochemical activity in vitro	Anti-inflammatory activity in vivo
Lipocortin I[a]			
Macrocortin	35-40 kDa, heat	Inhibition of	Carrageenan rat
Lipomodulin	stable	PLA_2[b,c,d]	paw and pleural
Renocortin			edema[a,b,c,d]
Uteroglobin-like protein[e,f]	15 kDa	Inhibition of PLA_2[g]	Carrageenan rat paw edema[e]
Vasocortin[b]	100 kDa heat labile	Not known	Dextran and sero-tonin rat paw edema[b,h,i]

[a]Flower, 1988.
[b]Koltai et al., 1987.
[c]Miele et al., 1988.
[d]Cirino et al., 1989.
[e]Volovitz et al., 1988.
[f]Dhanireddy et al., 1988.
[g]Miele et al., 1987.
[h]Carnuccio et al., 1987.
[i]Di Rosa et al., 1985.

be cloned and expressed in *E. coli* (Wallner et al., 1986). Based on that product, Cirino et al. (1989) could block the part of carrageenan-induced inflammation triggered via PLA_2. However, in the cell line U937 the inducibility by GCS of lipocortin I has been questioned (Bienkowski et al., 1989). Uteroglobin-like protein has been demonstrated in secretions from the tracheobronchial tree (Volovitz et al., 1988) and deserves further investigation in patients with asthma.

Vasocortin

Vasocortin is a separate entity from the lipocortins. It does not inhibit PLA_2 in vitro and in vivo it has shown an anti-inflammatory profile complementary to that of native lipocortin. Vasocortin reduces dextran and serotonin but not carrageenan-induced paw edema (Di Rosa et al., 1985; Carnuccio et al., 1987; Koltai et al., 1987), while lipocortin reportedly inhibits edema provoked by carrageenan but not by the other two mediators. Vasocortin is recovered in peritoneal lavage 1 h after GCS treatment. Anti-inflammatory activity has been shown (Koltai et al., 1987), even for small fragments of vasocortin (2 and 6 kDa). The sequence of these fragments or of the native protein has not yet been described.

GCS-Induced Receptors and Enzymes

The β-receptor and angiotensin-converting enzyme (ACE, kininase II) are examples of proteins whose synthesis is reported to be enhanced by GCS treatment. In lung cells in culture, GCS induces a doubling of the rate of β-receptor synthesis (Fraser and Venter, 1980). There is a latency time of several hours until the new β-receptors appear. After a few hours, GCS treatment enhances ACE activity in rabbit alveolar macrophages, and in rat lung (Di Rosa et al., 1985). ACE is one of the most important pathways for the inactivation of the inflammatory mediator bradykinin, and it may cleave this mediator during passage through the pulmonary vasculature (Bakhle et al., 1969). However, there are still no functional studies published that have investigated whether GCS pretreatment leads to a raised tolerance to exogenous bradykinin.

Current Status of GCS-Induced Proteins

Based on our knowledge of these proteins as mediators for GCS activity, it has been speculated that a more selective anti-inflammatory activity might be reached by using one of these proteins (produced by biotechnology) or even its active site (a small peptide produced by organic synthesis). However, much knowledge remains to be gained about which protein or which combination of proteins mediates the wanted and unwanted GCS actions, respectively, as well as the intra- and extracellular distribution of these proteins. The current thought is that an inflammation induced via released PLA_2 might be partially counteracted by recombinant lipocortin (Cirino et al., 1989), or by small peptides derived from lipocortinlike structures (Miele et al., 1988). However, because most types of inflammation are triggered via several signal transduction systems, it is not surprising that Ialenti et al. (1990) reported a better anti-inflammatory activity by combining lipocortinlike peptide with vasocortin than with each single agent. Even that combination would probably lack the receptor and enzyme-inducing potential of the GCS itself.

D. Effect on Secretion of IL-I and Tumor Necrosis Factor

The production of IL-1 seems to play a central role in the initiation of inflammatory responses in the lung (Bochner et al., 1987a). GCS can inhibit IL-1 production in vitro as well as in vivo (Staruch and Wood, 1985). Recent studies in monocytes demonstrate that the reduced IL secretion by a low concentration of GCS is mediated over the GCS-R and that there are blocks at several steps in the IL-1 processing: reduced mRNA formation, enhanced lability of the mRNA formed, and a blocked posttranscriptional processing (Knudsen et al., 1987; Kern et al., 1988; Lee et al., 1988). The last block could be demonstrated also when the GCS was not added until after the inflammatory stimulus. GCS also induces a block of TNF secretion. According to in vitro experiments, the block in TNF production requires a long coincubation time with GCS (48 h) (Waage et al., 1988).

IV. Effects of GCS on Selected Pathophysiological Mechanisms

A. IgE-Mediated Triggering

The initial trigger in the allergic response in atopic disease is generally believed to be the antigens acting on sensitized mediator cells, leading to an activation of these cells with subsequent release of proinflammatory mediators. It has been shown that prolonged treatment with topical glucocorticoids has an inhibitory effect on antigen-induced immediate reaction in vivo in human airways (Dahl and Johansson, 1982; Pipkorn, 1982a). Underlying mechanisms to this inhibition may theoretically involve a reduction of IgE production, reduction of IgE on the surface of the mediator cells, reduced responsiveness of the mediator cells (mast cells), reduced number or a redistribution of mast cells, reduced content of mediators in these cells, or perhaps a combination of these explanations. Systemic GCS treatment has minimal influence on the levels of circulating antibody levels (Settipane et al., 1987; Posey et al.,

1978). It is therefore highly unlikely that topical treatment with GCS would induce any reduction in the available amounts of circulating IgE. In vitro evidence (short-term incubation with glucocorticoids) indicates that there could be a reduction of IgE levels on the surface of mast cells due to GCS treatment (Yodoi et al., 1981). Local dermal GCS injection 90 min before local IgE injection protected rabbit skin against antigen challenge 3 days later via an immunological but not via an anti-inflammatory mechanism (Hellewell and Williams, 1989). Whether such a reduction in cell surface IgE is also present in humans in vivo is not known.

Effect on IgE-Mediated Mast Cell Release

Short-term in vitro GCS incubation of isolated human lung mast cells (Schleimer et al., 1983) or of human lung fragments (Bergstrand et al., 1986) does not to any great extent inhibit the anti-IgE or allergen-induced mediator release. This is in agreement with a minimal clinical influence on the immediate response by short-term GCS treatment. There are no in vitro studies on isolated mast cells using the prolonged treatment times required clinically to inhibit the immediate response to antigen challenge. After topical in vivo treatment for 1 week, a reduction of histamine release from human nasal tissue or from nasal secretion has, however, been clearly demonstrated (Pipkorn and Andersson, 1982; Pipkorn et al., 1987c) (Fig. 5).

Effects on Mast Cell Number and Tissue Histamine Content

In theory, the GCS-induced reduction of histamine release in vivo (Pipkorn, 1982a; Pipkorn et al., 1987c) could be explained by a reduction in the number of mediator cells in the tissue, besides making them less responsive to stimulation. This could be a crucial point since it has been shown that the density of mast cells near the epithelial surface is closely related to the reactivity of the airways in symptomatic disease (Flint et al., 1985; Pipkorn et al., 1989b). Also the immediate response in the skin is related to the density of mast cells in the dermis (Pipkorn et al., 1989a). On judging such studies, one should clarify if initially symptomatic individuals are studied. As an expression of the active disease, these cells may be present in altered number or location (Enerbäck et al., 1986, Flint et al., 1985). Furthermore, in active disease the activation of mast cells with subsequent mediator release might make these cells harder to detect using standard techniques for visualization. If allergic individuals are studied under baseline, nonsymptomatic conditions, a state under which it has been possible to show a glucocorticoid-induced reduction in the allergen-induced mediator generation (Pipkorn et al., 1987c), there appears to be no GCS-induced reduction of the number of mast cells in the airway mucosa (Pipkorn, 1983).

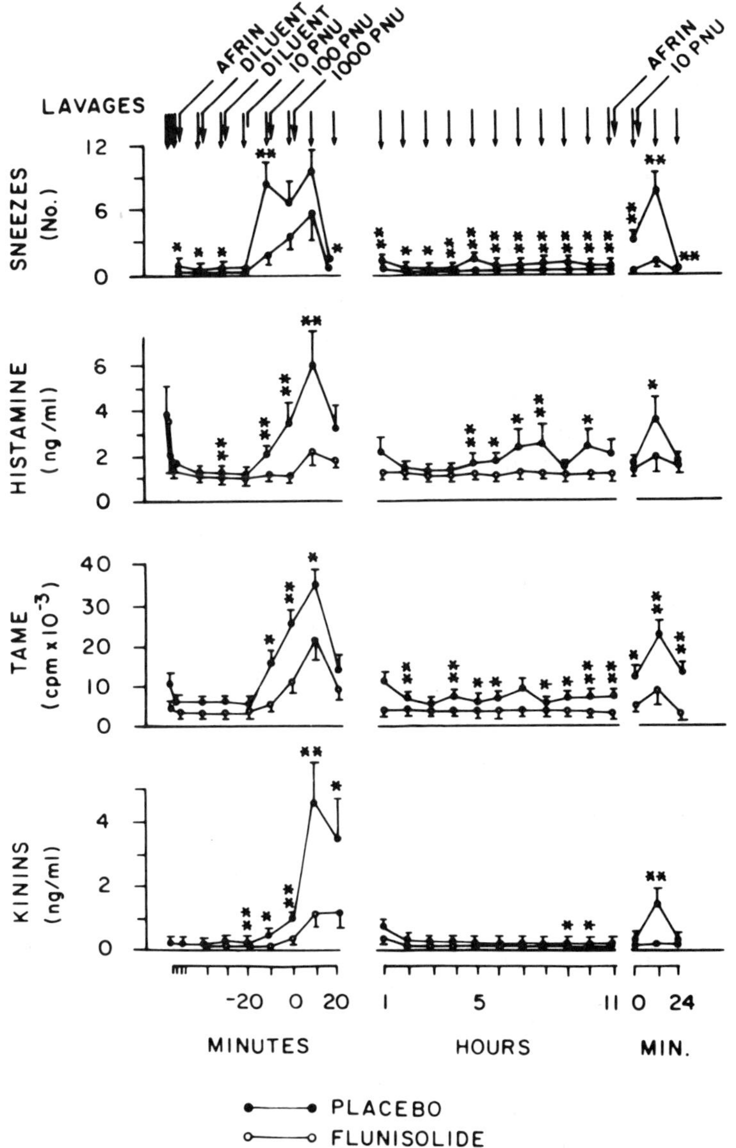

Figure 5 Nasal symptoms and levels of inflammatory mediators in nasal lavage following a nasal challenge with antigen after 1 week of placebo or flunisolide pretreatment. Shown are results obtained in the immediate phase after antigen challenge (0-20 min), in the protracted postallergen inflammatory phase (1-11 h), and the augmented postallergen increase in specific reactivity (last part). As shown, the active pretreatment inhibited symptoms and mediator generation in the immediate phase, ablated any increases in the protracted phase, and blocked the increase in reactivity (redrawn from Pipkorn et al., 1987b).

In studies investigating symptomatic patients, a much more conflicting picture is present, with some authors demonstrating an inhibition by GCS of the increased presence of mast cells (Okuda and Senba, 1980; Viegas et al., 1987) or no effect of GCS (Wihl et al., 1983; Orgel et al., 1986). Others fail to show an increase in mast cell number or GCS effects on this number (Pipkorn and Enerbäck, 1987). These discrepancies might be explained by differences in techniques used for sampling and visualization of the cells and/or differences in symptoms of the patients or timing of the samplings in relation to pollen exposure. Further studies that take all these factors into consideration must be done to clarify putative GCS effects on mast cell density in airways mucosa.

After 1 week of treatment with topical GCS, asymptomatic patients with hay fever showed only a minor reduction in histamine tissue levels (Pipkorn and Andersson, 1982). Even 3 weeks' treatment with topical glucocorticoids from the start of a pollen season did not drastically reduce the level of tissue histamine (Pipkorn and Enerbäck, 1987). Since histamine is stored mainly in mast cells, these findings are consistent with minimal GCS-induced changes in mast cell numbers (Pipkorn and Enerbäck, 1987). The GCS levels obtained in the mucosa of the upper airways would be much higher than those obtained in the tissue of the lower airways (the same GCS dosage is usually used in patients with rhinitis and asthma). It is, therefore, not unreasonable to suggest that topical GCS have limited actions on histamine-containing cells in the lower airways as well.

It becomes apparent that the target dosage and especially the duration of treatment are important for demonstrating an inhibitory effect of GCS on IgE-triggering events. Thus a high GCS dosage at the target site and a long duration of treatment appears crucial. However, the underlying mechanisms behind the inhibition remain to be clarified.

B. Other Triggers

Mast cells may also be activated through physical and resulting osmotic changes (Shaw et al., 1985; Eggleston et al., 1984). This has been confirmed in the upper airways, where cold dry air in selected individuals can trigger mast cells to release histamine, leading to symptoms of airway disease (Togias et al., 1985). So far, such an evidence for mast cell activation as a triggering event for reactions of the lower airways is limited (Iikura et al., 1988). However, given this background hypothesis, glucocorticoids may be effective via similar mechanisms as for the antigen-induced triggering events. Topical glucocorticoids are clinically effective in exercise-induced asthma as well as in nonallergic perennial (vasomotor) rhinitis (Henriksen, 1985; Lövkvist and Svensson, 1976). Furthermore, the latency time for demonstration of

GCS effects on non-IgE-mediated triggering events seems to be roughly similar to that for IgE-mediated events (Iikura et al., 1988), thus supporting similarities in protective mechanisms. For both types of events, the latency time to demonstrate GCS effects on the "habitual" changes in responsiveness appears to be even longer than for inhibiting the "immediate" responses, since improvement of such responsiveness might include a "normalization" of structurally changed airways (Woolcock et al., 1988).

C. Migration and Activation of Inflammatory Cells

Under experimental conditions, most proinflammatory mechanisms can be demonstrated to be reduced by GCS treatment (for review see Fahey et al., 1981; Kaliner, 1985; Ellul-Micallef, 1987; Schleimer et al., 1989). One should consider that several of these inhibitory activities are just putative for the therapeutic situation, since they have been demonstrated in vitro or in animals and often with supratherapeutic doses. Besides attenuating the principal inflammatory cells, GCS can also directly protect cells injured by the inflammatory process, such as endothelial and epithelial cells (see below) and fibroblasts.

Migration

Most evidence suggests that the target area for GCS treatment in asthma is the area outlined in Figure 2. Because inhaled GCS have minute GCS effect in the systemic circulation, many studies based on blood specimens may be less relevant. One such example is the effect on systemic redistribution of inflammatory cells. A single systemic dose of GCS results in marked change in the number of circulating cells. Most striking is the fall in the number of eosinophils, basophils, and monocytes to approximately 20% of the normal circulating quantity of each of these cell types (Saveedra-Delgado et al., 1980). The GCS effect is apparent within 4-6 h and abates by 24-48 h.

Since both the basophils and eosinophils are considered to be rather long-lived, the GCS effect is not thought to be a reduction of production of these cells in the bone marrow but a result of reversible sequestration of these cells in marrow or other tissues. The effect is transient when the treatment becomes continuous. This type of systemic redistribution is not seen after either short or prolonged inhalation of appropriate GCS dosages (Johansson et al., 1982; Lindqvist et al., 1986).

However, both oral and topical GCS can affect the influx of eosinophils into affected airway mucosa. Oral GCS treatment for 48 h prior to an allergen challenge has been shown to induce a blockage of the resulting influx of eosinophils (Bascom et al., 1989a). This was achieved without a concomitant reduction in the influx of neutrophils, but with a clinical improvment in the increase in responsiveness and late-occurring symptoms (Pipkorn et al., 1987a). Topically applied glucocorticoids, on the other hand, blocked the influx of most types of inflammatory cells (Fig. 6), thus suggesting a more general effect on cell recruitment.

The following discussion of GCS effects on cell recruitment and activation concentrates on human eosinophils and basophils. Even if there is only indirect evidence for these cells to be causative in airway inflammation and hyperresponsiveness, their presence in airway secretions is correlated with symptoms of asthma and rhinitis (Bascom et al., 1988, 1989a; Gibson et al., 1989). Thus, a reduction in their numbers or of their released products may at least indicate attenuation of allergic airway inflammation. The GCS-induced block of cellular influx into the target area may, theoretically, depend on reduced production of chemotactic stimuli, diminished responsiveness of inflammatory cells to these stimuli, or reduction of the inflammation-induced adhesiveness of the airway blood vessels. These putative mechanisms are discussed below.

In the allergic reaction, several chemotactic systems are activated and implicated for the recruitment of cells to the site of the allergic reaction (Kay, 1986; Venge et al., 1987). These systems include not only cell-specific chemo-

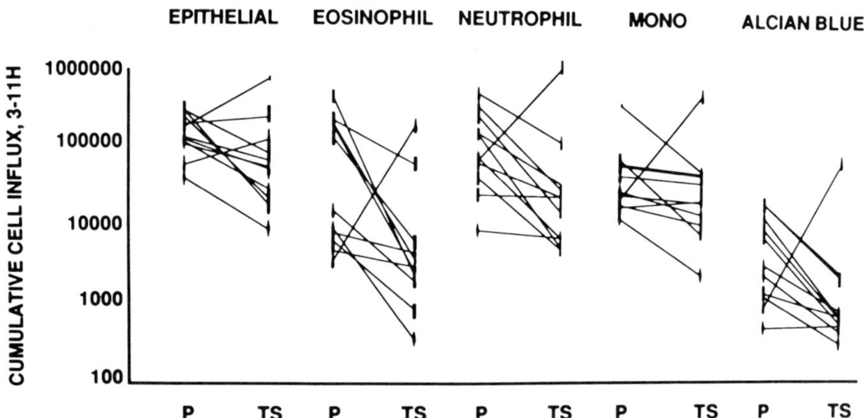

Figure 6 Effect of topical steroids on cumulative cell influx after a nasal antigen challenge. The cumulative influx is the sum of cells counted between 3 and 11 h after antigen challenge. Topical steroid treatment was associated with a significant reduction in the cumulative influx of eosinophils, neutrophils, and alcian-blue-stained cells (mast cells and basophils), but not mononuclear cells or epithelial cells (from Bascom et al., 1988; reproduced with permission from the *Journal of Allergy and Clinical Immunology*, **81**:580-589, 1988).

tactic activities but also substances that have been proposed to have an activity on several cell populations. Among the latter are the membrane-derived mediators, platelet-activating factor (PAF) and LTB_4. Both are produced by activation of the arachidonic acid through phospholipase A2. In vitro, GCS have been shown to decrease the activity of phospholipase A_2 via lipocortin formation (Flower, 1988). Thus, an attractive explanation is provided for the effect of GCS on the recruitment of cells to an inflammatory focus. GCS reduce the LTD_4, LTB_4, and PAF production of antigen-challenged guinea pig lung (Andersson et al., 1985, 1988). However, there are still no human data following challenge to show that GCS reduce the local release of arachidonic acid metabolites (Freeland et al., 1989). This lack of data is also substantiated by poor antiasthmatic efficacy of some tested leukotriene antagonists and lipoxygenase inhibitors.

A reduced cell influx may be secondary to a diminished responsiveness of the cells to chemotactic stimuli. When studied in Boyden chambers, GCS do not reduce the migratory response of human eosinophils (Venge et al., personal communication). However, GCS may reduce the adhesiveness of eosinophils (e.g., Altman et al., 1981) as well as inhibit the enhanced stickiness of inflamed vessels. A vascular site of action for the blocked cell recruitment by high GCS dosages is supported by the findings of Bascom et al. (1988). They demonstrated that topical treatment of nasal mucosa blocked the influx of most cell types. The underlying mechanism behind this broader activity is unclear but may putatively depend on modulation of adhesive proteins of the endothelial wall. Inflammatory mediators (e.g., IL-1) will induce expression in endothelial cells of adhesive proteins, which will trap cells as a first step in their migration to a localized inflammation (Rampart and Williams, 1989). Due to their high potency to reduce IL-1 formation also in lung (Bochner et al., 1987b), GCS would theoretically have the ability to reduce the formation of such adhesive proteins. If so, this may help to explain that the GCS-induced block of lymphocyte emigration depends on effects on the vessel wall and not on the lymphocyte itself (Chung et al., 1986).

Activation of Inflammatory Cells

In vitro incubation of human eosinophils with budesonide attenuates stimulus-induced release of the cytotoxic protein eosinophil catonic protein (ECP) (Venge and Dahl, 1989). With budesonide at 10^{-7} mol/L, which is a therapeutic concentration for the local site (see below), some reduction of ECP-release is seen after 30 min. Presumably due to combined effects through reduced influx and diminished degranulation, GCS attenuate the release of the eosinophil-derived cytotoxic proteins in human airways. When asthmatic patients inhaled budesonide for a 2-4 week period, a reduced ECP content

of bronchoalveolar lavage fluid has been demonstrated under basal conditions (Ådelroth et al., 1990) as well as after allergen challenge (De Monchy
et al., 1988). Oral GCS treatment of hospitalized patients reduced the eosinophil-derived major basic protein (MBP) content of sputum. In these patients
with more severe disease there was a latency time of several days to reach this
reduction (Friegas et al., 1981). Nasal inhalation of budesonide and flunisolide diminished the allergen-induced release of ECP, eosinophil-derived neurotoxin (EDN), or MBP (Bisgaard et al., 1990; Bascom et al., 1989b). Thus, a
reduced deposition of cytotoxic eosinophilic proteins in the airway mucosa
may be one important therapeutic action of GCS. A surprising finding is that
in asthmatic patients acute inhalation of budesonide will reduce the ECP levels
also in the systemic circulation (Venge et al., 1987). The underlying reason
for this is not clear, but may be either that blocking ECP release is one of
the most sensitive systemic actions of GCS or that the diminished blood content is secondary to the reduced ECP release in the airway and lung compartment. GCS do not reduce the formation of oxygen radicals of isolated
stimulated eosinophils (Stephanie Pincus, personal communications), so to
avoid that kind of cytotoxicity there must be a reduced influx of eosinophils.
Eosinophil products have been implicated in the genesis of the allergen-induced late-occurring symptoms (Friegas and Gleich, 1986; Gleich et al., 1988;
Wardlaw et al., 1988). A priming effect of eosinophil products on late airway obstruction is supported by the finding that the blood content of ECP
before challenge is correlated to the magnitude of the drop in FEV_1 during
the late bronchial obstruction (Venge et al., 1987). The relationship between
the postallergen hyperresponsiveness and eosinophil products has hitherto
been little studied in asthma. In the nose, this relationship is not conclusive
(Andersson et al., 1989c; Bascom et al., 1989b).

As studied by analyses of nasal washings, 1 week of topical GCS pretreatment can effectively block the allergen-challenge-induced influx of basophils (Bascom et al., 1988). Furthermore, there is clear evidence that GCS
reduce basophil degranulation (Schleimer et al., 1981; Bergstrand et al., 1984).
This reduced influx and activation of basophils may be a further mechanism
behind the GCS-induced reduction of late-occurring symptoms after allergen challenge.

D. Epithelial Integrity

Data from experimental animals as well as humans support the notion that
the function of the epithelium as a barrier to triggering events is a critical
function in the generation of changes in reactivity (Hogg and Eggleston,
1984). Activated eosinophils release cytotoxic agents that may participate in
sloughing of the epithelial lining (Friegas and Gleich, 1986; Gleich et al.,

1988; Dahl et al., 1988). Inhibition of eosinophils by GCS would be a logical explanation for a restored epithelial lining function. Although this is attractive as a hypothesis, functional human data linking epithelial morphology and degree of changed reactivity with the presence and activation of eosinophils are scarce. In the upper airways, where simultaneous monitoring of these parameters can be made, data have failed to demonstrate such a relationship (Bascom et al., 1989b; Andersson et al., 1989c). Furthermore, it is clear that a changed reactivity can occur following an allergen exposure without a visual disruption of the epithelial integrity (Enerbäck et al., 1986). Thus in topical GCS treatment of asthma a functional restoration of epithelium may well occur without evidence that the epithelial cells by themselves constitute a target for the GCS therapy.

E. Barrier Function of Microvascular Endothelium

The functional basis of inflammation-induced leakage of macromolecules into surrounding tissue is a reversible gap formation between endothelial cells of the postcapillary venules (for review, see Persson and Svensjö, 1985). What may be particular for airway inflammation is the presence of a huge vascular network in the submucosa, allowing it to deliver rapidly any extravasated components into the mucosa and even into the airway lumen. Of the released plasma components there are several systems with proinflammatory potential (e.g., the kallikrein, coagulation factors, plasminogen, proteases), which may contribute to and maintain edema of the airway wall, epithelial shedding, mucus thickening, and plugging (Persson, 1986; chap. 1): some of the signs characteristic for asthmatic airways. Hence, inhibition of plasma exudation was proposed as a major antiasthmatic action of GCS (Andersson and Persson, 1988).

In the upper airways, topical GCS have been shown to block any antigen-induced vascular leakage (Pipkorn et al., 1987a,b). The antipermeability efficacy of GCS in lower airways is supported by clinical studies based on sputum (see Chap. X) and by animal studies (Brattsand et al., 1987; Erjefält and Persson, 1986; Andersson and Persson, 1988). A direct action of GCS on the endothelial cell to stabilize them against contraction and resulting gap formation is probably central to this action. GCS receptors are present in endothelial cells (Johnson et al., 1982) and the antiedema action can be reversed by a GCS receptor antagonist (Peers et al., 1988). The latency time for appearance of the antiedema action can be as short as 1/2-1 h (Tsurufuji et al., 1980; Svensjö and Roempke, 1985; Miller-Larsson and Brattsand, 1990). Studies in the hamster cheek pouch show that GCS have a broad antiedema efficacy that is not limited to a single inflammatory mediator. Topical budesonide treatment can thus block leakage induced by "classic" mediators such as histamine and bradykinin, but also by oxidizing principles (tertiary butyl hydroperoxide) and by reperfusion after ischemia and by a PK-C activator (PMA) (Svensjö and Roempke, 1985; Persson et al., 1987). Both neutrophil-dependent (LTB_4-induced) and neutrophil-independent (histamine-induced) leakage is reduced (Björk et al., 1982). This suggests that GCS do not block leakage at the level of the triggering of the single inflammatory mediator but at some common later step in the activation process leading to the gap formation.

In a guinea pig model, budesonide blocked the late bronchial obstruction (Andersson et al., 1988) and the macromolecular extravasation into airway and lung tissue, but not the eosinophil number in BAL fluid (Andersson and Persson, 1988). The dose, which blocked the late obstruction, also reduced the extravasation, thus supporting a relationship between these two effects as proposed by Persson (1986) and O'Donnell (1988).

F. Bronchial Smooth Muscle Contraction

GCS have no direct bronchorelaxing activity on airway smooth muscle when added in vitro or given as in vivo pretreatment to healthy animals or humans (Andersson and Brattsand, 1982; Ramsdell et al., 1983). Even prolonged in vivo pretreatment does not affect the sensitivity of rat tracheal smooth muscle to contractile and relaxant drugs (Gustafsson and Persson, 1989). The early reports on a direct bronchorelaxing potential of GCS are dubious due to the vehicle used, lack of latency time, and difficulty in reproducing the relaxation with more potent synthetic GCS (for review see Ellul-Micallef, 1987).

However, GCS pretreatment blocks allergen-induced contraction of tracheal rings (Schleimer et al., 1987; Persson et al., 1989). The inhibitory activity probably depends on reduced release of anaphylactic mediators (Andersson and Brattsand, 1982; Andersson et al., 1985).

The importance of an effect of GCS on β-receptor-mediated bronchorelaxation in asthmatic persons is controversial. While prolonged treatment with β-agonists leads to a tolerance to the tremor-inducing action, there is much less tachyphylaxis to the bronchorelaxing activity of the β-agonist (Larsson et al., 1977). Therefore, in patients with light to moderate asthma restoration of the β-receptor function cannot be a major antiasthmatic mechanism of GCS. On the other hand, in patients with severe asthma, there seems to be a subset in whom subsensitivity to β-agonists develops (Ellul-Micallef, 1987). In such patients GCS administration restores the sensitivity to β-adrenergic bronchodilators (Ellul-Micallef, 1987; Brodde et al., 1988).

G. Nonspecific Hyperresponsiveness

It is not clear how the transitory hyperresponsiveness, which may be induced by acute allergen challenge, relates to the more persistent hyperresponsiveness seen in clinical asthma. It is reasonable to assume that there may be a continuum from acute hyperresponsiveness, to seasonal changes, and to the more long-standing changes observed in clinical asthma. Small changes of hyperresponsiveness may well start before symptomatic disease and structural changes eventually evolve.

One of the major novel findings with GCS therapy is its ability to suppress the nonspecific hyperresponsiveness. This ability has been demonstrated after acute allergen exposure, after seasonally altered responsiveness, as well as in asthmatic subjects with "habitual" hyperresponsiveness. The mechanisms behind this suppression are not known and may differ depending on the chronicity of hyperresponsiveness. Based on dose and time sequence studies, it has been shown that GCS-induced modulation of the transitory hyperresponsiveness after allergen exposure is at least partly different from the modulation of the late bronchial obstruction (Abraham et al., 1986). To suppress seasonal hyperresponsiveness, a treatment period of several weeks is essential (Borum et al., 1983; Sotomayor et al., 1984). To alleviate "habitual" hyperresponsiveness, months or even years of GCS treatment may be necessary (Woolcock et al., 1988) to reach the required functional and structural normalization of the airways. Such mechanistic studies are very hard to perform from an experimental point of view, but need clearly to be addressed in the clinic.

H. Airway Secretion

GCS reduce the amount of fluid lining the airways and this reduction is probably an important part of their unique therapeutic efficacy in severe asthma. The reduction probably depends on at least two mechanisms. There is accumulating evidence that plasma leakage is a crucial contributor to the fluid lining, including sputum (Persson, 1986). Since even short pulses of GCS have been shown to inhibit plasma leakage in animal models (cf. above), this effect explains the ability of GCS to reduce the amount of fluid as well as its albumin content (Moretti et al., 1984). There are also data from studies of the nose showing that systemic as well as topical GCS reduce the albumin content of airway secretions (Pipkorn et al., 1987a,b). Local production of mucus proteins may also be diminished by GCS. Incubation of feline and human airway mucosa in vitro with GCS reduced the glucoprotein production (Lundgren et al., 1988; Marom et al., 1984), which may contribute to a decreased viscosity of epithelial lining fluid. One report (Malm et al., 1982) proposes that topical GCS may inhibit metacholine-induced nasal secretions, but this finding has not been confirmed in upper or lower airways.

V. Pharmacological and Pharmacokinetic Aspects of GCS Development: Special Emphasis on Inhaled GCS

The most important step since GCS were introduced has been the development of GCS suitable for inhalation. The basis of local GCS therapy is that the therapeutic effect can be induced by triggering GCS receptors within the target area, reached by local GCS deposition, while the major side effects are provoked by GCS receptors located outside that area. In dermatology, the benefits of local GCS therapy were being used in the mid-1950s with application of topical hydrocortisone. For the treatment of asthma and rhinitis, it took nearly 20 years of further development to demonstrate the advantages of local treatment. In topical skin therapy there is a low risk of inducing general (systemic) GCS actions outside the treated area, because there is a restricted and retarded systemic absorption through the skin barrier (stratum corneum). This means that the rate of inactivation of absorbed GCS by biotransformation is normally not critical to avoid systemic actions. With inhalation therapy, on the other hand, there may be significant absorption of both the swallowed drug and that deposited in the airways (Ryrfeldt et al., 1982). This means that GCS optimal for inhalation must also be rapidly inactivated after absorption. The dilution occurring on uptake into the systemic circulation is not enough. Thus, inhalation of the potent and biostable (Tsuei et al., 1979) GCS dexamethasone produces antiasthmatic efficacy along with the side effects typical of oral therapy (Toogood and Lefcoe, 1965).

A. GCS Suitable for Inhalation

In the early 1970s it was shown that inhalation of selected GCS such as beclomethasone dipropionate, betamethasone valerate, and triamcinolone acetonide could alleviate the symptoms of asthma without depressing plasma cortisol levels or stunting the body growth to any appreciable extent (for review, see Mygind and Clark, 1980). An even better degree of differentiation between antiasthmatic efficacy and lack of systemic side effects was later shown for budesonide (for reviews see Brattsand et al., 1987; Barnes and Mygind, 1988; Brattsand, 1989). Flunisolide (Chaplin et al., 1980) is another GCS with favorable biotransformation, which has been developed for inhalational use. All five compounds mentioned above have an affinity for the GCS receptor that is at least 100 times higher than that of hydrocortisone (B, Axelsson, unpublished). This requirement is logical, since inhaled GCS are diluted over the vast airway surface, which explains the therapeutic failure with inhaled hydrocortisone, cortisone, and prednisolone (Mygind and Clark, 1980), all of which have a low receptor affinity.

Besides having high intrinsic potency, inhaled GCS need to be rapidly inactivated by liver biotransformation as demonstrated for BDP (Martin et al., 1973), flunisolide (Chaplin et al., 1980) and budesonide (Ryrfeldt et al., 1982; Andersson and Ryrfeldt, 1984). Selection of budesonide was based on work specifically designed to develop potent GCS with a low systemic activity due to rapid biotransformation (Brattsand et al., 1982b,c). This may explain why budesonide attains a better relationship between topical GCS activity and depression of plasma or urinary cortisol levels (Johansson et al., 1982; Löfdahl et al., 1984; Pedersen and Fuglsang, 1988) than is reached by BDP, which originally was developed for dermal use (Caldwell et al., 1968). The specificity of budesonide depends on the rapid biotransformation by human liver into metabolites with only 1/50-1/100 of the intrinsic GCS activity of budesonide (Edsbäcker et al., 1987; Dahlberg et al., 1984). This rapid and efficient inactivation explains the advantageous but unique low oral availability of budesonide (Table 2). Only 10% of the swallowed fraction of budesonide can contribute to systemic activity (Fig. 7). The fraction deposited in airway and lung (which is just a minor part of the dose reaching the patient) has a much higher bioavailability (Ryrfeldt et al., 1982), because there is no barrier to its absorption and no local inactivation. To avoid unwanted systemic activity, it is important that this fraction also will be efficiently inactivated by a high first-pass metabolism in the liver.

Table 2 Oral Bioavailability of GCS in Humans

GCS	Oral bioavailability %: Range of published data
Hydrocortisone	40-71
Prednisolone	60-100
Methylprednisolone	49-99
Dexamethasone	53-83
Flunisolide	21
Budesonide	11-13

No figure is available for beclomethasone dipropionate.
Source: Summarized from Edsbäcker, 1986.

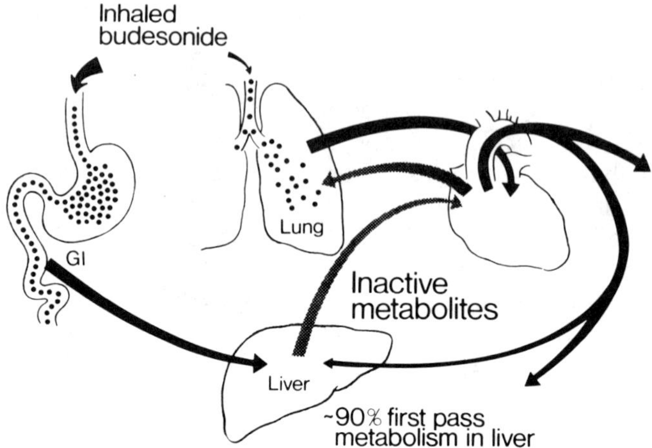

Figure 7   Pharmacokinetic properties of inhaled budesonide in humans: a schematic overview.

B. "Hit-and-Run" Action of Inhaled GCS

Animal experiments performed with budesonide in vivo (Brattsand et al., 1982a) and in vitro with perfused lung (Ryrfeldt et al., 1989) show that about 50% of a GCS dose instilled into the airways is absorbed within 10-30 min into the systemic circulation. Thirty minutes after instillation of a clinically relevant dose (1 μg to rat airways), the budesonide concentration in the studied tissue compartment (airways plus lung) was approximately 1 μmol/L (Ryreldt et al., 1989). For the first minutes after application, the local airway concentration can be anticipated to be higher still.

That this budesonide concentration is sufficiently large and persists long enough to induce a strong local anti-inflammatory response at the site of application has been verified in functional models, such as the hamster cheek pouch (Svensjö and Roempke, 1985) and the rat trachea (Miller-Larsson and Brattsand, 1990). In these models budesonide was topically perfused for defined periods and with different concentrations and the subsequent block of inflammation-induced macromolecular extravasation was determined. When superfused for a restricted period, a budesonide concentration of 1 μmol/L was needed to block the extravasation. On the other hand, with such a concentration a superfusion lasting for just 5-10 min (Fig. 8) was sufficient to trigger a strong antipermeability activity, which was still local for the superfusion site. With regard to the basic mechanism of GCS (induction of mediator proteins; cf. Fig. 3), the triggered response is protracted. In the tracheal

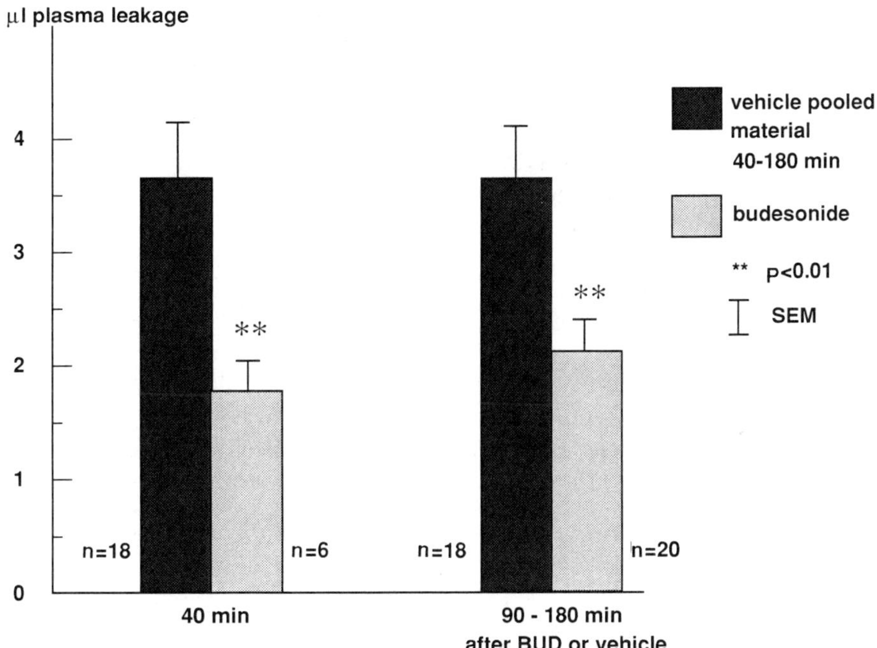

Figure 8 Inhibition of bradykinin-induced macromolecular leakage from rat trachea by 10 min of local perfusion with budesonide 3×10^{-6} mol/L. Budesonide or vehicle was perfused for the first 10 min and bradykinin challenges were performed (for 10 min periods each) at 40 min as well as later (between 90 and 180 min).

model 10 min of budesonide superfusion reduced extravasation for at least 5 h (Miller-Larsson and Brattsand, 1990, unpublished). Therefore, at least for one important type of antiasthmatic activity, inhaled GCS may be considered as "hit-and-run" drugs, distinct from the other types of antiasthmatic agents.

A minor fraction of airway deposited GCS adheres for a much longer time to airway and lung tissue. The fraction is larger than the very small pool bound to the GCS receptors. Protease treatment is needed for its quantitative release (Ryrfeldt et al., 1989). As studied with dexamethasone, it resides in endothelial cells, alveolar type 2 cells, fibroblasts, and smooth muscle cells (Beer et al., 1983). The biological activity of this fraction, when bound or when released, is currently unknown, but it may markedly prolong the GCS trigger period in the target organ for those GCS actions that may need a longer trigger time than discussed above. Hence, depending on the type of anti-inflammatory action induced in airway mucosa, inhalational GCS can be both "hit-and-run" drugs (for actions triggered by a high but brief GCS pulse) and sustained drugs (for actions in which a prolonged trigger time is much more important than a high tissue concentration of GCS). The relative importance of these two types of action has still to be determined. However, the improved therapeutic potency of inhalational GCS suggests that the "hit-and-run" type may be important for antiasthmatic efficacy.

VI. Concluding Remarks

Based on the latency time required for their induction, Figure 9 summarizes two major antiasthmatic effects of GCS: improved basal respiration and decreased bronchial responsiveness. The figure also presents proposals for GCS mechanisms underlying these effects. There is a temporal correspondence

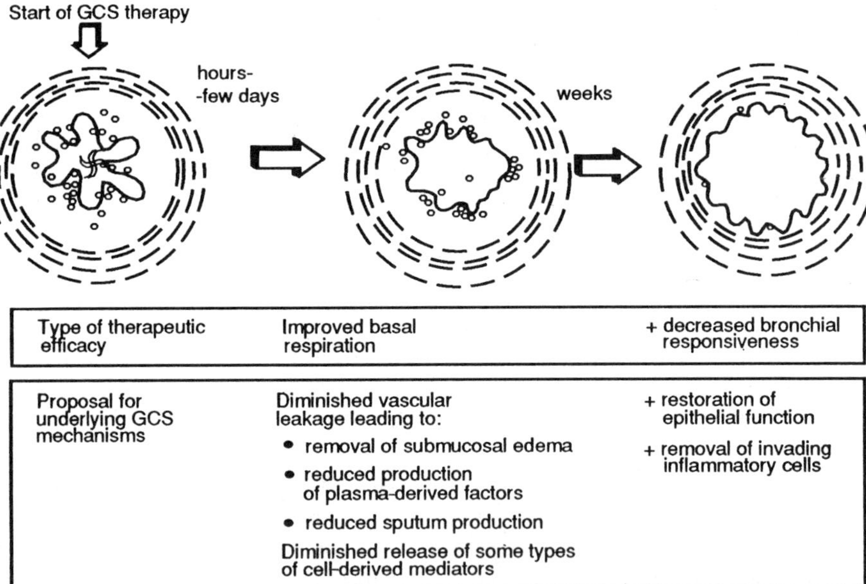

Type of therapeutic efficacy	Improved basal respiration	+ decreased bronchial responsiveness
Proposal for underlying GCS mechanisms	Diminished vascular leakage leading to: • removal of submucosal edema • reduced production of plasma-derived factors • reduced sputum production Diminished release of some types of cell-derived mediators	+ restoration of epithelial function + removal of invading inflammatory cells

Figure 9 Two main therapeutic effects of GCS in clinical asthma: improved basal respiration and decreased bronchial responsiveness, and proposed underlying anti-inflammatory mechanisms. The cross-section of the airways symbolizes start of therapy: smooth muscle, swollen submucosa with foci of infiltrated inflammatory cells, strongly folded mucosa due to the swollen submucosa, airway lumen with recruited inflammatory cells and mucus plugs.

between the improvement of basal respiration, experienced by asthmatic patients within a few hours (Ellul-Micallef and Johansson, 1983), and the rapid reduction in inflammation-induced vascular leakiness of airways in the experimental setting. That reduction may promptly alleviate submucosal edema and the vascular part of sputum production, and by that counteract some of the obstruction of asthmatic airways. Furthermore, reduced vascular leakage would diminish the production of plasma-derived inflammatory mediators. The release of some proinflammatory mediators from, for example, eosinophils and basophils, might be rapidly blocked by GCS.

The other important therapeutic action—the decreased responsiveness to specific and nonspecific stimuli—needs a much longer latency time to be achieved. In the experimental setting this is mimicked by a prolonged latency time for demonstration of a GCS-induced block of, for example, the immediate phase after allergy, exercise, or nonspecific challenge. It is not known whether the extended latency time means that other protective mechanisms must be involved as well, such as removal of invading inflammatory cells with a sluggish turnover. Because a substantial part of mucosal and submucosal space can be occupied by invading inflammatory cells in chronic asthma (cf. Chap. 3), removal of these cells will increase the free airway caliber. Furthermore, a gradual restoration of epithelial function may decrease the responsiveness.

To achieve reduction of inflammation-induced vascular leakiness, GCS do not need to be present for the whole latency period. In fact, it is sufficient to pulse airway tissue for just a few minutes with GCS concentrations relevant for inhalational use. After such a pulse the GCS can be absorbed from the airways and inactivated by biotransformation, while the local antipermeability action persists for hours. This property of selected GCS may partially explain the unmatched clinical efficacy of inhalational GCS in the treatment of asthma and rhinitis.

Discussion

Kaliner: Can you tell us which cells or tissues are most responsive to GCS?

Brattsand: For the vascular antipermeability action, I believe the most important mechanism is a direct effect on endothelial cells.

Capron: My comment is related to the heterogeneity of eosinophil susceptibility to corticosteroids. We have noticed that in some patients with hypereosinophilia resistant to corticosteroid therapy, the proportion of hypodense eosinophils was increased. Recently we have shown that eosinophils from such patients lack glucocorticoid receptors and there is a correlation between the absence of receptors and the lack of sensitivity to glucocorticoid therapy. (Pim et al., *Clin. Dermatol.*, in press).

Brattsand: It would be of great interest to know if also the steroid-resistant asthma may depend on a downregulation of glucocorticoid receptors. However, I am surprised that there are so few problems with reduced sensitivity in chronic asthma therapy with glucocorticoids.

Kay: The T cell seems to be a particularly sensitive target for corticosteroids. Many actions have been described, including inhibition of IL2 receptor upregulation and of signal transduction following T-cell receptor activation. Low doses (10^{-9} M or lower) are often sufficient for these effects. Higher concentration of steroids are needed to inhibit inflammatory cells.

Venge: The sensitivity also depends on which function of the cell is examined. It is true that neutrophils are remarkably steroid insensitive. However, with the eosinophil it depends on the function you are studying. Thus, granule protein secretion is very potently inhibited by budesonide at doses of 10^{-9}-10^{-10} M, depending on the time of preincubation.

Brattsand: I think that evolution has given glucocorticoids the ability to induce different types of attenuation of different cells. These drugs have selective cellular actions through concentration- and time-dependent mechanisms.

Kaliner: Can anyone relate which cells or tissues are most steroid responsive? Are eosinophils, lymphocytes, or macrophages more responsive to glucocorticoids than blood vessels?

Schleimer: Among the leukocytes, the best indicators are that neutrophils are relatively steroid unresponsive while basophils, eosinophils, lymphocytes, and monocytes/macrophages are steroid responsive. This seems to be true both in vivo and in vitro.

Persson: If plasma exudation is effectively reduced by glucocorticoid (by any significant anti-inflammatory mechanism) treatment, this will prevent the appearance in airways of activated plasma protein systems such as complement, kinins, coagulation, and others. Active peptides from these systems and other factors in exuded plasma may cause migration, priming, and activation of inflammatory cells. In turn this means that an antiexudative effect hypothetically can explain both the acute and the long-term (cellular-dependent) anti-inflammatory effects of glucocorticoids in patients with asthma.

Barnes: Endogenous steroids may be very important in regulating inflammatory responses. Thus, adrenalectomy will enhance microvascular leak in rat skin and airways. This suggests that the very low endogenous levels of steroids may suppress inflammation.

Brattsand: I can confirm the pulmonary anti-inflammatory importance of the endogenous glucocorticoid tone. Also, Carl Persson has reminded us that the cold bath is an ancient cure for asthma and suggested that the effect is secondary to enhanced cortisol secretion. In mice we find that cold exposure increases by 10-fold the level of corticosterone in plasma.

Fuller: Do you think that under some circumstances you need systemic steroids, such as in patients with acute asthma?

Brattsand: In patients with acute asthma, several systemic proinflammatory systems may be involved and systemic glucocorticoids are required.

Acknowledgment

The secretarial assistance of M. Broman is kindly acknowledged.

References

Abraham, W. M., Laues, S., Stevenson, J. S., and Yerger, L. D., (1986). Effect of an inhaled glucocorticosteroid (budesonide) on post-antigen induced increases in airway responsiveness. *Bull Eur. Physiopathol. Respir.* **22**:387-392.

Addison, T. (1855). *On the Constitutional and Local Effects of Disease of the Suprarenal Capsules.* London, Samuel Highley.

Ädelroth, E., Rosenhall, L., Johansson, S.-Å., Linden, M., and Venge, P. (1990). Inflammatory cells and eosinophil activity in asthmatics investigated by bronchoalveolar lavage. The effect of anti-asthmatic treatment with budesonide or terbutaline. *Am. Rev. Respir. Dis.* (in press).

Altman, L. C., Hill, J. S., Harfield, W. M., and Mullarkey, M. F. (1981). Effects of corticosteroids on eosinophil chemotaxis and adherence. *J. Clin. Invest.* **67**:28-36.

Altounyan, R. E. C. (1970). Changes in histamine and atropine responsiveness as a guide to diagnosis and evaluation of therapy in obstructive airways disease. In *Disodium Cromoglycate in Allergic Airways Disease.* Edited by J. Pepys and A. W. Frankland. London, Butterworth, pp. 47-53.

Andersson, M., and Pipkorn, U. (1987). Inhibition of the dermal immediate allergic reaction by topically applied glucocorticosteroids. *J. Allergy Clin. Immunol.* **77**:345-349.

Andersson, M., von Kogerer, B., Andersson, P., and Pipkorn, U. (1987). Allergen induced nasal hyperreactivity appears unrelated to the size of the nasal and dermal immediate allergic reaction. *Allergy* **42**:631-637.

Andersson, M., Andersson, P., and Pipkorn, U. (1988). Topical glucocorticosteroids and allergen-induced increase in nasal reactivity; relationship between treatment time and inhibitory effect. *J. Allergy Clin. Immunol.* **82**:1019-1026.

Andersson, M., Andersson, P., and Pipkorn, U. (1989a). Allergen-induced specific and non-specific nasal hyperreactivity; reciprocal relationship and inhibition by topical glucocorticosteroids. *Acta Otolaryngol. (Stockh.)* **107**:270-277.

Andersson, M., Svensson, C., Andersson, P., and Pipkorn, U. (1989b). Objective monitoring of the inflammatory response of the nasal mucosa in hay fever patients during natural allergen exposure. *Am. Rev. Respir. Dis.* **139**:911-914.

Andersson, M., Andersson, P., Venge, P., and Pipkorn, U. (1989c). Eosinophils and eosinophil cationic protein (ECP) in nasal lavages during allergen-induced hyperresponsiveness. Effect of topical glucocorticosteroid treatment. *Allergy* **44**:342-348.

Andersson, P. H., and Ryrfeldt, Ä. (1984). Biotransformation of the topical glucocortiocids budesonide and beclomethasone dipropionate in human liver and lung homogenate. *J. Pharm. Pharmacol.* **36**:763-765.

Andersson, P. T., and Brattsand, R. (1982). Protective effects of the glucocorticoid budesonide on lung anaphylaxis in actively sensitized guinea-pigs: inhibition of IgE- but not IgG-mediated anaphylaxis. *Br. J. Pharmacol.* **76**:139-147.

Andersson, P. T., and Persson, C. G. A. (1988). Developments in anti-asthma glucocorticoids. In *Directions for New Anti-Asthma Drugs*. Edited by S. R. O'Donnell and C. G. A Persson. Basel, Birhäuser Verlag, pp. 239-260.

Andersson, P., Chignard, M., Brange, C., Nilsson, T., Juhlin, M., and Le-Couedic, L. P. (1985). Effect of glucocorticosteroid treatment on antigen-induced mediator release from sensitized guinea-pig lungs. In *Glucocorticosteroids, Inflammation and Bronchial Hyperreactivity*. Edited by J. C. Hogg, R. Ellul-Micallef, and R. Brattsand. Amsterdam, Excerpta Medica, pp. 132-135.

Andersson, P. T., Brange, C., von Kogerer, B., Sonmark, B., and Stahre, G. (1988). Effect of glucocorticosteroid treatment on ovalbumin-induced IgE-mediated and late allergic response in guinea-pig. *Int. Arch. Allergy Appl. Immunol.* **87**:32-39.

Bakhle, Y. S., Reynard, A. M., and Vane, J. R. (1969). Metabolism of the angiotensins in isolated perfused tissues. *Nature* **222**:956-959.

Barnes, P., and Mygind, N. (1988). *Budesonide, Clinical Experience in Asthma and Rhinitis*. Manchester, ADIS Press.

Bascom, R., Wachs, M., Naclerio, R. M., Pipkorn, U., Galli, S., and Lichtenstein, L. M. (1988). Basophil influx occurs after nasal antigen challenge: effects of topical corticosteroid pretreatment. *J. Allergy Clin. Immunol.* **81**:580-589.

Bascom, R., Pipkorn, U., Lichtenstein, L. M., and Naclerio, R. M. (1989a). The influx of inflammatory cells into nasal washings during the late response to antigen challenge: effect of systemic corticosteroid. *Am. Rev. Respir. Dis.* **138**:406-412.

Bascom, R., Pipkorn, U., Proud, D., Donette, S., Gleich, G. J., Lichtenstein, L. M., and Naclerio, R. M. (1989b). Major basic protein and eosinophil-derived neurotoxin concentrations in nasal lavage fluid after antigen challenge. Effect of systemic corticosteroids and relationship to eosinophil influx. *J. Allergy Clin. Immunol.* **84**:338-346.

Baxter, J. D., and Rousseau, G. G. (1979). Glucocorticoid Hormone action: an overview. In *Glucocorticoid Hormone Action.* Edited by J. D. Baxter and G. G. Rousseau. New York, Springer Verlag.

Beer, D, Cunha, G., and Malkinson, A. (1983). Autoradiographic demonstration of the specific binding and nuclear localization of ^{3}H-dexamethasone in adult mouse lung. *Lab. Invest.* **49**:725-734.

Bergstrand, H., Björnson, A., Lundquist, B., Nilsson, A., and Brattsand, R. (1984). Inhibitory effect of glucocorticosteroids on anti-IgE-induced histamine release from human basophilic leukocytes: evidence for a dual mechanism of action. *Allergy* **39**:217-230.

Bergstrand, H., Lindquist, B., and Petersson, B.-Å. (1986). The glucocorticosteroid budesonide partially blocks histamine release from human lung tissue in vitro. *Allergy* **41**:319-329.

Besedovsky, J., Del Rey, A., Sorkin, E., and Dinarello, C. (1986). Immunoregulatory feedback between IL-1 and glucocorticoid hormones. *Science* **233**:652-654.

Bienkowski, J. M., Petro, M. A., and Robinson, L. J. (1989). Inhibition of thromboxane A synthesis in U937 cells by glucocorticoids. Lack of evidence for lipocortin 1 as the second messenger. *J. Biol. Chem.* **264**:6536-6544.

Bisgaard, H., Grönborg, H., Mygind, N., Dahl, R., Lindqvist, N., and Venge, P. (1990). Allergen-induced increase of eosinophil cationic protein in nasal lavage fluid: effect of the glucocorticoid budesonide. *J. Allergy Clin. Immunol.* in press.

Björk, J., Hedqvist, P., and Arfors, K.-E. (1982). Increase in vascular permeability induced by leukotriene B$_4$ and the role of polymorphonuclear leukocytes. *Inflammation* **6**:189-200.

Blackwell, G., Carnuccio, R., Di Rosa, M., Flower, R., Parente, L., and Persico, P. (1980). Macrocortin: a polypeptide causing the anti-phospholipase effect of glucocorticoids. *Nature* **287**:147-149.

Bochner, B. S., Lady, S. D., Plaut, M., Dinarello, C. A., and Schleimer, R. P. (1987a). Interleukin 1 production by human lung tissue. I Identification and characterization. *J. Immunol.* **139**:2297-2302.

Bochner, B. S., Rutledge, B. K., and Schleimer, R. P. (1987b). Interleukin 1 production by human lung tissue. II Inhibition by human lung tissue. *J. Immunol.* **139**:2303-2307.

Booij-Nord, K., DeVries, K., Sluiter, H. J., and Orie, N. G. M. (1972). Late bronchial reaction to experimental inhalation of house dust mite. *Clin. Allergy* **2**:43-61.

Borum, P., Grønborg, H., Brofelt, S., and Mygind, N. (1983). Nasal reactivity in rhinitis. *Eur. J. Respir. Dis.* **64** (suppl 128):65-71.

Brattsand, R. (1989). Development of glucocorticoids with lung selectivity. In *Clinical and Experimental Aspects.* Edited by F. E. Hargreave, J. C. Hogg, J.-L., Malo, and J. H. Toogood. Amsterdam, Excerpta Medica, pp. 17-38.

Brattsand, R., Källström, L., Nilsson, E., Ryrfeldt, Å., and Tönnesson, M. (1982a). The lung disposition of budesonide in guinea pig and rat. *Eur. J. Respir. Dis.* **63** (suppl 122):263-265.

Brattsand, R., Thalén, A., Roempke, K., Källström, L., and Gruvstad, E. (1982b). Influence of 16α, 17α-acetal substitution and steroid nucleus fluorination on the topical to systemic activity ratio of glucocorticoids. *J. Steroid Biochem.* **16**:779-786.

Brattsand, R., Thalén, A., Roempke, K., Källström, L., and Gruvstad, E. (1982c). Development of new glucocorticosteroids with a very high ratio between topical and systemic activities. *Eur. J. Respir. Dis.* **63** (suppl 122):62-73.

Brattsand, R., Andersson, P., Edsbäcker, S., and Ryrfeldt, Å. (1987). Developments of glucocorticosteroids with lung selectivity. In: *Advances in the Use of Inhaled Corticosteroids.* Edited by R. Ellul-Micallef, W. K. Lam, and J. H. Toogood. Amsterdam, Excerpta Medica, pp. 60-78.

Brodde, O. E., Howe, U., Egerzegi, S., Konietzko, N., and Michel, M. C. (1988). Effect of prednisolone and ketotifen on beta-2-adrenoceptors in asthmatic patients receiving beta-2-bronchodilators. *Eur. J. Clin. Pharmacol.* **34**:145-150.

Brönnegård, M. (1988). Studies on the structure and function of the human and the rat glucocorticoid receptor. Stockholm, Karolinska Institutet, Dissertation, pp. 1-57.

Burge, P. S. (1982). The effect of corticosteroids on the immediate asthmatic reaction. *Eur. J. Respir. Dis.* **63** (suppl 122):163-166.

Caldwell, I. W., Hall-Smith, S. P., Main, R. A., Ashurst, P. J., Kirton, V., Simpson, W. T., and Williams, G. W. (1968). Clinical evaluation of a new topical corticosteroid beclomethasone dipropionate. *Br. J. Dermatol.* **80**:111-117.

Carnuccio, R., Di Rosa, M., Flower, R., and Pinto, A. (1981). The inhibition by hydrocortisone of prostaglandin biosynthesis in rat peritoneal leukocytes is correlated with intracellular macrocortin levels. *Br. J. Pharmacol.* **74**:322-324.

Carnuccio, R., Di Rosa, M., Cuerrasio, B., Luvone, T., and Sautebin, L. (1987). Vasocortin—a novel glucocorticoid-induced anti-inflammatory protein. *Br. J. Pharmacol.* **90**:443-445.

Chaplin, M., Rooks, W., Swensson, E., Cooper, W., Nerenberg, C., and Chu, J. (1980). Flunisolide metabolism and dynamics of a metabolite. *Clin. Pharmacol. Ther.* **27**:402-413.

Chung, H.-T., Samlowski, W. E., and Daynes, R. A. (1986). Modification of the murine immune system by glucocorticosteroids: alterations of the tissue localization properties of circulating lymphocytes. *Cell. Immunol.* **101**:571-585.

Cirino, G., Peers, S. H., Flower, R. J., Browing, J. L., and Pepinsky, R. B. (1989). Human recombinant lipocortin 1 has acute local anti-inflammatory properties in the rat paw edema. *Proc. Natl. Acad. Sci. USA* **86**: 3428-3432.

Cockcroft, D. W., and Murdock, K. Y. (1987). Comparative effects of inhaled salbutamol, sodium cromoglycate, and beclomethasone dipropionate on allergen-induced early asthmatic responses, late asthmatic responses, and increased bronchial responsiveness to histamine. *J. Allergy Clin. Immunol.* **79**:734-740.

Connell, J. T. (1969). Quantitative intranasal pollen challenges: the priming effect in allergic rhinitis. *J. Allergy* **43**:33-44.

Crabtree, G. R., Gillis, S., Smith, K., and Munck, A. (1979). Glucocorticoids and immune responses. *Arthritis Rheum.* **22**:1246-1256.

Dahl, R., and Johansson, S.-Å. (1982). Importance of duration of treatment with inhaled budesonide on the immediate and late bronchial reaction. *Eur. J. Respir. Dis.* suppl 122:167-175.

Dahl, R., Fredens, K., and Venge, P. (1988). The eosinophil. In *Asthma, Basic Mechanisms and Clinical Management.* Edited by P. J. Barnes, I. Rodger, and N. Thomsom. London: Academic Press, pp. 115-130.

Dahlberg, E., Thalén, A., Brattsand, R., Gustafsson, J.-Å., Johansson, U., Roempke, K., and Saartok, T. (1984). Correlation between chemical structure, receptor binding and biological activity of some novel, highly active 16α, 17α-acetal-substituted glucocorticoids. *Mol. Pharmacol.* **25**:70-78.

deMonchy, J. G. R., Kauffman, H. F., Venge, P., Koeter, G. H., Jansen, H. M., Sluiter, H. J., and de Vries, K. (1985). Bronchoalveolar eosinophilia during allergen-induced late asthmatic reactions. *Am. Rev. Respir. Dis.* **131**:373-376.

deMonchy, J. G. R., Postma, D. S., Kauffman. H. F., Venge, P., Weeke, F. W., and de Vries, K. (1988). Pretreatment with inhaled corticosteroids reduces eosinophil chemotaxis of BAL fluid following house dust mite challenge. *N. Engl. Allergy Proc.* p. 249 (abstract).

Dhanireddy, R., Kikukawa, T., and Mukherjee, A. B. (1988). Detection of a rabbit uteroglobin-like protein in human neomatal tracheobronchial washings. *Biochem. Biophys. Res. Commun.* **152**:1447-1454.

Di Rosa, M., Calignario, A., Carnuccio, R., Ialenti, A., and Sautebin, L. (1985). Multiple control of inflammations by glucocorticoids. *Agents Actions.* **17**:284-288.

Easton, J. G. (1981). Effect of an inhaled corticosteroid on methacholine airway reactivity. *J. Allergy Clin. Immunol.* **67**:388-390.

Edsbäcker, S. (1986). Studies on the metabolic fate and human pharmacokinetics of budesonide. Lund, Lund University Dissertation, pp. 1-43.

Edsbäcker, S., Andersson, P., Lindberg, C., Paulson, J., Ryrfeldt, Å., and Thalén, A. (1987). Liver metabolism of budesonide in rat, mouse and man. *Drug Metab. Dispos.* **15**:403-411.

Eggleston, P. E., Kagey-Sobotka, A., Schleimer, R. P., and Lichtenstein, L. M. (1984). Interaction between hyperosmolar and IgE-mediated histamine release from basophils and mast cells. *Am. Rev. Respir. Dis.* **130**:86-91.

Ellul-Micallef, R. (1987). Pharmacokinetics and pharmacodynamics of glucocorticosteroids. In *Drug Therapy for Asthma, Research and Clinical Practice.* Edited by J. W. Jenne and S. Murphy. New York, Marcel Dekker, pp. 463-516.

Ellul-Micallef, R., and Johansson, S.-Å. (1983). Acute dose-response studies in bronchial asthma with a new corticosteroid, budesonide. *Br. J. Clin. Pharmacol.* **15**:419-422.

Enerbäck, L., Pipkorn, U., and Granerus, G. (1986). Intraepithelial migration of nasal mucosal mast cells in hay fever. *Int. Arch. Allergy Appl. Immunol.* **80**:44-51.

Erjefält, I., and Persson, C. G. A. (1986). Anti-asthma drugs attenuate inflammatory leakage of plasma into airway lumen. *Acta Physiol. Scand.* **128**:653-654.

Fahey, J. V., Guyre, P. M., and Munck, A. (1981). Mechanisms of anti-inflammatory actions of glucocorticoids. In: *Advances in Inflammation Research* vol. 2. Edited by G. Weissman. New York, Raven Press, pp. 21-51.

Flint, K. C., Leung, K. B. P., Hudspith, B. N., Brostoff, J., Pearce, F. L., and Johnson, N. M. (1985). Bronchoalveolar mast cells in extrinsic asthma: a mechanisms for the initiation of antigen specific bronchoconstriction. *Br. Med. J.* **291**:923-926.

Flower, R. J. (1988). Lipocortin and the mechanisms of action for glucocorticoids. *Br. J. Pharmacol.* **94**:987-1015.

Flower, R. J., Parente, L., Persico, P., and Salmon, J. A. (1986). A comparison of the acute inflammatory response in adrenalectomised and sham-operated rats. *Br. J. Pharmacol.* **87**:57-62.

Fraser, C. M., and Venter, J. C. (1980). The synthesis of β-adrenergic receptors in cultured human lung cells: induction by glucocorticoids. *Biochem. Biophys. Res. Commun.* **94**:390-397.

Freeland, H., Pipkorn, U., Proud, D., Bascom, R., Naclerio, R. M., Lichtenstein, L. M., and Peters, S. P. (1989). Leukotriene B4 as a mediator of early and late reactions to antigen in humans. The effect of systemic glucocorticoid treatment in vivo. *J. Allergy Clin. Immunol.* **83**:634-642.

Friegas, E., and Gleich, G. J. (1986). The eosinophil and the pathophysiology of asthma. *J. Allergy Clin. Immunol.* **77**:527-537.

Friegas, E., Loegering, D., Solley, G., et al. (1981). Elevated levels of the eosinophil granule major basic protein in the sputum of patients with bronchial asthma. *Mayo. Clin. Proc.* **56**:345-353.

Gibson, P. G., Girgis-Gabardo, A., Morris, M. M., Mattoli, S., Kay, J. M., Dolovich, J., Denburg, J., and Hargreave, F. E. (1989). Cellular characteristics of sputum from patients with asthma and chronic bronchitis. *Thorax*, in press.

Gleich, G. J., Flavahan, N. A., Fujisawa, T., and Van Houtte, P. M. (1988). The eosinophil as a mediator of damage to respiratory epithelium. A model for bronchial hyperreactivity. *J. Allergy Clin. Immunol.* **81**:776-781.

Gustafsson, B., and Persson, C. G. A. (1989). Effect of three weeks' treatment with budesonide on in vitro contractile and relaxant airway effects in the rat. *Thorax* **44**:24-27.

Hammarlund, A., Olsson, P., and Pipkorn, U. (1989). Blood flow in dermal allergen-induced immediate and late phase reactions. *Clin. Exp. Allergy* **19**:197-202.

Hargreave, F. E., Ramsdale, E. H., Kirby, J. G., and O'Byrne, P. M. (1986). Asthma and the role of inflammation. *Eur. J. Respir. Dis.* **69** (suppl 147):16-31.

Hartley, J. P. R., and Walters, E. H. (1982). Role of airway reactivity in pathogenesis of asthma. *Eur. J. Respir. Dis.* **63** (suppl 122):29-35.

Hellewell, P., and Williams, T. J. (1989). An anti-inflammatory steroid inhibits tissue sensitization by IgE in vivo. *Br. J. Pharmacol.* **96**:5-7.

Henriksen, J. M. (1985). Effect of inhalation of corticosteroid on exercise-induced asthma: randomized double-blind, cross over study of budesonide in asthmatic children. *Br. Med. J.* **291**:248-249.

Hirschmann, R., Böhm, V., and Funke, T. (1988). Hydrogen peroxide production ex vivo by peritonitis exudate leukocytes of rats and influence of dexamethasone and glucocorticoid antagonist. *Agents Actions* **23**:101-102.

Hogg, J. C., and Eggleston, P. A. (1984). Is asthma an epithelial disease? *Am. Rev. Respir. Dis.* **129**:207-208.

Holmberg, K., Bake, B., and Pipkorn, U. (1988). Nasal mucosal blood flow after nasal allergen challenge. *J. Allergy Clin. Immunol.* **81**:541-547.

Ialenti, A., Doyle, P. M., Hardy, G. W., Simpkin, D. S. E.,and Di Rosa, M. (1990). Anti-inflammatory effects of vasocortin and nonapeptide fragments of uteroglobin and lipocortin I. *Agents Actions* **29**(½):48-49.

Iikura, Y., Nagakura, T., Walsh, G. M., Akimoto, K., Kisida, M., Kondou, T., Odajima, Y., Okuma, M., Akazawa, A., and Yukishita, T. (1988). Role of chemical mediators after antigen and exercise in children with asthma. *J. Allergy Clin. Immunol.* **81**:1050-1055.

Johansson, S.-Å., Andersson, K.-E., Brattsand, R., Gruvstad, E., and Hedner, P. (1982). Topical and systemic glucocorticoid potencies of budesonide and beclomethasone dipropionate in man. *Eur. J. Clin. Pharmacol.* **22**:523-529.

Johnson, L. K., Longenecker, J. P., Baxter, J. D., Dallmann, M. F., Widmaier, E. P., and Eberhardt, N. L. (1982). Glucocorticoid action: a mechanism involving nuclear and non-nuclear pathways. *Br. J. Dermatol.* **107** (suppl. 23):6-23.

Kaliner, M. (1985). Mechanism of glucocorticosteroid action in bronchial asthma. *J. Allergy Clin. Immunol.* **76**:321-329.

Kay, A. B. (1986). Cells causing airway inflammation. *Eur. J. Respir. Dis.* **69** (suppl 147):38-43.

Kern, J. A., Lamb, R. J., Reed, J. C., Daniele, R. P., and Nowell, P. C. (1988). Dexamethasone inhibition of interleukin I beta production by human monocytes. *J. Clin. Invest.* **81**:237-244.

Knudsen, P. J., Dinarello, C. A., and Strom, T. B. (1987). Glucocorticoids inhibit transcriptional and posttranscriptional expression of interleukin I in U937 cells. *J. Immunol.* **139**:4129-4134.

Koltai, M., Kovács, Z., Nemecz, G., Mécs, I., and Szekeres, L. (1987). Glucocorticoid-induced low molecular mass anti-inflammatory factors which do not inhibit phospholipase A_2. *Eur. J. Pharmacol.* **134**:109-112.

Konno, A., Togawa, K., and Hishira, S. (1981). Seasonal variation of sensitivity of nasal mucosa in pollinosis. *Arch. Otorhinolaryngol.* **232**:253-261.

Larsson, R., Svedmyr, N., and Thiringer, G. (1977). Lack of bronchial β-adrenoreceptor resistance in asthmatics during long term treatment with terbutaline. *J. Allergy Clin. Immunol.* **59**:93-100.

Laue, L., Kawai, S., Brandon, D. D., Brightwell, D., Barnes, K., et al. (1988). Receptor-mediated effects of glucocorticoids on inflammation: enhancement of the inflammatory response with a glucocorticoid antagonist. *J. Steroid Biochem.* **29**:591-598.

Lee, S. W., Tsou, A. P., Chan, H., Thomas, J., Petrie, K., Eugui, E., and Allison, A. C. (1988). Glucocorticoids selectively inhibit the transcription of the interleukin I β gene and decrease the stability of interleukin I βmRNA. *Proc. Natl. Acad. Sci.* **85**:1204-1208.

Lindqvist, N., Balle, V., Karma, P., Karje, J., Lindström, D., Mäkinen, J., Pukander, J., Ruoppio, P., Suonpää, J., Östlund, W., and Pipkorn, U. (1986). Long term safety and efficacy of budesonide nasal aerosol in perennial rhinitis—a 12 month multicentre study. *Allergy* **41**:179-186.

Löfdahl, C.-G., Mellstrand, T., and Svedmyr, N. (1984). Glucocorticoids and asthma. Studies of resistance and systemic effects of glucocorticoids. *Eur. J. Respir. Dis.* **65**:(suppl 136):69-79.

Lövkvist, T., and Svensson, G. (1976). Treatment of vasomotor rhinitis with intranasal beclomethasone dipropionate (Becotide) *Acta Allerg.* **31**:227-238.

Lundgren, J. D., Hirata, F., Marom, Z., Logun, C., Steel, L., Kaliner, M., and Shelhamer, J. (1988). Dexamethasone inhibits respiratory glycoconjugate secretion from feline airways in vitro by the induction of lipocortin (lipomodulin) synthesis. *Am. Rev. Respir. Dis.* **137**:353-357.

Malm, L., Wihl, J.-Å., Lamm, C. J., and Lindqvist, N. (1982). Reduction of metacholine induced nasal secretions by the treatment with a new topical steroid in perennial nonallergic rhinitis. *Allergy* **36**:209-214.

Marom, Z., Shelhamer, J., Alling, D., and Kaliner, M. (1984). The effects of corticosteroids on mucous glycoprotein secretion from human airways in vitro. *Am. Rev. Respir. Dis.* **129**:62-65.

Martin, G. L., Atkins, P. C., Dunsky, E. H., and Zweiman, B. (1980). Effect of theophylline, terbutaline, and prednisolone on antigen-induced bronchospasm and mediator release. *J. Allergy Clin. Immunol.* **66**:204-212.

Martin, L., Tanner, R., Clark, T., and Cochrane, G. (1973). Absorption and metabolism of orally administered beclomethasone dipropionate. *Clin. Pharmacol. Ther.* **15**:267-275.

Miele, L., Cordella-Miele, E., and Mukhurjee, A. T. S. (1987). Uteroglobin: structure, molecular biology and perspectives on its function as a phospholipase inhibitor. *Endocr. Rev.* **8**:474-490.

Miele, L., Cordella-Miele, E., Facchiano, A., and Mukherjee, A. T. S. (1988). Novel anti-inflammatory peptides from the region of highest similarity between uteroglobin and lipocortin. *Nature* **335**:726-730.

Miller-Larsson, A., and Brattsand, R. (1990). Topical anti-inflammatory activity of the glucocorticoid budesonide on airway mucosa. Evidence for a hit and run type of activity. *Agents Actions* **29**(½):127-129.

Moretti, M., Giannico, G., Marchioni, C. F., and Bisetti, A. (1984). Effects of methyl prednisolone on sputum biochemical components in asthmatic bronchitis. *Eur. J. Respir. Dis.* **65**:365-370.

Munch, A., Guyre, P. M., and Holbrook, N. J. (1984). Physiological functions of glucocorticoids in stress and their relation to pharmacological actions. *Endocr. Rev.* **5**:25-44.

Mygind, N., and Clark, T. J. H. (1980). *Topical Steroid Treatment for Asthma and Rhinitis.* London, Balliére Tindall.

Naclerio, R. M., Meier, H. L., Kagey-Sobotka, A., Adkinson Jr., N. F., Meyers, D. A., Norman, P. S.. and Lichtenstein, L. M. (1984). Mediator release after nasal airway challenge with allergen. *Am. Rev. Respir. Dis.* **128**:597-602.

Naclerio, R. M., Proud, D., Togias, A. G., Adkinson, Jr., N. F., Meyers, D. A., Kagey-Sobotka, A., Plaut, M., Norman, P. S., and Lichtenstein, L. M. (1987). Inflammatory mediators in late antigen-induced rhinitis. *N. Engl. J. Med.* **313**:65-70.

Nakamura, H., Motoyoshi, S., and Kadokawa, T. (1988). Anti-inflammatory action of IL-I through the pituitary-adrenal axis in rats. *Eur. J. Pharmacol.* **151**:67-73.

O'Donnell, S. R. (1988). Airway microvascular permeability in asthma: a target for drug action? In *Directions for New Anti-Asthma Drugs.* Edited by S. R. O'Donnell and C. G. A. Persson. Basel, Birshäuser Verlag, pp. 217-238.

Okuda, M., and Senba, O. (1980). Effects of beclomethasone dipropionate nasal spray on subjective and objective findings in perennial rhinitis. *Clin. Otolaryngol.* **53**:15-21.

Orgel, H. A., Heltzer, E. O., Kemp, J. P., and Welch, M. J. (1986). Clinical, rhinomanometric, and cytological evaluation of seasonal allergic rhinitis treated with beclomethasone dipropionate as aqueous nasal spray or pressurized aerosol. *J. Allergy Clin. Immunol.* **77**:858-864.

Pedersen, S., and Fuglsand, G. (1988). Urine cortisol excretion in children treated with high doses of inhaled corticosteroids: a comparison of budesonide and beclomethasone. *Eur. Respir. J.* **1**:433-435.

Peers, S. H., Moon, D., and Flower, R. (1988). Reversal of the anti-inflammatory effects of dexamethasone by the glucocorticoid antagonist RU 38436. *Biochem. Pharmacol.* **37**:556-557.

Pepys, J., and Huthcroft, B. J. (1975). Bronchial provocation test in etiologic diagnosis and analysis of asthma. *Am. Rev. Respir. Dis.* **112**:829-858.

Persson, C. G. A. (1986). Role of plasma exudation in asthmatic airways. *Lancet* **2**:1126-1129.

Persson, C. G. A., and Svensjö, E. (1985). Vascular responses and their suppression: drug interferring with venular permeability. In *Handbook of Inflammation,* volume 5. *The Pharmacology of Inflammation.* Edited by I. L. Bonta, M. A. Bray, and M. J. Parnham. Amsterdam, Elsevier, pp. 61-81.

Persson, N. H., Erlansson, M., Bergqvist, D., Takolander, R., and Svensjö, E. (1987). Terbutaline and budesonide as inhibitors of postischaemic permeability increase. *Acta Physiol. Scand.* **129**:517-524.

Persson, C. G. A., Andersson, P., and Gustafsson, B. (1989). Budesonide reduces sensitivity to antigen but does not alter base-line tone or responsiveness to carbachol, terbutaline or enprofylline in IgE-sensitized guinea-pig tracheae. *Int. Arch. Allergy. Appl. Immunol.* **88**:381-385.

Pipkorn, U. (1982a). Budesonide and nasal allergen challenge testing in man. *Allergy* **37**:129-134.

Pipkorn, U. (1982b). Budesonide and nasal histamine challenge. *Allergy* **37**:359-363.

Pipkorn, U. (1983). Effect of topical glucocorticoid treatment on nasal mucosal mast cells in allergic rhinitis. *Allergy* **38**:125-129.

Pipkorn, U. (1988). Nasal provocation. *Clin. Rev. Allergy* **6**:285-302.

Pipkorn, U., and Andersson, P. (1982). Budesonide and nasal mucosal histamine content and anti-IgE induced histamine release. *Allergy* **37**:591-595.

Pipkorn, U., and Enerbäck, L. (1987). Nasal mucosal mast cells and histamine in hay fever: effect of topical glucocorticoid treatment. *Int. Arch. Allergy Appl. Immunol.* **84**:123-128.

Pipkorn, U., and Karlsson, G. (1988). Methods for obtaining specimens from the nasal mucosa for morphological and biochemical analysis. *Eur. Respir. J.* **1**:856-862.

Pipkorn, U., Bisgaard, H., and Wihl, J.-Å. (1987a). Nasal provocation testing and lavage technique. In *Pathophysiological Aspects of Allergic and Vasomotor Rhinitis.* Edited by N. Mygind and U. Pipkorn. Copenhagen, Munksgaard, pp. 149-164.

Pipkorn, U., Proud, D., Schleimer, R. P., Peters, S. P., Adkinsson, N. F., Kagey-Sobotka, A., Norman, P. S., Lichtenstein, L. M., and Naclerio, R. M. (1987b). Effects of short term systemic glucocorticoid treatment on human nasal mediator release after antigen challenge. *J. Clin. Invest.* **80**:957-961.

Pipkorn, U., Proud, D., Lichtenstein, L. M., Kagey-Sobotka, A., Norman, P. S., and Naclerio, R. M. (1987c). Inhibition of mediator release in allergic rhinitis by pretreatment with topical glucocorticosteroids. *N. Engl. J. Med.* **316**:1506-1510.

Pipkorn, U., Pukander, J., Suonpää, J., Mäkinen, J., and Lindqvist, N. (1988a). Long-term safety of budesonide nasal aerosol—a 5 1/2 year follow up study. *Clin. Allergy* **18**:253-259.

Pipkorn, U., Karlsson, G., and Enerbäck, L. (1988b). Cellular response of the human allergic nasal mucosa to natural allergen exposure. *J. Allergy Clin. Immunol.* **82**:1046-1054.

Pipkorn, U., Hammarlund, A., and Enerbäck, L. (1989a). Prolonged treatment with topical glucocorticoids results in an inhibition of the allergen-induced weal and flare response and a reduction in skin mast cell numbers and histamine content. *Clin. Exp. Allergy* **19**:19-25.

Pipkorn, U., Karlsson, G., and Enerbäck, L. (1989b). Secretory activity of nasal mucosa mast cells and histamine release in hay fever. *Int. Arch. Allergy Appl. Immunol.* **87**:349-360.

Poothullil, J., Umemoto, L., Dolovich, J., Hargreave, F. E., and Day, R. P. (1976). Inhibition by prednisone of late cutaneous allergic responses induced by antiserum to human IgE. *J. Allergy Clin. Immunol.* **57**:164-167.

Posey, W. C., Nelson, H. S., Branch, B., and Perlman, D. S. (1978). The effects of acute corticosteroid therapy for asthma on serum immunoglobulin levels. *J. Allergy Clin. Immunol.* **62**:340-340.

Rampart, M., and Williams, T. (1989). Evidence that neutrophil accumulation induced by interleukin-1 requires both local protein biosynthesis and neutrophil CD18 antigen expression in vivo. *Br. J. Pharmacol.* in press.

Ramsdell, J. W., Berry, C. C., and Clausen, J. L. (1983). The immediate effects of cortisol and pulmonary function in normals and asthmatics. *J. Allergy Clin. Immunol.* **71**:69-74.

Ryan, G., Latimer, K. M., Juniper, E. F., Roberts, R. S., and Hargreave, F. E. (1985). Effect of beclomethasone dipropionate on bronchial responsiveness to histamine in controlled non-steroid-dependent asthma. *J. Allergy Clin. Immunol.* **75**:25-30.

Ryrfeldt, Å., Andersson, P., Edsbäcker, S., Tönnesson, M., Davies, D., and Pauwels, R. (1982). Pharmacokinetics and metabolism of budesonide a selective glucocorticoid. *Eur. J. Respir. Dis.* **63** (suppl 122):86-95.

Ryrfeldt, A., Persson, G., and Nilsson, E. (1989). Pulmonary disposition of the potent glucocorticoid budesonide, evaluated in an isolated perfused rat lung model. *Biochem. Pharmacol.* **38**:17-22.

Saavedra-Delgado, A. M. P., Mathews, K. P., Pan, P. M., Kay, D. R., and Muilenberg, M. L. (1980). Dose response studies of whole blood histamine and basophil counts by prednisone. *J. Allergy Clin. Immunol.* **66**: 464-471.

Schleimer, R. P., Lichtenstein, L. M., and Gillespie, E. (1981). Inhibition of basophil histamine release by anti-inflammatory steroids. *Nature* **292**: 454-457.

Schleimer, R. P., Schulman, R. P., McGlashan, D. W., Peters, S. P., Hayes, E. C., Adams, G. K., Lichtenstein, L. M., and N. S. Adkinson (1983). Effects of dexamethasone on mediator release from human lung fragments and purified human lung mast cells. *J. Clin. Invest.* **71**:1830-1835.

Schleimer, R. P., Undem, B. J., Meeker, S., Bollinger, M. E., Adkinson, N. F., Lichtenstein, L. M., and Adams, G. K. (1987). Dexamethasone inhibits the antigen-induced contractile activity and release of inflammatory mediators in isolated guinea-pig lung. *Am. Rev. Respir. Dis.* **135**:562-566.

Schleimer, R. P., Claman, H., and Oronsky, H. (1989). *Anti-Inflammatory Steroid Action*: *Clinical and Basic Aspects*. San Diego, Academic Press.

Settipane, G. A., Pudupakkam, R. K., and McGowan, J. H. (1987). Corticosteroid effect on immunoglobulins. *J. Allergy Clin. Immunol.* **62**:162-166.

Shaw, R. J., Andersson, R. D., Durham, S. R., Taylor, K. M., Shoeffel, R. E., Green, W., Torzillo, P., and Kay, A. B. (1985). Mediators of hypersensitivity and 'fog'-induced asthma. *Allergy* **40**:48-57.

Solley, G. O., Gleich, G. J., Jordan, R. E., and Schroeter, A. L. (1976). The late phase of the immediate wheal and flare skin reaction: its dependence upon IgE antibodies. *J. Clin. Invest.* **58**:408-420.

Sotomayor, H., Badier, M., Verrloet, D., and Orehek, J. (1984). Seasonal increase of carbachol airway responsiveness in patients allergic to grass pollen. *Am. Rev. Respir. Dis.* **130**:56-58.

Staruch, M. J., and Wood, D. D. (1985). Reduction of serum interleukin-1-like activity after treatment with dexamethasone. *J. Leukocyte Biol.* **37**:193-207.

Stefanovic, D. S. (1972). Corticosteroid-induced atrophy of the skin with teleangiectasia. *Br. J. Dermatol.* **87**:548-553.

Svensjö, E., and Roempke, K. (1985). Time-dependent inhibition of bradykinin and histamine-induced increase in microvascular permeability by local glucocorticosteroid treatment. In *Glucocorticosteroids, Inflammation and Bronchial Hyperreactivity*. Edited by J. C. Hogg, R. Ellul-Micallef, and R. Brattsand. Amsterdam, Excerpta Medica, pp. 136-144.

Svensson, C., Pipkorn, U., Baumgarten, C. R., Alkner, U., and Persson, C. G. A. (1989). Reversibility and reproducibility of histamine-induced plasma leakage of the human nasal airways. *Thorax* **44**:13-18.

Talbot, S., Atkins, P. C., and Zweiman, B. (1987). In vivo effects of corticosteroids on human allergic responses. I. Effects of systemic administration of steroids. *Ann. Allergy* **58**:363-365.

Togias, A. G., Naclerio, R. M., Proud, D., Fish, J. E., Adkinson Jr, N. F., Kagey-Sobotka, A., Norman, P. S., and Lichtenstein, L. M. (1985). Nasal challenge with cold, dry air results in release of inflammatory mediators: Possible mast cell involvement. *J. Clin. Invest.* **76**:1375-1381.

Toogood, J., and Lefcoe, N. (1965). Dexamethasone aerosol for the treatment of steroid dependent chronic bronchial asthmatic patients. *J. Allergy* **36**:321-332.

Tsuei, S., Moore, R., Ashley, J., and McBride, W. (1979). Disposition of synthetic glucocorticoids I Pharmacokinetics of dexamethasone in healthy adults. *J. Pharmacokinet. Biopharmacol.* **7**:249-265.

Tsurufuji, S., Sugia, K., Takemasa, F., and Yoshizawa, S. (1980). Blockade by antiglucocorticoids, actinomycin D and cycloheximide of anti-inflammatory action of dexamethasone against bradykinin. *J. Pharmacol. Exp. Ther.* **212**:225-231.

Venge, P., and Dahl, R. (1989). Are blood eosinophil number and activity important for the development of the late asthmatic reaction after allergen challenge? *Eur. Respir. J.* **2** (suppl 6):430S-434S.

Venge, P., Dahl, R., and Håkansson, L. (1987). Heat-labile neutrophil chemotactic activity in subjects with asthma after allergen inhalation: relation to the late asthmatic reaction and effects of asthma medication. *J. Allergy Clin. Immunol.* **80**:679-688.

Viegas, M., Gomez, E., Brooks, J., Gatland, D., and Davies, R. J. (1987). Effect of the pollen season on nasal mast cells. *Br. Med. J.* **294**:414.

Vilsviik, J. S., Jensen, A. O., and Walstad, R. (1975). The effect of beclomethasone dipropionate aerosol on allergen induced nasal stenosis. *Clin. Allergy* **5**:291-294.

Volovitz, B., Nathanson, I., De Castro, G., Kikukawa, T., Mukherjee, A. B., Brodsky, L., Fox, M. J., and Ogra, P. L. (1988). Relationship between leukotriene C_4 and uteroglobin-like protein in nasal and tracheobronchial mucosa of children. *Int. Arch. Allergy. Appl. Immunol.* **86**: 420-425.

Voris, B. P., and Young, D. A. (1981). Glucocorticoid-induced proteins in rat thymus cells. *J. Biol. Chem.* **256**:11319-11329.

Waage, A., and Bakke, O. (1988). Glucocorticoids suppress the production of tumour necrosis factor by lipopolysaccharide-stimulated human monocytes. *Immunology* **63**:299-302.

Wallner, B., Mattaliano, R., Hession, R., et al. (1986). Cloning and expression of human lipocortin, a phospholipase A_2 inhibitor with potential antiinflammatory activity. *Nature* **320**:77-81.

Wardlaw, A. J., Dunnette, S., Gleich, G., et al. (1988). Eosinophils and mast cells in bronchoalveolar lavage in subjects with mild asthma. *Am. Rev. Respir. Dis.* **137**:62-69.

Wihl, J.-Å., Brofelt, S., Grønberg, H., Borum, P., and Mygind, N. (1983). Blind study of basophilic cells in nasal smears from patients with grass pollen hay fever. *Eur. J. Respir. Dis.* **64** (suppl 128):383-386.

Wikström, A.-N., Bakke, O., Okret, S., et al. (1987). Intracellular localization of the glucocorticoid receptor: evidence for cytoplasmic and nuclear localization. *Endocrinology* **120**:1232-1242.

Woolcock, A. J., Yan, K., and Salome, C. M. (1988). Effect of therapy on bronchial hyperresponsiveness in the long-term management of asthma. *Clin. Allergy* **18**:165-176.

Yodoi, J., Hirashima, M., and Ishizaka, K. (1981). Lymphocytes bearing Fc receptors for IgE. Vi. Suppressive effect of glucocorticoids on the expression on Fc2 receptors and glycosylation of IgE binding factors. *J. Immunol.* **127**:471-476.

AUTHOR INDEX

Italic numbers give the page on which the complete reference is listed.

A

Aalberse, R. C., 598, 599, 602, 610, *624, 625*

Aarden, L. A., 258, *265*

Aarhus, L. L., 136, 137, 138, 139, 144, 145, 146, 149, 150, 151, 153, 154, 158, 175, 177, *178, 181,* 368, *379*

Abbey, H., 8, 9, 15, 16, *44*

Abboud, R., 344, *353*

Abdel-Latif, A., 363, *377*

Abdel-Latif, A. A., 301, *317*

Abraham, K. M., 252, *264*

Abraham, W., 510, *520*

Abraham, W. M., 286, *289, 299,* 529, *555,* 575, 576, *578, 582,* 687, *695*

Ackerman, G. L., 642, *655*

Ackerman, S. J., 104, 111, *127,* 249, *261,* 413, *435,* 479, 480, 481, 484, 485, 487, *494, 495, 496, 497*

Adams, G. K., 678, 686, *707*

Adams, G. K., III, 145, 149, *187,* 303, *322,* 423, *437*

Adamus, W. S., 283, *289, 290*

Addis, G. J., 508, *517*

Addison, T., 667, *695*

Adelroth, E., 60, *63,* 312, 314, *317,* 684, *695*

Adelson, A. M., 562, *585*

Adkinson, N. F., 233, *244,* 270, *298,* 423, 425, *437, 438,* 602, 604, 607, 608, 610, 616, 618, *630, 631,* 648, 649, 661, 686, *707*

Adkinson, N. F., Jr., 145, 149, *187,* 669, 672, 680, *704, 708*

Adkinson, N. S., 678, *707*

Adkinsson, N. F., 672, 679, 685, 687, *706*

Adler, K. B., 143, 146, 149, 156, 159, 160, 170, 171, 173, 175, *180,* 279, *290*

Adolphson, C. R., 111, *128,* 167, *182,* 251, *262,* 466, 468, *473,* 477, 478, 482, 484, 486, *497*

Adrian, T. E., 396, *402*

Advenier, C., 142, 145, 150, 156, 159, *179, 180,* 391, *400,* 426, *429*

Agarwal, M. K., 602, *630*

Ahlman, H., 106, *131*

Ahrens, R. C., 523, 526, 527, 532, *547, 551*

M